PEDIATRIC PRACTICE

Cardiology

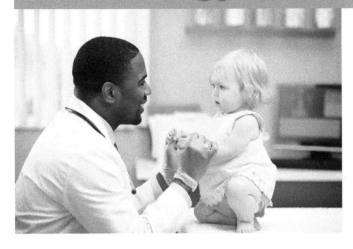

NOTICE

Medicine is an ever-changing science. As new research and clinical experience broaden our knowledge, changes in treatment and drug therapy are required. The authors and the publisher of this work have checked with sources believed to be reliable in their efforts to provide information that is complete and generally in accord with the standards accepted at the time of publication. However, in view of the possibility of human error or changes in medical sciences, neither the authors nor the publisher nor any other party who has been involved in the preparation or publication of this work warrants that the information contained herein is in every respect accurate or complete, and they disclaim all responsibility for any errors or omissions or for the results obtained from use of the information contained in this work. Readers are encouraged to confirm the information contained herein with other sources. For example and in particular, readers are advised to check the product information sheet included in the package of each drug they plan to administer to be certain that the information contained in this work is accurate and that changes have not been made in the recommended dose or in the contraindications for administration. This recommendation is of particular importance in connection with new or infrequently used drugs.

PEDIATRIC PRACTICE

Cardiology

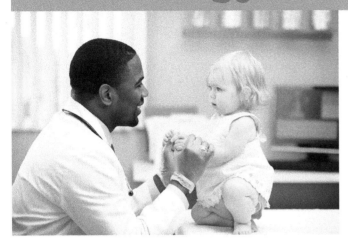

Marie Murphy Gleason
Division of Cardiology
The Children's Hospital of Philadelphia
Philadelphia, Pennsylvania

Jack Rychik
Division of Cardiology
The Children's Hospital of Philadelphia
Philadelphia, Pennsylvania

Robert Shaddy
Division of Cardiology
The Children's Hospital of Philadelphia
Philadelphia, Pennsylvania

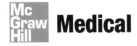 **Medical**

New York Chicago San Francisco Lisbon London Madrid Mexico City
Milan New Delhi San Juan Seoul Singapore Sydney Toronto

1 2 3 4 5 6 7 8 9 0   CTP/CTP   17 16 15 14 13 12

ISBN 978-0-07-176320-2
MHID 0-07-176320-1

This book was set in Minion by Cenveo Publisher Services.
The editors were Alyssa Fried and Brian Kearns.
The production supervisor was Sherri Souffrance.
Project management was provided by Anupriya Tyagi, Cenveo Publisher Services.
The designer was Janice Bielawa; the cover designer was David Dell'Accio.
The cover image of a doctor listening to the chest sounds of a 5-month-old patient using a stethoscope is credit of Ian Hooten/Photo Researchers, Inc.
China Translation & Printing Services, Ltd. was printer and binder.

Library of Congress Cataloging-in-Publication Data

Gleason, Marie Murphy.
    Pediatric practice. Cardiology/Marie Murphy Gleason, Robert Shaddy, Jack Rychik.
      p. ; cm.
    Cardiology
    Includes bibliographical references and index.
    ISBN 978-0-07-176320-2 (hardcover : alk. paper)
    I. Shaddy, Robert E.   II. Rychik, Jack, 1959-   III. Title.   IV. Title:
    Cardiology.
    [DNLM: 1. Cardiovascular Diseases.   2. Adolescent.   3. Child.
    4. Diagnostic Techniques, Cardiovascular.   5. Infant.   WS 290]
      618.92'1—dc23
                                                                   2011053188

This book is dedicated to the patients and families
who deal with cardiac disease every day.
We also dedicate it to the medical professionals in all areas
who contribute to their care, no matter how big or small.

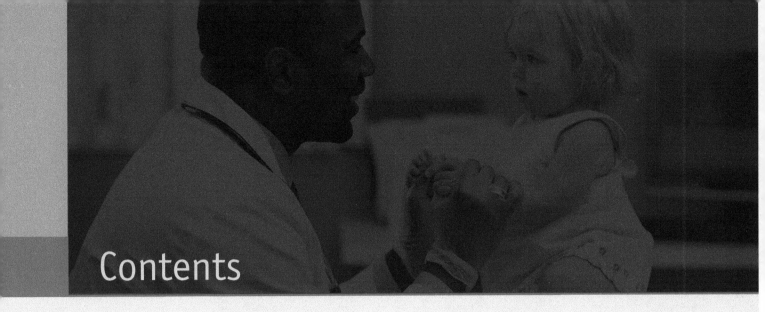

Contents

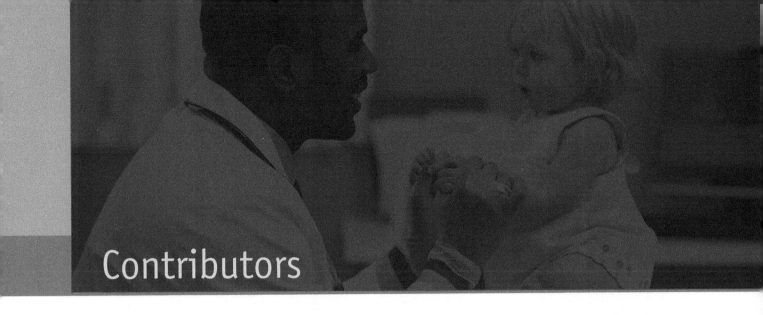

Contributors

Anirban Banerjee, MD
Clinical Associate Professor of Pediatrics
The University of Pennsylvania School of Medicine
Attending Cardiologist
The Children's Hospital of Philadelphia
Philadelphia, Pennsylvania

Katherine Bates, MD
Instructor in Pediatrics
The University of Pennsylvania School of Medicine
Fellow in Cardiology
The Children's Hospital of Philadelphia
Philadelphia, Pennsylvania

Thomas Bernadzikowski, MS, MSN, CRNP
Certifed Registered Nurse Practitioner
Cardiology, Cardiomyopathy and
   Heart Failure Program
The Children's Hospital of Philadelphia
Philadelphia, Pennsylvania

William Bonney, MD
Assistant Professor of Pediatrics
The University of Pennsylvania School of Medicine
Staff Cardiologist
Section of Electrophysiology
Division of Cardiology
The Children's Hospital of Philadelphia
Philadelphia, Pennsylvania

Jeffrey R. Boris, MD
Clinical Associate Professor of Pediatrics
The University of Pennsylvania School of Medicine
Staff Cardiologist
The Children's Hospital of Philadelphia
Philadelphia, Pennsylvania

Julie Brothers, MD
Assistant Professor of Pediatrics
The University of Pennsylvania School of Medicine
Director, Lipid Heart Clinic, Division of Cardiology
The Children's Hospital of Philadelphia
Philadelphia, Pennsylvania

Meryl Cohen, MD
Medical Director
Echocardiography Laboratory
Associate Director, Cardiology Fellowship Program
The Children's Hospital of Philadelphia
Associate Professor of Pediatrics
University of Pennsylvania School of Medicine
Philadelphia, Pennsylvania

Lisa C.A. D'Alessandro, MD
Instructor in Pediatrics
The University of Pennsylvania School of Medicine
Fellow in Cardiology
The Children's Hospital of Philadelphia
Philadelphia, Pennsylvania

Brooke Davey, MD
Cardiology Fellow
The Children's Hospital of Philadelphia
Instructor in Pediatrics
University of Pennsylvania School of Medicine
Philadelphia, Pennsylvania

Alex Davidson, MD
Professor of Clinical Pediatrics and Medicine
The University of Pennsylvania School of Medicine
Staff Cardiologist
Philadelphia Adult Congenital Cardiac Center
The Children's Hospital of Philadelphia and Hospital
   of the University of Pennsylvania
Philadelphia, Pennsylvania

Michael V. Di Maria, MD
Instructor in Pediatrics
The University of Pennsylvania School of Medicine
Fellow, Pediatric Cardiology
The Children's Hospital of Philadelphia
Philadelphia, Pennsylvania

Aaron Dorfman, MD
Assistant Professor of Clinical Pediatrics
The University of Pennsylvania School of Medicine
Staff Cardiologist, Division of Cardiology
The Children's Hospital of Philadelphia
Voorhees, New Jersey

David Drajpuch, MSN, RN, CRNP
Nurse Practitioner
Philadelphia Adult Congenital Cardiac Center
The Children's Hospital of Philadelphia and Hospital
   of the University of Pennsylvania
Philadelphia, Pennsylvania

Paul Farrell Jr, MD
Clinical Professor of Pediatrics
The University of Pennsylvania School of Medicine
Staff Cardiologist
The Children's Hospital of Philadelphia
Philadelphia, Pennsylvania

Mark Fogel, MD
Director of Cardiac Magnetic Resonance Imaging
The Children's Hospital of Philadelphia
Professor of Pediatrics and Radiology
University of Pennsylvania School of Medicine
Philadelphia, Pennsylvania

Stephanie Fuller, MD
Assistant Professor of Surgery
The University of Pennsylvania School of Medicine
Staff Surgeon
Philadelphia Adult Congenital Cardiac Center
The Children's Hospital of Philadelphia and Hospital
   of the University of Pennsylvania
Philadelphia, Pennsylvania

Therese M. Giglia, MD
Associate Professor of Clinical Pediatrics
The University of Pennsylvania School of Medicine
Staff Cardiologist
Division of Cardiology
The Children's Hospital of Philadelphia
Philadelphia, Pennsylvania

Matthew J. Gillespie, MD
Assistant Professor of Pediatrics
The University of Pennsylvania School of Medicine
Staff Cardiologist
Division of Cardiology
Section of Interventional Cardiology
The Children's Hospital of Philadelphia
Philadelphia, Pennsylvania

Andrew C. Glatz, MD
Assistant Professor of Pediatrics
The University of Pennsylvania School of Medicine
The Children's Hospital of Philadelphia
Philadelphia, Pennsylvania

Marianne Glanzman, MD
Division of Child Development
Rehabilitation and Metabolic Disease and Center for
   Management of ADHD
Clinical Associate Professor of Pediatrics
The Children's Hospital of Philadelphia
The University of Pennsylvania School of Medicine
Philadelphia, Pennsylvania

Marie M. Gleason, MD
Clinical Professor of Pediatrics
The University of Pennsylvania School of Medicine
Director, Outpatient and Community Cardiology
Associate Chief, Division of Cardiology
The Children's Hospital of Philadelphia
Philadelphia, Pennsylvania

Donna Goff, MD
Instructor in Pediatrics
University of Pennsylvania School of Medicine
Senior Cardiology Imaging Fellow
The Children's Hospital of Philadelphia
Philadelphia, Pennsylvania

David J. Goldberg, MD
Assistant Professor of Pediatrics
The University of Pennsylvania School of Medicine
Department of Pediatrics, Division of Cardiology
The Children's Hospital of Philadelphia
Philadelphia, Pennsylvania

Elizabeth Goldmuntz, MD
Associate Professor in Pediatrics
The University of Pennsylvania School of Medicine
Attending Cardiologist
The Children's Hospital of Philadelphia
Philadelphia, Pennsylvania

Brian D. Hanna, MDCM, PhD
Clinical Professor of Pediatrics
Section of Pediatric Pulmonary Hypertension
The University of Pennsylvania School of Medicine
Philadelphia, Pennsylvania

Ramesh Iyer, MD
Clinical Associate Professor of Pediatrics
The University of Pennsylvania School of Medicine
Attending Electrophysiologist
The Children's Hospital of Philadelphia
Philadelphia, Pennsylvania

Beth Kaufman, MD
Assistant Professor of Pediatrics
The University of Pennsylvania School of Medicine
Director, Cardiomyopathy and Heart Failure Program
Division of Cardiology
The Children's Hospital of Philadelphia
Philadelphia, Pennsylvania

Yuli Y. Kim, MD
Assistant Professor of Medicine
The University of Pennsylvania School of Medicine
Director, Philadelphia Adult Congenital Cardiac
  Center
The Children's Hospital of Philadelphia and Hospital
  of the University of Pennsylvania
Philadelphia, Pennsylvania

Roxanne E. Kirsch, MD, FRCPC, FAAP
Staff Cardiac Intensivist
Division of Anesthesiology and Critical Care Medicine
The Children's Hospital of Philadelphia
Philadelphia, Pennsylvania

Javier J. Lasa, MD
Instructor in Pediatrics
The University of Pennsylvania School of Medicine
Fellow, Division of Cardiology
The Children's Hospital of Philadelphia
Philadelphia, Pennsylvania

Daniel Licht, MD
Director of Neurovascular Imaging
Assistant Professor of Neurology and Pediatrics
The Children's Hospital of Philadelphia
The University of Pennsylvania School of Medicine
Philadelphia, Pennsylvania

Kimberly Y. Lin, MD
Assistant Professor of Pediatrics
The University of Pennsylvania School of Medicine
Section of Heart Failure and Transplant
The Children's Hospital of Philadelphia
Philadelphia, Pennsylvania

Camila Londono-Obregon, MD
Instructor in Pediatrics
The University of Pennsylvania School of Medicine
Cardiology Fellow
The Children's Hospital of Philadelphia
Philadelphia, Pennsylvania

Lisa M. Montenegro, MD
Assistant Professor of Anesthesiology and Critical
  Care Medicine
The University of Pennsylvania School of Medicine
Staff Cardiac Anesthesiologist
The Children's Hospital of Philadelphia
Philadelphia, Pennsylvania

Shobha Natarajan, MD
Assistant Clinical Professor of Pediatrics
The University of Pennsylvania School of Medicine
Division of Cardiology
The Children's Hospital of Philadelphia
Philadelpha, Pennsylvania

Matthew J. O'Connor, MD
Instructor in Pediatrics
The University of Pennsylvania School of Medicine
Senior Cardiology Imaging Fellow
Division of Cardiology
The Children's Hospital of Philadelphia
Philadelphia, Pennsylvania

Stephen Paridon, MD
Medical Director
Exercise Laboratory
The Children's Hospital of Philadelphia
Professor of Pediatrics
The University of Pennsylvania School of Medicine
Philadelphia, Pennsylvania

Aimee Parnell, MD
Instructor in Pediatrics
The University of Pennsylvania School of Medicine
Senior Fellow
Division of Cardiology
The Children's Hospital of Philadelphia
Philadelphia, Pennsylvania

Akash Patel, MD
Assistant Professor of Pediatrics
The University of Pennsylvania School of Medicine
Staff Cardiologist
Section of Electrophysiology, Division of Cardiology
The Children's Hospital of Philadelphia
Philadelphia, Pennsylvania

Shabnam Peyvandi, MD
Instructor in Pediatrics
The University of Pennsylvania School of Medicine
Fellow in Cardiology
The Children's Hospital of Philadelphia
Philadelphia, Pennsylvania

Michael Quartermain, MD
Assistant Professor of Pediatrics
University of Pennsylvania School of Medicine
Cardiology Attending
The Children's Hospital of Philadelphia
Philadelphia, Pennsylvania

Chitra Ravishankar, MBBS
Assistant Professor of Pediatrics
The University of Pennsylvania School of Medicine
Staff Cardiologist
The Children's Hospital of Philadelphia
Philadelphia, Pennsylvania

Lindsay S. Rogers, MD
Instructor in Pediatrics
The University of Pennsylvania School of Medicine
Cardiology Fellow
The Children's Hospital of Philadelphia
Philadelphia, Pennsylvania

Jonathan J. Rome, MD
Professor of Pediatrics
The University of Pennsylvania School of Medicine
Associate Chief, Division of Cardiology
The Children's Hospital of Philadelphia
Philadelphia, Pennsylvania

Jack Rychik, MD
Professor of Pediatrics
The University of Pennsylvania School of Medicine
Associate Chief
Division of Cardiology
The Children's Hospital of Philadelphia
Philadelphia, Pennsylvania

Shyam K. Sathanandam, MD
Interventional Cardiology Fellow
Division of Cardiology
The Children's Hospital of Philadelphia
Philadelphia, Pennsylvania

Susan Schachtner, MD
Clinical Associate Professor of Pediatrics
University of Pennsylvania School of Medicine
Attending Cardiologist
The Children's Hospital of Philadelphia
Philadelphia, Pennsylvania

Matthew C. Schwartz, MD
Instructor in Pediatrics
The University of Pennsylvania School of Medicine
Senior Cardiology Fellow
The Children's Hospital of Philadelphia
Philadelphia, Pennsylvania

Maully Shah, MBBS
Associate Professor of Pediatrics
The University of Pennsylvania School of Medicine
Section Head, Electrophysiology, Division of
  Cardiology
The Children's Hospital of Philadelphia
Philadelphia, Pennsylvania

Anita Szwast, MD
Assistant Professor of Pediatrics
The University of Pennsylvania School of Medicine
Cardiology Attending
The Children's Hospital of Philadelphia
Philadelphia, Pennsylvania

Joseph W. Turek, MD, PhD
Cardiothoracic Surgery Fellow
Department of Surgery
The Children's Hospital of Philadelphia
Philadelphia, Pennsylvania

Victoria L. Vetter, MD, MPH
Professor of Pediatrics
The University of Pennsylvania School of Medicine
Senior Cardiologist
The Children's Hospital of Philadelphia
Philadelphia, Pennsylvania

R. Lee Vogel, MD
Attending Cardiologist
Clinical Associate Professor
The Children's Hospital of Philadelphia
University of Pennsylvania School of Medicine
Philadelphia, Pennsylvania

Stephen H. Walker, MS, CRNP
Nurse Practitioner
Division of Cardiology
The Children's Hospital of Philadelphia
Philadelphia, Pennsylvania

Shari L. Wellen, MD
Instructor in Pediatrics
The University of Pennsylvania School of Medicine
Fellow, Pediatric Cardiology
The Children's Hospital of Philadelphia
Philadelphia, Pennsylvania

Gil Wernovsky, MD
Medical Director
NeuroCardiac Care Program
Associate Chief
Division of Pediatric Cardiology
Professor of Pediatrics
The Children's Hospital of Philadelphia
The University of Pennsylvania School of Medicine
Philadelphia, Pennsylvania

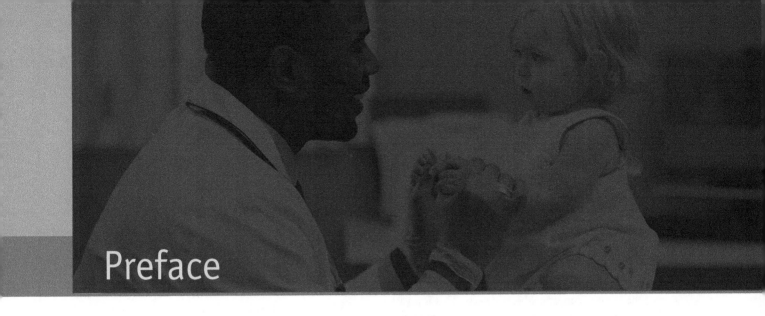

Preface

Pediatric cardiology is one of the oldest of the pediatric subspecialties. The last half of the 20th century showed a remarkable change in the focus of cardiologists from the treatment of acquired cardiac disease, like rheumatic fever, to the diagnosis and treatment of congenital heart defects of increasing complexity. Since the 1960s, each decade has brought new tools and medications to aid pediatric cardiologists in their care of children with heart disease. Arguably, one of the greatest tools, 2-dimensional and Doppler echocardiography, allows cardiologists to rapidly and accurately obtain vital anatomic and physiologic information noninvasively on patients of all ages. This tool was extended to prenatal diagnosis late in the 20th century. In the 1970s and 1980s, advances in surgical techniques and equipment that allowed surgery on small infants and children changed our management strategies for complex congenital heart disease from palliative to "corrective" therapies. Advances in cardiac catheterization and the birth of interventional cardiac procedures have allowed pediatric cardiologists the ability to offer nonsurgical options to many patients, where none existed before.

These remarkable therapeutic changes have resulted in several shifts of focus in pediatric cardiology. In clinical care, there is continued effort in determining the best management strategies for patients, including early diagnosis and the use of clinical guidelines. Importantly, the number of survivors with congenital heart disease of all types has grown exponentially, including patients with very complex disease who never lived to adulthood before the current era. This mandates that all primary care practitioners become well-versed in the wide range of diseases that now exist in the pediatric and young adult population. This book provides multiple chapters with information to allow primary care providers to become familiar with the tools used in the care of pediatric cardiology patients and the opportunity to review the different types of congenital heart defects in detail. Each chapter describes the cardiac anatomy and physiology, but also includes the management strategies that we use.

The management focus has also shifted from the postnatal diagnosis of congenital heart disease to prenatal diagnosis. This book provides a chapter for primary care physicians to become more familiar with the information gathered by fetal cardiologists from fetal echocardiography and how fetal diagnosis has impacted upon the care of patients and families with serious congenital heart disease. On the opposite end of the spectrum, the growing population of adults with congenital heart disease is an emerging and problematic issue. Here we face our greatest unknowns and challenges. Additionally, as this patient pool expands, it will mandate the need for more adult cardiac specialists with specific knowledge of congenital heart disease and the various management strategies that have allowed their survival. Currently, there are a relatively small number of adult specialists with this expertise, compared to the number of adult patients. This will prove to be a vital area of need in the future. This book provides a chapter that reviews some of these critical adult congenital heart issues.

In the current era, the likelihood that an infant with complex congenital heart disease will survive is very high. An area of growing research is how these children are doing from a neurocognitive perspective. It is not enough that a child survives heart surgery and goes to school. What is also important is how the child functions in the world with his or her peers. This is of critical importance to the family, and it is very important that primary care providers know what to be on the alert for, whether it be learning disabilities or other psychosocial issues that strain the child and family. This unique area is covered in a chapter that should be of interest to all readers.

Although congenital heart disease is a common form of birth defect in the general population, it is not the only type of heart problem approached in this book. The different forms of acquired inflammatory heart disease are reviewed here. Additionally, there is an important chapter that addresses the risk factors for acquired adult heart disease (atherosclerosis, hypertension, and obesity) during childhood. Given the epidemic of childhood obesity, this is a matter of high concern both to physicians and families, and this chapter should be of special interest to all primary care providers.

In the research realm, there is continued growth and interest in understanding the genetics and pathophysiology of the various congenital heart defects. This is a vast and complex area and cannot be reviewed in detail here. We have, however, included a chapter that reviews the current tools available to assess the genetics of congenital heart disease, as well as the forms of congenital heart disease that are associated with certain known syndromes. Perhaps in a different decade, the results of research efforts will allow us to intervene and either modify or alleviate some forms of congenital heart disease.

It is important to remember that the care of the pediatric heart patient is a joint effort between the subspecialist and the primary care practitioner. When physicians work with a shared knowledge base, then the care of the patient will be enhanced. It is our hope that this book will provide valuable information about all aspects of congenital and acquired heart disease to our colleagues in primary care medicine. It should also be helpful to medical students and pediatric or family practice residents in learning more about this important subspecialty. Whether you are a physician in the office, a nurse practitioner in a clinic, an emergency medicine physician, a dentist, or an obstetrician-gynecologist, there is no doubt that patients with congenital and acquired heart disease will cross your path. Given the variety of types of cardiac disease that exist, this can be an overwhelming concern. Our goal is that this book be an easy and reliable resource for obtaining up-to-date and accurate information as rapidly as possible. In that way, we can hope to ensure excellent care of these complex patients in the future.

Marie M. Gleason
Jack Rychik
Robert Shaddy

Acknowledgments

We would like to thank our spouses, Edward Gleason, Susan Rychik, and Jamee Roberts, for their continued support of our daily work as pediatric cardiologists, as well as their support of our extra endeavors, like this book. They understand the importance of education for patients, families, and other medical caretakers when it comes to patients with cardiac disease. We also want to recognize the hard work and effort demonstrated by our senior cardiology fellows who served as co-authors on most of the chapters in this book. Their ownership of the project, along with the attending physicians, was a valuable learning experience for all. We are proud to say that they will be the next generation of pediatric cardiologists.

Marie M. Gleason
Jack Rychik
Robert Shaddy

CHAPTER 1

Normal Cardiac Physiology and the Cardiac Exam

Michael V. Di Maria,
Jeffrey R. Boris and Victoria L. Vetter

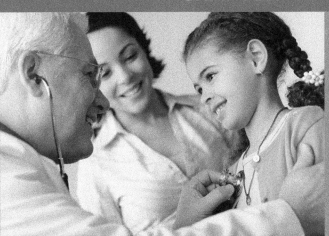

NORMAL CARDIAC ANATOMY

The normal heart is composed of two ventricles that circulate blood through the pulmonary and systemic capillary beds in series, providing a means of delivering oxygen and nutrients to the tissues and removing carbon dioxide and metabolic waste. Deoxygenated blood is received in the right atrium and pumped from the right ventricle through the pulmonary capillary bed, where carbon dioxide is exchanged for oxygen in the alveoli. Pulmonary venous return to the left atrium is circulated through the systemic capillary bed by the left ventricle (Figure 1-1).

NORMAL CARDIAC PHYSIOLOGY

The term "cardiac cycle" refers to the events that occur in 1 heartbeat. By convention, the cycle is said to begin with the onset of systole. Notably, the events in the right and left heart occur in parallel, in the same sequence and at roughly the same time, although at different pressures. These events are tied to the electrical activities of the heart in a process described as electromechanical coupling. Figure 1-2 depicts the events of the cardiac cycle, including the surface electrocardiogram (ECG) and intracardiac pressures and volumes.

Ventricular Diastole

In diastole, the ventricles fill with blood, which occurs in two phases. In the first phase, the ventricle fills passively as the ventricular myocardium relaxes and blood is drawn into the ventricles through the atrioventricular (AV) valves as the pressure in the ventricle drops below that of the atria. Next, depolarization of the sinus node, located in the superior portion of the right atrium, initiates atrial contraction. On the surface ECG, atrial systole inscribes a P wave. As the atria contract, additional blood is pumped into the ventricles—the second phase of diastole. Meanwhile, the wave of depolarization travels along the atrial wall toward the ventricles. It ultimately reaches the AV node near the medial aspect of the tricuspid valve. The AV node funnels the impulse into the bundle of His, which rapidly conducts the impulse into the ventricles.

Ventricular Systole

On the surface ECG, ventricular depolarization results in the inscription of the QRS complex. As the ventricles start to contract, the ventricular pressure begins to rise, and the AV valves close when the pressure in the ventricle exceeds that of the atria. A period called isovolumetric contraction follows, as the ventricular pressure increases without a change in volume, as both the AV valves and the semilunar valves are closed. As the pressure in the ventricles increases, it soon exceeds the aortic and pulmonary artery pressure and causes the aortic and pulmonary valves to open, ejecting blood through the great arteries. As the blood is ejected, the ventricular pressure falls. At this point, the ventricular myocardium has begun to repolarize. Ventricular repolarization results in the inscription of the T wave on the surface ECG. When the ventricular pressure drops below that of the great artery, the semilunar valve closes. As the ventricular pressure continues to fall and becomes lower than the atrial pressure, the AV valve opens. The cycle then begins anew.

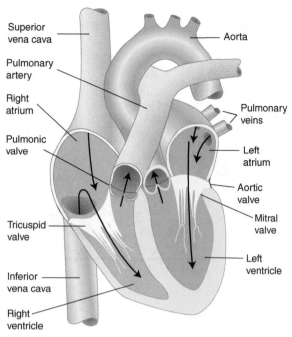

FIGURE 1-1 ■ The normal heart. (*Modified, with permission, from Mohrman DE, Heller LJ. Cardiovascular Physiology. 7th ed. New York, NY: McGraw-Hill; 2010.*)

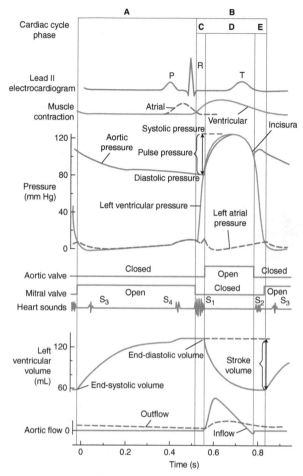

FIGURE 1-2 ■ The Wiggers diagram depicts the events taking place during the cardiac cycle. (*Modified, with permission, from Mohrman DE, Heller LJ. Cardiovascular Physiology. 7th ed. New York, NY: McGraw-Hill; 2010.*)

Cardiac Output

Cardiac output is determined by several factors. The term stroke volume has been used to describe the amount of blood that is ejected in 1 cardiac cycle. Thus, the stroke volume multiplied by the heart rate will yield a volume per unit time. Traditionally, cardiac output is described in liters per minute. The cardiac index is the cardiac output divided by body surface area, a common way of correcting or normalizing the cardiac output for patient size, and is reported as liters per minute per meter squared. This is useful in that a normal adolescent may have a cardiac output many times that of an infant, but the cardiac index would be similar when adjusted for body size.

Determinants of Stroke Volume

Preload

Starling's law states that stroke volume will vary as a function of the amount of blood that fills the heart during diastole. The ventricular filling pressure is referred to as preload. The unfilled ventricle cannot generate any pressure because it must be filled in order to squeeze. The increased stroke volume ejected during systole in response to increased preload is a property of the myocytes themselves. Increasing preload increases stroke volume by increasing the end-diastolic volume, keeping the end-systolic volume the same. Under normal loading conditions, increases in end-diastolic volume do not result in drastically increased end-diastolic pressure;

however, when stretched to near-maximum length, the myocytes reach a threshold at which they are unable to accommodate additional volume without relatively large increases in pressure. The relationship between pressure and volume is illustrated in Figure 1-3.

Diastolic dysfunction occurs when relatively normal end-diastolic volumes are associated with high end-diastolic pressures. Diastolic dysfunction is characterized by a stiff, poorly distensible ventricle. Clinically, poor left ventricular compliance results in left atrial hypertension, which results in high pressures in the pulmonary veins. This, in turn, results in elevated hydrostatic pressure in the pulmonary capillaries and subsequent pulmonary edema, tachypnea, increased work of breathing, and respiratory insufficiency or failure.

Afterload

The resistance in the systemic arteries, against which the left ventricle pumps, has been referred to as afterload. Stroke volume changes in response to alterations

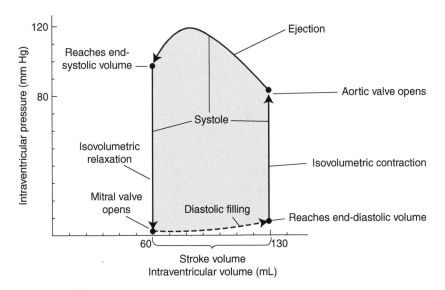

FIGURE 1-3 ■ The pressure-volume curve illustrates the relationship between pressure, along the *y*-axis, and volume, on the *x*-axis. (*Modified, with permission, from Mohrman DE, Heller LJ.* Cardiovascular Physiology. *7th ed. New York, NY: McGraw-Hill; 2010.*)

in afterload. Afterload can be thought of as the amount of work the heart muscle performs. As the afterload increases, the ventricle squeezes until the amount of pressure that it can generate equals the workload imposed by the vascular resistance. At a higher afterload, the stroke volume decreases because contraction stops when the pressure-generating capacity of the ventricle has been reached and the end-systolic volume is increased. Clinically, the hypertensive patient, with high systemic vascular resistance, will manifest a lower stroke volume. This would result in decreased cardiac output, as described earlier.

Contractility

The ventricular myocytes shorten during contraction as a result of the actin-myosin cross-bridge formation. Under the influence of increased sympathetic tone, the pressure-generating capacity of the ventricle increases related to the availability of intracellular calcium. This results in a more vigorous squeeze and a lower end-systolic volume, increasing the stroke volume. Exercise results in a high catecholamine state, which leads to increased contractility. This augments both heart rate and stroke volume, leading to increased cardiac output in response to the increased metabolic need. Conversely, an excessively high or prolonged catecholamine state can increase the stiffness of the ventricle and ultimately reduce contractility. In addition, decreased contractility can result from metabolic derangements, such as acidosis or myocardial ischemia.

Pressure, Flow, and Resistance

Although described in relation to electrical circuits in terms of voltage, resistance, and current, Ohm's law

applies to hydraulic circuits as well. Ohm's law states that pressure is equal to resistance multiplied by flow. Importantly, it is not the preload, afterload, or contractility of the ventricle that determines the pressure in a vascular bed. The flow, typically described in liters per minute, and the resistance, measured in Wood units, dictates the pressure. The resistance in a vascular bed is determined by both the muscular tone in the arteries and the downstream resistance to flow through the capillary bed. For example, in pulmonary hypertension, it is not right ventricular contractility that causes the elevated pulmonary artery pressures; the elevated pulmonary vascular resistance is the primary derangement, and the elevated right ventricular pressure is a necessary compensation. In pulmonary hypertension, due to increased blood flow in the pulmonary arteries from intracardiac shunting, an increase in smooth muscle mass in the pulmonary arterial walls occurs. With prolonged exposure to high rates of flow, the increased smooth muscle mass and tone becomes irreversible, and a permanent state of pulmonary hypertension ensues. This clinical scenario occurs in the setting of a large, unrepaired ventricular septal defect (VSD) and results in Eisenmenger syndrome.

HISTORY AND PHYSICAL EXAMINATION

Birth History

When gathering the history of a patient with suspected cardiac disease, the importance of both the antenatal and birth history should not be underestimated; any such history is invaluable. Many pregnant women undergo a screening ultrasound at around 20 weeks gestation, which may prompt a fetal echocardiogram if any concerning anomalies are detected; similarly, any history of fetal arrhythmias should be noted. Details, such as a history of taking prenatal vitamins, and any complications during the pregnancy should be investigated. Especially in the newborn period, the circumstances surrounding the birth should be elicited in detail. Information, including Apgar scores, the need for resuscitation in the delivery room, birth weight, nursery course, duration of stay, and discharge medications should all be ascertained in the course of a first office visit. Any perinatal respiratory distress, cyanosis, murmur, or difficulty feeding should be explored for possible cardiac etiologies.

History of Present Illness

Commonly, cardiac disease in the infant or child will present with respiratory symptoms, cyanosis, or shock. In the first several months of life, tachypnea and increased work of breathing can be signs of heart failure, although the mechanism is very different from that of the adult with heart failure due to ischemic cardiomyopathy. Sweating when nursing or bottle-feeding can be a sign of heart failure in infants. Cyanosis or shock should prompt rapid evaluation in the emergency room setting to rule out life-threatening problems, such as cyanotic heart disease, severe pulmonary disease, or foreign-body aspiration.

Other elements of the history that can be helpful when screening patients for potential cardiac pathology include reports of chest pain, fainting or dizzy spells, palpitations, heart murmur, or other cardiac diagnosis.

Past Medical History

A complete understanding of the medical history informs the diagnostician and allows the necessary exchange of relevant information with other practitioners. Likewise, important clues to systemic illnesses or genetic conditions that may be associated with cardiac diseases or defects can be revealed.

Family History

The etiology of congenital heart disease continues to be a topic of much investigation. Congenital heart disease in a sibling or parent increases the chances of congenital heart disease in an individual. A family history of genetic syndromes should also be explored. Sudden death can have heritable causes, such as hypertrophic cardiomyopathy, long QT syndrome, or Marfan syndrome. An initial history should include questions about relatives who have died suddenly or unexpectedly, such as those who might have died of sudden infant death syndrome or while swimming or driving alone, especially when unexplained death occurs under age 35 years. Other family history to be ascertained includes syncope, seizures, arrhythmias, and other cardiac diseases presenting under the age of 50 years.

Vital Signs

Growth parameters

Poor growth can be a manifestation of cardiac pathology. Infants with congestive heart failure do not grow well, due to a diversion of metabolic resources to maintaining systemic cardiac output, rather than somatic growth.

Temperature

Fever can cause tachycardia, increase the intensity of an innocent murmur, or accompany infectious or inflammatory diseases that can affect the heart, such as infectious endocarditis, rheumatic fever, or rheumatoid arthritis.

Heart rate

Heart rate should be noted and compared to established normal ranges for age, taking into account the patient's emotional and physical state. Anxiety, fear, and agitation commonly cause sinus tachycardia in the examination room and prevent an accurate assessment of the resting heart rate. Resting sinus tachycardia has a long differential diagnosis that cannot be fully explored here but should raise concern for underlying disease. Supraventricular tachycardia generally occurs at heart rates greater than 150 to 180 beats per minute and is often too fast to count accurately.

Bradycardia occurs in the setting of excellent physical conditioning, as well as with eating disorders, heart block, elevated intracranial pressure, sinus node dysfunction after a history of cardiac surgery, and hypothyroidism.

Blood pressure

Blood pressure should be measured in the seated position, with the patient's feet on the ground, the patient's back supported, and the patient resting quietly and calmly for 5 minutes. The use of electronic blood pressure monitoring devices is commonly used in practice, but measuring blood pressure using a manual cuff to confirm abnormal results should be performed. The blood pressure cuff should be the appropriate size for the patient's arm, and the sphygmomanometer should be calibrated every 6 months. The blood pressure in the right upper extremity should be measured and compared to the blood pressure in either leg. The right upper extremity blood pressure will likely be equivalent to, or less than, that of the leg. However, if the right upper extremity blood pressure is greater than the blood pressure in the leg, a diagnosis of coarctation of the aorta should be entertained. Normal values for blood pressure are based on sex, age, and height percentiles and are widely published for comparison.[1,2]

Respiratory rate

Respiratory rate should also be noted and compared to age-related normal values. Historical data should also be taken into account when tachypnea is present, as in the case of an ongoing viral respiratory tract infection. Tachypnea, as mentioned earlier, can be a sign of congestive heart failure in infants resulting from pulmonary overcirculation and edema.

Oxygen saturation

Oxygen saturation should be part of the routinely measured vital signs. In the newborn period, desaturation can be a sign of cyanotic congenital heart disease and should prompt urgent referral. Additionally, differential desaturation between the upper and lower extremities, which refers to decreased saturations in the lower extremities compared to the upper, is due to deoxygenated blood entering the descending aorta via a patent ductus arteriosus (PDA) and requires further evaluation.

Inspection

General appearance

The examiner should regard the patient overall, noting any indication that the patient is distressed or agitated. Separate from behavioral causes, agitation may be a sign of distress in all age groups. The nutritional status of the patient also should be assessed, as well as the interaction between patient and parent or guardian.

Dysmorphisms. Dysmorphic features may signal the presence of a genetic abnormality. Associations between genetic anomalies and congenital heart disease are discussed elsewhere.

Color: Cyanosis. Cyanosis indicates the presence of at least 5 g/dL of deoxygenated hemoglobin, regardless of the amount of oxygenated hemoglobin. Patients with high hemoglobin concentrations need a smaller fraction of their total hemoglobin to be deoxygenated to appear cyanotic. Conversely, a patient who is anemic would require a large percentage of their total hemoglobin to be deoxygenated to have the same appearance. For example, a chronically hypoxemic patient with a total hemoglobin of 20 g/dL would require only 25% of their hemoglobin to be deoxygenated to be cyanotic, whereas an anemic patient with a hemoglobin of 7 g/dL would require greater than 50% deoxyhemoglobin to be cyanotic. Cyanosis is best evaluated in a well-lit room. The oral mucous membranes, gums, and tongue should be inspected because they will not be affected by peripheral vasoconstriction due to temperature or elevated vascular tone or be obscured by skin pigmentation.

Respiration

Labored respirations and tachypnea may result from pulmonary overcirculation and pulmonary edema in the infant with a large left-to-right shunt. Pulmonary edema may also result from left heart failure or from hypoplastic structures in the left heart with inadequate systemic blood flow. Additionally, hypoxemia from severe cyanosis or acidosis can cause respiratory distress.

Neck veins

Jugular venous distention is a rare finding in pediatrics. In the newborn, the neck is relatively short and not easily visible. In older children, even those with elevated right atrial pressures and hepatomegaly, jugular venous distention may not be evident. The hepatojugular reflex, compressing the liver during inspection of the neck veins to see if they become more prominent, should be performed with the patient in the supine position with the head elevated to 30 degrees.

Chest wall asymmetry and defects

Prominence of the left chest can indicate the presence of right ventricular enlargement. An absence of muscle mass in the left chest can also indicate Poland anomaly, or hypoplasia of the pectoralis minor, which can be associated with congenital cardiac defects. Pectus deformities, such as pectus excavatum and scoliosis, can be associated with Marfan syndrome. Kyphosis and scoliosis can lead to restrictive lung disease and pulmonary hypertension.

Visualization of the point of maximal impulse

The point of maximal impulse (PMI) can often be seen in the normal child and should be located in the fourth to fifth intercostal space, at the midclavicular line. If it is displaced to the left or inferiorly, it can indicate cardiomegaly.

Edema

Peripheral edema is caused by systemic venous congestion and is a rare finding in young children. Elevated systemic venous pressure is a feature of advanced right heart dysfunction. Typically, edema in children is due to renal or hepatic disease, although patients with decompensated, postoperative single-ventricle physiology may exhibit this finding due to elevated central venous pressure.

Diaphoresis

Diaphoresis is another term for perspiration. Infants in heart failure can become diaphoretic when feeding, which is related to the increased adrenergic tone that results from chronic, low cardiac output. If related to heart failure, other signs of distress, such as tachypnea and poor growth, should accompany this. Diaphoresis secondary to environmental factors in the absence of other findings does not indicate the presence of occult heart disease. For example, sweating occurs normally during periods of high vagal tone, such as sleeping.

Clubbing

Prolonged hypoxemia and polycythemia result in engorgement of the capillaries beneath the nail beds in the fingers and toes. As a result, the concavity formed by the eponychium (cuticle) disappears, giving the appearance of a thick, wide distal phalanx. Clubbing also occurs secondary to disease in other organ systems; cirrhosis and cystic fibrosis are two examples.

Palpation

When palpating the pediatric chest to assess for the PMI, the examiner should use the most sensitive part of the hand. The patient should be in the upright position. Many find the volar surface of the proximal fingers (metacarpal heads and proximal phalanges) to be the most sensitive. Others find that the fingertips are adequate. If the PMI is palpated in the right chest, dextrocardia should be considered.

Point of maximal impulse
Right ventricle impulse.
Often, a hyperdynamic right ventricle is associated with an indistinct impulse. A hypertrophied right ventricle, associated with elevated pressure, produces a relatively short "tap" that can be appreciated at the left lower sternal border. An enlarged right ventricle due to increased volume loading, on the other hand, results in a more diffuse "lift," or "heave," that is gradual in onset.

Left ventricle impulse.
As stated earlier, the examiner palpates a normal PMI at the left lower sternal border, in the fourth to fifth intercostal space, at the midclavicular line. If the left ventricle is dilated, the PMI is shifted inferiorly and leftward. A hyperdynamic PMI in the correct location may be a sign of increased cardiac output.

Thrills

When the turbulent blood flow that results in a murmur can be palpated on the chest wall, this is called a thrill. Thrills can be felt in the precordial, suprasternal, and carotid areas and result from significant cardiac pathology. If a murmur is low grade but a thrill is palpated, then the finding is more likely a pulsation and not a thrill. Any child with a murmur loud enough to result in a true thrill should be referred to a cardiologist.

Pulses

Peripheral pulses should be assessed for their presence, strength, and regularity. The prominence of the pulses is important. Pulses are classically graded on a scale of 0 to 4: 0 = absent pulses; 1 = barely palpable pulses; 2 = easily palpable pulses; 3 = full pulses; and 4 = bounding pulses. A pulse that feels "bounding" may be the result of a "run-off" lesion, such as aortic insufficiency or PDA. This finding results from a very wide pulse pressure; in the case of aortic insufficiency, the backflow of blood into the ventricle lowers the diastolic pressure. This has been referred to as a "water-hammer" pulse, so named for the Victorian-era toy. A diminished pulse in the setting of clinical instability can be a sign of low cardiac output, indicating that urgent resuscitation is needed.

Pulsus paradoxus. The term pulsus paradoxus refers to an exaggeration of the normal reduction in pulse pressure seen during inspiration from conditions that limit the size of the pericardial space, such as cardiac tamponade and constrictive pericardial disease. The normal difference in systolic pressure during respiration should be less than 10 mm Hg; values greater than this should raise concern for tamponade.

Variation. Sinus arrhythmia is the physiologic increase in heart rate during inspiration and decrease in expiration and is a response to increased preload generated when the intrathoracic pressure decreases during inspiration. This is a normal finding and should disappear with breath holding. Long pauses between pulsations or early pulsations require further investigation.

Comparison between upper and lower extremities. Coarctation of the aorta, a constriction that develops distal to the left subclavian artery, results in upper extremity hypertension and diminished pulses in the lower extremities. Blood pressures in all four extremities should be checked in any pediatric patient with upper extremity hypertension to rule out coarctation of the aorta. Simultaneous palpation of the right radial and either femoral pulse should be performed to assess for pulse lag and for the presence of a femoral pulse. Lag between the upper and lower extremities or absence of the femoral pulse is suggestive of a coarctation.

Percussion

Cardiomegaly can be detected in severe cases by percussing the thorax. Similarly, pleural effusions or pulmonary consolidation can be identified. Percussion is used to augment the cardiac examination in determining the span of the liver. In cases where the lungs are hyperinflated, as in reactive airways disease, inferior displacement of the diaphragm can allow palpation of the liver edge below the costal margin. Percussion of a normal liver span can reassure the examiner that the liver is not enlarged, such as in congestive heart failure, but simply displaced. Enlargement of the spleen typically does not occur without enlargement of the liver; however, isolated splenomegaly can occur in endocarditis.

Auscultation

The patient

Auscultation of the heart in a child is often easier to do compared with adolescents or adults, because the chest wall is thinner and there is less space between the chest wall and the heart. This results in clearer auscultation and easier recognition of heart sounds. Conversely, it can be more difficult in younger patients due to poor patient cooperation and higher heart rates. Because auscultation is dependent on the patient being calm and quiet, it is recommended that the provider perform this early in the examination, to ensure improved likelihood of having an accurate and complete cardiac assessment.

The stethoscope

A stethoscope should be comfortable for the examiner to use. Using the same stethoscope consistently will eliminate inconsistencies in the acoustic qualities of different stethoscopes. The tubing should also be less than 18 inches in length to avoid attenuation of sound transmission. The bell of the stethoscope lets in all sounds, whereas the diaphragm is a high-pass filter, letting in higher pitched sounds. Therefore, sounds heard with the bell alone are considered low pitch; those heard solely with the diaphragm are high pitched; and those heard with both are considered medium pitched. The bell should be applied lightly to the chest wall so as not to cause the skin to act as a diaphragm. The diaphragm should be applied with more pressure to eliminate apposition abnormalities. In addition, the diaphragm should not be too large for the chest, which will also cause auscultated apposition artifacts.

Heart sounds

S_1. The first heart sound coincides with the AV valves closing and can be best heard at the left lower sternal border. Although the tricuspid and mitral valves close at this time, S_1 is usually heard as a single sound. Compared with the second heart sound, S_1 is typically lower pitched and longer. If there is any confusion as to which heart sound is which, palpating the carotid pulse while auscultating can be helpful; S_1 precedes the pulsation, and S_2 follows it.

S_2. The second heart sound results from closure of the 2 semilunar valves, the pulmonic and aortic valves. Splitting of the second heart sound, the ability to discern that there are 2 sounds as opposed to 1, occurs normally with respiratory variation. The sounds are abbreviated A_2, for aortic valve closure, which is best heard in the right second intercostal space, and P_2 for the sound of pulmonic valve closure, which is heard at the left second intercostal space. A_2 normally occurs prior to P_2. With inspiration, the downward movement of the diaphragm creates negative intrathoracic pressure. Blood is pulled from the vena cavae into the right atrium and pumped into the right ventricle. During ventricular contraction, the larger volume of blood in the right ventricle, compared with the left ventricle, takes longer to eject. This prolongation in ejection time results in delayed closure of the pulmonic valve and splitting of the second heart sound. Other alterations in intensity and timing of the second heart sounds are summarized in Table 1-1.

Gallops

S_3. The third heart sound occurs during the rapid ventricular filling phase during early diastole and is heard in normal children. It is a low-pitched sound that is best heard at the apex. The cadence of an S_3 rhythm has been described as "Ken-tuck-y."

S_4. The fourth heart sound has a much more foreboding association with ventricular dysfunction and is nearly always pathologic. It can be heard in late diastole, after atrial contraction, and results from decreased ventricular compliance. Alternately, an S_4 rhythm shares the same cadence as the word "Ten-nes-see." It is associated with congestive heart failure and diastolic dysfunction.

Gallops can be heard separately over the right and left ventricles. S_3 and S_4 can be heard separately, or they can occur together as an intense "summation" gallop.

Clicks and snaps

Click. An ejection click is a high-pitched noise that closely follows the first heart sound and occurs in the setting of semilunar valve stenosis or dilation of the great arteries. It is also appreciated in the setting of a bicuspid aortic valve, an abnormal common semilunar valve (such as in truncus arteriosus), and Ebstein anomaly of the tricuspid valve (in which there can be multiple clicks). It is often considered to be associated with turbulence downstream from an abnormal valve. A midsystolic click, heard slightly later in systole, occurs with mitral valve prolapse.

Snap. In the setting of congenital mitral valve stenosis or rheumatic mitral valve disease, a diastolic opening snap can be heard at the left sternal border but is rare in pediatric patients.

Rub

A friction rub occurs in the setting of pericardial inflammation, such as pericarditis, and results from the

Abnormalities in the Second Heart Sound

Finding	Structural Causes	Functional Causes
Widely split	■ Idiopathic dilation of the PA ■ Secundum atrial septal defect	■ RV volume overload ■ RV pressure overload ■ Conduction delay, especially right bundle branch block
Narrowly split	■ Aortic stenosis	■ Pulmonary hypertension
Single	■ Single semilunar valve ■ Severe aortic stenosis ■ Transposition of the great arteries (prior to repair) ■ Tetralogy of Fallot	■ Pulmonary hypertension
Paradoxically split	■ Severe aortic stenosis	■ LBBB/WPW
Increased intensity		■ Pulmonary hypertension
Decreased intensity	■ Pulmonary stenosis ■ Tetralogy of Fallot ■ Tricuspid atresia	

LBBB, left bundle branch block; PA, pulmonary artery; RV, right ventricle; WPW, Wolff-Parkinson-White.

visceral and parietal layers of the pericardium rubbing against each other. A rub is best heard at the left sternal border and has an alternating or creaking leather quality. Notably, a large effusion may not produce a friction rub due to the separation between the two layers of pericardium; however, in a small effusion, the layers are more closely approximated and more likely to generate a rub.

Knock

A pericardial knock occurs in the setting of chronic constrictive pericarditis. These knocks are uncommon in pediatric patients.

Murmurs

Murmurs result from turbulent intracardiac or intravascular blood flow. A murmur can be appreciated in roughly two thirds of all normal children and three quarters of normal newborns. Thus, the presence of a murmur does not indicate pathology. The accurate description of a murmur should include the following characteristics: timing, location and radiation, pitch, intensity, and the response to diagnostic maneuvers. Every patient should be examined in both the supine and either standing or sitting positions. Infants can be held in an upright position by a seated parent, facing the examiner, to simulate standing. Asking patients to perform certain tasks during the physical examination

can be helpful in making diagnoses based on how the activity changes the heart sounds.

Innocent murmurs, also called benign, normal, or functional murmurs, occur in the setting of normal intracardiac anatomy. A familiarity with innocent murmurs allows the practitioner to reliably differentiate them from pathologic murmurs, without needing to know the specific lesion or defect associated with the abnormal heart sounds. The features of the 6 common innocent murmurs are summarized in Table 1-2. Notably, many innocent murmurs may be audible until the patient reaches young adulthood.

Pathologic murmurs are sounds produced by turbulent flow due to abnormal intracardiac or intravascular obstructions or connections. Features that make a murmur more likely to be associated with a pathologic lesion include loudness, a "harsh" quality, an associated thrill or click, an abnormal second heart sound, abnormal femoral pulses or radial-femoral pulse delay, or an active precordium. Visual representations of common murmurs are depicted in Figure 1-4.

Systolic murmurs

Systolic murmurs can be divided into two groups, ejection and holosystolic; notably, holosystolic murmurs arise from two distinct sources: VSDs and regurgitant AV valves.

Ejection murmurs. Ejection murmurs begin a short period of time after the first heart sound (closure

		Innocent/Functional Murmurs		
Type	Age	Location	Sound	Maneuvers
Still murmur	2-8 years, can occur in infants or adolescents	Hockey stick distribution (apex, LLSB, LMSB, RUSB)	Vibratory, buzzing, "cooing dove," "guitar-string twang," occurring as a systolic ejection murmur	Have patient sit up or stand up: murmur should disappear or localize to LLSB
Venous hum	2-6 years, rarely younger	RUSB, LUSB, occasionally RMSB	Blowing, roaring, wheezing, distant-sounding continuous murmur with diastolic accentuation	Lay patient down, compress jugular vein, or turn head: murmur should disappear
Physiologic peripheral pulmonary stenosis	Infants 0-6 months	Parasternal, precordium, louder in the axillae and back	Short, systolic ejection murmur	Murmur sounds the same across the precordium and back and does not change with position; should be gone by age 6 months
Carotid bruit	8-14 years	Anterolateral neck, supraclavicular area	Somewhat harsh, short, systolic ejection murmur	Have patient hyperextend their shoulders: murmur should disappear
Innocent pulmonary systolic murmur	8-14 years	LMSB, LUSB	Short, soft, flowing or somewhat grating ejection murmur	Have patient sit or stand up: murmur should disappear or become quieter and localize to LUSB
Mammary souffle	Adolescent girls with active breast development, pregnancy (third trimester), or lactating	Over the breasts	Blowing sound, breath-like, continuous murmur with systolic accentuation and diastolic spillover	Compress breast tissue under the stethoscope or between fingers to suppress the murmur

LLSB, left lower sternal border; LMSB, left midsternal border; LUSB, left upper sternal border; RMSB, right midsternal border; RUSB, right upper sternal border.

of the AV valves). The ventricle contracts before the semilunar valve opens, called the isovolumetric contraction time. When the pressure in the ventricle exceeds that of the great artery, the semilunar valve opens. The murmur coincides with ejection of blood via the outflow tract. The murmur begins as a low-intensity sound, increases in intensity to a peak, and then decreases in intensity and usually ends before S_2 (crescendo-decrescendo type).

Holosystolic murmurs. Holosystolic murmurs, unlike ejection murmurs, begin immediately after S_1. These murmurs result from either insufficient AV valves or VSDs, beginning as soon as the ventricle starts contracting. Typically, these murmurs last throughout systole and do not vary considerably in intensity like ejection murmurs.

Timing. In the case of ejection murmurs, the severity of obstruction influences the timing of onset and completion of the murmur. Mild stenosis causes an earlier, shorter murmur. More severe obstruction causes a more prolonged murmur, because the ejection time is increased in the setting of profound outflow tract obstruction; this is the same reason that the second heart sound splits more widely when there is pulmonary valve stenosis. However, in cases of decreased cardiac contractility, such as severe or critical aortic stenosis, the murmur duration and intensity may be actually diminished.

Location and radiation. Many murmurs are loud enough to be heard throughout the precordium, but defining the point where the murmur is loudest can help to identify its etiology. The point where the murmur is loudest corresponds with the proximity of the head of the stethoscope to the origin of the lesion. This is illustrated in Figure 1-5. Similarly, murmurs propagate through vascular structures. An ejection murmur of pulmonary valve stenosis radiates to the back and axillae, where the branch pulmonary arteries are directing the sound. Importantly, if there are significant anatomic abnormalities, then structures may not be located where one would expect; thus, the origin of the heart sounds may be shifted as well. In an extreme

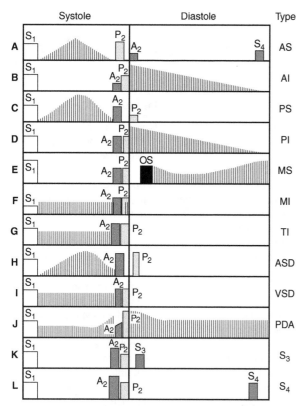

FIGURE 1-4 ■ Graphic representation of common heart murmurs. Height of box indicates intensity of heart sound; hatched lines indicate pattern of murmur. S_1: Occurs at beginning of systole and is closure of the mitral (M_1) and tricuspid (T_1) valves. Normally, T_1 is heard only at the left lower sternal border. S_1 is loudest at the apex. S_2: Occurs at end of systole and is closure of the aortic (A_2) and pulmonic valves (P_2). P_2 is best heard at the left second intercostal space (ICS). S_2 is loudest at the right second ICS. The left second ICS is where to listen for splitting of A_2 and P_2. At end inspiration with tidal breathing, there is more pronounced splitting of the A_2 and P_2 sounds (they are farther apart than at end expiration). With normal physiology, M_1 occurs before T_1, and A_2 occurs before P_2. AI, aortic insufficiency; AS, aortic stenosis; ASD, atrial septal defect; MI, mitral inflow; MS, mitral stenosis; PDA, patent ductus arteriosus; PI, pulmonary insufficiency; PS, pulmonary stenosis; TI, tricuspid inflow; VSD, ventricular septal defect. (*Modified, with permission, from Gomella LG, Haist SA.* Clinician's Pocket Reference. *11th ed. New York, NY: McGraw-Hill; 2007.*)

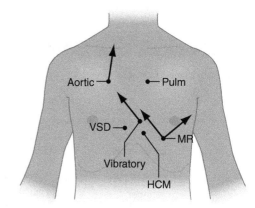

FIGURE 1-5 ■ Sites of auscultation. The aortic valve listening areas are at the left second and right fourth intercostal space. The pulmonic valve listening area is at the left second intercostal space. The tricuspid valve listening area is at the left, parasternal sixth intercostal space, and the mitral valve listening area is also in the sixth intercostal space, at the midclavicular line. HCM, hypertrophic cardiomyopathy; Pulm, pulmonary; MR, mitral regurgitation; VSD, ventricular septal defect. (*Reproduced, with permission, from Fauci AS, Kasper DL, Braunwald E, et al.* Harrison's Principles of Internal Medicine. *17th ed. New York, NY: McGraw-Hill; 2008.*)

example, dextrocardia, the heart is in the right side of the chest, and physical examination findings would be left-right inverted as well.

Quality. The pitch or character of a murmur helps identify the etiology of the murmur as well. The most common innocent murmur, a Still murmur, has been described as vibratory or twangy. Ejection murmurs occurring in the setting of semilunar valve stenosis sound harsh. Most regurgitant murmurs have a high-pitched, blowing nature. Murmurs arising from a VSD also have a harsh, roaring quality. Small VSD murmurs may have a more expulsive or squirty quality. PDA murmurs are described as having a machine-like sound.

Intensity. Systolic murmurs are graded on a scale of 1 to 6 in intensity, and diastolic murmurs are graded on a scale of 1 to 4 as early, mid, or late. The descriptions are as follows:

■ Grade 1 murmur = barely audible, or intermittent
■ Grade 2 murmur = soft but easily audible, identified readily by all examiners, and equally loud as the breath sounds
■ Grade 3 murmur = louder than the breath sounds
■ Grade 4 murmur = accompanied by a thrill, as are louder murmurs
■ Grade 5 murmur = audible with the head of the stethoscope held on end against the chest
■ Grade 6 murmur = appreciated with the stethoscope held away from the chest or with the naked ear

Maneuvers. Table 1-3 lists several maneuvers that can be useful in evaluating cardiac murmurs. Some examiners will also listen after a period of brief, light exercise (such as running in place) to exaggerate clicks and murmurs by increasing cardiac output. Squatting increases systemic vascular resistance and initially increases systemic venous return and, hence, stroke volume. Standing up decreases afterload, systemic venous return, and stroke volume. The Valsalva maneuver (expiring against a closed glottis) causes a rise in intrathoracic pressure and a rise in intracardiac pressure as well. Because systemic vascular resistance is not affected by this maneuver, the increased ventricular pressure causes a decrease in any outflow tract gradient.

Maneuvers Used in Evaluating Heart Murmurs

Maneuver	Effect	Useful for Evaluating
Squatting	↑ SVR Some ↑ venous return	HCM: ↓ murmur
Standing	↓ afterload ↓ stroke volume ↓ venous return	HCM: ↑ murmur
Valsalva	↑ intrathoracic pressure ↑ ventricular pressure No change in SVR	HCM: ↓ murmur
Exercise: running in place	↑ cardiac output	↑ most murmurs
Isometric handgrip	↑ SVR ↑ cardiac output	↑ regurgitant murmurs, VSDs AS, HCM: ↓ murmur
Position: left lateral decubitus	Brings apex of the heart closer to the chest well	↑ aortic murmurs
Leaning forward		↑ mitral murmurs
Compression of left jugular vein or turning the head	↓ great vein return to the heart	Abolish venous hums
Shoulder extension	Subclavian artery compression	Abolish supraclavicular bruits
Breath holding (end expiration)	Decreased lung volume	Easier to hear soft aortic and mitral murmurs
Deep inspiration	↑ systemic venous return	↑ TR, PS, PI murmurs
Lower extremity elevation	↑ systemic venous return	↑ murmurs and gallops

AS, aortic stenosis; HCM, hypertrophic cardiomyopathy; PI, pulmonary insufficiency; PS, pulmonary stenosis; SVR, systemic vascular resistance; TR, tricuspid regurgitation; VSD, ventricular septal defect.

Diastolic murmurs

Early diastolic murmurs. Early diastolic murmurs are generally due to aortic or pulmonary valve leakage. They begin immediately after S_2 as high-intensity sounds that decrease through the early part of diastole (decrescendo murmur). Because the aorta normally has a higher diastolic pressure than the pulmonary artery, the murmur of aortic insufficiency will be higher pitched. An early diastolic murmur of pulmonary valve insufficiency can be medium to low pitched, in the case of normal pressures, or high pitched if there is pulmonary hypertension.

Mid-diastolic murmurs. Mid-diastolic murmurs are the result of turbulent blood flow through the mitral or tricuspid valves during the passive filling phase of the ventricle. Also referred to as a "rumble," this sound is low pitched and is therefore best heard with the bell of the stethoscope. Mitral inflow murmurs are loudest at the apex and usually related to increased pulmonary venous return to the left atrium due to a left-to-right shunt. Tricuspid inflow murmurs usually are associated with atrial septal defects and partially anomalous pulmonary venous return; they are best heard at the left or right lower sternal border.

Late diastolic murmurs. Late diastolic murmurs occur during atrial systole, when blood moves through

the AV valves more forcefully. This occurs with mitral or tricuspid stenosis.

Continuous murmurs

As the name implies, continuous murmurs are heard throughout systole and into diastole. They result from continuous turbulent blood flow, which may be arterial or venous. The classic example of a continuous murmur in pediatrics results from a PDA. The murmur of a PDA is loudest at the left upper sternal border. The murmur increases in intensity during systole and becomes less intense but continues into diastole. There are times when a loud systolic murmur and a loud diastolic murmur can occur sequentially but should not be thought of as a continuous murmur. As in the case of aortic stenosis and insufficiency, there is a systolic ejection murmur followed by an early diastolic decrescendo murmur, and such combinations are often referred to as "to-and-fro" murmurs.

Sample Description of a Cardiac Examination

With practice, combining the various terms used to describe the cardiac examination can give an accurate clinical assessment of the heart. For example, a description of the examination of a Still murmur would include the following: "The precordium is quiet with a normal

S_1 and S_2. There are no clicks or gallops. There is a grade 2/6 short, medium-pitched, vibratory midsystolic murmur heard loudest at the apex and left lower sternal border, which radiates to the left middle and right upper sternal borders. It disappears in the upright position. Diastole is silent." This provides a picture of the pertinent positive and negative points associated with the cardiac examination that, in this case, clearly illustrates this patient's definitive clinical findings.

COMMON CARDIOVASCULAR CHIEF COMPLAINTS SEEN IN GENERAL PEDIATRIC CLINICS

Common indications for referral to pediatric cardiology clinics include palpitations, syncope, and chest pain. A thorough understanding of the cardiac history and physical examination is essential to determine the likely importance of a murmur or of these common symptoms. The following section will review the most common complaints, their differential diagnosis, and the approach to diagnosis. A discussion of treatments is also included.

Palpitations

Definition and epidemiology

Palpitations refer to the sensation of irregular, unusual, forceful, or strong heartbeats and can be associated with either slow, rapid, or irregular heart rates or rhythms. Determining the presence of palpitations in the pediatric population has many challenges; primarily, children often do not accurately report palpitations to their parents. Additionally, no large population-based studies in children describe the incidence or prevalence of these symptoms.

Pathogenesis

Palpitations have many causes, and the etiologies are quite heterogeneous. The perception of an abnormal heart rhythm may or may not correlate with an actual abnormal heart rhythm.

Clinical presentation

An important goal of the history is to discern whether the palpitations are isolated, intermittent, clustered, or sustained. This helps to differentiate between single ectopic beats, bursts of ectopy, or sustained runs of tachycardia. For younger children, it may be helpful to tap or clap a rhythm, giving examples of both a regular rhythm with a premature beat and a sustained tachycardia or bradycardia. Another goal of the interview

should be to establish whether the potential arrhythmia has hemodynamic effects. The association of dizziness or syncope with the palpitations suggests a decreased cardiac output with a low blood pressure and indicates that further evaluation to rule out an arrhythmia should not be delayed.

Children sometimes report sinus tachycardia as palpitations. Increased heart rate due to sinus tachycardia typically has a gradual onset and offset, which occurs most commonly in the setting of exercise, anxiety, fever, or other normal physiologic conditions. On the other hand, supraventricular and ventricular tachycardia typically begin abruptly. It may be difficult to distinguish abrupt onset and offset due to the usual presence of sinus tachycardia during exercise.

Although isolated premature atrial or ventricular beats occur in children, they are uncommon, but increase in adolescence. Even isolated premature beats can be bothersome, especially if the patient is very conscious of them or if they occur frequently, particularly if they comprise over 20% to 30% of the rhythm.

Sustained palpitations should raise concern for tachyarrhythmia. In addition, other systemic or exogenous causes should be considered in the differential diagnosis. This includes abnormal electrolytes, anemia, hyperthyroidism, excessive catecholamines, or ingestion of substances such as caffeine, tobacco, or sympathomimetic medications. Children on stimulant medications for attention deficit disorder or asthma may have increased heart rates while taking those medications.

Differential diagnosis

Table 1-4 lists the differential diagnosis of palpitations.

Making the diagnosis

See the algorithm in Figure 1-6.

Diagnostic tests

An ECG should be obtained to demonstrate the baseline rhythm and to evaluate the corrected QT interval. If ectopy is frequent, it can be assessed in real time by obtaining a continuous ECG or "rhythm strip." If the palpitations occur on a daily basis, a 24-hour ambulatory Holter monitor may be useful. The goal is to document abnormal rhythms during symptoms, either linking them or disproving an association. When palpitations occur very intermittently, other types of rhythm-recording devices are more useful. An ambulatory event recorder works by monitoring the heart rhythm, either continuously if connected by leads or intermittently when applied to the chest. These can be useful for capturing events that need evaluation. In both cases, the results can be sent via telephone, wireless, or satellite transmission to a central processing agency and forwarded to the ordering physician.

Differential Diagnosis of Palpitations

- Primary arrhythmia
  - Premature atrial contraction
  - Premature ventricular contraction
  - Supraventricular tachycardia
  - Ventricular tachycardia
  - Bradycardia or AV block
- Fever
- Anemia
- Dehydration
- Exercise
- Intense emotional response
- Anxiety, fear, panic attack
- Drug or toxin ingestion
- Hyperthyroidism
- Pheochromocytoma
- Structural congenital heart disease
- Myocarditis or cardiomyopathy
- Intracardiac tumor

Treatment

The management of palpitations depends on the underlying causes, which are addressed in detail in other chapters of this book.

Referral guidelines

Exogenous causes (listed in Table 1-4) may result in palpitations. When appropriate, testing for those conditions should be performed. There should be a heightened level of concern when palpitations occur in the presence of structural or functional heart disease or electrical heart conditions or when underlying arrhythmias are known to be present. Further evaluation should be sought in the presence of those aforementioned conditions as well as with the occurrence of sustained tachycardia. The presence of associated syncopal events, ischemic chest pain, or sustained or symptomatic palpitations that interfere with daily activity should raise concern, as should a family history of early sudden death (<35 years of age), sudden infant death syndrome, sudden unexpected infant death, or other inherited conditions, including long QT syndrome, that are associated with sudden cardiac death.

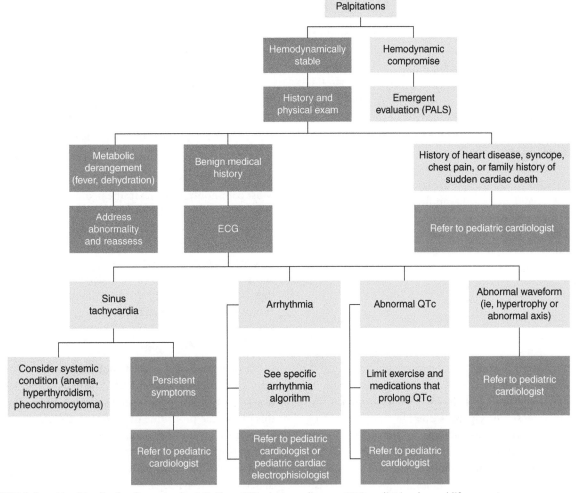

FIGURE 1-6 ■ Algorithm for the diagnosis of palpitations. ECG, electrocardiogram; PALS, pediatric advanced life support.

Syncope

Definition and epidemiology

Syncope, the medical term for fainting, is a brief, sudden, usually temporary loss of consciousness, resulting from a lack of blood flow and oxygen to the brain, most commonly from low arterial blood pressure, with spontaneous recovery. The incidence of syncope throughout childhood is approximately 15%, with the highest occurrence in adolescence.[3,4]

Pathogenesis

The various causes of syncope represent a heterogeneous spectrum of pathologies that culminate in temporary hypoperfusion of the brain.

Clinical presentation

The history is of particular importance, especially in identifying the cases with a potentially life-threatening etiology. The history should emphasize the precise sequence of events leading up to and during the loss of consciousness, sometimes from the viewpoint of a bystander if the child cannot remember. If the patient has multiple episodes, the frequency, timing, and duration of each event should be detailed. The patient's posture (supine, sitting, or standing) during the event is important. All associated signs and symptoms should be reviewed, including pallor, diaphoresis, visual or auditory changes, dizziness, palpitations, hyperventilation, nausea, incontinence, seizure-like activity (including timing of seizure activity as to before or after loss of consciousness), and the presence of confusion or a postictal state after the syncopal event. The length of time to complete recovery should be noted.

Prodromal symptoms of diaphoresis; pallor; dizziness; blurry vision; nausea; and the sensation of feeling hot or cold, of hearing muffled sounds, or of having blurred vision, tunnel vision, or visual black spots that precede a syncopal event favor a diagnosis of neurally mediated syncope (NMS). This is associated with autonomic imbalance and increased vagal tone. Similarly, the characteristics of the environment in which the event occurred are important, such as the ambient temperature or crowding of the area. Other important factors include prolonged standing and rapid rising from sitting or kneeling to standing, as in church. Prolonged crying or temper tantrums often precede a breath-holding spell. If syncope occurs with exercise, one should determine the timing of the events with respect to the level or intensity of vigorous exercise (early on during warm-up, during peak activity, or immediately after stopping exercise). Syncope that occurs with vigorous exercise suggests a much more dangerous mechanism than an event that occurs several minutes after exercise, although both can occur in association with serious cardiac conditions. Similarly, syncope that occurs in association with emotional or psychological stress can be due to an arrhythmia or to a neurally mediated mechanism and requires further evaluation. Pain can often result in a marked vagal autonomic nervous system output and can be associated with NMS. Dietary habits should be explored, including skipped meals and total fluid and salt intake for the day. Based on the fact that dehydration results in decreased urination, the frequency of urination should be assessed. The color of the urine can also be a helpful; very infrequent, dark-colored urine may signal inadequate fluid intake. Caffeine (eg, coffee, tea, soda, energy drinks) and alcohol are diuretics and may cause negative fluid balance; daily caffeine or other diuretic intake should be quantified.

Any family history of sudden cardiac death may be an indicator of a heritable disease such as long QT syndrome or hypertrophic cardiomyopathy, especially if this occurs in very young (<35 years of age) or moderately young (<50 years of age) family members.

The physical examination should include orthostatic vital signs, in addition to the standard cardiac physical examination. Orthostatic vital signs should particularly note the changes in heart rate and blood pressure from the supine to the immediate standing position and after standing for 3 to 5 minutes. An increase in heart rate or decrease in blood pressure can suggest that the individual is hypovolemic and needs to increase his or her daily fluid (and possibly salt) intake. Particular attention should be paid to any left ventricular outflow tract murmurs (harsh systolic ejection murmurs along the left sternal border and at the apex), which may be a sign of hypertrophic cardiomyopathy or aortic stenosis.

Neurally mediated syncope

Most commonly, syncope in the pediatric population is due to a neurally mediated mechanism in children. The term "reflex syncope" has been used synonymously to describe loss of consciousness resulting from episodic, inappropriate vasodilatation or bradycardia related to autonomic nervous system imbalance.[5] The peak incidence occurs between 15 and 19 years of age and is more common in females than males.

Vasodepressor syncope

In vasodepressor syncope, hypotension occurs in the setting of autonomic dysfunction, with a compensatory heart rate increase prior to the syncopal event. During this phase, the prodrome of dizziness, pallor, diaphoresis, nausea, or auditory or visual symptoms may occur. The patient may report a rapid heart rate in the pre-event period, but bradycardia is most common immediately after the syncopal event with increased heart rate returning after return of consciousness.

Cardioinhibitory syncope

By contrast, in cardioinhibitory syncope, the heart rate slows or stops for several seconds, resulting in a fall in blood pressure. High vagal tone is thought to be responsible, along with increased sensitivity of the sinus node. A very slow heart rate may be noted following a cardio-inhibitory event.

Postural orthostatic tachycardia syndrome

Patients with postural orthostatic tachycardia syndrome (POTS) have an impaired ability to appropriately increase peripheral vascular tone in response to orthostatic stress. This syndrome is characterized by exaggerated sinus tachycardia in response to postural changes, such as standing upright. There is accompanying systemic hypotension and clinical orthostasis. In the older child or adolescent, the diagnosis is made by an increase in heart rate from supine to standing of at least 30 beats per minute or by an increase in heart rate to at least 120 beats per minute in the first 10 minutes of upright position. This is considered to be a dysautonomia, which is felt to be a different pathophysiologic mechanism from typical NMS.

Arrhythmias

Any rhythm that causes low cardiac output and a decrease in blood pressure and cerebral blood flow may cause a loss of consciousness. This can include supraventricular tachycardia (SVT) and ventricular tachycardia (VT) or abrupt bradycardia. Most children and adolescents tolerate SVT well depending on the rate and the underlying baseline structure and function of the myocardium. With the onset of SVT, the blood pressure often falls, and the person can feel lightheaded or faint. VT is more often associated with underlying cardiac abnormalities and, thus, more likely to be poorly tolerated and associated with syncope. If a rhythm-related cause of syncope is suspected based on history, various etiologies causing tachycardia should be considered. These include Wolff-Parkinson-White syndrome with atrial fibrillation and rapid ventricular response; torsades de pointes, a type of VT associated with long QT syndrome; short QT syndrome; Brugada syndrome; catecholaminergic polymorphic VT; arrhythmogenic right ventricular cardiomyopathy/dysplasia (ARVC/D); and hypertrophic and dilated cardiomyopathies. In association with congenital heart disease, both SVT and VT may result in syncope.

Bradyarrhythmias may also cause syncope and include sinus node dysfunction or high-grade AV block with long pauses in the rhythm. This is most likely to occur in the setting of congenital heart disease or acquired heart disease such as Lyme disease with complete heart block or with myocarditis.

Structural or functional heart disease

Hypertrophic cardiomyopathy is associated with syncope secondary to a variety of mechanisms. The abnormal myocardial structure characteristic of hypertrophic cardiomyopathy is most commonly arrhythmogenic. When present, outflow tract obstruction can lead to coronary ischemia, resulting in secondary ventricular arrhythmias.

Other diagnoses to consider include valvar aortic stenosis; anomalous origin of the left coronary artery from the wrong sinus; postoperative congenital heart defects, especially in patients having ventricular surgery or with single ventricle physiology (Fontan palliations); dilated cardiomyopathy; right ventricular cardiomyopathy; acute myocarditis; and pulmonary hypertension.

Noncardiac causes

Other entities in the differential diagnosis include seizure, atypical migraine, drug ingestion, vertigo, narcolepsy, cataplexy, hypoglycemia, vertebrobasilar vasospasm, hyperventilation syndrome, metabolic causes such as severe hypoglycemia, and psychogenic causes/conversion reaction.

Differential diagnosis

Important causes of syncope are listed in Table 1-5.

Differential Diagnosis of Syncope

- Long QT syndrome
- Brugada syndrome
- Short QT syndrome
- Polymorphic catecholaminergic ventricular tachycardia (CPVT)
- WPW, SVT, atrial fibrillation
- Heart block
- Sinus node dysfunction
- Arrhythmogenic right ventricular cardiomyopathy/dysplasia
- Hypertrophic cardiomyopathy
- Coronary abnormalities
- Severe aortic stenosis
- Dilated cardiomyopathy
- Pulmonary hypertension
- Myocarditis
- Neurocardiogenic syncope
- Orthostatic hypotension
- Hyperventilation syndrome
- Breath holding spell
- Drug or toxin exposure
- Hypoglycemia
- Seizure

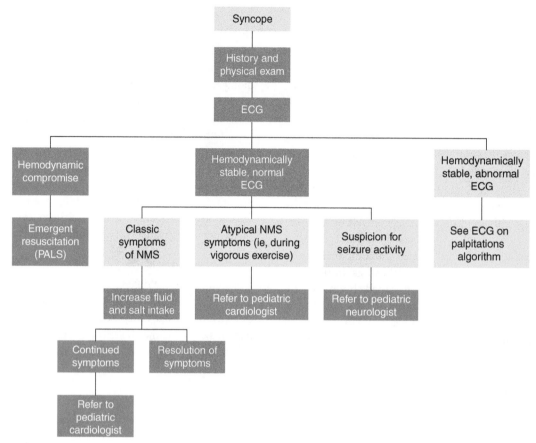

FIGURE 1-7 ■ Algorithm for the diagnosis of syncope. ECG, electrocardiogram; NMS, neurally mediated syncope; PALS, pediatric advanced life support.

Making the diagnosis

See the algorithm in Figure 1-7.

Diagnostic tests

An ECG should be obtained, especially in the patient without a prior study, to calculate the corrected QT interval and rule out long or short QT syndromes, Brugada syndrome, or other rhythm or conduction abnormalities such as pre-excitation (Wolff-Parkinson-White) or AV block. Additionally, one should evaluate the ECG for evidence of myocardial ischemia or inflammation, right or left ventricular hypertrophy, or findings of right ventricular conduction delay seen in ARVC/D or left ventricular conduction delay seen in dilated cardiomyopathy.

Other laboratory studies can be helpful, including a blood glucose level, complete blood count, electrolytes, urine pregnancy, or urine toxin screen. In the appropriate clinical setting, selected tests can rule out hypoglycemia, anemia, pregnancy, or ingestion. Electrolytes can be helpful in further exploring intravascular volume status.

In situations where history and physical examination cannot differentiate between NMS and other causes of loss of consciousness and symptoms are atypical or potentially threatening, tilt-table testing may be helpful.

However, because there can be up to a 40% false-positive rate with head-up tilt-table testing in adolescents, patients at this level of complexity can benefit from referral to a pediatric cardiologist or pediatric electrophysiologist. If arrhythmia is suspected, additional testing such as a 24-hour Holter monitor or event recorder may be warranted. Implantable event loop recorders may be helpful in extreme cases where serious recurrent symptoms cannot be explained and persist over long periods of time or result in serious injury.

Treatment

Often, vasodepressor syncope can be managed by increasing fluid and salt intake. Current recommendations include drinking at least four 8- to 12-oz glasses of noncaffeinated fluid per day. Another way of estimating necessary fluid intake would be to attempt 1.5 to 2 oz of fluid per kilogram. Patients should be advised never to allow themselves to feel thirsty. If there are known triggers, these should be avoided when possible. Similarly, high-risk activities like swimming alone or other activities in which loss of consciousness could result in severe injury should be avoided. Blood drawing is often a trigger and should be accomplished in a supine position when the patient is known to be well hydrated. Most states will not allow driving within 6 to 12 months of loss of consciousness, and many states require the physician to report syncope or events that result in loss of consciousness to the motor vehicle department.

Increasing the salt in the diet can be extremely helpful if the blood pressure is low or normal at baseline. Practically speaking, this means eating nonfatty, salty snacks, such as pretzels or pickles, as well as salting meat and vegetables. Most patients with NMS have spontaneous resolution of their symptoms or learn to accommodate to their fluid intake needs by adulthood. If the above measures are ineffective, then medications may be considered and may be recommended by a cardiology consultation.

Abortive maneuvers can be helpful in some cases. Lying down with the feet elevated is most useful. If this is not possible, squatting or sitting down and placing one's head between the knees may abort an episode of impending syncope, increasing systemic vascular resistance and bringing the head to heart level. Isometric maneuvers, such as pushing the hands together or tightly crossing the legs, or moving in place may prove helpful to some patients in aborting impending syncope.

Referral guidelines

Patients with syncope that occurs during or immediately after exercise raise greatest concern for a cardiac etiology, although NMS can occur after exercise in the face of extreme dehydration and vasodilatation. Recurrent symptoms or a worrisome family history should result in referral in most cases. Symptoms associated with the syncopal event such as chest pain, cyanosis, shortness of breath, or palpitations should prompt referral.

Chest Pain

Definition and epidemiology

Importantly, chest pain due to myocardial ischemia or other cardiac conditions is rare in a pediatric patient. Diagnosing the rare case of angina is dependent on taking a meticulous history. Rapid identification of myocardial ischemia in the pediatric patient can be life saving. The differential diagnosis of chest pain in pediatrics can be categorized by organ system: musculoskeletal, pulmonary, gastrointestinal, psychogenic, and cardiac. The causes of chest pain by organ system are summarized in Table 1-6.

Clinical presentation

Young children have difficulty in localizing pain and may point to the chest when the pain originates in the abdomen or vice versa. Despite this ambiguity, the history alone may lead to the diagnosis in most cases. Using the alphabetical pneumonic in Table 1-7 helps to generate a complete and organized history.

Causes of Pediatric Chest Pain	
Idiopathic	12%-85%
Musculoskeletal	15%-31%
Pulmonary	12%-21%
Psychiatric	5%-17%
Gastrointestinal	4%-7%
Cardiac	4%-6%
Other	4%-21%

Data from Eslick GD. Epidemiology and risk factors of pediatric chest pain: a systematic review. Pediatr Clin North Am. 2010;57:1211-1219.

On physical examination, chest pain that the examiner can reproduce by gently palpating the chest wall can be diagnostic of a musculoskeletal etiology; for example, pain on palpation of the sternum or costochondral joints strongly suggests a diagnosis of costochondritis. Tachypnea, wheezing, increased work of breathing, and respiratory distress may be signs of a pulmonary etiology. In the correct clinical setting, absent or distant breath sounds can be a sign of consolidation or air leak syndrome, such as pneumothorax. The acutely ill child with lethargy, fever, and a gallop rhythm or a pericardial rub requires emergent evaluation for myocarditis or pericarditis.

Musculoskeletal causes

Traumatic pain should be considered and can be ruled out easily by history. This should include overuse injuries, which are sometimes seen in adolescents who have had a recent increase in their activity level (eg, starting a weight-lifting regimen or a new sport). **Idiopathic chest wall pain**, also called "precordial catch" or "Texidor's twinge," refers to brief, episodic, sharp chest pain that is worse with inspiration and occurs at rest. It can occur anywhere around the precordium and is typically not reproducible with palpation. Inflammation of the costochondral joint can occur in the setting of a viral illness or an overuse injury and results in **costochondritis.** Chest pain associated with costochondritis has been classically described as pain that can be reproduced on palpation of the costochondral joint.

Pulmonary causes

Chest pain of a pulmonary nature generally has been described as pleuritic, worsening with deep inspiration. Asthma or **reactive airways disease** is a frequent cause of chest pain in children.[6] Spontaneous **pneumothorax** (or pneumomediastinum) classically occurs in tall, thin teenage males. It presents as sudden-onset, sharp chest pain. There is a high recurrence risk of primary spontaneous pneumothorax in the general population, somewhere

Alphabetical Pneumonic for Evaluating Pediatric Chest Pain

L: Location	Ask the patient to point with one finger to the place it hurts the most.
M: Movement/motion	Recall activities that have produced the pain, such as heavy lifting, repetitive motions, new athletic activities, chronic cough/emesis.
N: Notable associated symptoms	Rule out dyspnea, diaphoresis, nausea or vomiting, dizziness, syncope, palpitations, rash, fever, cough, hyperventilation including carpal-pedal spasm, and perioral numbness.
O: Onset	Establish the circumstances surrounding the onset of pain.
P: Provocation/palliation	Ask what makes the pain better and worse.
Q: Quality	Determine the nature of the pain, particularly whether the pain is sharp, dull, or burning. Children may need additional descriptors or demonstrations, such comparing the pain to a pin stick or someone sitting on their chest.
R: Radiation	Establish whether the pain spreads to the left arm, epigastrium, or neck/jaw, which tends to be suggestive of angina.
S: Severity	Specify the severity of the pain on a scale of 1 to 10. This also requires qualification: "where 1 is no pain and 10 is the worst pain you could imagine."
T: Timing	Ask about the frequency and duration, and create a timeline detailing the pain chronologically.

around 50%.[7] It worsens with inspiration and can be associated with dyspnea. If present, connective tissue disease, such as Marfan syndrome, should be explored. **Pulmonary embolism** is rare in pediatrics but has a higher incidence in select populations. Patients at high risk include the immobile postoperative patient; hypoproteinemic children with protein-losing enteropathy, persistent pulmonary effusions, or chylothorax; those with other hypercoagulable disorders; patients with autoimmune disease; or patients with a history of intravenous drug abuse. Oral contraceptives can increase the risk. **Pulmonary hypertension** can present with chest pain, although it more commonly presents with dyspnea on exertion, fatigue, or syncope with exercise. **Pneumonia**, bronchitis, or empyema can cause pain and should be considered in the setting of fever and cough.

Gastrointestinal causes

Gastroesophageal reflux causes retrosternal, burning or squeezing chest pain. Older patients may complain of belching or bloating, sometimes with an acid taste in the mouth, especially when supine. Antacids will provide temporary relief and can be useful as a diagnostic test. Eating will generally cause the pain to dissipate, only to return shortly thereafter. **Esophageal dysmotility** leading to achalasia is a rare cause of chest pain. An esophageal foreign body should also be considered in the appropriate setting. **Epigastric pain** may be reported as chest pain in children and may be due to gastritis, hepatitis, pancreatitis, or biliary tract disease.

Psychogenic causes

Anxiety or stress may result in symptoms of chest pain, particularly common in adolescents.[8] Indeed, anxiety

has been reported as both cause and effect of chest discomfort in this age group.

Cardiac or pericardial causes

Pericarditis causes a sharp, retrosternal pain that can be referred to the left shoulder. Classically, it is less severe when leaning forward and worsened when supine. A viral prodrome may be present on history. Examination findings may include a pericardial friction rub, muffled heart sounds, and pulsus paradoxus if a large pericardial effusion is present causing pericardial tamponade. Chest pain due to **myocardial ischemia** has been described as severe, sometimes "squeezing" or "pressure," which may radiate to the neck, jaw, or left shoulder. Patients typically appear to be in distress and are diaphoretic or dyspneic. ECG changes include ST-segment elevation or depression, T-wave inversion, or Q waves. Cardiac enzymes are elevated, specifically troponin I and CK-MB fraction. In the pediatric age group, congenital coronary anomalies or coronary involvement from Kawasaki disease should be considered in the differential diagnosis. Severe left ventricular outflow tract obstruction can cause decreased coronary perfusion pressure with increased myocardial oxygen demand, producing angina. This can be seen in severe aortic stenosis and hypertrophic cardiomyopathy. Myocardial bridging refers to cases where the coronary artery dives beneath the epicardium briefly before returning to the surface of the heart, creating a bridge of muscle over the vessel. If this is present, then as myocardial oxygen demand increases, the ability of the bridged coronary to provide adequate tissue oxygenation may be inadequate, creating a state of relative ischemia; however, there is some debate surrounding the clinical significance of myocardial bridging.[9] **Coronary**

vasospasm is rare in the pediatric population, but similar conditions of inadequate tissue oxygen delivery can occur. In the absence of specific triggers, this is referred to as Prinzmetal angina. Cocaine or other sympathomimetics can cause coronary vasospasm and myocardial ischemia; vasospasm is compounded in this setting by increased contractility and myocardial oxygen demand.

Anatomic anomalies of the coronaries, such as the origin of both coronaries from the same sinus of Valsalva, can cause angina pectoris.[10,11] A recent survey of sudden death in young athletes revealed that coronary anomalies are the third most common cause of death, accounting for 13.6% of sudden cardiac deaths.[12] With the origin of the left coronary from the right sinus of Valsalva, the left main coronary may pass between the aortic root and the main pulmonary artery; patients with this anomaly are at high risk for sudden death or acute myocardial infarction.[10] The mechanism of ischemia in this circumstance remains controversial.

Arrhythmias can cause a sensation that may be perceived or related as pain in younger patients. Alternately, arrhythmia with elevated heart rates may cause a lower blood pressure or decreased coronary perfusion, leading to chest pain. **Myocarditis** can cause a dull, substernal chest pain but is typically associated with respiratory distress, fatigue, or cardiovascular collapse. Examination findings will include a gallop rhythm and tachycardia. ECG findings will reflect ischemia by manifesting ST-segment changes, Q waves, or T-wave abnormalities including inversion. In the normal child, **aortic dissection** is quite rare; however, in the subset of patients with Marfan syndrome presenting with chest pain, dissection should be strongly considered and evaluated because it is a life-threatening complication. Bicuspid aortic valve, the most common congenital cardiac anomaly, also leads to dilation of the ascending aorta in many cases; the prevalence of ascending aortic dilation in persons with a bicuspid aortic valve varies based on the population studied, but has been estimated as 56% in those less than 30 years of age and as high as 88% in those greater than 80 years of age.[13] The lifetime risk of dissection in the presence of a bicuspid aortic valve has been estimated as 6%, 9-fold higher than the general population.[13] Although aortic dissection and rupture very rarely occur in children, dilation of the aortic root begins early in life.[14]

Other Causes

Several other causes of potentially life-threatening chest pain do not fit into the previous categories. For example, chest wall tumors can present with chest pain and may go undiagnosed if dismissed as being due to idiopathic musculoskeletal pain; acute chest syndrome in the patient with sickle cell disease should be considered when appropriate.

Differential Diagnosis of Chest Pain

- Trauma
- Idiopathic chest wall pain
- Costochondritis
- Asthma
- Spontaneous pneumothorax
- Pulmonary embolism
- Pulmonary hypertension
- Pneumonitis, bronchitis, or empyema
- Gastroesophageal reflux
- Esophageal dysmotility
- Gastritis
- Acute chest syndrome
- Chest wall tumor
- Sympathomimetic use
- Myocarditis
- Pericarditis
- Aortic dissection
- Aortic stenosis
- Hypertrophic cardiomyopathy
- Coronary or Prinzmetal's angina
- Anatomic coronary anomalies

Differential diagnosis

The differential diagnosis of chest pain is listed in Table 1-8.

Making the diagnosis

See the algorithm in Figure 1-8.

Diagnostic tests

Evaluating the degree of gastroesophageal reflux may include empiric antacid, where relief of retrosternal pain may be both diagnostic and therapeutic. In the inpatient setting, pH or impedance probe testing can confirm a diagnosis of gastroesophageal reflux disease.

Chest x-ray is useful in diagnosing gross, anatomic causes of chest pain, such as chest wall tumors and traumatic injuries, and pneumonia or pneumothorax. An enlarged cardiac silhouette may signal pericarditis or myocarditis. A widened mediastinum could suggest an aortic dissection. An **ECG** may show signs of myocardial ischemia, inflammation, arrhythmia, decreased voltages as in myocarditis, or ventricular hypertrophy as in hypertrophic cardiomyopathy. Diffuse ST-segment or T-wave changes may be a sign of pericarditis, myocarditis, or coronary ischemia. Q waves usually indicate the presence of prior ischemic injury. Rarely, an emergent **ECG** may be needed, particularly to evaluate cardiac causes of hemodynamic instability, to rule out myocarditis with decreased ventricular function, or to assess for cardiac tamponade, aortic root dissection, coronary anomalies, and pulmonary hypertension.

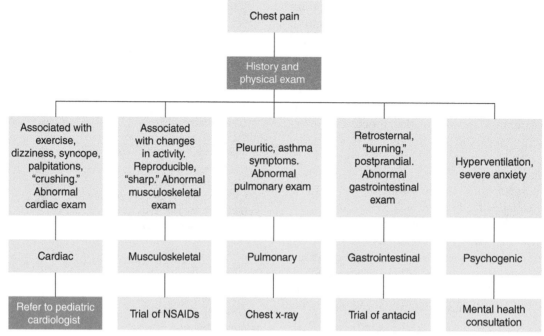

FIGURE 1-8 ■ Algorithm for the diagnosis of chest pain. NSAIDs, nonsteroidal anti-inflammatory drugs.

Treatment

Due to the degree of anxiety that often accompanies the chief complaint of chest pain, reassurance should be foremost in most cases where the etiology is found to be benign. Management must be tailored to the individual disease state.

Referral guidelines

Further evaluation should occur when chest pain begins suddenly; is brought on by exertion or excitement; is associated with dizziness, syncope, or palpitations; awakens the patient from sleep; is described as crushing; or is associated with a history of cardiac disease.

Clinical Pearls

- Cardiac output is determined by preload, afterload, and stroke volume.
- Diastolic murmurs are always abnormal.
- Familiarizing oneself with the normal cardiovascular findings in children, including knowledge of the innocent murmurs, allows for more accurate discernment of abnormal findings and, hence, appropriate referrals for evaluation.
- Most chest pain in children is noncardiac, but ruling out a cardiac etiology is important and can typically be done with a thorough history and examination.
- Neurally mediated syncope can usually be treated successfully with increased fluid and salt intake.
- Syncope or presyncope that occurs during exercise requires prompt evaluation, and exercise should be restricted until that evaluation can take place.
- Sustained palpitations should raise concern for nonsinus tachycardia and merit evaluation.

REFERENCES

1. Sinaiko AR, Gomez-Marin O, Prineas RJ. Prevalence of "significant" hypertension in junior high school-aged children: the Children and Adolescent Blood Pressure Program. *J Pediatr*. 1989;114:664-669.
2. Sorof JM, Lai D, Turner J, Poffenbarger T, Portman RJ. Overweight, ethnicity, and the prevalence of hypertension in school-aged children. *Pediatrics*. 2004;113: 475-482.
3. Pratt JL, Fleisher GR. Syncope in children and adolescents. *Pediatr Emerg Care*. 1989;5:80-82.
4. McHarg ML, Shinnar S, Rascoff H, Walsh CA. Syncope in childhood. *Pediatr Cardiol*. 1997;18:367-371.
5. Wieling W, Ganzeboom KS, Saul JP. Reflex syncope in children and adolescents. *Heart*. 2004;90:1094-1100.
6. Wiens L, Sabath R, Ewing L, Gowdamarajan R, Portnoy J, Scagliotti D. Chest pain in otherwise healthy children and adolescents is frequently caused by exercise-induced asthma. *Pediatrics*. 1992;90:350-353.
7. Sadikot RT, Greene T, Meadows K, Arnold AG. Recurrence of primary spontaneous pneumothorax. *Thorax*. 1997;52:805-809.
8. Pantell RH, Goodman BW Jr. Adolescent chest pain: a prospective study. *Pediatrics*. 1983;71:881-887.
9. Alegria JR, Herrmann J, Holmes DR Jr, Lerman A, Rihal CS. Myocardial bridging. *Eur Heart J*. 2005;26: 1159-1168.
10. Roberts WC. Major anomalies of coronary arterial origin seen in adulthood. *Am Heart J*. 1986;111:941-963.
11. Angelini P, Walmsley RP, Libreros A, Ott DA. Symptomatic anomalous origination of the left coronary artery from the opposite sinus of Valsalva. Clinical presentations, diagnosis, and surgical repair. *Tex Heart Inst J*. 2006;33:171-179.

12. Maron BJ. Sudden death in young athletes. *N Engl J Med.* 2003;349:1064-1075.

13. Tadros TM, Klein MD, Shapira OM. Ascending aortic dilatation associated with bicuspid aortic valve: pathophysiology, molecular biology, and clinical implications. *Circulation.* 2009;119:880-890.

14. Warren AE, Boyd ML, O'Connell C, Dodds L. Dilatation of the ascending aorta in paediatric patients with bicuspid aortic valve: frequency, rate of progression and risk factors. *Heart.* 2006;92:1496-1500.

CHAPTER 2

Cardiac Testing

Brooke T. Davey, R. Lee Vogel,
Meryl S. Cohen, Mark A. Fogel and
Stephen M. Paridon

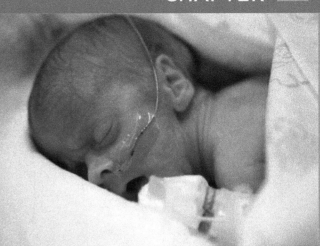

INTRODUCTION

Evaluation of the infant, child, or young adult with cardiovascular symptoms may require the application of a variety of cardiac tests. Each of these tests has specific indications that provide unique information for characterization of a particular problem, but these tests also have limitations. Adding various tests allows for the layering of information until a rich composite model of the cardiovascular structure and function is built. This allows for optimal understanding of the condition and the implementation of the most appropriate and efficient care.

In this chapter, we review 4 fundamental types of noninvasive cardiac testing: electrocardiography, exercise/cardiopulmonary stress testing, echocardiography, and cardiac magnetic resonance imaging.

ELECTROCARDIOGRAPHY TESTING

The Pediatric Electrocardiogram

Introduction to the pediatric electrocardiogram

Electrocardiography has always been one of the fundamental procedures used in the diagnosis and treatment of cardiac disease ever since Einthoven first recorded the heart's electrical activity in 1901 using a string galvanometer. Information gained from the electrocardiogram (ECG) can be used to help determine the cardiac anatomy, the cardiac rhythm and electrical conduction, and the effect of therapeutic interventions on cardiac electrical activity. Since the advent of echocardiography, a pediatric cardiologist rarely depends on the ECG to accurately predict the cardiac anatomy. However, the ECG is indispensable in the evaluation of a child with a suspected cardiac rhythm abnormality. It is now well recognized that some medications may significantly alter the heart's electrical properties to the point that it places the patient at increased risk for sudden cardiac death, usually from a form of polymorphic ventricular tachycardia known as torsade de pointes. As such, screening and serial ECGs are indicated. Although still an area of controversy in the United States, there are proponents who say that an ECG should be included in the preparticipation sports evaluation and before the initiation of stimulant medication for attention-deficit hyperactivity disorder.[1-4] Although today's ECG machines are smaller, portable, and readily available, the waveforms they produce are not different than those seen by Einthoven over a century ago.

Basic concepts and the approach to the pediatric ECG

For a complete description of the ECG, the reader is referred to the many textbooks devoted exclusively to ECG interpretation. The basic 12-lead ECG includes the limb leads I, II, III, aVR, aVL, and aVF plus the precordial leads V_1 to V_6. Because most pediatric cardiologists see children with anatomically abnormal hearts, the typical pediatric ECG records 15 leads, the additional 3 being lead V_3R, V_4R, and V_7 (Figure 2-1). The different leads that are used in the ECG provide unique perspectives for the evaluation of the electrical system of the heart as a whole. This concept is represented by the hexaxial reference system and the horizontal reference system (Figure 2-2). In the hexaxial system, the limb leads represent different degrees of orientation in relationship to the vertical plane of the heart from 0 to ±180 degrees. The positive or negative deflections created by

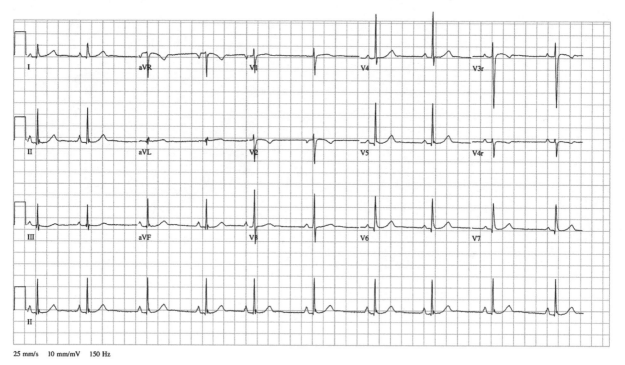

25 mm/s   10 mm/mV   150 Hz

FIGURE 2-1 ■ This is a pediatric 15-lead ECG in a 9-year-old female.

the depolarization forces in these different leads may be interpreted using this vector system to identify the cumulative direction of the electrical stimulus within the myocardium. Meanwhile, the horizontal reference system represents the precordial leads V_1 to V_7, as well as V_3R and V_4R. This system provides information about the anteroposterior and left to right aspects of the horizontal plane of the heart.[5] The pediatric leads V_3R and V_4R allow for a more thorough evaluation of the right ventricle, whereas V_7 allows for a more thorough evaluation of the left ventricle.

As with all parameters in pediatrics, the ECG also has a wandering baseline of normal for nearly all measurements. One must know the age and the clinical condition of the patient before any meaningful interpretation of the ECG can be made. Davignon's published normative data by age in 1979 is still used, but many institutions have subsequently developed their own standards.[6] A systematic approach to ECG interpretation is recommended. Heart rate; QRS and P-wave axis; PR, QRS, and corrected QT intervals; evidence of right or left ventricular hypertrophy; ST and T-wave patterns; and assessment for cardiac rhythm abnormalities should be evaluated sequentially. Some ECG machines have an automated interpretation function that should only be used as a preliminary read of the study.

Average heart rates at rest should generally be below 100 beats per minute (bpm) after age 5 years. Neonatal heart rates above 235 bpm are usually not secondary to sinus tachycardia but are more typical of a true cardiac

tachydysrhythmia. Similarly, a 6-year-old with a fever and a heart rate of 130 bpm may simply have sinus tachycardia secondary to the fever with no evidence of cardiac disease. Again, the age and clinical condition of the child must be known to accurately interpret the ECG.

The QRS axis is measured using leads I and aVF. It is a limited element of the ECG that can assist in the diagnosis of congenital heart disease. Typically, newborns have a mean QRS axis that is rightward, negative in lead I and positive in lead aVF. The mean QRS axis drifts leftward after birth generally assuming the normal adult QRS axis of 0 to 90 degrees by 1 month of age. Children with trisomy 21 associated with a complete common atrioventricular (AV) canal cardiac defect usually have an ECG that demonstrates a superior mean QRS axis. In leads I and aVF, the QRS is negative, whereas in leads aVR and aVL, it is positive. It must be remembered, however, that all children with Down syndrome should have a formal cardiac evaluation and echocardiogram performed in the neonatal period, even if the ECG is normal. Children with tricuspid atresia may have cyanosis and an ECG with left axis deviation. Right axis deviation with right ventricular hypertrophy can be seen in children with pulmonary hypertension. Most types of congenital cardiac defects do not have a unique QRS axis, but an abnormal QRS axis for age should raise the possibility that a cardiac abnormality may be present.

Measurement of the P-wave axis is performed using the same leads as the measurement of the QRS axis. In a normal heart, it falls between 0 and 90 degrees,

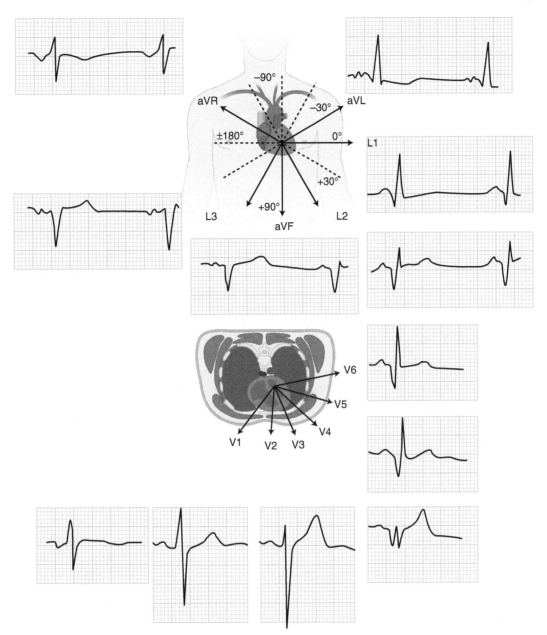

FIGURE 2-2 ■ Hexaxial and horizontal reference systems. The ECG records the net sum of the heart's electrical activity over time. Lead placement in relation to the heart determines whether a potential difference between the heart and the electrode is a positive or negative deflection. (*Reproduced, with permission, from Tintinalli JE, Stapczynski JS, Ma OJ, Cline DM, Cydulka RK, Meckler GD. Tintinalli's Emergency Medicine: A Comprehensive Study Guide. 7th ed. New York, NY: McGraw-Hill; 2011.*)

indicating that the atrial activity is originating in the high right atrium, the location of the sinus node. A P-wave axis outside of that quadrant is consistent with an ectopic atrial rhythm, limb lead reversal, or dextrocardia. P and QRS right axis deviation associated with decreasing QRS amplitudes from V_1 to V_6 is strongly suggestive of mirror-image dextrocardia. These are minor points, but it is something a cardiologist looks for in a child with a murmur or history of palpitations.

Variations in the PR interval are typically seen in healthy, athletic adolescents, especially during sleep.

The pattern seen varies from isolated prolonged PR intervals known as first-degree AV block, more accurately described as prolonged AV conduction, to Mobitz type I, second-degree AV block with progressively lengthening PR intervals, also known as Wenckebach phenomenon. With Wenckebach phenomenon, there is progressive prolongation of the PR interval until there is a loss of conduction to the ventricle. The cause is usually increased vagal tone. More pathologic manifestations of AV nodal conduction occur with Mobitz type II, second-degree AV block when the PR interval stays constant but P waves are conducted to the ventricle in various conduction ratios such as 2:1, 3:1, and 4:1. This condition may progress to complete heart block, in which the P waves and QRS complexes are completely dissociated from one another. PR prolongation may also be seen after ingesting drugs that affect AV conduction or as an effect of increased intracranial pressure, such as an obstructed central nervous system shunt used in hydrocephalus. Conversely, short PR intervals are seen in patients with Wolff-Parkinson-White syndrome due to pre-excitation of the ventricle through an accessory pathway. The ECG in Pompe disease characteristically demonstrates a short PR interval associated with biventricular hypertrophy.

The QRS duration varies with age. In most children, it is less than 90 ms. In infants, it is somewhat less than that. This is important because in the neonatal period, ventricular tachycardia may be mistaken for supraventricular tachycardia. The location of open heart surgery increases the risk of either right bundle-branch block or left bundle-branch block, both having a characteristic wide QRS pattern. Surgery that involves closure of a ventricular septal defect, such as in tetralogy of Fallot, may injure the right bundle branch of the conduction system, which results in a right bundle-branch block pattern. Left ventricular outflow tract surgery may injure the left bundle branch, causing left bundle-branch block. Other causes of a wide QRS interval are a premature ventricular depolarization, a premature atrial depolarization with aberrant conduction, a ventricular paced depolarization, and ventricular pre-excitation as seen in Wolff-Parkinson-White syndrome. Certain anti-arrhythmic medications and hyperkalemia may prolong the QRS duration. Dilated cardiomyopathy, arrhythmogenic right ventricular dysplasia, and Kearns-Sayre syndrome may demonstrate wide QRS patterns.

Measurement of the corrected QT interval is important for any child presenting with syncope or a seizure. Long QT syndrome is a cardiac repolarization abnormality that makes the heart vulnerable to a form of polymorphic ventricular tachycardia known as torsade de pointes. In some cases, the ventricular tachycardia degenerates into ventricular fibrillation and death. Measurement of the corrected QT interval must be made on a clean, high-quality original or photocopied ECG using the Bazett formula: QT corrected = QT interval ÷ √Preceding R-R interval. The proper measurements cannot be made from a faxed copy of the ECG. The upper limit of normal varies among cardiologists, but 460 ms is probably a reasonable number.[7] If a patient has a history of dizziness, palpitations, syncope, or seizures and a prolonged corrected QT interval, consultation with a cardiologist is recommended. There is a growing list of medications that may cause prolongation of the corrected QT interval. This information is readily available from a pharmacist or hospital formulary and available online at www.qtdrugs.org.[8]

Before echocardiography, cardiac chamber enlargement and hypertrophy were routinely assessed by ECG. Tall, pointed P waves in lead II suggested right atrial enlargement, or P pulmonale, and biphasic P waves in lead V_1 suggested left atrial enlargement, or P mitrale. Similarly, there are many different rules for determining the presence or absence of left and right hypertrophy based on ECG findings. Unfortunately, in children with structurally abnormal hearts, some of the rules do not apply. The same can occur in children with chest wall deformities such as pectus excavatum or carinatum and scoliosis. It is not uncommon to see an ECG pattern of left ventricular hypertrophy in a healthy, lean child only to find out that an echocardiogram demonstrates no hypertrophy. An R wave greater than 30 mm in V_1 is a good marker of probable right ventricular hypertrophy in a child greater than 4 years old. A Q wave in V_1 also suggests right ventricular hypertrophy, in addition to a prominent S wave in V_6 greater than 5 mm in patients over 1 year of age. In the pediatric ECG, the T wave in V_1 is upright immediately after birth but subsequently becomes inverted within the first week of life until adolescence. An upright T wave in V_1 from 1 week of age to the beginning of puberty suggests right ventricular hypertrophy. R waves greater than 25 mm in V_6, Q waves greater than 5 mm in V_6, and S waves greater that 20 mm in V_1 suggest left ventricular hypertrophy.

ST-segment abnormalities and T-wave inversions are commonly seen in adult medicine in the setting of ischemia and infarction of the myocardium secondary to coronary artery disease. Compromise to coronary perfusion is much less common in the pediatric population but can occur in certain settings. During ischemia, T waves become inverted. ST-segment elevations develop with acute infarction of the myocardium, and Q waves develop with tissue necrosis.[9] The inferior leads II, III, and aVF represent the inferior region of the myocardium perfused by the right coronary artery. Leads V_1 to V_4 represent the anterior region of the myocardium supplied by the left anterior descending artery, whereas leads I, aVL, V_5, and V_6 represent the lateral region of the heart supplied by the circumflex artery. In patients with dextro-transposition of the great arteries, a perfusion defect may develop after the arterial switch operation due to complications from the transfer of the coronary arteries. Cases of anomalous origin of the coronary arteries may also produce ST and T-wave changes, as well as prominent Q waves, whereas Prinzmetal angina may show abnormalities secondary to coronary vasospasm. Thrombi compromising the coronary circulation can occur with aneurysms of the coronary arteries secondary to Kawasaki disease.

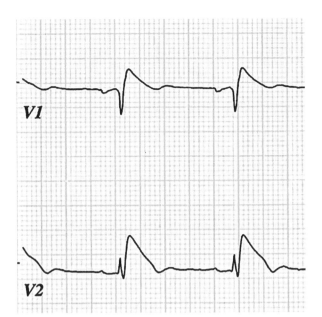

FIGURE 2-3 ■ Brugada syndrome. This tracing shows a right bundle-branch pattern and ST elevation. (*Reproduced, with permission, from Koop KJ, Stack LB, Storrow AB, Thurman RJ. The Atlas of Emergency Medicine. 3rd ed. New York, NY: McGraw-Hill; 2009.*)

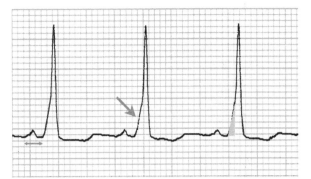

FIGURE 2-4 ■ Wolff-Parkinson-White (WPW) syndrome. This tracing shows evidence of an accessory pathway that is seen in patients with WPW. The PR interval is shortened (double arrow) and a delta wave (upsloping initial QRS segment) is seen (arrow, shaded area). (*Reproduced, with permission, from Koop KJ, Stack LB, Storrow AB, Thurman RJ. The Atlas of Emergency Medicine. 3rd ed. New York, NY: McGraw-Hill; 2009.*)

If there are diffuse ST-segment elevations that do not follow a pattern of coronary ischemia, pericarditis should be considered. In addition, early repolarization, also known as J point elevation, is a type of ST-segment elevation pattern that is a variant of normal. An ECG with a right bundle-branch block pattern with ST-segment elevations in V_1 to V_3 suggests Brugada syndrome, an inherited disease caused by a mutation in cardiac sodium channels that places the patient at risk for sudden cardiac death (Figure 2-3). A pattern of diffuse T-wave inversions with signs of left ventricular hypertrophy is commonly seen in patients with hypertrophic cardiomyopathy.

Cardiac Rhythm Detection

Fifteen-lead ECG with rhythm strip

The 15-lead ECG with a rhythm strip is the test of choice for documenting and diagnosing cardiac rhythm abnormalities if the cardiac dysrhythmia is occurring at the time the tracing is being obtained. Premature atrial and ventricular depolarizations, supraventricular and ventricular tachydysrhythmias, and all forms of heart block can be readily identified. In a person with a history of supraventricular tachycardia, the characteristic short PR interval with a delta wave denoting ventricular pre-excitation or Wolf-Parkinson-White syndrome can be seen during sinus rhythm (Figure 2-4). Long rhythm strips recording the lead with the clearest P wave can be very helpful when interpreting complex dysrhythmias.

Continuous ambulatory ECG or Holter monitoring

For patients who have daily episodes of palpitations or other suspected cardiac rhythm problems intermittently throughout the day, a 24- to 48-hour ambulatory ECG should be considered. Norman Jefferis Holter developed the technology in 1949. The recorders are small and lightweight and can be worn inconspicuously. A 5-lead cable is attached to the chest by snap-on lead patches. Three ECG leads are monitored continuously, and every depolarization is stored on a digital chip (Figure 2-5). The patient is encouraged to keep a diary noting the time of the palpitations and any associated symptoms. During playback, an accurate correlation between the symptom and cardiac rhythm can be made. For children who are not verbal, the parent enters their observations on the diary. The only major disadvantage to the 24-hour ambulatory ECG is that the patient cannot swim or bathe during the recording period.

Event recorders: looping and nonlooping

Patients who have intermittent episodes throughout the month are better served using one of the cardiac event monitors known as transtelephonic event recorders. These recorders are about the size of a cellular phone and come in 2 varieties: nonlooping and looping. In a nonlooping recorder, the patient places the recorder over the heart when he or she experiences palpitations. The patient-activated recorder then records for about 30 to 90 seconds storing the tracing in the unit's memory. The patient then calls the monitoring company's central station at his convenience and downloads the stored ECG tracing directly over the telephone. The receptionist receives the call and forwards the tracing to the physician for review (Figure 2-6). In a looping recorder, the recorder is similar to a 24-hour ambulatory ECG monitor

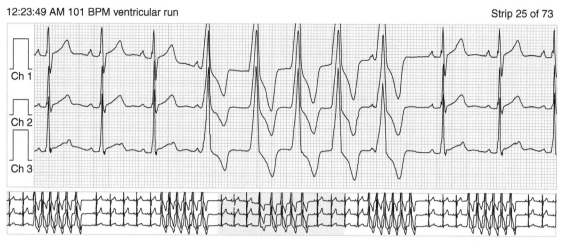

FIGURE 2-5 ■ This is a 24-hour ambulatory ECG tracing showing an accelerated ventricular rhythm/slow ventricular tachycardia in an 8-year-old male.

but uses only a 2-lead cable. The unit contains a memory chip that continuously stores about 90 seconds of data. After 90 seconds, the stored data are written over with another 90 seconds of new data. The monitor is worn continuously. The patient simply presses a button when he or she experiences any symptoms. The recorder then stores the data that were recorded about 30 seconds before the button was pressed and for about 60 seconds after activation.

A nonlooping recorder should be used for patients who have episodes that last for at least 2 minutes, the time it would take to get the recorder, place it on the chest in a private location because it has to placed directly on the skin, and activate the recorder. Looping recorders are useful in patients who have very brief episodes or

in cases where it would be useful to examine the cardiac rhythm just before the onset of palpitations. In both the looping and nonlooping forms, usually more than one episode can be stored in the unit's memory. At this time, the data can only be uploaded to the central station by a landline phone.

External cardiac ambulatory telemetry and insertable cardiac monitors

For more rigorous, ambulatory, long-term monitoring, there are continuous monitoring systems that work in concert with a dedicated cellular phone. These systems use a 3–chest lead array that connects to a small recorder that has the capability of analyzing the data. If it detects an irregular heart rhythm, it

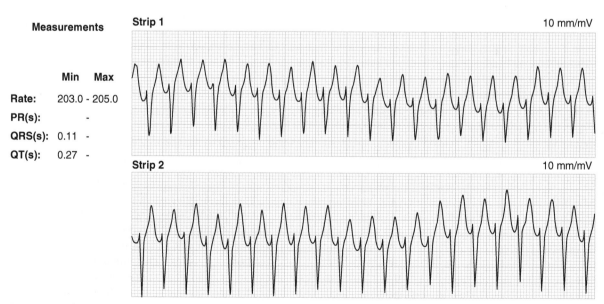

Measurements		
	Min	Max
Rate:	203.0	205.0
PR(s):	-	
QRS(s):	0.11	-
QT(s):	0.27	-

Strip 1   10 mm/mV

Strip 2   10 mm/mV

FIGURE 2-6 ■ This example is a nonlooping transtelephonic event recorder tracing showing a narrow QRS tachycardia consistent with supraventricular tachycardia in a 9-year-old female.

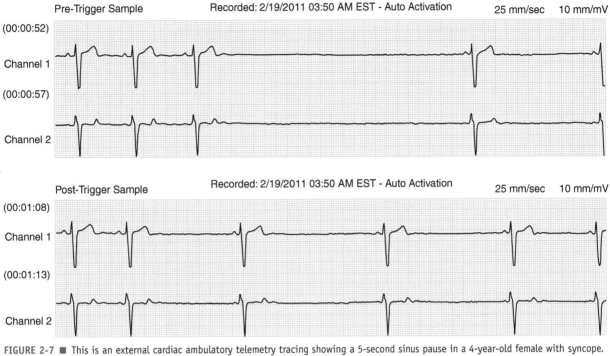

Pre-Trigger Sample   Recorded: 2/19/2011 03:50 AM EST - Auto Activation   25 mm/sec   10 mm/mV

(00:00:52)

Channel 1

(00:00:57)

Channel 2

Post-Trigger Sample   Recorded: 2/19/2011 03:50 AM EST - Auto Activation   25 mm/sec   10 mm/mV

(00:01:08)

Channel 1

(00:01:13)

Channel 2

FIGURE 2-7 ■ This is an external cardiac ambulatory telemetry tracing showing a 5-second sinus pause in a 4-year-old female with syncope.

sends the data wirelessly to a dedicated cellular phone, which, in turn, sends the data to a central receiving station. These external cardiac ambulatory telemetry (ECAT) systems operate automatically and do not need patient activation. They are most useful in patients having recurrent syncopal episodes that are believed to be secondary to a cardiac dysrhythmia and for infants or young children with a suspected, intermittent significant dysrhythmia such as supraventricular tachycardia, ventricular tachycardia, or heart block with long pauses (Figure 2-7). For them to work properly and effectively, the dedicated cellular phone must be within 90 feet of the recorder and the patient must wear the recorder continuously except when showering, bathing, or swimming.

Finally, there are insertable cardiac monitors (ICMs) that are small, Band-Aid size recorders that are placed subcutaneously on the chest over the heart. These devices can be patient activated or can be automatically triggered. When activated, data are stored in the device and interrogated noninvasively by a programmer similar to that used for pacemaker interrogation. These monitors can function for up to 3 years. They are probably most useful for patients with syncope thought to be secondary to significant but infrequent dysrhythmias. Table 2-1 summarizes the recommendations for the various cardiac rhythm recording equipment.

Additional testing for rhythm disturbances

For patients who experience palpitations during or after physical activity, a cardiac exercise test may be

indicated. During the study, the patient's ECG is constantly monitored and may provide useful clinical information. Lastly, an invasive cardiac electrophysiology study may be necessary to define the mechanism of a diagnosed cardiac dysrhythmia. In these studies, electrode catheters are placed within the heart to map the electrical impulses within the conduction system and myocardium. Programmed electrical stimulation is used to initiate arrhythmias to establish or confirm the diagnosis and locate the source of the abnormal rhythm. Once the mechanism is understood, catheter ablation techniques may be curative.[10]

ECG Testing Pearls

- Although not useful for accurately defining cardiac anatomy and function, the ECG and other noninvasive cardiac rhythm–recording modalities are necessary to properly diagnose a cardiac rhythm abnormality.
- The ECG can demonstrate potentially dangerous cardiac interval changes secondary to medication or electrolyte disturbances.
- The role of the ECG in preparticipation sports screening or before initiating certain stimulant medications is evolving.
- Ultimately, the usefulness and importance of the ECG and its interpretation lie in knowing what question about the patient's cardiac condition needs to be answered.[11]
- If an arrhythmia occurs infrequently, there are a variety of options for monitoring that can be used to capture the abnormal rhythm.

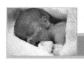

Recommendations for Assessing Cardiac Electrical Properties

	15-Lead Electrocardiogram	24- to 48-Hour Ambulatory Electrocardiogram	Nonlooping Event Recorder	Looping Event Recorder	External Cardiac Ambulatory Telemetry	Insertable Cardiac Monitor
Cardiac intervals	First choice	Not recommended	Not recommended	Not recommended	Not recommended	Not recommended
Heart rate range	Obtain as baseline	First choice	Second choice	Second choice	Second choice	Not recommended
Daily dysrhythmia	Obtain as baseline	First choice	Second choice	Second choice	Second choice	Not recommended
Weekly/monthly dysrhythmia, >2 minutes duration	Obtain as baseline	Second choice	First choice	Second choice	Second choice	Not recommended
Weekly/Monthly dysrhythmia, <2 minutes duration	Obtain as baseline	Second choice	Not recommended	First choice	Second choice	Not recommended
Syncope	Obtain as baseline	Second choice	Not recommended	First choice	First choice	Third choice

CARDIOPULMONARY STRESS TESTING

Introduction

Exercise testing has become an integral part of the evaluation of children with congenital and acquired cardiovascular disease. Children are seldom sitting or lying quietly during waking hours. The evaluation of the patient in the exercise physiology laboratory allows the clinician to assess the cardiovascular system in a state that is more likely to be reflective of the normal daily physical activities. Although most exercise laboratories in children's hospitals were originally designed primarily for cardiac patients, their role is expanding and now includes testing of many noncardiac symptoms and diseases.

Basic Exercise Physiology

Optimal exercise performance requires a continuous meshing of multiple systems of organs.[12,14] The roles of the heart and lungs are to provide adequate energy substrates to working skeletal muscle and to remove the end products of aerobic and anaerobic metabolism during exercise. Assuring proper exercise performance requires the seamless and continuous meshing of multiple systems of organs.[13,14] Working together, the muscular, cardiovascular, and pulmonary systems must produce mechanical energy from chemical energy at the cellular level, with subsequent delivery and removal of substrates for energy production and by-products of muscle metabolism. All of this is accomplished while maintaining chemical and thermal homeostasis within narrow ranges.

At the cellular level, adenosine triphosphate is the chief source of chemical energy for the exercising muscle. The stores of adenosine triphosphate and phosphocreatine in the myocytes are sufficient only for 10 to 15 seconds of activity and thus must continuously be replenished anaerobically in the cytosol or aerobically in the mitochondria.[13,15] Anaerobic activities use glucose, which is metabolized to pyruvate. Pyruvate is converted into lactic acid and excreted into the blood stream, where it is buffered by sodium bicarbonate converting it to lactate. This reaction results in the production of carbon dioxide and water, which are excreted in the lungs. The other fate of pyruvate, as well as fats, is aerobic metabolism in the Krebs cycle. Adenosine triphosphate is produced in large quantities via the electron transport chain, with oxygen functioning as the terminal electron acceptor, again producing carbon dioxide and water as by-products.[14,15]

During any activity, the availability and use of substrates will vary depending on the type, intensity, and duration of activity. The ratio of carbon dioxide production to oxygen consumption, abbreviated V_{CO_2}/

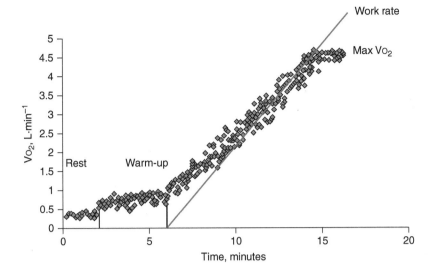

FIGURE 2-8 ■ The relationship between consumption of oxygen Vo$_2$ and rate of work during progressive exercise in a healthy and well-conditioned adolescent. Note that, with the onset of exercise, there is an essentially linear relationship between these 2 features. Close to the peak of exercise, the consumption of oxygen levels off, despite the continued rise in rate of work. (*Reproduced with permission, from Stephens P Jr, McBride MG, Paridon SM. Cardiopulmonary Stress Testing. In: Paediatric Cardiology. 3rd ed. edited by Anderson RH et al. (Philadelphia, PA: Churchill Livingstone/Elsevier, 2010), 415-436.*)

VO$_2$, is called the respiratory exchange ratio (RER) or, if in a steady state, the respiratory quotient. In a state of high use of fat, the ratio is approximately 0.7. Conversely, during pure carbohydrate metabolism, the ratio is 1.0, reflecting the lower amount of oxygen needed to oxidize carbohydrates. The resting RER in the well-fed state will usually range from 0.8 to 0.9.

During a typical graded maximal exercise test, the work rate is gradually increased over the course of 10 to 15 minutes. Production of adenosine triphosphate will need to increase as mechanical work increases, and at low levels of work, this increase is met predominantly by increased aerobic metabolism. As work rate increases, consumption of oxygen increases in a linear fashion (Figure 2-8). Near peak work rates, consumption will tend to plateau, as maximal Vo$_2$ is achieved. This phenomenon is often absent in children.[14,16,17]

As Vo$_2$ increases in response to increased work rate, there is a gradual rise in the RER with a gradual shift in use of carbohydrates as an energy source, allowing for more efficient use of oxygen. Second, the rise in the ratio occurs as a result of increased levels of lactate in the blood. At approximately 50% to 60% of the maximal Vo$_2$, levels of lactate begin to rise in the serum. This point is known as the lactate threshold and is the onset of anaerobic metabolism by the exercising muscles. Above the threshold, levels of lactate rise exponentially as work rate increases, necessitating increased buffering by sodium bicarbonate in order to maintain blood pH homeostasis. The by-product of the buffering process, carbon dioxide, must be removed in order to maintain levels within the normal range. This causes a significant rise in production of carbon dioxide out of proportion to the rise in consumption of oxygen, resulting in the RER increasing to greater than 1.0. The RER in adults at peak exercise may be as high as 1.2 to 1.4 but is usually somewhat lower in children.[16-21] The increase in production of carbon dioxide associated with the buffering of lactate allows for measurement of a noninvasive surrogate of the lactate threshold. This surrogate, known as the ventilatory anaerobic threshold, is defined as the point where production of carbon dioxide and minute ventilation begin to rise out of proportion to the consumption of oxygen (Figure 2-9). Unfortunately, the ventilatory anaerobic threshold can be difficult to measure accurately in smaller children who tend to have erratic patterns of breathing.[16-21]

The Heart and Lung as Service Organs

The rise in Vo$_2$ during exercise is dependent on increases in stroke volume, heart rate, and widening of the difference in the content of oxygen in arterial and mixed venous blood. During strenuous exercise, cardiac output may rise as much as 5-fold over resting levels, with both stroke volume and heart rate contributing to this increase[15,21-25] (Figure 2-10). By a combination of autonomic and metabolic vasoregulatory mechanisms, blood flow is preferentially shunted to the exercising muscles (Figure 2-11). At peak exercise, blood flow to exercising muscle may be 80% or more of the total cardiac output.[26-28] Because of the difficulties in measuring cardiac output during exercise and the linear relationship of Vo$_2$ with cardiac output over a wide range, it is the most commonly used surrogate of cardiac output during exercise testing.[14,26,29,30]

Consumption of oxygen and removal of carbon dioxide require that the cardiovascular and pulmonary systems work together as a single integrated unit. For this reason, there is a very tight relationship between minute ventilation (VE), Vo$_2$, and Vco$_2$. Such a relationship is demonstrated in ventilatory equivalents for carbon dioxide and oxygen, namely VE/Vco$_2$ and VE/Vo$_2$. The typical relationship of minute ventilation to increasing

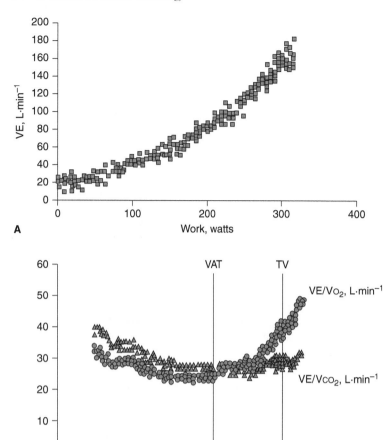

A

B

FIGURE 2-9 ■ **A.** The relationship of minute ventilation (VE) to rate of work in the same subject as in Figure 2-8. Note there is a steady rise in minute ventilation as rate of work increases. **B.** The ventilatory equivalents of oxygen (VE/V_{O_2}) and carbon dioxide (VE/V_{CO_2}) for the same subject. The onset of the ventilatory anaerobic threshold (VAT) is marked. (*Reproduced with permission, from Stephens P Jr, McBride MG, Paridon SM. Cardiopulmonary Stress Testing. In: Paediatric Cardiology. 3rd ed. edited by Anderson RH et al. (Philadelphia, PA: Churchill Livingstone/ Elsevier, 2010), 415-436.*)

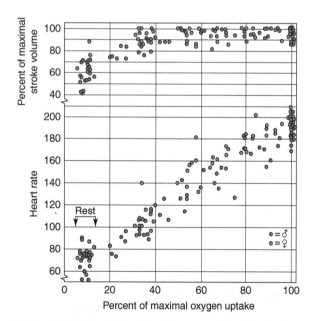

FIGURE 2-10 ■ The relationship of heart rate and stroke volume to increasing consumption of oxygen during cycle ergometry in 23 male and female subjects. Note that stroke volume reaches its maximal value at approximately 30% to 40% of the maximal uptake of oxygen. Heart rate continues to rise in a linear fashion throughout exercise. (*Reprinted, with permission, from Astrand P, Rodahl K. The Muscle and Its Contraction. Textbook of Work Physiology, Physiological Bases of Exercise. 3rd ed., Vol. 2. New York, NY: McGraw-Hill, Inc.; 1986:12-53.*)

work rate and the relationship of VE/V_{CO_2} and VE/V_{O_2} to work rate are depicted in Figure 2-9.[14,18-20]

Laboratory Requirements

Environment

Adequate space and environmental controls are important in order to ensure a successful exercise test. Sufficient space is needed to accommodate the various ergometers and monitoring equipment, including emergency resuscitation equipment, while maintaining adequate space to access the patient in emergency situations.[31] The climate of the laboratory must be well controlled for temperature and humidity to allow proper thermoregulation during the exercise test.[32]

Safety precautions

Exercise testing has been performed in children with very low risk, even in those who have complex disease.[33,34] Although significant complications of exercise testing are rare, proper safety precautions are essential. Key staff usually include at least one physician who is well trained in pediatric exercise testing. A physician does not need to be present for testing patients deemed to be at low risk or healthy[32,35] but

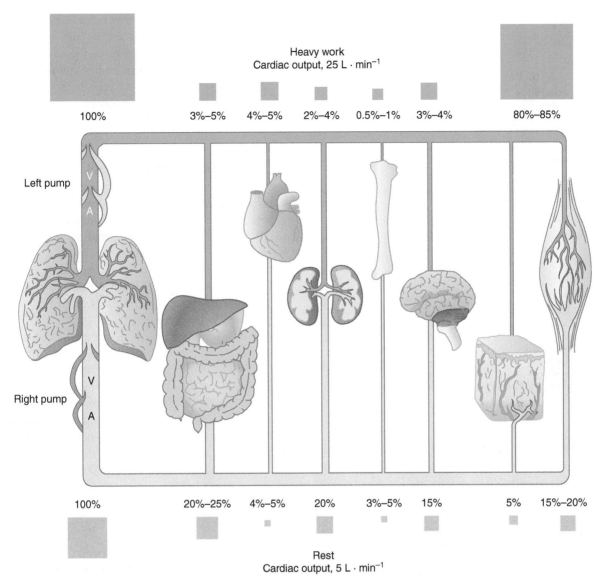

Heavy work
Cardiac output, 25 L · min⁻¹

$$\text{Heavy work, Cardiac output, } 25\ \text{L}\cdot\text{min}^{-1}$$

100%   3%–5%   4%–5%   2%–4%   0.5%–1%   3%–4%   80%–85%

Left pump

Right pump

100%   20%–25%   4%–5%   20%   3%–5%   15%   5%   15%–20%

Rest
Cardiac output, 5 L · min⁻¹

FIGURE 2-11 ■ The parallel circuits of flow through the various systems of organs, both at rest and during peak exercise. Note that the cardiac output increases by approximately 5-fold from rest to strenuous exercise. The relative distribution of flow to the various systems, in contrast, is significantly different from rest to peak exercise. In both states, the red squares are proportional to the percentage of cardiac output received by the particular system. Note that the flow of blood to the muscle increases from approximately 15% to 20% of cardiac output at rest to 80% to 85% of the cardiac output at peak exercise. (*Reprinted, with permission, from Astrand P, Rodahl K.* The Muscle and Its Contraction. Textbook of Work Physiology, Physiological Bases of Exercise. *3rd ed., Vol. 2. New York, NY: McGraw-Hill, Inc.; 1986:12-53.*)

should be present at the testing of any child deemed to be at increased risk of a complication, such as a child with a life-threatening arrhythmia or syncope. The American Heart Association published guidelines for patients who are at low risk for exercise complications that require a physician to be available, but not physically present (Table 2-2).[35] The risk for each patient must be individually assessed.

Equipment

Ergometers. In most pediatric exercise laboratories, testing is primarily directed toward measuring aerobic capacity. Therefore, ergometers should generate work in the large muscle groups. The 2 types of ergometers most commonly used are the motorized treadmill and the upright cycle ergometer. The choice of ergometer depends on the type of information desired, but there are both advantages and disadvantages to each modality (Table 2-3).[36-38] Therefore, it is best that a laboratory be equipped to perform testing using either type of ergometer.

ECG recorders. Many high-quality commercial ECG recording systems are currently available. No system currently available is designed specifically for pediatric use, but all are generally acceptable without

Indications for Exercise Testing That May Not Require a Physician's Presence

- Assessment of working capacity in healthy children for research.
- Evaluations of chest pain of noncardiac origin.
- Postoperative follow-up of patients with good hemodynamics to assess working capacity or rehabilitation screen.
- Evaluation of isolated PACs or PVCs in a healthy child with a normal QTc.
- Routine follow-up of known arrhythmias or pacemakers.
- Kawasaki disease or other coronary abnormalities without a known history of ischemia.
- Asymptomatic mild aortic stenosis.
- Evaluation of asymptomatic mild congenital or acquired cardiac malformations.

Data from Washington RL, Bricker JT, Alpert BS, et al. Guidelines for exercise testing in the pediatric age group. From the Committee on Atherosclerosis and Hypertension in Children, Council on Cardiovascular Disease in the Young, the American Heart Association. Circulation. 1994;90:2166-2179.
Data from Stephens P Jr, McBride MG, Paridon SM. Exercise Testing in Pediatric Cardiology. Philadelphia, PA: Lippincott, Williams & Wilkins; 2010:415-436.
PACs, premature atrial contractions; PVCs, premature ventricular contractions.

modification. Minimization of distortion of signals is accomplished with computer digitization of the analog electrical signal. The printer should use a direct writer mechanism.[36]

Respiratory gases analyzers. The use of these analyzers has become routine in laboratories studying pediatric exercise physiology. Measurements of consumption of oxygen, production of carbon dioxide, and pulmonary functions such as minute ventilation, tidal volume,

Treadmill Versus Cycle Ergometer

Features	Treadmill	Cycle
Patient familiarity	+	
Higher work rates and oxygen consumption	+	
Greater pediatric experience		+
Quantification of work performed		+
ECG and blood pressure artifact		+
Safety		+
Expense		+
Noise		+

Reproduced with permission, from Stephens P Jr, McBride MG, Paridon SM. Cardiopulmonary Stress Testing. In: Paediatric Cardiology. 3rd ed. edited by Anderson RH et al. (Philadelphia, PA: Churchill Livingstone/Elsevier, 2010), 415-436.

and respiratory rate are easily obtainable. Several systems at reasonable prices are commercially available. In addition to measuring expired gases, these systems are frequently equipped to perform resting spirometry and to receive input from other sources, such as an ECG recorder. This allows a single system to generate complete and final reports.

Protocols

The Bruce protocol and its modifications are the most commonly used treadmill protocols in the pediatric exercise laboratory, consisting of 3-minute stages with an increase in both speed and grade of the treadmill at each stage.[38] In the last decade, protocols with shorter stages, usually of 1 or 2 minutes, and smaller incremental increases in rates of work have gained popularity. These protocols, such as the Balke treadmill protocol, may use a fixed speed, with increases only in grade, or may increase both speed and grade.

The most commonly used cycle protocol is that devised by James, which consists of 10 stages, each lasting 3 minutes.[39] The incremental increases for each stage vary depending on body surface area. Collection of expired gas is such a common occurrence that many laboratories are now using ramp cycle protocols. In this protocol, the rate of work is increased in small, frequently single-watt increments, thus producing a smooth continuous rise throughout the test.[31,37,38] Protocols are shown in Figures 2-12 and 2-13.

Indications for Exercise Testing

Indications for exercise testing depend on symptoms and/or the presence of a particular disease. The American Heart Association issued guidelines for indications for stress testing in children (Table 2-4).[37] Although these guidelines were designed primarily for cardiovascular disease, they are in most cases applicable to conditions involving other organ systems. Regardless of the disease process, the goals of exercise testing are primarily identification of potential causes of exercise intolerance, stratification of risk for patients for exercise, and assessment of the physical capacity of patients. The data obtained may be helpful in the decision process regarding therapeutic intervention, restriction of physical activity, and programs for rehabilitation or conditioning.

Reasons for exercise testing in patients with congenital heart disease are often multiple. A comprehensive exercise test should routinely evaluate cardiovascular capacity and pulmonary capacity, assess for rhythm disturbances and ischemia, and help assess for ability and risk for participation in competitive and recreational activities.[40-50] Exercise testing is also useful in diagnostic evaluation and assessing therapeutic response

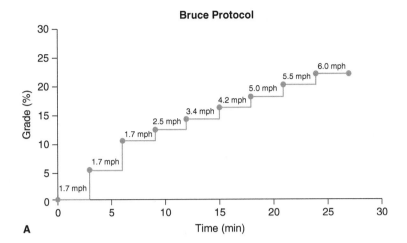

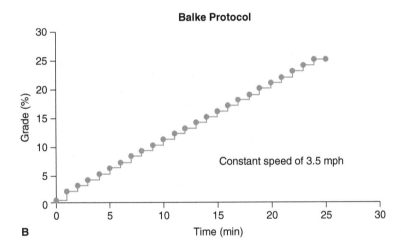

FIGURE 2-12 ■ The panels show the protocols for testing using a treadmill. **A.** The Bruce protocol consists of 3-minute stages with an increase in both speed and grade. The first 2 stages are often omitted in healthy adult testing. **B.** In the Balke protocol, the grade is increased from 0% to 2% after the first minute and increased 1% in each subsequent minute. The speed of the treadmill is held constant at 3.5 mph. (*Reproduced with permission, from Stephens P Jr, McBride MG, Paridon SM. Cardiopulmonary Stress Testing. In: Paediatric Cardiology. 3rd ed. edited by Anderson RH et al. (Philadelphia, PA: Churchill Livingstone/Elsevier, 2010), 415-436.*)

to therapy for various acquired heart diseases, such as cardiomyopathy and Kawasaki disease, or as part of ongoing evaluation of cardiac transplantation. Its utility in the screening and risk stratification of certain causes of sudden death, such as anomalous coronary arteries, is less certain.[45,47,51-60]

Exercise testing is often extremely useful in the diagnosis and evaluation of many pulmonary conditions. These tests frequently require specific pretesting such as spirometry and special protocols. A treadmill sprint protocol is usually used to assess exercise-induced asthma.[61-63] Patients with pulmonary hypertension are usually tested using a 6-minute walk protocol, which can be safely performed even in this quite ill population.[64-69] Standard protocols are useful in the evaluation of chronic pulmonary disease such as cystic fibrosis or to assess the effects of chest wall abnormalities such as pectus deformities.[70]

Less common reasons for exercise testing include evaluation of diseases involving the gastrointestinal, renal, hematologic, or neurologic systems. In most cases, exercise testing is used to help with risk stratification and

Exercise Testing Pearls

■ Exercise testing demonstrates aspects of a patient's physiology that may be more reflective of his or her daily activities compared with that of a sedentary office visit.

■ Basic exercise physiology encompasses the interaction between the musculoskeletal, pulmonary, and cardiovascular systems in order to generate mechanical energy from chemical energy and to remove the end products of aerobic and anaerobic metabolism.

■ Maximal oxygen consumption (Vo_2) and the ventilatory anaerobic threshold are data points that are useful in the analysis of exercise capacity.

■ An exercise test protocol, using a treadmill or cycle ergometer, is used to perform an exercise test, whereas an ECG recorder and a respiratory gas analyzer generate data for analysis.

■ Exercise testing not only provides important information about patients with cardiovascular disease, but can also provide data for patients with diseases affecting other organ systems or for those who have unexplained exercise intolerance.

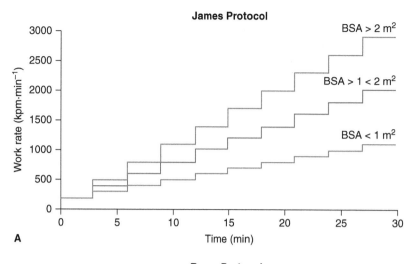

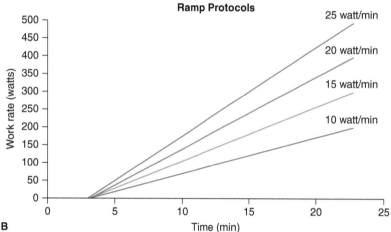

FIGURE 2-13 ■ Protocols for use with an upright cycle ergometer. **A.** The James protocol. The initial rate of work is 200 kpm/min. The rate is increased every 3 minutes by different amounts, depending on the body surface area (BSA) of the patient. **B.** The ramp protocol. The patient initially pedals for 3 minutes with unloaded cycling to establish a baseline metabolic state. The rate of work is then increased continuously at a chosen level based on the physical condition, age, and size of the patient. (*Reproduced with permission, from Stephens P Jr, McBride MG, Paridon SM. Cardiopulmonary Stress Testing. In: Paediatric Cardiology. 3rd ed. edited by Anderson RH et al. (Philadelphia, PA: Churchill Livingstone/Elsevier, 2010), 415-436.*)

Indications for Performing an Exercise Test

- Evaluate specific symptoms or signs induced by exercise.
- Identify abnormal adaptive responses to exercise in cardiac or noncardiac disorders.
- Assess the effectiveness of medical or surgical interventions.
- Assess functional capacity for vocational, recreational, and athletic recommendations.
- Discover prognosis for a specific disorder.
- Evaluate overall physical fitness levels.
- Establish baseline data for follow-up of rehabilitation programs.

Data from Washington RL, Bricker JT, Alpert BS, et al. Guidelines for exercise testing in the pediatric age group. From the Committee on Atherosclerosis and Hypertension in Children, Council on Cardiovascular Disease in the Young, the American Heart Association. Circulation. 1994;90:2166-2179.
Data from Stephens P Jr, McBride MG, Paridon SM. Exercise Testing in Pediatric Cardiology. Philadelphia, PA: Lippincott, Williams & Wilkins; 2010:415-436.

assessment of the severity of the disease. Use of exercise testing to help design and monitor physical rehabilitation programs is becoming increasingly common for these types of chronic disease as well as for obesity and weight management.[60,68,71-76]

Finally, one of the largest groups of patients seen in the exercise physiology laboratory is children who have various exercise-induced symptoms without a clearly identifiable source. Exercise testing may be useful in identifying potential etiologies of symptoms. Exercise-induced dyspnea or new onset of exercise intolerance and fatigue may be due to noncardiac causes, such as pulmonary, musculoskeletal, or hematologic disorders. Evaluation of exercise-induced syncope or near syncope may result in the diagnosis of neutrally mediated syncope or, more rarely, cardiac arrhythmias.

Contraindications

There are both absolute and relative reasons not to perform exercise testing. Many of these reasons are listed

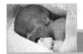

Contraindications to Exercise Testing

Absolute
- Active inflammatory heart disease
- Active hepatitis
- Acute myocardial infarction
- Active pneumonia
- Severe systemic hypertension for age
- Acute orthopedic injury to an exercise muscle group

Relative
- Severe left ventricular outflow obstruction
- Severe right ventricular outflow obstruction
- Congestive heart failure
- Pulmonary vascular obstructive disease
- Severe mitral stenosis
- Ischemic coronary artery disease
- Advanced ventricular arrhythmias

Reproduced with permission, from Stephens P Jr, McBride MG, Paridon SM. Cardiopulmonary Stress Testing. In: Paediatric Cardiology. 3rd ed. edited by Anderson RH et al. (Philadelphia, PA: Churchill Livingstone/Elsevier, 2010), 415-436.

in Table 2-5. As a rule, absolute contraindications result from an acute ongoing process affecting one or more of the major organ systems, such as myocarditis or hepatitis.[38,41]

Relative contraindications require that the physician supervising the laboratory evaluate the relative risk and benefit for exercise testing for that particular patient.[32,35] Occasionally, a relatively high risk during exercise testing may be acceptable. For example, routine exercise testing in patients with advanced pulmonary vascular obstructive disease is not appropriate because of the high risk of exercise-induced sudden death. Nonetheless, exercise testing may be warranted as part of an evaluation to make a difficult decision concerning the timing of lung or heart–lung transplantation.

ECHOCARDIOGRAPHY IMAGING TESTING

Basic Principles

History

The field of echocardiography arose from observations in animal behavior. Abbe Lazzaro Spallanzani, described as the "father of ultrasound," discovered in the early 1700s that bats are able navigate in complete darkness using echo reflection of sound inaudible to the human ear. Contributions in the 19th century included the work of Christian Johann Doppler, who demonstrated that a

moving sound source created variability in the pitch of that sound (the Doppler effect), and the discovery by Pierre and Jacques Curie of piezoelectricity, which could be converted into ultrasound waves. In the early 20th century, sonar was developed to detect enemy submarines during World War I.

In 1953, Dr. Helmut Hertz and Dr. Inge Edler studied methods described by Floyd Firestone in the 1940s to detect metal flaws in machinery using reflected sound waves. Pairing this information with a commercial ultrasonoscope, they were able to record movement of the mitral valve and portions of the myocardium.[77] Inge Edler, considered the "father of echocardiography," was later able to detect mitral stenosis and other clinical entities using this technique. Thus, echocardiography emerged as a clinical, noninvasive tool to detect heart disease.

M-mode

M-mode (motion mode) echocardiography became one of the first clinically useful methods to obtain ultrasound images of the heart. M-mode has excellent temporal and spatial resolution, allowing for an assessment of subtle motion abnormalities and accurate measurement of cardiac structures. An ultrasound transducer sends out ultrasound energy along a single line of interrogation and receives waves reflected back from the cardiac structure of interest[78] (Figures 2-14 and 2-15). In this manner, M-mode echocardiography provides an "ice pick" view of the heart over time. In the past, M-mode was used to identify valvular disease and even some forms of congenital heart disease. However, it was displaced by 2-dimensional imaging for most uses. Presently, M-mode is most commonly used to measure

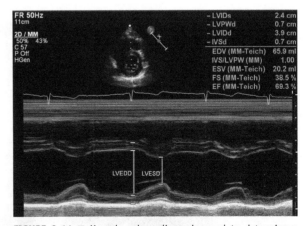

FIGURE 2-14 ▪ M-mode echocardiography used to determine a patient's shortening fraction. LVEDD represents left ventricular end-diastolic dimension, while LVESD represents the left ventricular end systolic dimension. These values are used to calculate the shortening fraction, a quantitative measure of left ventricular function commonly used in pediatric echocardiography.

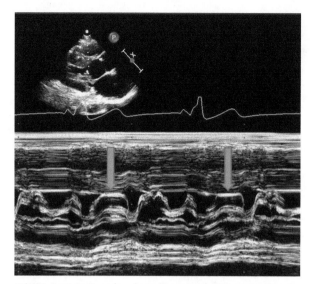

FIGURE 2-15 ■ M-mode echocardiography depicting systolic anterior motion of the mitral valve leaflet. The blue arrows show the mitral valve leaflet contacting a hypertrophied ventricular septum during systole. This phenomenon is seen in patients with hypertrophic cardiomyopathy and suggests that left ventricular outflow tract obstruction is present. It is often associated with mitral regurgitation.

cardiac dimensions and left ventricular shortening (see Assessment of Cardiac Function).

Two-dimensional sector scanning

M-mode is limited in its ability to define the relationship of cardiac structures to each other. Thus, 2-dimensional echocardiography was developed as a method of imaging along a series of lines typically spread into a 90-degree arc. A grayscale is used to measure amplitude of the reflected wave; these waves are then constructed in real time (multiple frames per second) to create an

image. Two-dimensional echocardiography has now become the basis of the evaluation of cardiac function and morphology (Figure 2-16). The images obtained by 2-dimensional echocardiography allow for instantaneous anatomic and functional assessment of the heart. In addition, quantitative measurements of the dimensions, areas, and volumes of cardiac structures can also be performed using this modality.

Doppler imaging

Doppler imaging came into clinical use in the 1970s. This modality transformed echocardiography into a tool that could characterize intracardiac blood flow patterns in addition to assessment of morphology and function. Doppler interrogation uses changes in frequency of transmitted ultrasound waves. The Doppler equation is applied via an ultrasound beam with a known frequency transmitted and reflected back by red blood cells in motion.[79] The change in frequency of the transmitted sound compared with that of the reflected sound produces a frequency shift that can then be converted into a velocity. There are 3 types of Doppler imaging performed in routine echocardiography: pulsed wave Doppler, continuous wave Doppler, and color flow mapping.

Pulsed wave Doppler uses a single crystal to sample the blood flow velocity at a site of interest. The Nyquist limit represents the maximum velocity that can be obtained using this modality. Pulsed wave Doppler is used to assess normal blood flow patterns in the heart (ie, AV valve inflow, outflow tracts). The advantage of this modality is that it can sample a volume of blood in a specific location (eg, proximal or distal to a valve). The disadvantage of this modality is that aliasing occurs after the Nyquist limit is reached; thus at this limit, the true

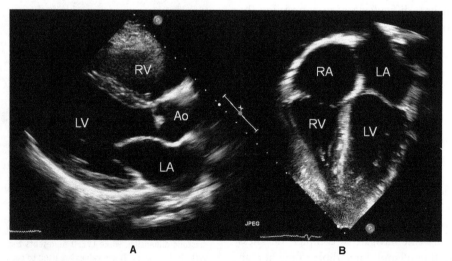

FIGURE 2-16 ■ **A.** Two-dimensional echocardiographic image from a parasternal long axis view in a normal heart. **B.** Two-dimensional echocardiographic image from an apical 4-chamber view in a normal heart. Ao, aorta; LA, left atrium; LV, left ventricle; RA, right atrium; RV, right ventricle.

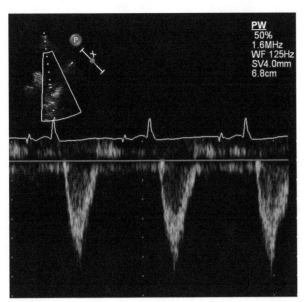

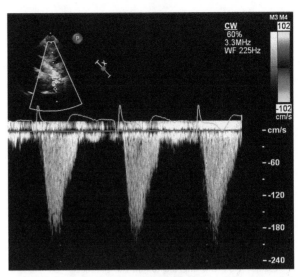

FIGURE 2-18 ■ Continuous wave Doppler pattern of the descending aorta. This is normal spectral pattern using continuous wave Doppler for the descending aorta. Continuous wave Doppler shows flow velocities across the entire sampled beam. Thus, some blood cells have faster velocities than others.

FIGURE 2-17 ■ Pulsed wave Doppler pattern of the descending aorta. This is a normal spectral pattern of the descending aorta that shows laminar flow (all blood cells accelerate and decelerate at similar velocities) with no evidence of obstruction or diastolic run-off. Pulsed wave Doppler samples the blood flow velocity at a particular location within the field of interest.

maximal velocity at the site of interrogation cannot be determined. Pulsed wave Doppler is displayed as a spectrogram (Figure 2-17). Laminar flow is best displayed using pulsed wave Doppler.

Continuous wave Doppler uses 2 crystals to continuously transmit and receive an ultrasound signal, allowing for detection of the highest blood flow velocity across the sampled beam path. This modality is not limited by the Nyquist phenomenon and can be used to determine a true maximal velocity. However, it cannot determine the precise location of the site of obstruction because it has no range resolution. It is also displayed using a spectrogram (Figure 2-18). Continuous wave Doppler is ideal to measure high-velocity blood flow jets in the heart such as AV valve regurgitation and flow across restrictive septal defects.

Using the blood flow velocities obtained by Doppler interrogation, pressure gradients may be determined across valves and vessels. A modification of the Bernoulli equation is applied to blood flow transiting a narrowed orifice (Figure 2-19). The flow acceleration and viscous friction components of the equation are eliminated because of their minimal impact in the heart; convective acceleration is used alone. In addition, flow velocity proximal to a fixed orifice is much lower than the peak flow velocity and can also be ignored. As a result, the modified Bernoulli equation is:

$$\text{Pressure gradient} = 4 \times v^2 = (2v)^2$$

where v = peak flow velocity. This modified equation has been validated and has a fairly accurate correlation

with direct invasive measurements performed in the cardiac catheterization laboratory.[80] The maximal Doppler velocity measured by the modified Bernoulli equation is a maximal instantaneous gradient, whereas the gradient measured in the catheterization laboratory represents a peak to peak gradient and is typically less than that of the maximal instantaneous gradient. The mean gradient represents an average of the pressure gradients. Pressure gradients obtained using the modified Bernoulli equation provide clinically useful information including right ventricular systolic pressure, aortic stenosis maximal gradient, pulmonary artery diastolic and systolic pressure, and pressure gradients across septal defects.

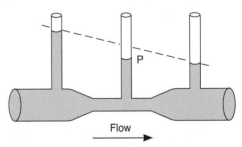

FIGURE 2-19 ■ Bernoulli's principle. When fluid flows through the narrow portion of the tube, the kinetic energy of flow is increased as the velocity increases, and the potential energy is reduced. Consequently, the measured pressure (P) is lower than it would have been at that point if the tube had not been narrowed. The dashed line indicates what the pressure drop due to frictional forces would have been if the tube had been of uniform diameter. (*Reproduced, with permission, from Barrett KE, Barman SM, Boitano S, Brooks H:* Ganong's Review of Medical Physiology. *23rd ed. New York, NY: McGraw-Hill; 2010.*)

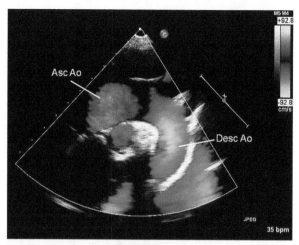

FIGURE 2-20 ■ Color flow image of the aortic arch. The red color represents blood flow directed toward the transducer (the point of the sector) as it flows into the ascending aorta (Asc Ao) in systole, whereas the blue color represents blood flow directed away from the transducer as it flows down the descending aorta (Desc Ao).

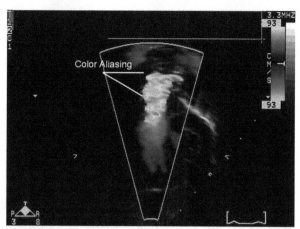

FIGURE 2-21 ■ Aliasing of color flow. Color aliasing occurs at a site of turbulence. In this example, aliasing is seen as blood flows across a stenotic pulmonary valve when the Nyquist limit is reached. The blood going at the maximum velocity of the scale is designated as yellow. Once the blood goes faster than the maximum on the scale (0.93 m/s), the color reverts to the opposite color (in this case, turning from blue to red). Therefore, color Doppler identifies that there is a pressure gradient across this valve but does not identify the severity of the gradient.

Color flow imaging

Color flow was developed in the late 1970s to visualize the direction of blood flow on a 2-dimensional image. Since then, it has become an essential part of the echocardiographic evaluation of hemodynamics. A color scale is designated and applied to each frequency shift detected within the color sector. Color flow Doppler is a variation of pulsed wave Doppler and therefore is also susceptible to the Nyquist phenomenon. By convention, blood flow directed toward the transducer is red, whereas blood flow directed away from the transducer is blue (Figure 2-20). When the Nyquist limit is reached, color aliasing occurs. Aliasing occurs at sites of turbulence and may appear green or yellow in color depending on the color flow map that is used (Figure 2-21). The colorized image represents the velocity, direction, and turbulence of the flow of blood within the cardiac structures. An assessment of valvular stenosis and/or regurgitation and septal shunting is often determined using this technique.

Tissue Doppler imaging

Tissue Doppler imaging (TDI) measures myocardial tissue velocities rather than red blood cell velocities using very low scales. The myocardium and fibrous skeleton of the heart have greater reflectivity and diminished motion compared to red blood cells. As a result, specific filters are used on the echo machine in order to exclude red blood cell flow and properly record myocardial tissue. The tissue velocities are also encoded with color (again, red is toward the transducer, and blue is away from the transducer).

This technology has several important applications. The velocity and movement of the myocardium is determined by the underlying systolic and diastolic

cardiac function. Mitral annular motion and tricuspid annular motion as measured by TDI can be used to assess ventricular diastolic function[81] (Figure 2-22). The advantage of using AV valve annular motion is that it is relatively preload independent.

During systole, the AV valve annulus is displaced toward the apex. The annulus is then displaced away from the apex in diastole. The recoil of the ventricle after the release of contraction is appreciated in the early diastolic motion of the annulus and reflects diastolic function. Late diastolic motion of the annulus reflects both diastolic ventricular function and atrial systolic function. Annulus motion is evaluated by sampling the velocities at the septal–annular junction of the mitral valve, the lateral–annular junction of the mitral valve, and the medial–annular junction of the tricuspid valve. These samples create 2 diastolic waveforms called the E' wave, seen in early diastole, and the A' wave, seen in late diastole with atrial contraction. There is also a systolic waveform, the S' wave, that can be measured. Measurements comparing the E wave of mitral inflow to E' are useful for evaluation of diastolic function. TDI can also be used to assess regional ventricular performance by measuring tissue velocities of particular wall segments. This is useful in patients with dyssynchrony or regional dysfunction.

Contrast echocardiography

Contrast echocardiography using agitated saline is commonly used in the pediatric population to evaluate intracardiac shunts that are difficult to visualize by conventional echocardiography (ie, small patent

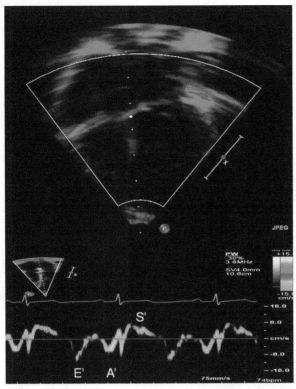

FIGURE 2-22 ■ Tissue Doppler imaging (TDI) with pulsed wave Doppler of the septal annular junction. TDI targets the myocardial fibers to create a spectral pattern. The E′ wave occurs during the initial filling of the ventricle during early diastole. The A′ wave occurs with the filling of the ventricle during atrial contraction in late diastole. The S′ wave occurs with ventricular systole.

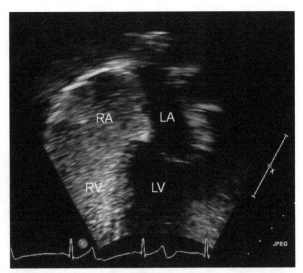

FIGURE 2-23 ■ Four-chamber 2-dimensional view of a bubble study. Agitated saline is often used to identify intracardiac shunts that are difficult to see using other modalities (ie, foramen ovale). In this example, agitated saline fills the right chambers of the heart with no evidence of an intracardiac communication. LA, left atrium; LV, left ventricle; RA, right atrium; RV, right ventricle.

foramen ovale, unroofed coronary sinus, or pulmonary arteriovenous malformations). Air is very reflective to ultrasound beams. When saline solution is infused, the microbubbles do not pass through the pulmonary capillary bed. As a result, they should not appear on the left side of the heart unless there is a direct or indirect communication between the right and left chambers of the heart (Figure 2-23). A negative contrast effect may be seen if there is left to right shunting.[82] In adults, other contrast agents that do pass through the pulmonary vascular bed are used to assess myocardial perfusion and to enhance left ventricular endocardial borders.

Three-dimensional echocardiography

Three-dimensional (3D) echocardiography is a newer modality that allows the echocardiographer to view the heart from any angle. Color flow mapping also has 3D capability. Initial 3D images were created using multiple 2-dimensional images.[83] In recent years, technology has improved to produce real-time 3D pyramidal images. Data sets are typically obtained using several cardiac cycles. As this technology continues to evolve, the clinical application of 3D echo is expanding. It is currently used to evaluate ventricular volume and mass measurements, regional

wall motion abnormalities, and the morphologic evaluation of valvular disease and septal defects (Figure 2-24).

Pediatric Echocardiography

Indications for referral

All patients who have suspected cardiac abnormalities should be referred to a cardiologist prior to undergoing echocardiography. A comprehensive history and physical examination are essential tools that cardiologists use to determine if an echocardiogram is an appropriate test to answer a clinical question. Appropriate referrals for transthoracic and transesophageal echocardiography are listed in Tables 2-6 and 2-7, respectively. A detailed history and interpretation of cardiac examination findings is also helpful to echocardiographers interpreting the study, in order to properly address the clinical questions at hand.

Standard views for a normal pediatric echocardiogram

The initial echocardiographic evaluation of a child should be a complete study, if possible, using an examination protocol devised by the echocardiography laboratory. This protocol should include standard views, modalities used at each view, and methods for displaying, recording, and storing the information.[84] Acoustic views are used that best display the cardiac anatomy, allow for proper Doppler interrogation of valves and other structures, and target any abnormalities detected during the echocardiogram. If the patient has unusual cardiac anatomy or chest wall deformities, variations

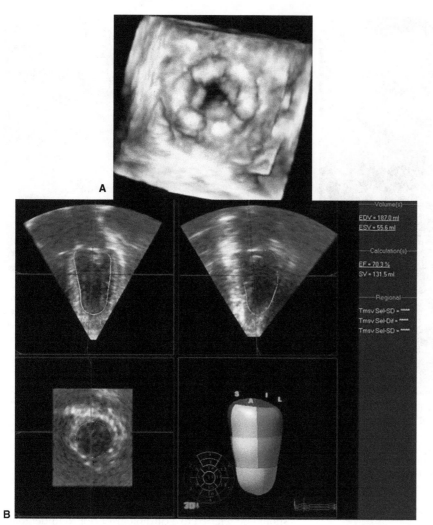

FIGURE 2-24 ■ **A.** Three-dimensional imaging of a bioprosthetic tricuspid valve. This image is taken from the undersurface of the tricuspid valve within the right ventricle. The outer ring has 3 prominent struts attached to the annulus of the valve. There are 3 leaflets that are in the open position in this image. **B.** Three-dimensional assessment of left ventricular function. Using the 3 different views shown, a 3-dimensional model is created of the left ventricle that can be used to evaluate ventricular function.

of these views may be used to obtain adequate images for interpretation. Image optimization should be performed at the start of the echocardiogram to obtain the best quality study. In addition to the technical adjustments, the appropriate size probe and transducer frequency should be used.

The American Society of Echocardiography recommends 5 standard views in pediatric echocardiography (Figure 2-25). These are the subcostal or subxiphoid view, the apical view, the left parasternal view, the suprasternal notch view, and the right parasternal view. While working within these windows, images can be obtained from different planes of examination, including the frontal or transverse plane, the sagittal plane, the right anterior oblique plane, and the left anterior oblique plane.

Measurement adjustments for growth

A challenge within pediatric imaging is to determine normal values for anatomic structures during different stages of growth and development. In pediatric cardiac assessment, body surface area is commonly used to index various measures such as cardiac output.[85] For

cardiac structures, z-scores are generally used to compare a particular patient to the normal population and to determine if a structure is increasing in size out of proportion to normal growth. The z-score represents a standard deviation relative to the mean of the values of the population that may be used to adjust for age or body size. Using this method, a z-score of 0 represents the mean of the population for that particular value, whereas a z-score of +2 or −2 represents a value that is 2 standard deviations above or below the mean of the population. Z-scores greater than 2 or less than −2 are considered abnormal. Many echocardiographic reports have the capability to track a particular measure over time in the same patient; this is quite useful in making determinations about timing of some cardiac interventions. For example, mitral valvuloplasty may be considered when the left ventricle begins to dilate out of proportion to normal growth.

Assessment of cardiac function

Systolic performance reflects contractile function of the heart, allowing the ventricles to eject blood to the vascular beds. There are many modalities used to assess

Common Indications for Pediatric Transthoracic Echocardiography

Clinical Concerns/Diagnosis	Focus of Evaluation
Exam findings concerning for congenital heart disease: ■ Pathologic murmur ■ Neonatal cyanosis with failed hyperoxia test	Structural heart disease
Kawasaki disease	Coronary artery aneurysm
Connective tissue disorders: ■ Marfan syndrome ■ Ehlers-Danlos syndrome	Aortopathy, valvular disease
Muscular dystrophies	Dilated or hypertrophic cardiomyopathy
Noonan syndrome	Pulmonary valve stenosis, septal defects, hypertrophic cardiomyopathy
William syndrome	Supravalvar stenosis, branch pulmonary artery stenosis
Down syndrome	Ventricular septal defects, endocardial cushion defects, patent ductus arteriosus, atrial and/or tetralogy of Fallot
DiGeorge syndrome	Aortic arch anomalies, tetralogy of Fallot, truncus arteriosus, ventricular septal defects with arch obstruction
Signs/symptoms of heart failure	Cardiomyopathy, pulmonary hypertension, structural heart disease
Exposure to anthracycline medications	Cardiomyopathy
Prolonged arrhythmia	Diminished cardiac function, structural heart disease
Cardiogenic syncope	Hypertrophic cardiomyopathy, dilated cardiomyopathy, coronary artery anomalies, diminished cardiac function, arrhythmogenic right ventricular dysplasia
Prematurity with continuous murmur	Patent ductus arteriosus

left ventricular systolic performance. The 2 most commonly used methods are the shortening fraction and ejection fraction. The percent fractional shortening (SF) is defined as the change in dimension of the left ventricle from end-diastole to end-systole using the equation:

$$SF = \frac{\text{left ventricular end-diastolic dimension} - \text{left ventricular end-systolic dimension} \times 100}{\text{left ventricular end-diastolic dimension}}$$

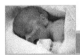

Common Indications for Pediatric Transesophageal Echocardiography

Inadequate images by transthoracic imaging
Evaluation for intracardiac shunt in patients who have had stroke event
Examination for thrombus prior to cardioversion of arrhythmia
Evaluation for evidence of intracardiac endocarditis
Preoperative evaluation to confirm cardiac anatomy
Intraoperative or postoperative evaluation to visualize a surgical repair and to assess hemodynamics and volume status
Guidance for interventional cardiac catheterization procedures

SF is assessed in M-mode at the level of the papillary muscles in the parasternal short view. This view shows the ventricular septum and inferolateral wall of the left ventricle contracting and relaxing in systole and diastole. A normal SF ranges from 28% to 38%.[85] A SF below 28% suggests left ventricular systolic dysfunction, and a SF above 38% suggests hyperdynamic systolic function. There are limitations to this measure with regard to global ventricular performance because it only measures circumferential shortening and is geometry dependent; however, it is readily reproducible and easy to measure.

It is important to recognize that SF cannot be accurately measured in the setting of paradoxical septal wall motion (frequently seen after heart transplantation or tetralogy of Fallot repair). Ejection fraction (EF) represents the fraction of change between the left ventricular volume in diastole compared with systole (Figure 2-26). Using an apical 4-chamber view as well as an apical 2-chamber view with 2-dimensional echocardiography, the modified Simpson's method may be applied to the left ventricle. The chamber is divided into disks of equal height in order to estimate the left

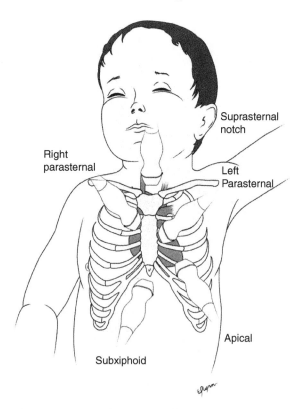

Right
parasternal

Suprasternal
notch

Left
Parasternal

Apical

Subxiphoid

FIGURE 2-25 ■ American Society of Echocardiography pediatric echocardiography views and sweeps. Transducer locations for standard imaging windows. 1. Subxiphoid or subcostal. 2. Apical. 3. Left parasternal. 4. Suprasternal notch. 5. Right parasternal. (*Reproduced, with permission, from Lai WW, Mertens L, Cohen M, Geva T, eds. Echocardiography in Pediatric and Congenital Heart Disease: From Fetus to Adult. New York, NY: Wiley-Blackwell Publishing; 2009.*)

ventricular volume in systole and diastole. The equation for EF is as follows:

$$EF = \frac{\text{left ventricular end-diastolic volume} - \text{left ventricular end-systolic volume} \times 100}{\text{left ventricular end-diastolic volume}}$$

A normal EF ranges between 55% and 75%. 3D echocardiography can now be used to measure EF as well.

Maximal dP/dt is a measure of ventricular contraction and is obtained using the continuous wave Doppler pattern of AV valve regurgitation. This measure assesses the mean rate of pressure generation by the ventricle during isovolumic contraction. Maximal dP/dt is determined by the time interval between a velocity of 1 m/s and 3 m/s (Figure 2-27). The difference in pressure is approximately 32 mm Hg, as determined by the Bernoulli equation, and is divided by the time interval. Normal values of dP/dt for the left ventricle are 1200 mm Hg/s and above. Limitations to this technique are as follows: AV valve regurgitation must be present in order to determine the value, it is preload dependent, and it requires an excellent envelope to accurately determine the values. In addition, severe AV valve regurgitation alters the value because it affects preload.

Assessment of right ventricular performance has been more challenging using echocardiography. Geometric assumptions made about the left ventricle cannot be applied to the right ventricle, which is a complex tripartite structure rather than elliptical in shape. Subjective assessment of ventricular performance is frequently used but is not ideal because of interobserver variability and reproducibility. New software has been developed to

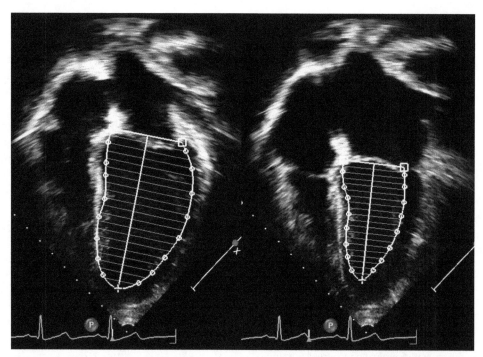

FIGURE 2-26 ■ Assessment of the left ventricular ejection fraction. Using the apical 4-chamber view, the left ventricle is outlined in systole and diastole. The ventricle may also be outlined in systole and diastole in a 2-chamber view. Using the modified Simpson's method, the ejection fraction is calculated and may be used as another quantitative measure of left ventricular function.

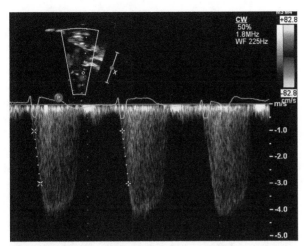

FIGURE 2-27 ■ Measurement of left ventricular dp/dT. This image depicts continuous wave Doppler of the left atrioventricular valve regurgitation jet. The difference in pressure divided by the time interval between 1 m/s and 3 m/s are used to determine the value. This particular patient has a low dp/dT of 713 mm Hg/s (normal, 1200 mm Hg/s), suggesting impairment of ventricular contraction.

measure 3D right ventricular EF. Good correlation has been found between the 3D echocardiographic measure of EF and similar measures made by cardiac magnetic resonance imaging.

Myocardial performance index (MPI) is a method that can be used to assess global ventricular function because it uses systolic and diastolic time intervals for its calculation (Figure 2-28). MPI is not geometry dependent and therefore can be used to assess performance of both the right and left ventricles. Using either blood pool Doppler or TDI, MPI is calculated as follows:

$$MPI = \frac{\text{isovolumic contraction time} + \text{isovolumic relaxation time}}{\text{ventricular ejection time}}$$

Normal MPI for the left ventricle is ≤0.35, whereas normal MPI for the right ventricle is ≤0.28. As a ventricle begins to fail, isovolumic times increase and ejection times decrease; thus MPI increases. MPI does not distinguish between systolic and diastolic dysfunction, and similar to SF and EF, it is preload and afterload dependent. When using the blood pool to make the calculation, error can occur if the heart rate changes significantly during the acquisition. MPI is generally used to follow ventricular function in a patient serially over time.

Diastolic dysfunction occurs in children with congenital and acquired heart disease and may affect long-term outcome. Evaluation of diastolic dysfunction may be performed using spectral Doppler flow patterns. The mitral valve inflow pattern demonstrates an E and an A wave. The E wave represents the initial rapid filling of the ventricle during diastole following the opening of the mitral valve, whereas the A wave represents the flow across the mitral valve with atrial contraction. The normal ratio of E wave velocity to A wave velocity is approximately 2.3. As the myocardium develops abnormal relaxation, the E and A wave patterns change; typically the E/A ratio becomes ≤1. The inflow E/A ratio continues to change with worsening diastolic dysfunction. Other measures of diastolic function that complement use of E/A ratio include E-wave deceleration time, pulmonary venous flow patterns, TDI velocities, and color M-mode flow propagation.

Myocardial deformation imaging, also known as strain imaging, is a technique that is used to evaluate both systolic and diastolic function. Myocardial deformation can be measured in radial, longitudinal, and circumferential planes. Calculations of strain and strain

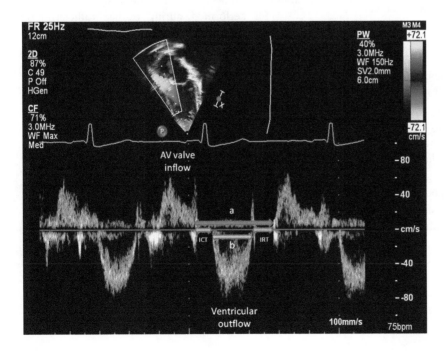

FIGURE 2-28 ■ Calculation of the myocardial performance index (MPI). This pulsed wave Doppler pattern demonstrates an antrioventricular (AV) valve inflow pattern above the baseline and a ventricular outflow pattern below the baseline. MPI can be calculated using this tracing by adding isovolemic contraction time (ICT) to isovolemic relaxation time (IRT) and dividing the two by the ejection time (b). An analogous method of calculating MPI is (a − b)/b, where "a" represents the total systolic time.

rate from myocardial deformation reflect regional function. Strain rate is calculated as follows:

$$\text{Strain rate} = \frac{\text{myocardial velocity at segment 2 (V2)} - \text{myocardial velocity at segment 1 (V1)}}{\text{distance between segments 1 and 2}}$$

Applications of this modality in pediatrics are just emerging but will be particularly useful for regional wall motion abnormalities seen in diseases such as tetralogy of Fallot, single ventricle, and cardiomyopathies.

Transesophageal Echocardiography

Indications and contraindications

Transesophageal imaging began in the 1970s when an M-mode transducer was placed on a transesophageal probe. Since that time, transesophageal echocardiography (TEE) technology has improved significantly and has become an important component of cardiac testing. The availability of pediatric-sized probes has also expanded the use of TEE to the field of pediatric cardiology. Indications for performance of TEE are listed in Table 2-7. Most importantly, this modality is used in the operating room to evaluate cardiac surgical repair, in the cardiac catheterization laboratory to guide interventions, and when the quality of transthoracic imaging is inadequate to answer an important clinical question.[86] Contraindications to TEE relate to patient sedation, airway control, severe coagulopathies, and esophageal abnormalities. A TEE cannot be performed properly and effectively on patients who are not adequately sedated. In the pediatric population, general anesthesia is generally used to perform these studies. Thus, TEE is an invasive procedure with anesthesia risk. Complications of the procedure include esophageal injury or perforation, compression of left atrium or airway, bleeding, and arrhythmia.

TEE in the operating room and cardiac catheterization lab

In the operating room, TEE can be useful both before and after surgical intervention (Figure 2-29). Once the patient is sedated in preparation for surgery, TEE is often performed to confirm the cardiac anatomy and establish spatial relationships between particular structures not fully visualized by transthoracic echocardiography. Cardiac physiology can also be evaluated under general anesthesia. The degree of valvular regurgitation and velocity through regions of obstruction may be altered under these conditions. This information is useful for comparison purposes during the postoperative TEE examination.

Evaluation of a surgical repair prior to chest closure by TEE provides the surgical team with an intraoperative assessment of cardiac anatomy and hemodynamics. If there is an identified hemodynamic issue such as a significant shunt through a residual defect,

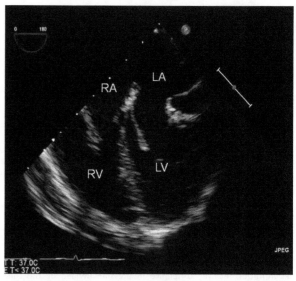

FIGURE 2-29 ■ Transesophageal image from a 4-chamber view. The 4-chamber view is useful to evaluate the atrioventricular valves and to assess ventricular function. LA, left atrium; LV, left ventricle; RA, right atrium; RV, right ventricle.

inadequate flow through a conduit or shunt, or important AV valve regurgitation, the surgeon has the opportunity to return to bypass and address the problem. It is important to note that there are limitations with this assessment because the hemodynamic condition of the patient often changes after they emerge from anesthesia and sedation. In addition to the assessment of the repair, postoperative TEE is helpful to identify residual air within the cardiac chambers or within the myocardium; intracardiac air can cause arrhythmias and myocardial dysfunction. TEE can also evaluate the patient's volume status and filling of the ventricles once cardiopulmonary bypass has been terminated.

TEE performed during cardiac catheterization assists in interventions. It augments the information provided by cardiac catheterization alone and also provides instantaneous assessment of ventricular performance and valvular function. TEE is used during cardiac catheterization most frequently for device placement, as well as other catheter-directed interventions such as atrial septostomy (typically for transposition of the great arteries), atrial septal defect device placement, stent placement in vascular structures, and dilation of valves.

CARDIAC MAGNETIC RESONANCE IMAGING TESTING

Introduction

Cardiac magnetic resonance (CMR), which uses magnetism and radiofrequency pulses to image the heart, is and function in congenital heart disease.[87-91] The CMR volume at The Children's Hospital of Philadelphia has grown in double digits in 8 of the last 11 years and serves as a resource for both clinical and research endeavors; it is complementary to both echocardiography and cardiac catheterization.

Uses of CMR in Congenital Heart Disease

Anatomy

Unrestrained by acoustic windows as in echocardiography and lacking ionizing radiation as in cardiac catheterization, CMR can be used in the very large or the very small patient serially. Defining anatomy is a major strength of this imaging modality; static bright and dark blood imaging (Figures 2-30 and 2-31) are used to demonstrate the salient points of the cardiovascular system in nearly any plane. This can be accomplished with a set of 2-dimensional images or "dynamic" 3D imaging where magnetic resonance "dye" (gadolinium) is injected and followed through the cardiovascular system with subsecond resolution (Figures 2-32 and 2-33); each "phase" of these images is a 3D image in itself and can be reconstructed into a volume-rendered display (Figure 2-33). This heart can be manipulated by software in any direction or cut in any plane to give the physician the view needed to understand the anatomy. In addition

a not a "new" or "novel" imaging technique in infants, children, and adolescents; it has been practiced for over 30 years and has evolved into a vibrant, dynamic imaging modality in the evaluation of anatomy, physiology,

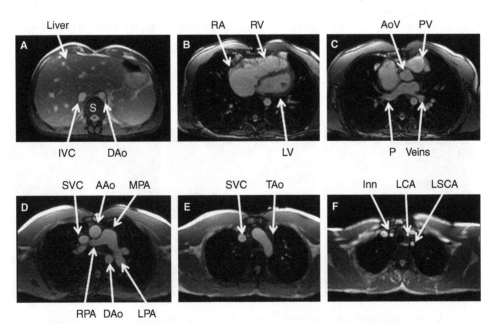

FIGURE 2-30 ■ Stack of static axial bright blood images. This set of selected images is taken from a patient with tetralogy of Fallot after repair. The images are in the axial plane where the top of the image is anterior, the bottom is posterior, the left of the image is the patient's right, and the right of the image is the patient's left. Images progress from inferior to superior as they go up the alphabet (from **A** to **F**). In **A**, the liver, inferior vena cava (IVC), and descending aorta (DAo) to the left (patient's left) of the spine (S) are easily seen. In **B**, a number of millimeters superiorly, the right atrium (RA) and right ventricle (RV) are now clear along with the left ventricle (LV). Even further superiorly in **C**, the aortic (AoV) and pulmonic valves (PV) are visualized along with the pulmonary veins (P Veins). In **D**, the ascending (AAo) and DAo are seen along with their relationships to the main (MPA), right (RPA), and left (LPA) pulmonary arteries. The superior vena cava (SVC) is clearly seen to the right (patient's right) and anterior to the RPA. At the level of the transverse aortic arch (TAo) in **E**, the SVC is still seen. At the most superior level shown (**F**), the branches of the Ao are seen—the innominate artery (Inn), the left carotid artery (LCA), and the left subclavioan artery (LSCA).

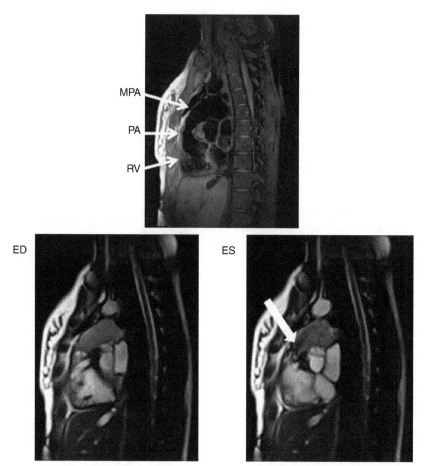

FIGURE 2-31 ■ Dark blood imaging and cine. The top panel is a dark blood image of a patient with pulmonary stenosis in the right ventricular outflow tract view. Note how clearly the right ventricle (RV), pulmonary annulus (PA), and main pulmonary artery (MPA) are seen. Bottom images are 2 frames from a steady-state free precession cine in the same view as in the dark blood image; to the left is a frame at end-diastole (ED), and to the right is a frame at end-systole (ES). Note the turbulence (arrow) demonstrated by the loss of signal (dark on the image) in the MPA.

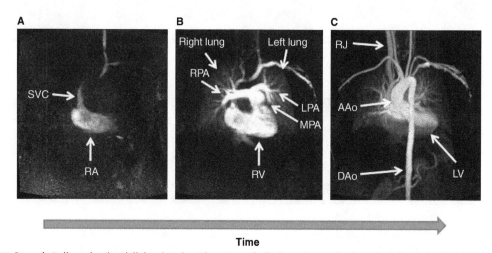

FIGURE 2-32 ■ Dynamic 3-dimensional gadolinium imaging. These 3 panels depict 3 phases of a dynamic 3-dimensional gadolinium administration in a patient after tetralogy of Fallot repair. Gadolinium is injected by power injector peripherally and followed through the cardiovascular system. A 3-dimensional slab is acquired at each phase and can be made into a volume-rendered display (see Figure 2-33). Time after injection proceeds from left to right (**A** through **C**). In **A**, gadolinium is injected in the left arm and is seen in the superior vena cava (SVC) and the right atrium (RA). In **B**, a few seconds later, the gadolinium has traversed the right ventricle (RV) and right (RPA) and left pulmonary arteries (LPA) to enter the lungs. A few more seconds later in **C**, the gadolinium has entered the left ventricle (LV), ascending aorta (AAo), and descending aorta (DAo); some gadolinium is seen recirculating into the right jugular vein (RJ) most prominently. MPA, main pulmonary artery.

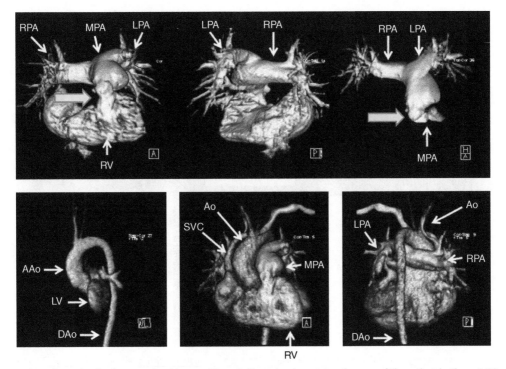

FIGURE 2-33 ■ Three-dimensional volume-rendered images. These 3-dimensional reconstructions are of the patient in Figure 2-32 who has right ventricular (RV) outflow tract obstruction (yellow arrow). Upper left and upper middle panels are 3-dimensional images of the right side of the circulation looking from anterior (left) and posterior (middle). The main (MPA), right (RPA), and left pulmonary arteries (LPA) are clearly seen. The upper right panel has the RV removed so that the MPA and branch pulmonary arteries can be seen from the superior aspect of the chest. The left lower panel demonstrates the left side of the heart from the left lateral view where the left ventricle (LV), ascending aorta (AAo), and descending aorta (DAo) are clearly seen in the candy cane view. The lower middle and lower right panels combine both right and left sides of the heart into one reconstruction. SVC, superior vena cava.

to large cardiovascular structures, small structures can be imaged as well. For example, coronary imaging by CMR came into practical clinical use in the mid-1990s; it uses a free breathing technique using a "navigator" that monitors diaphragmatic motion to ensure little blurring from respiratory motion (Figure 2-34). The technique uses specialized radiofrequency pulses to destroy signal from fat (fat saturation) and the myocardium (T_2 preparation). It is very accurate with regard to the detection of anomalous coronary lesions and Kawasaki disease and is very good at detecting coronary artery narrowing.

Physiology and function

By those not familiar with the imaging modality, magnetic resonance imaging (MRI) is generally thought of as a "static" imaging modality with no movement; this could not be farther from the truth. Besides anatomy, a huge strength of CMR is the ability to image ventricular function and blood flow. By using very fast pulse sequences termed *cine MRI* (2 types: steady-state free precession and gradient echo), high temporal resolution motion of the heart is captured over a number of heartbeats (Figure 2-35) as opposed to the "instantaneous" imaging of echocardiography and cardiac catheterization.

In this way, the heart function is "averaged" into the image as opposed to needing to view multiple heartbeats and having the imager "average" it in his or her mind. Nevertheless, CMR can also be used as "real-time" imaging as well capable and able to perform interactive "sweeps" of the cardiovascular system. In addition, with CMR, the ventricle can be "sliced" into cubes of magnetization, and those cubes can be observed for their deformation to determine if regional wall motion abnormalities are present (called myocardial tagging). Indeed, for ventricular volumes and mass, CMR has become the "gold standard" even in the echocardiography community; between 1997 and 2005, a search of the literature revealed 51 published studies where 3D echocardiography was compared to CMR as gold standard. Because of its inherent 3D nature, CMR can assess ventricular volumes and mass independent of geometric assumptions.

Not only can heart motion be visualized, but also blood flow can be evaluated through a technique called phase contrast (also called phase-encoded) velocity mapping (Figures 2-36 to 2-39). The distinction between blood velocities measured by echocardiography and those measured by CMR is that in the latter, velocities can be measured into and out of the imaging

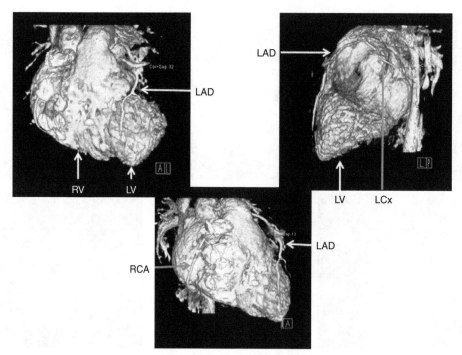

FIGURE 2-34 ■ Coronary imaging. The 3-dimensional whole-heart images are of a patient with a left ventricular (LV) fibroma. The upper left panel demonstrates the left anterior descending coronary artery (LAD) running down the interventricular groove between the LV and right ventricle (RV) in a nearly frontal view. The upper right panel demonstrates both the LAD and the left circumflex coronary artery (LCx), which courses over the tumor; the tumor itself is invisible in this type of imaging because it is not perfused, which is what coronary imaging in this technique depends on. The lower image demonstrates the right coronary artery (RCA) coursing in the right atrioventricular groove.

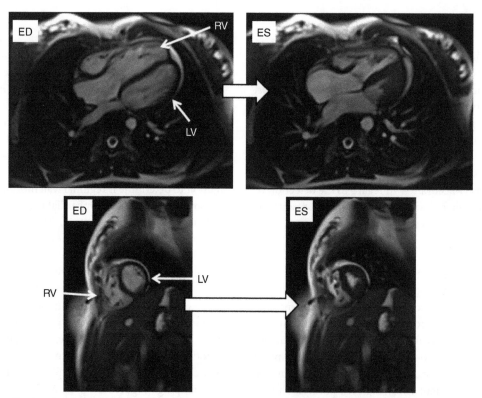

FIGURE 2-35 ■ Cine imaging. The 4-chamber (top) and short axis (bottom) views are from a patient after tetralogy of Fallot repair demonstrating ventricular shortening. Images are shown at end-diastole (ED) on the left and end-systole (ES) on the right. Note how the right (RV) and left ventricles (LV) contract, with the cavity getting smaller and the myocardial walls thickening.

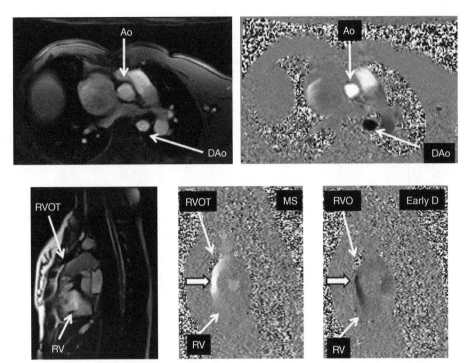

FIGURE 2-36 ■ Phase-encoded velocity mapping. The top panels are an example of through plane phase-encoded velocity mapping through the aortic valve (Ao), where velocity is measured into and out of the plane of the image and flow can be measured. The left upper panel is the anatomic (magnitude) image, and the right upper image is the phase image where the velocity is measured. Directionality is coded as white toward the head and black toward the feet; note how in the right phase image, the Ao velocities are white (blood flow toward the head), whereas the descending aortic (DAo) velocities are black. The lower panels are an example of in-plane phase-encoded velocity mapping across the right ventricular outflow tract (RVOT) in the patient in Figures 2-32 and 2-33. The left panel is the anatomic image for orientation, whereas the middle and right panels are phase images at midsystole (middle, MS) and early diastole (right, Early D). As in the through-plane example, directionality is coded as white toward the head and black toward the feet. Note the white flow through the RVOT (arrow) in MS and the pulmonary insufficiency (arrow) jet toward the feet into the right ventricle (RV) in Early D.

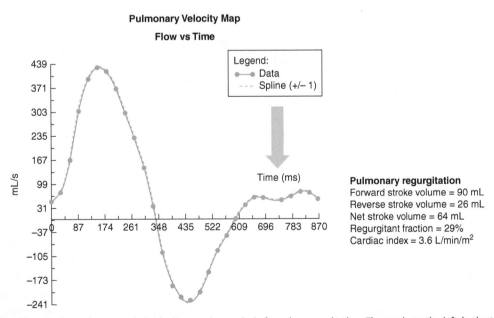

FIGURE 2-37 ■ Through plane phase-encoded velocity mapping analysis for valve regurgitation. The graph on the left is the through plane phase-encoded velocity map of the pulmonary valve in a patient after tetralogy of Fallot repair. The y-axis measures flow in milliliters per second (mL/s), and the x-axis measures time in milliseconds (ms). Forward flow is above the baseline, and reverse flow is below the baseline. Note the antegrade diastolic flow, which is classic for a patient after tetralogy of Fallot repair (arrow). By integrating the area above the baseline and below the baseline of the curves, forward and reverse stroke volumes can be calculated; from that, the net stroke volume and regurgitant fraction can be calculated. Cardiac index (measured in liters per minute per meter^2 [L/min/m^2]) is calculated by multiplying the stroke volume by the heart rate recorded during the acquisition of the images. On the right are the calculations.

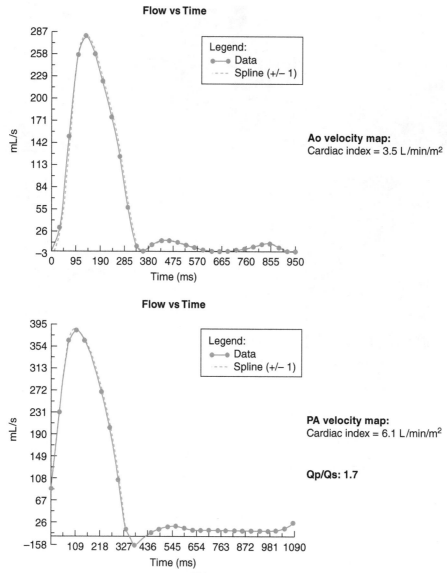

FIGURE 2-38 ■ Through plane phase-encoded velocity mapping analysis for pulmonary to systemic flow ratio (Qp/Qs). The data are taken from a patient with a moderate-size atrial septal defect. The top graph is the through plane phase-encoded velocity map of the aortic (Ao) valve, whereas the bottom graph is from the pulmonary artery (PA). The y-axis measures flow in milliliters per second (mL/s), and the x-axis measures time in milliseconds (ms). Forward flow is above the baseline, and reverse flow is below the baseline. By integrating the area above the baseline and below the baseline of the curves, forward and reverse stroke volumes can be calculated; from that, the net stroke volume can be calculated, and multiplication by the heart rate recorded during the acquisition of the images will yield the cardiac index (measured in liters per minute per meter^2 [L/min/m^2]). By dividing the cardiac output of the pulmonary artery by the aorta, Qp/Qs can be calculated.

plane ("through plane mapping"); if a blood vessel is imaged in cross-section, blood flow (not just velocities) can be measured in this manner (Figures 2-36 to 2-38). Directionality is coded on the image as either signal intense (white) or signal poor (black) or by color. By focusing on the region of interest (eg, the cross-section of the blood vessel) and multiplying the velocity in each pixel by the area of the pixel, the flow in that pixel is obtained. If all the pixels within the cross-section are summed and undergo the same multiplication by their respective velocities, the flow at one phase of the cardiac cycle is obtained. By obtaining multiple phases across the cardiac cycle and integrating the data over all the phases, flow in one heartbeat is obtained; multiply this by the heart rate over the course of imaging will yield cardiac output. Similar to cine, velocity mapping images can be created over many heartbeats and "averaged" into the image or can be "real time," similar to echocardiography and cardiac catheterization. There are multiple applications of this including measuring cardiac output (Figures 2-36 and 2-38), valve regurgitation (Figure 2-37), pulmonary to systemic flow ratio (Qp/Qs; Figure 2-38; relative flow to the lungs and the systemic circulation, which is necessary to assess in, for example, an atrial septal defect), and regional lung perfusion (see below).

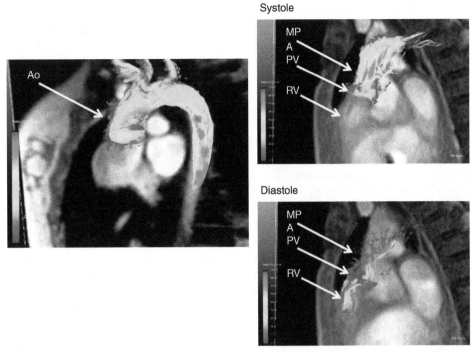

FIGURE 2-39 ■ Four-dimensional flow mapping. By obtaining a 3-dimensional phase-encoded velocity slab, 4-dimensional flow imaging can be performed. The vectors show the direction of flow, and the color codes velocity (faster flow in red and yellow, slower flow in green and blue). The panel on the left is 4-dimensional flow imaging in the normal aorta (Ao) in the candy cane view. The panels on the right are the right ventricular outflow tract from a patient after tetralogy of Fallot repair with pulmonary insufficiency; images are in systole (top) and diastole (bottom). Note the flow back into the right ventricle (RV) from the main pulmonary artery (MPA) in the bottom image. PV, pulmonary valve.

There are other types of phase-encoded velocity mapping with different applications. In plane velocity mapping measures blood flow in the plane of the image as in echocardiography (Figure 2-36); this is useful for detecting stenosis, regurgitation, and other forms of flow visualization (eg, the direction of flow across an atrial septal defect). Four-dimensional flow imaging acquires 3D velocities in a "slab" of tissue and is useful in visualization of flow characteristics as well (Figure 2-39). Finally, velocity mapping can be used to detect the small velocities of myocardial tissue, similar to Doppler tissue imaging in echocardiography (called myocardial velocimetry in CMR) to assess regional wall motion.

Measurement of CMR parameters of physiology and function are very accurate. One of the ways this is accomplished is by "internal checks" on the data. For example, flows in the branch pulmonary arteries should equal to flow in the main pulmonary artery. This, in turn, should equal to flow in the aorta in the absence of intracardiac shunts, which in turn, should equal the sum of the flow in the inferior and superior vena cava in the absence of aortic to pulmonary collateral flow. Cardiac output as measured by velocity mapping in the aorta should equal to flow as measured by cine of the left ventricle in the absence of mitral insufficiency or intracardiac shunts.

By injecting gadolinium and imaging very quickly, the myocardium on CMR will turn from signal poor to signal intense (black to white). In myocardial wall regions, which are either ischemic or infarcted, little or no gadolinium will traverse these regions on first pass of the blood, and this principle is used in CMR to determine myocardial perfusion defects. Gadolinium is administered with and without adenosine (which is a coronary vasodilator), and armed with that data, both qualitative and quantitative information regarding blood flow to the myocardium can be obtained. This is useful in cases such as anomalous origins of coronaries, patients with chest pain, or patients who have undergone surgical manipulation of the coronaries such as after the Ross procedure or transposition of the great arteries after arterial switch operation.

Tissue characterization

The most common form of tissue characterization referred to CMR in congenital heart disease is to assess for myocardial scarring (also called "viability" or "delayed enhancement"). After gadolinium is injected, the heart is imaged 5 to 15 minutes later as gadolinium is distributed in the extravascular space; infarcted, fibrosed, or scarred myocardium will avidly take up this magnetic contrast dye, which will appear white on the image. Normal myocardium will have coronary flow to "wash out" the contrast agent so it will be dark on the image. This technique has revolutionized many areas and is useful in postoperative patients (eg, single-ventricle patients after Fontan procedure), in chest pain, and in characterizing ventricular tissue such as in myocarditis, hypertrophic cardiomyopathy, and arrhythmogenic right ventricular dysplasia. It is a very sensitive technique; contrast ratios of close to 500 times have been achieved between scarred and nonscarred tissue. The amount of scarred tissue can also be measured.

Characterizing myocardial masses such as tumors and thrombus by CMR uses a number of different types of techniques. Using viability imaging along with other images such as T1 weighting (with and without fat saturation as well as prior to and after gadolinium administration), T2 weighting, gradient echo imaging (a form of cine), myocardial tagging, and perfusion, the type of mass or tumor can be diagnosed with a relatively high degree of accuracy. For example, a hemangioma will demonstrate perfusion very similar to the myocardial cavity. A fibroma will "light up" on delayed-enhancement imaging, and a lipoma will show up bright on T1-weighted imaging and then "disappear" when performing the same imaging in the same plane using a fat saturation.

The measurement of T2* in the relaxation process of the protons can be used to assess the amount of myocardial iron present. Obtaining multiple images at various times when radiofrequency pulses are emitted and using a gradient echo sequence, the myocardium and liver can be seen to become increasingly dark. Because iron is ferromagnetic, it changes the magnetic properties of the myocardium, and increasing iron concentration decreases the measured T2* and makes the myocardium even darker. Values below 20 ms are at risk for poor ventricular function, and chelation therapy in cases of thalassemia and sickle cell disease can be modified.

Indications for CMR

Presently, CMR is used in conjunction with other imaging modalities such as echocardiography or cardiac catheterization; however, in a number of areas such as vascular rings and ventricular volumes and mass, CMR has become the imaging modality of choice and the gold standard. As mentioned, CMR offers several advantages over other imaging modalities including freely selectable imaging planes without limitations to "windows" (as in echocardiography) or overlapping structures (as

Cardiac Magnetic Resonance Indications for Anatomy

Indication	Examples
Great vessels ■ Aorta ■ Pulmonary artery	Transposition of the great arteries Truncus arteriosus Vascular rings Coarctation of the aorta
Venous connections ■ Systemic ■ Pulmonary	Total anomalous pulmonary venous connection Left superior vena cava
Extracardiac conduits	Fontan procedure
Intracardiac baffles	Rastelli operation
Valve morphology	Bicuspid aortic valve
Complex congenital heart disease	Heterotaxy
Spatial relationships ■ Within cardiovascular system ■ Cardiovascular system with extracardiac structures	Double outlet right ventricle Heterotaxy
Pericardial disease	Restrictive cardiomyopathy Partial absence of the pericardium
Ventricle characterization	Arrhythmogenic right ventricular dysplasia Hypertrophic cardiomyopathy Myocarditis
Coronary arteries	Anomalous origin of the left coronary artery from the right sinus Anomalous coronary artery from the pulmonary artery Kawasaki disease
Cardiac tumor presence	Myxoma Fibroma Rhabdomyoma

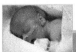

Cardiac Magnetic Resonance Indications for Physiology/Function and Tissue Characterization

Indication	Examples
Ventricular function ■ Global (ejection fraction, end-diastolic volume, ventricular mass) ■ Regional	Ventricular volumes after Fontan or tetralogy of Fallot repair Regional wall motion abnormalities after arterial switch operation for transposition of the great arteries
Cardiac output	Cardiomyopathy Single ventricles
Valve regurgitation	Pulmonary insufficiency after tetralogy of Fallot repair
Valve stenosis	Bicuspid aortic valve
Vessel stenosis	Coarctation of the aorta
Collateral flow	Single ventricles Coarctation of the aorta
Shunts (Qp/Qs)	Atrial septal defect Ventricular septal defect
Flow directionality/visualization	Atrial septal defect Isolated left subclavian artery
Regional perfusion of organ (eg, lungs)	Fontan procedure Residual branch pulmonary artery stenosis after tetralogy of Fallot repair
Viability (myocardial scarring)	After repair of anomalous origin of the left coronary artery from the pulmonary artery
Myocardial perfusion	Chest pain Fontan procedure Hypertrophic cardiomyopathy
Tumor characterization (ie, what type of tumor the mass is)	Myxoma Fibroma Rhabdomyoma
Myocardial iron assessment	Thalassemia Sickle cell disease
Pressure gradients	Pulmonary stenosis Coarctation of the aorta

in angiography), lack of ionizing radiation (as in computerized tomography), excellent soft tissue contrast, a capacity for true 3D imaging of both anatomy and physiology/function, accurate flow quantification using phase contrast velocity mapping, noninvasive labeling of the myocardium or blood (myocardial tagging), assessment of myocardial viability and perfusion, and coronary imaging (Figure 2-34). Because of this capability to be a "one-stop shop," CMR is indicated in many areas for specific and global assessments. Tables 2-8 and 2-9 list the indications for anatomy, physiology, function, and tissue characterization.

Pushing the Envelope and Future Developments

New CMR techniques and applications are always being developed. The combination of CMR and cardiac catheterization called XMR pushes the imaging envelop and is being performed in only a few centers around the world, such as The Children's Hospital of Philadelphia. This involves techniques such as fusion of CMR and cardiac catheterization imaging by creating 3D images by CMR and superimposing them on fluoroscopy in the catheterization lab to use as a "road map" for the cardiologist performing the catheterization. Placing catheters in the catheterization lab and then moving the patient to the CMR suite to obtain simultaneous pressures, flows, and anatomy is another approach. Finally, performing the catheterization solely in the CMR suite has been performed at some centers. CMR has some obvious advantages in this regard; for example, electrophysiologists can actually see the "burn" they are creating for the first time by CMR and can use that in their practice.

Other developments are currently on their way to becoming routine. Exercise CMR uses a CMR-compatible ergometer for the patient to exercise with, and imaging takes place immediately after the exercise is finished. "3D printing," or stereolithography, allows for creation of physical 3D models from CMR data sets that cardiologists or surgeons can hold in their hands. Combining CMR with computational fluid mechanics and the ability to do "virtual surgery" allows cardiologists and surgeons to predict the result of an intervention. Finally, anatomic and functional fetal CMR is now able to visualize the beating fetal heart in utero and obtain ventricular performance parameters unable to be obtained by echocardiography well.

Conclusion

CMR is a vibrant, dynamic, multifaceted field within congenital heart disease that allows for "one-stop shopping" for cardiovascular anatomy, physiology, function, and tissue characterization. It has myriad utilities in congenital heart disease and holds the future promise of many more developments.

CMR Clinical Pearls

- Referral for CMR in congenital heart disease should be performed by a pediatric cardiology specialist after a full cardiac evaluation.
- The CMR examination is a very specialized procedure and requires the selected application of multiple techniques within the imaging modality to accomplish the diagnosis.
- There are numerous techniques within CMR for anatomy such as bright blood imaging (steady-state free precession and gradient echo imaging), dark blood imaging (T1- and T2-weighted imaging) and 3D gadolinium imaging.
- There are numerous techniques within CMR for physiology and function such as cine imaging (steady-state free precession and gradient echo imaging), phase-encoded velocity mapping, and myocardial perfusion. Cine and phase-encoded velocity mapping act as internal checks on each other, making ventricular performance parameters very accurate.
- Ejection fraction, ventricular volumes and mass, cardiac index, Qp/Qs, regurgitant fraction, and relative flows to both lungs are some of the many physiology and function parameters assessed by CMR.
- There are numerous techniques within CMR for tissue characterization such as viability, tumor characterization, and T2* for myocardial iron assessment. Diseases such as myocardial infarction, myocarditis, hypertrophic cardiomyopathy, and arrhythmogenic right ventricular dysplasia are just some of the applications for these techniques.
- Multiple developments are under way to make future novel applications of CMR a reality, such as XMR, exercise CMR, 3D printing of physical models from CMR images, surgical planning, and fetal CMR.

REFERENCES

1. Pelliccia A, Corrado D. Can ECG screening prevent sudden death in athletes? *BMJ.* 2010;341:c4923.
2. Bahr R. Can ECG screening prevent sudden death in athletes? *BMJ.* 2010;341:c4914.
3. Chaitman BR. Should an electrocardiogram be included in routine preparticipation screening of young athletes? *Circulation.* 2007;116:2610-2615.
4. Myerburg RJ, Vetter VL. Should an electrocardiogram be included in routine preparticipation screening of young athletes? *Circulation.* 2007;116:2616-2626.
5. Myung P, Guntheroth WG. *How to Read Pediatric ECGs.* 4th ed. Philadelphia, PA: Mosby Elsevier; 2006.
6. Davignon A, Rautaharju P, Barselle E, Soumis F, Megelas M. Normal ECG standards for infants and children. *Pediatr Cardiol.* 1979/80;1:123-134.
7. Johnson JN, Ackerman MJ. QTc: how long is too long? *Br J Sports Med.* 2009;43:657-662.
8. Arizona Center for Education and Research on Therapeutics. QT drug lists by risk groups. Available at: http://www.qtdrugs.org. Accessed September 15, 2011.
9. Dubin D. *Rapid Interpretation of EKGs.* 6th ed. Tampa, FL: COVER Publishing Company; 2000.
10. Fogoros R. *Electrophysiology Testing.* 4th ed. Pittsburgh, PA: Blackwell Publishing Ltd.; 2006.
11. Benson DW: The normal electrocardiogram. In: Emmanouilides GC, Allen HD, Riemenschneider TA, Gutgesell HP, eds. *Heart Disease in Infants, Children and Adolescents.* Baltimore, MD: Williams & Wilkins; 1995:163.
12. Stephens P Jr, McBride MG, Paridon SM. Cardiopulmonary Stress Testing. In: *Paediatric Cardiology.* 3rd ed. edited by Anderson RH et al. Philadelphia, PA: Churchill Livingstone/Elsevier, 2010; 415-436.
13. Wasserman K, Hansen JE, Sue DY, Whipp BJ, Casaburi R. Exercise testing and interpretation: an overview. In: *Principles of Exercise Testing and Interpretation.* 2nd ed. New York, NY: Lea & Febiger; 1994:1-8.
14. Wasserman K, Hansen JE, Sue DY, Whipp BJ, Casaburi R. Physiology of exercise. In: *Principles of Exercise Testing and Interpretation.* 2nd ed. New York, NY: Lea & Febiger; 1994:9-51.
15. Astrand P, Rodahl K. The muscle and its contraction. In: *Textbook of Work Physiology, Physiological Bases of Exercise.* 3rd ed. New York, NY: McGraw-Hill, Inc.; 1986:12-208.
16. Wilmore JH, Costill DL. *Physiology of Sport and Exercise.* Champaign, IL: Human Kinetics; 1994.
17. Braden DS, Strong WB. Cardiovascular responses to exercise in childhood. *Am J Dis Child.* 1990;144:1255-1260.
18. Wasserman K, McIlroy MB. Detecting the threshold of anaerobic metabolism in cardiac patients during exercise. *Am J Cardiol.* 1964;14:844-852.
19. Davis JA. Anaerobic threshold: review of the concept and directions for future research. *Med Sci Sports Exerc.* 1985;17:6-18.
20. Anderson GS, Rhodes EC. A review of blood lactate and ventilatory methods of detecting transition thresholds. *Sports Med.* 1989;8:43-55.
21. Inbar O, Bar-Or O. Anaerobic characteristics in male children and adolescents. *Med Sci Sports Exerc.* 1986;18:264-269.
22. Rowland TW. Response to endurance exercise: cardiovascular system. *Dev Exerc Physiol.* 1996;8:117-140.

23. Bar-Or O, Shephard RJ, Allen CL. Cardiac output of 10- to 13-year-old boys and girls during submaximal exercise. *J Appl Physiol.* 1971;30:219-223.

24. Protas EJ. Normal cardiovascular anatomy, physiology, and responses at rest and during exercise. In: Hasson SM, ed. *Clinical Exercise Physiology.* St. Louis, MO: CV Mosby; 1994:101-120.

25. Holmgren A, Linderholm H. Oxygen and carbon dioxide tensions of arterial blood during heavy and exhaustive exercise. *Acta Physiol Scand.* 1958;44:203-215.

26. Astrand P, Rodahl K. Body fluids, blood and circulation. *Textbook of Work Physiology, Physiological Bases of Exercise.* 3rd ed. New York, NY: McGraw-Hill, Inc.; 1986:127-208.

27. Paridon SM. Exercise physiology and capacity. In: Rychik J, Wernovsky G, eds. *Hypoplastic Left Heart Syndrome.* New York, NY: Springer; 2003:329-346.

28. Green JH. *The Autonomic Nervous System and Exercise.* London, UK: Chapman and Hall; 1990.

29. Freedson PS, Goodman TL. Measurement of consumption of oxygen. In: Rowland TW, ed. *Pediatric Laboratory Exercise Testing, Clinical Guidelines.* Champaign, IL: Human Kinetics Publishers; 1993:91-113.

30. Wasserman K, Hansen JE, Sue DY, Whipp BJ, Casaburi R. *Measurements During Integrative Cardiopulmonary Exercise Testing. Principles of Exercise Testing and Interpretation.* 2nd ed. New York, NY: Lea & Febiger; 1994:52-79.

31. Barber G. Paediatric exercise testing—methodology, equipment, and normal values. *Prog Pediatr Cardiol.* 1993;2:4-10.

32. Tomassoni TL. Conducting the pediatric exercise test. In: Rowland TW, ed. *Pediatric Laboratory Exercise Testing, Clinical Guidelines.* Champaign, IL: Human Kinetics Publishers; 1993;1-17.

33. Alpert BS, Verrill DE, Flood NL, et al. Complications of ergometer exercise in children. *Pediatr Cardiol.* 1983;4:91-96.

34. Freed M. Exercise testing in children: a survey of techniques and safety [abstract]. *Circulation.* 1981;64(suppl IV): IV-278.

35. Washington RL, Bricker JT, Alpert BS, et al. Guidelines for exercise testing in the paediatric age group. *Circulation.* 1994;90:4;2166-2179.

36. Stephens P, Paridon SM. Exercise testing in pediatrics. *Pediatr Clin North Am.* 2004;51:1569-1587.

37. Wasserman K, Hansen JE, Sue DY, et al. Protocols for exercise testing. In: *Principles of Exercise Testing and Interpretation.* Philadelphia, PA: Lea & Febiger; 1994:96-111.

38. Rowland TW. Aerobic exercise testing protocols. In: Rowland TW, ed. *Pediatric Laboratory Exercise Testing, Clinical Guidelines.* Champaign, IL: Human Kinetics Publishers; 1993:19-41.

39. James FW, Kaplan S, Glueck CJ, et al. Responses of normal children and young adults to controlled bicycle exercise. *Circulation.* 1980;61:902-912.

40. Akkerman M, van Brussel M, Bongers BC, Hulzebos EH, Helders PJ, Takken T. Oxygen uptake efficiency slope in healthy children. *Pediatr Exerc Sci.* 2010;22:431-441.

41. Fahey JT, Bryant NJ, Karas D, Goldberg B, Destefano R, Gracco LC. Exercise-induced stridor due to abnormal movement of the arytenoid area: videoendoscopic diagnosis and characterization of the "at risk" group. *Pediatr Pulmonol.* 2005;39:51-55.

42. Giardini A, Specchia S, Gargiulo G, Sangiorgi D, Picchio FM. Accuracy of oxygen uptake efficiency slope in adults with congenital heart disease. *Int J Cardiol.* 2009;133:74-79.

43. Goldberg S, Schwartz S, Izbicki G, Hamami RB, Picard E. Sensitivity of exercise testing for asthma in adolescents is halved in the summer. *Chest.* 2005;128:2408-2411.

44. Macucci F, Guerrini L, Strambi M. Asthma and allergy in young athletes in Siena Province. Preliminary results. *J Sports Med Phys Fitness.* 2007;47:351-355.

45. McBride MG, Schall JI, Zemel BS, Stallings VA, Ittenbach RF, Paridon SM. Clinical and genetic correlates of exercise performance in young children with cystic fibrosis. *Percept Mot Skills.* 2010;110:995-1009.

46. Paridon SM, Mitchell PD, Colan SD, et al. A cross-sectional study of exercise performance during the first 2 decades of life after the Fontan operation. *J Am Coll Cardiol.* 2008;52:99-107.

47. Pasquali SK, Marino BS, Pudusseri A, et al. Risk factors and comorbidities associated with obesity in children and adolescents after the arterial switch operation and Ross procedure. *Am Heart J.* 2009;158:473-479.

48. Siddiqui S, Patel DR. Cardiovascular screening of adolescent athletes. *Pediatr Clin North Am.* 2010;57:635-647.

49. van der Cammen-van Zijp MH, Ijsselstijn H, Takken T, et al. Exercise testing of pre-school children using the Bruce treadmill protocol: new reference values. *Eur J Appl Physiol.* 2010;108:393-399.

50. Wong JA, Gula LJ, Klein GJ, Yee R, Skanes AC, Krahn AD. Utility of treadmill testing in identification and genotype prediction in long-QT syndrome. *Circ Arrhythm Electrophysiol.* 2010;3:120-125.

51. Brothers J, Carter C, McBride M, Spray T, Paridon S. Anomalous left coronary artery origin from the opposite sinus of Valsalva: evidence of intermittent ischemia. *J Thorac Cardiovasc Surg.* 2010;140:e27-e29.

52. Brothers J, Gaynor JW, Paridon S, Lorber R, Jacobs M. Anomalous aortic origin of a coronary artery with an interarterial course: understanding current management strategies in children and young adults. *Pediatr Cardiol.* 2009;30:911-921.

53. Brothers JA, McBride MG, Marino BS, et al. Exercise performance and quality of life following surgical repair of anomalous aortic origin of a coronary artery in the pediatric population. *J Thorac Cardiovasc Surg.* 2009;137: 380-384.

54. McBride MG, Binder TJ, Paridon SM. Safety and feasibility of inpatient exercise training in pediatric heart failure: a preliminary report. *J Cardiopulm Rehabil Prev.* 2007;27:219-222.

55. Osaki M, McCrindle BW, Van Arsdell G, Dipchand AI. Anomalous origin of a coronary artery from the opposite sinus of Valsalva with an interarterial course: clinical profile and approach to management in the pediatric population. *Pediatr Cardiol.* 2008;29:24-30.

56. Pasquali SK, Marino BS, McBride MG, Wernovsky G, Paridon SM. Coronary artery pattern and age impact exercise performance late after the arterial switch operation. *J Thorac Cardiovasc Surg.* 2007;134:1207-1212.

57. Pasquali SK, Marino BS, Powell DJ, et al. Following the arterial switch operation, obese children have risk factors for early cardiovascular disease. *Congenit Heart Dis.* 2010;5:16-24.

58. Raisky O, Bergoend E, Agnoletti G, et al. Late coronary artery lesions after neonatal arterial switch operation: results of surgical coronary revascularization. *Eur J Cardiothorac Surg.* 2007;31:894-898.

59. Sethna CB, Salerno AE, McBride MG, et al. Cardiorespiratory fitness in pediatric renal transplant recipients. *Transplantation.* 2009;88:395-401.

60. Weaver DJ Jr, Kimball TR, Knilans T, et al. Decreased maximal aerobic capacity in pediatric chronic kidney disease. *J Am Soc Nephrol.* 2008;19:624-630.

61. Joyner BL, Fiorino EK, Matta-Arroyo E, Needleman JP. Cardiopulmonary exercise testing in children and adolescents with asthma who report symptoms of exercise-induced bronchoconstriction. *J Asthma.* 2006;43:675-678.

62. Lex C, Dymek S, Heying R, Kovacevic A, Kramm CM, Schuster A. Value of surrogate tests to predict exercise-induced bronchoconstriction in atopic childhood asthma. *Pediatr Pulmonol.* 2007;42:225-230.

63. Paridon SM, Alpert BS, Boas SR, et al. Clinical stress testing in the pediatric age group: a statement from the American Heart Association Council on Cardiovascular Disease in the Young, Committee on Atherosclerosis, Hypertension, and Obesity in Youth. *Circulation.* 2006;113:1905-1920.

64. Barst RJ, Mubarak KK, Machado RF, et al. Exercise capacity and haemodynamics in patients with sickle cell disease with pulmonary hypertension treated with bosentan: results of the ASSET studies. *Br J Haematol.* 2010;149:426-435.

65. Garofano RP, Barst RJ. Exercise testing in children with primary pulmonary hypertension. *Pediatr Cardiol.* 1999;20:61-64.

66. Lesser DJ, Fleming MM, Maher CA, Kim SB, Woo MS, Keens TG. Does the 6-min walk test correlate with the exercise stress test in children? *Pediatr Pulmonol.* 2010;45:135-140.

67. Smith G, Reyes JT, Russell JL, Humpl T. Safety of maximal cardiopulmonary exercise testing in pediatric patients with pulmonary hypertension. *Chest.* 2009;135:1209–1214.

68. Takken T, Engelbert R, van Bergen M, et al. Six-minute walking test in children with ESRD: discrimination validity and construct validity. *Pediatr Nephrol.* 2009;24:2217-2223.

69. Yetman AT, Taylor AL, Doran A, Ivy DD. Utility of cardiopulmonary stress testing in assessing disease severity in children with pulmonary arterial hypertension. *Am J Cardiol.* 2005;95:697-699.

70. Castellani C, Windhaber J, Schober PH, Hoellwarth ME. Exercise performance testing in patients with pectus excavatum before and after Nuss procedure. *Pediatr Surg Int.* 2010;26:659-663.

71. Burkhardt BE, Fischer PR, Brands CK, et al. Exercise performance in adolescents with autonomic dysfunction. *J Pediatr.* 2011;158:28-32.

72. Haley SM, Fragala-Pinkham M, Ni P. Sensitivity of a computer adaptive assessment for measuring functional mobility changes in children enrolled in a community fitness programme. *Clin Rehabil.* 2006;20:616-622.

73. Hayman LL, Williams CL, Daniels SR, et al. Cardiovascular health promotion in the schools: a statement for health and education professionals and child health advocates from the Committee on Atherosclerosis, Hypertension, and Obesity in Youth (AHOY) of the Council on Cardiovascular Disease in the Young, American Heart Association. *Circulation.* 2004;110:2266-2275.

74. Painter P, Krasnoff J, Mathias R. Exercise capacity and physical fitness in pediatric dialysis and kidney transplant patients. *Pediatr Nephrol.* 2007;22:1030-1039.

75. Ten Harkel AD, Takken T. Exercise testing and prescription in patients with congenital heart disease. *Int J Pediatr.* 2010:791980.

76. Williams CL, Hayman LL, Daniels SR, et al. Cardiovascular health in childhood: a statement for health professionals from the Committee on Atherosclerosis, Hypertension, and Obesity in the Young (AHOY) of the Council on Cardiovascular Disease in the Young, American Heart Association. *Circulation.* 2002;106:143-160.

77. Oh KJ, Seward JB, Tajik AJ, eds. How to obtain a good echocardiography examination: ultrasound physics, technique, and medical knowledge. In: *Echo Manual.* Philadelphia, PA: Lippincott Williams & Wilkins; 2007:1-6.

78. Armstrong WF, Ryan T. Specialized echocardiographic techniques and methods. In: *Feigenbaum's Echocardiography.* 7th ed. Philadelphia, PA: Lippincott Williams & Wilkins; 2010:1-8.

79. Oh KJ, Seward JB, Tajik AJ, eds. Doppler echocardiography and color flow imaging: comprehensive noninvasive hemodynamic assessment. In: *Echo Manual.* Philadelphia, PA: Lippincott Williams & Wilkins; 2007:59-79.

80. Armstrong WF, Ryan T, eds. Hemodynamics. In: *Feigenbaum's Echocardiography.* 7th ed. Philadelphia, PA: Lippincott Williams & Wilkins; 2010:217-240.

81. Frommelt PC. Diastolic ventricular function assessment. In: Lai WW, Mertens LL, Cohen MS, Geva T, eds. *Echocardiography in Pediatric and Congenital Heart Disease: From Fetus to Adult.* Hoboken, NJ: Blackwell Publishing Ltd.; 2009:95-116.

82. Oh KJ, Seward JB, Tajik AJ, eds. Contrast echocardiography. In: *Echo Manual.* Philadelphia, PA: Lippincott Williams & Wilkins; 2007:99-108.

83. Oh KJ, Seward JB, Tajik AJ, eds. Transthoracic echocardiography: M-mode, two-dimensional, and three-dimensional. In: *Echo Manual.* Philadelphia, PA: Lippincott Williams & Wilkins; 2007:7-28.

84. Lai WW, Ko, HH. The normal pediatric echocardiogram. In: Lai WW, Mertens LL, Cohen MS, Geva T, eds. *Echocardiography in Pediatric and Congenital Heart Disease: From Fetus to Adult.* Hoboken, NJ: Blackwell Publishing Ltd.; 2009:34-50.

85. Sluysmans T, Colan SD. Structural measurements and adjustments for growth. In: Lai WW, Mertens LL, Cohen MS, Geva T, eds. *Echocardiography in Pediatric and Congenital Heart Disease: From Fetus to Adult.* Hoboken, NJ: Blackwell Publishing Ltd.; 2009:53-62.

86. Stevenson JG. Transesophageal echocardiography. In: Lai WW, Mertens LL, Cohen MS, Geva T, eds. *Echocardiography in Pediatric and Congenital Heart Disease: From Fetus to Adult.* Hoboken, NJ: Blackwell Publishing Ltd.; 2009: 671-686.

87. Fogel MA, ed. *Principles and Practice of Cardiac Magnetic Resonance in Congenital Heart Disease: Form, Function and Flow.* Oxford, UK: Wiley-Blackwell; 2010.

88. Whitehead MA, Ewing S, Fogel MA. Complex congenital heart disease. In: Ho V, Reddy G, eds. *Imaging of the Cardiovascular System.* New York, NY: Elsevier Publishing Company; 2011.

89. Fogel MA. Complex congenital heart disease. In: Kramer C, Hundley WG, eds. *Atlas of Cardiovascular Magnetic Resonance Imaging. An Imaging Companion to Braunwald's Heart Disease.* New York, NY: Saunders/Elsevier; 2010.

90. Fogel MA. Cardiac magnetic resonance in congenital heart disease. In: Cetta F, O'Leary P, Eidem B. *Echocardiography in Pediatric and Adult Congenital Heart Disease.* Philadelphia, PA: Wolters Kluwer/Lippincott Williams & Wilkens; 2010.

91. Fogel MA. Special considerations: cardiac magnetic resonance in infants and children. In: Manning WJ, Pennell DJ, eds. *Cardiovascular Magnetic Resonance.* 2nd ed. Philadelphia, PA: Saunders/Elsevier; 2010.

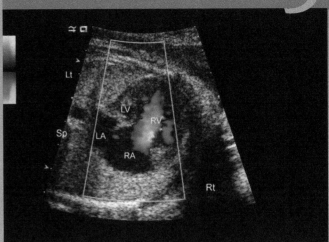

CHAPTER 3

Fetal Cardiology

Donna Goff,
Michael Quartermain and
Anita Szwast

Congenital heart disease comprises the most common form of congenital anomaly found in humans, affecting 8 of every 1000 live births and 10 to 12 out of every 1000 pregnancies. Over the past 20 years, fetal echocardiography has emerged as a reliable and accurate means to diagnose these problems associated with cardiac structure and function prior to birth. As imaging technologies continue to improve, a higher percentage of congenital heart defects and abnormalities of fetal cardiovascular function can be detected prior to birth, allowing practitioners to counsel parents about their unborn child's expected outcome and to implement prenatal and perinatal management strategies in order to maximize postnatal outcome.

THE FETAL CARDIOVASCULAR SYSTEM

In contrast to postnatal circulation, in which the pulmonary and systemic circulation are arranged in series, the fetal circulation is arranged in parallel because the placenta, rather than the lungs, serves as the site of oxygenation and ventilation. As a consequence, the right ventricle pumps approximately 55% to 60% of the combined cardiac output, whereas the left ventricle pumps approximately 40% to 45%.[1] As shown in Figure 3-1, the fetal blood flow patterns are optimized to deliver oxygen and nutrition to vital organs, while shunting blood away from less important structures. Indeed, the placenta has extremely low resistance in order to promote blood flow to this site. Within the capillary bed of the placenta, oxygen is exchanged for carbon dioxide. A single umbilical vein then leaves the placenta carrying richly oxygenated blood back to the fetus through the umbilical cord. To

bypass most of the liver, the umbilical vein inserts into the ductus venosus, which then connects with the inferior vena cava to enter the right atrium. The angle at which the ductus venosus inserts into the inferior vena cava–right atrium junction directs most of the richly oxygenated blood across the foramen ovale and into the left atrium and left ventricle. The left ventricle, in turn, perfuses the coronary arteries and the cerebral vasculature. These fetal physiologic adaptations ensure that the most richly oxygenated blood is delivered to the most vital structures in need of oxygen, namely the myocardial and cerebral circulations. Similarly, the most deoxygenated blood returning from the superior vena cava is directed to the tricuspid valve and into the right ventricle, which pumps blood into the main pulmonary artery and across the ductus arteriosus to return to the descending aorta and ultimately to the umbilical arteries. Because the fetal lungs are compressed and not responsible for oxygenation and ventilation prior to birth, the resistance within the pulmonary vasculature is quite high to ensure that deoxygenated blood crosses the ductus arteriosus rather than entering the fetal lungs, to return deoxygenated blood to the site of oxygenation within the fetus, namely the placenta.

UNIQUENESS OF THE FETAL MYOCARDIUM

Compared to the adult myocardium, the fetal myocardium demonstrates unique myocardial properties. Fetuses have impaired myocardial relaxation, secondary to a greater percentage of noncontractile elements[2] and less efficient removal of calcium from troponin C within the cardiac myocyte.[3] As a result, ventricular filling

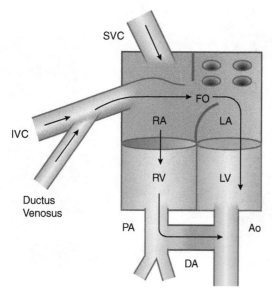

FIGURE 3-1 ■ The fetal circulation. The ductus venosus carries the most highly oxygenated blood across the foramen ovale (FO) to the left atrium (LA), the left ventricle (LV), and then out of the aorta (Ao) to supply the coronary arteries and brain. The superior vena cava (SVC) directs the most deoxygenated blood across the tricuspid valve into the right ventricle (RV) and then out the pulmonary artery (PA) and ductus arteriosus (DA) to return to the lower half of the body and the placenta. IVC, inferior vena cava; RA, right atrium.

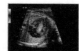

Indications for Fetal Echocardiography

Maternal Indications
- Family history of congenital cardiac disease
- Metabolic disorders, such as phenylketonuria or diabetes
- Exposure to teratogens
- Exposure to inhibitors of prostaglandin synthetase, such as ibuprofen, salicylic acid, or indomethacin
- Infection with rubella
- Autoimmune disease, such as systemic lupus erythematosus or Sjögren syndrome
- Familial inherited disorders, such as Ellis-van Creveld syndrome, Marfan syndrome, or Noonan syndrome
- Artificial fertilization

Fetal Indications
- Abnormal obstetrical ultrasound screening
- Extracardiac abnormality
- Chromosomal abnormality
- Arrhythmia
- Hydrops
- Increased nuchal translucency in first trimester
- Multiple gestation and twin–twin transfusion syndrome

in the fetus is accomplished predominantly by active atrial contraction rather than passive ventricular filling. Inherent stiffness of the fetal myocardium underlies the mechanism for fetal hydrops. Any disease process that results in a slight increase in atrial pressure is poorly tolerated, leading to the findings of hydrops fetalis, characterized by fluid in any two extravascular spaces, such as ascites, peripheral or scalp edema, pleural effusions, or pericardial effusions.

SCREENING WITH FETAL ECHOCARDIOGRAPHY

Screening fetal echocardiograms are typically performed between 18 and 22 weeks of gestation. At these gestational ages, there is adequate amniotic fluid volume to allow good visualization of the cardiac structures and vasculature for an accurate diagnosis. After 30 weeks of gestation, the increase in fetal body mass and the shadowing effects of the fetal ribs may make image acquisition more difficult. However, early transabdominal and transvaginal fetal echocardiography may be performed as early as 11 to 14 weeks of gestation in high-risk pregnancies, such as those with aneuploidy, those with increased nuchal translucency during scanning at 10 to 14 weeks, and those with a family history of congenital heart disease.[4]

Current indications for fetal echocardiography, as recommended by the American Society of Fetal Echocardiography, are outlined in Table 3-1.[5] These indications are broken down into maternal and fetal indications. Twenty years ago, the most common indications for fetal echocardiography were family history of congenital heart disease, a 2-vessel cord, maternal diabetes mellitus, or maternal exposure to teratogens. However, less than 10% of these referrals actually had congenital heart defects. In contrast, as imaging technologies have continued to improve, the most common indication for referral today is an abnormal obstetrical ultrasound evaluation, yielding congenital heart defects and abnormalities of fetal cardiovascular function in approximately half of these referrals.[6] Novel, emerging indications for fetal echocardiography include a nuchal translucency measuring greater than 3 mm between 10 and 14 weeks of gestation[7] and in vitro fertilization, particularly if the procedure includes intracytoplasmic sperm injection.[8] Table 3-2 summarizes maternal medical conditions and medication exposures with associated congenital heart lesions.

FETAL CARDIOVASCULAR IMAGING

Cross-sectional imaging remains the gold standard for the diagnosis of structural cardiac disease during fetal life. The Pediatric Council of the American Society of Echocardiography recommends obtaining multiple cross-sectional tomographic views of the heart in order to make an accurate diagnosis.[5] Curvilinear ultrasound

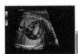

Maternal Conditions and Medication Exposures with Known Congenital Heart Disease (CHD) Associations

Maternal Medical Condition/ Medication Exposure	CHD
Diabetes	Conotruncal defects/ cardiomyopathy
Phenylketonuria	TOF, VSD, PDA, LVOTO
Autoimmune–lupus	Complete heart block
Rubella infection	PS, PDA
Lithium	Ebstein anomaly
Retinoic acid	Severe and complex CHD, conotruncal defects

LVOTO, left ventricular outflow tract obstruction; PDA, patent ductus arteriosus; PS, pulmonic stenosis; TOF, tetralogy of Fallot; VSD, ventricular septal defect.

transducers, using ultrasound frequencies between 3 and 7 MHz, allow for better image acquisition on the gravid uterus. Fetal echocardiography should include an apical 4-chamber view of the heart, an apical 5-chamber view, a long axis view of the left ventricular outflow tract, a right ventricular outflow tract view, a short axis view at the outflow tracts, a short axis view at the level of the ventricles, a long axis view of the superior and inferior vena cavae, a view of the ductal arch, and a view of the aortic arch[5] (Figure 3-2). The fetal heart rate should be documented, and any arrhythmia confirmed with M-mode imaging. The diameters of all valves should be measured in systole at right angles to the plane of flow.[5] Reference ranges for the diameters of all valves over the

course of gestation have been published.[9] Cardiac dysfunction may be assessed by cross-sectional interrogation by the presence of ascites, pleural or pericardial effusions, skin edema, and cardiomegaly, as defined by a ratio of cardiothoracic areas of greater than 0.36.[10] A cardiothoracic area ratio greater than 0.6 is associated with an extremely poor outcome.[11]

Color Doppler interrogation adds to the assessment of fetal cardiovascular well-being by establishing the degree of valvular stenosis and regurgitation, if present. Mild tricuspid regurgitation may be seen throughout gestation and is frequently a benign finding,[12,13] but tricuspid regurgitation detected during early scanning, from 11 to 14 weeks, may be a marker for aneuploidy, even in the absence of structural heart disease.[14] In contrast, regurgitation across the mitral, pulmonic, or aortic valves is usually not a normal finding and suggests pathology, secondary to underlying structural cardiac disease or fetal cardiac failure. Cardiovascular physiology can also be assessed by color Doppler echocardiography by determining the direction of blood flow. In the normal fetal circulation, the direction of shunting is right to left at both the patent foramen ovale and the ductus arteriosus. Abnormal directions of flow at these sites may suggest cardiac disease. For example, left-to-right flow at the patent foramen ovale or bidirectional shunting through the ductus arteriosus with reversal of flow in the transverse arch may indicate inadequacy of the left ventricle.[15,16]

Doppler echocardiography adds tremendous value to the assessment of the fetal cardiovascular system. Expected Doppler flow patterns for the umbilical artery, umbilical vein, middle cerebral artery, ductus venosus,

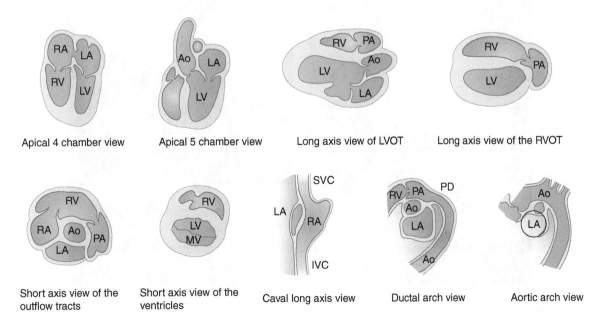

FIGURE 3-2 ■ The fetal imaging views. Ao, aorta; IVC, inferior vena cava; LA, left atrium; LV, left ventricle; MV, mitral valve; PA, pulmonary artery; PDA, patent ductus arteriosus; RA, right atrium; RV, right ventricle; SVC, superior vena cava.

atrioventricular valve inflow, and ductus arteriosus have been well described in the literature at each gestational age. In fetuses with altered hemodynamics secondary to congenital heart disease, intrauterine growth retardation, twin to twin transfusion syndrome, or significant extracardiac anomalies known to impact the fetal cardiovascular system, Doppler echocardiography may help to quantify the degree of cardiac compromise that otherwise may not be evident with 2-dimensional and color Doppler techniques alone.

Umbilical Artery and Vein

The umbilical cord, usually containing 2 arteries and 1 vein, is a vital structure linking the fetus to the placenta. The presence of a single umbilical artery may be an isolated finding or may be associated with growth retardation or chromosomal abnormalities, particularly when there are multiple congenital anomalies detected on fetal ultrasonography.[17] Pulsed wave Doppler interrogation of the umbilical cord is best performed parallel to flow within the midportion of the cord during fetal apnea. Doppler sampling within the umbilical artery reflects downstream resistance within the placenta. As discussed earlier, the resistance within the umbilical artery is generally quite low in order to promote blood flow to the placenta so that nutrients and gases may be effectively exchanged. As shown in the top left-hand panel of Figure 3-3, the Doppler flow pattern within the

umbilical artery is characterized by continuous forward flow both in systole and in diastole. In cases of intrauterine growth retardation, the diastolic velocity within the umbilical cord decreases and may even be absent—see top right-hand panel of Figure 3-3. Fetuses with diastolic flow reversal within the umbilical artery, as shown in the bottom left-hand panel of Figure 3-3, are at risk for an in utero demise.

Conversely, Doppler assessment of the umbilical vein reflects central venous pressure. As central venous pressure rises on account of heart failure, complete atrioventricular block, or severe tricuspid regurgitation, changes within the Doppler flow patterns are first seen in the inferior vena cava, then in the ductus venosus, and finally in the umbilical vein. The umbilical venous Doppler flow pattern is usually described as phasic, low-velocity flow—see the top left-hand panel of Figure 3-3. Respiratory variation may be seen if the Doppler sample is not acquired during fetal apnea. With increases in central venous pressure, notching is first seen at end-diastole. In cases of severe compromise, venous pulsations—consisting of *s*, *d*, and *a* waves, may be seen—as shown in the bottom right-hand panel of Figure 3-3.

Ductus Venosus

The ductus venosus is a key structure in fetal life that enables most of the highly oxygenated blood returning from the umbilical vein to enter the inferior vena

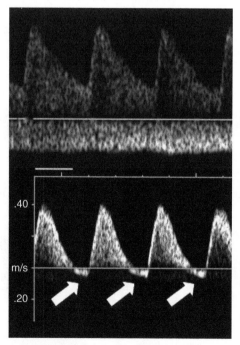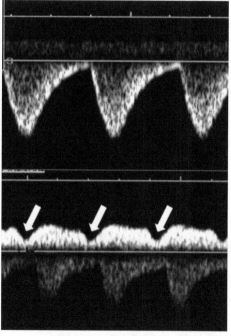

FIGURE 3-3 ■ The umbilical artery and vein Doppler tracings. The top left panel demonstrates normal umbilical artery (UA) and umbilical vein (UV) Doppler flow patterns; the top right panel demonstrates diminished diastolic flow, which returns to baseline in the UA. The bottom left panel demonstrates reversal of flow in the UA with atrial contraction, as illustrated with the arrows. The bottom right panel demonstrates venous pulsations, as illustrated with the arrows.

Normal Decreased flow with atrial contraction Reversal of flow with atrial contraction

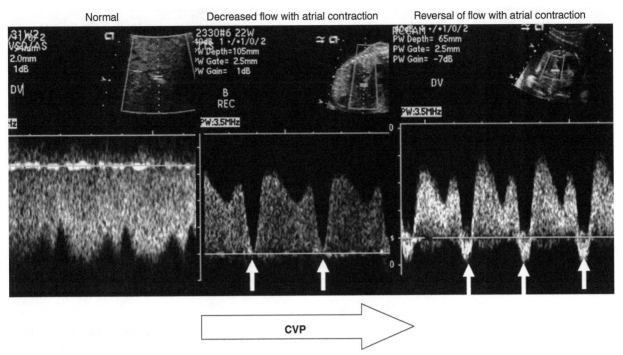

CVP

FIGURE 3-4 ■ The ductus venosus (DV) Doppler flow patterns. The left panel demonstrates the normal flow pattern. As central venous pressure (CVP) increases, flow returns to baseline with atrial contraction first, and then there is reversal of flow with atrial contraction.

cava, thereby bypassing the liver. Absence of the ductus venosus is associated with an increased incidence of fetal anomalies, including congenital heart disease, chromosomal anomalies, and fetal hydrops—especially in cases where the liver is bypassed entirely and all umbilical venous return is directed into the right atrium. Given its proximity to the heart, abnormalities in the ductus venosus Doppler flow pattern may be seen prior to any changes within the umbilical vein. The ductus venosus Doppler flow pattern is compromised of *s*, *d*, and *a* waves (Figure 3-4). After 14 weeks of gestation, flow within the ductus venosus should be all antegrade with no reversal with atrial contraction. Over the course of gestation, resistance within the ductus venosus in normal fetuses progressively declines. In fetuses with hemodynamic abnormalities associated with elevated central venous pressure, the *a*-wave velocity, corresponding to atrial contraction, decreases initially and then becomes reversed as shown in Figure 3-4. Pathologic conditions associated with *a*-wave reversal in the ductus venosus include complete atrioventricular block and severe tricuspid regurgitation, as seen in Ebstein anomaly and in the recipient twins of the twin–twin transfusion syndrome.

Middle Cerebral Artery

Doppler assessment of the middle cerebral artery provides vital information about overall fetal health as well as about the cerebrovascular resistance. Figure 3-5 demonstrates the normal Doppler flow pattern of the middle cerebral artery. Generally, most of the flow occurs during systole with only a small amount of flow in diastole. The peak systolic velocity within the middle cerebral artery increases over the course of gestation, although an elevated peak systolic velocity within the middle cerebral artery may suggest an underlying diagnosis of fetal anemia. In fetuses with normal hemodynamics, the resistance within the cerebral vasculature is greater than the placental resistance. However, in fetuses with chronic hypoxia or inadequate cardiac output, there may be "cephalization" of flow characterized by a ratio of resistance in the middle cerebral artery compared to the umbilical artery of less than 1, otherwise known as the "brain-sparing effect."

Altered flow patterns within the fetal brain have also been well described in fetuses with congenital heart disease. Compared to normal fetuses, fetuses with left-sided obstructive lesions, such as hypoplastic left heart syndrome, have decreased resistance within the middle cerebral artery, likely as a mechanism to improve flow to the fetal brain.[18] Whether this abnormal flow pattern impacts fetal brain development is an ongoing area of investigation, although abnormalities of the brain have been described in neonates with congenital heart disease even prior to any surgical palliation.[19-21] Conversely, in fetuses with increased blood flow to the fetal brain secondary to right-sided obstructive lesions, the cerebrovasculature vasoconstricts in an attempt to limit cerebral blood flow.[18] As a consequence, the resistance

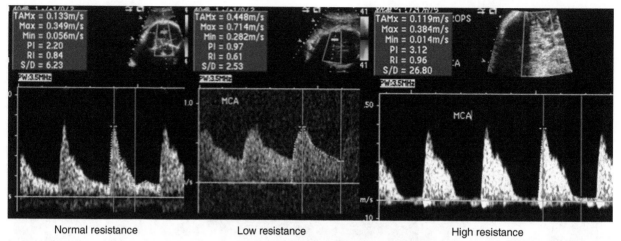

Normal resistance   Low resistance   High resistance

FIGURE 3-5 ■ The middle cerebral artery (MCA) Doppler flow patterns. The left panel demonstrates normal cerebrovascular resistance, the middle panel demonstrates low cerebrovascular resistance with increased diastolic flow, and the right panel demonstrates high cerebrovascular resistance with decreased diastolic flow.

within the middle cerebral artery is increased in these fetuses compared to normal fetuses.

Tricuspid and Mitral Inflow

As previously discussed, the fetal myocardium is comprised of greater noncontractile elements compared to the mature myocardium.[2] As a consequence of this inherent diastolic dysfunction, there is decreased passive ventricular filling and a greater percentage of ventricular filling during atrial contraction. This, in part, explains why fetuses with complete heart block may develop hydrops fetalis. Without the contribution of atrial contraction to ventricular filling, preload may become compromised, resulting in an overall decreased cardiac output.

Figure 3-6 demonstrates the normal biphasic inflow pattern in the fetus. As shown below, there is a lower E-wave velocity, representing passive ventricular filling, and a dominant *a*-wave velocity, representing active atrial contraction. The ratio of the E wave to the *a* wave increases over the course of gestation as the relaxation properties of the fetal myocardium improve. With altered ventricular compliance secondary to ventricular hypertrophy, as seen in the recipient twin of the twin–twin transfusion syndrome, or endocardial fibroelastosis, as seen in critical aortic stenosis and evolving hypoplastic left heart syndrome, the normal biphasic inflow pattern may fuse into a single peak inflow, as shown in Figure 3-6.

Ductus Arteriosus

The ductus arteriosus enables the oxygen-poor blood pumped by the right ventricle to bypass the fetal lungs and return to the placenta via the descending aorta. The

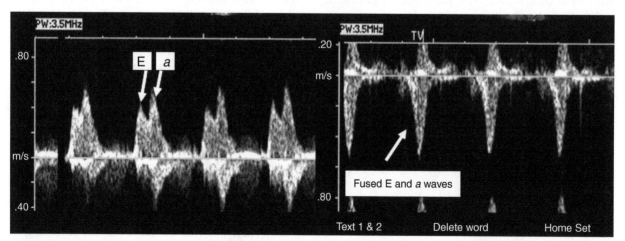

FIGURE 3-6 ■ The atrioventricular valve inflow patterns. The left panel demonstrates the normal biphasic inflow pattern characterized by a smaller E wave, representing passive ventricular filling, and a dominant *a* wave, characterized by active atrial contraction. The right panel demonstrates a monophasic inflow pattern with fusion of the E and *a* waves.

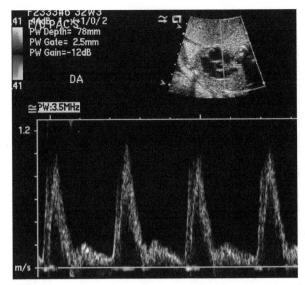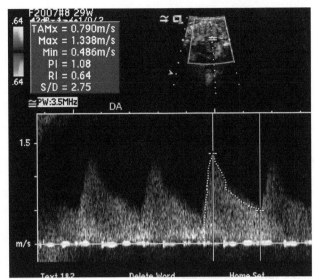

FIGURE 3-7 ■ The ductus arteriosus Doppler flow patterns. The left panel illustrates the normal Doppler flow pattern in the ductus arteriosus (DA). The right panel demonstrates a fetus with ductal constriction. Note the increased diastolic flow and the pulsatility index of less than 1.9.

Doppler flow pattern, as shown in Figure 3-7, is laminar with predominantly systolic flow and a smaller amount of diastolic flow. The ductus arteriosus should be large and unrestrictive to avoid passage through the fetal lungs, which are under high resistance during fetal life. Indeed, significant constriction of the ductus arteriosus, as shown in Figure 3-7, imposes greater afterload on the right ventricle, which can lead to right ventricular hypertrophy, tricuspid regurgitation, and ultimately, right ventricular failure and intrauterine fetal demise. Numerous medications, most notably corticosteroids, high-dose aspirin, and prostaglandin synthetase inhibitors, have been implicated as causing ductal constriction. Figure 3-7 shows the Doppler flow pattern of the ductus arteriosus in a fetus with severe ductal constriction. Closure of the ductus arteriosus in utero with evidence for right ventricular failure should prompt clinicians to strongly consider delivery of the baby to prevent an in utero fetal demise.

COMMON EXTRACARDIAC ANOMALIES AND THEIR EFFECTS ON THE FETAL CARDIOVASCULAR SYSTEM

A variety of extracardiac anomalies have the potential to negatively impact the fetal cardiovascular circulation. The fetal circulation and myocardium are inherently different from the adult cardiovascular system and have limited mechanisms to respond to hemodynamic stressors.[22] With the development of ultrasound technology, fetal echocardiography is now a vital part of the evaluation and management of the fetus with an extracardiac anomaly. The following section will review the most common extracardiac anomalies that affect the fetal cardiovascular system.

Sacrococcygeal Teratoma

Sacrococcygeal teratoma (SCT) is the most common tumor presenting in newborn humans. This highly vascularized tumor can grow very large, sometimes larger than the fetus itself. An SCT acts as an arteriovenous shunt, producing a large volume load to the fetal heart with subsequent development of high-output cardiac failure. With increasing use of prenatal ultrasound, antenatal diagnosis of SCT has dramatically increased. Fetal SCT is associated with a variable clinical pattern; a small SCT may not be detectable until after birth and have no physiologic effect on the fetus, whereas a large SCT may lead to cardiac failure, hydrops, and fetal death.[23] As the arteriovenous shunt and volume load increases, the cardiac chambers dilate, and cardiac output increases as a compensatory response (Figure 3-8). Fetal echocardiography with the use of Doppler techniques can estimate fetal cardiac outputs, which can aid in management decisions.[24-26] Normal fetal cardiac outputs are in the 425 to 550 mL/min/kg range but can be as high as 1000 mL/min/kg or greater. Our protocol for assessing fetuses with volume-loading lesions such as an SCT is shown in Table 3-3.

Congenital Cystic Adenomatoid Malformation

Space-occupying intrathoracic lesions may have significant impact on the fetal heart. Congenital cystic adenomatoid malformation (CCAM) is a benign cystic

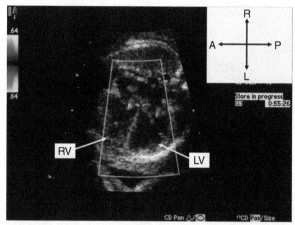

FIGURE 3-8 ■ A 4-chamber view of a fetus with a large sacrococ-cygeal teratoma in the vertex position. There is cardiomegaly, mitral and tricuspid valve regurgitation, and a small pericardial effusion. LV, left ventricle; RV, right ventricle.

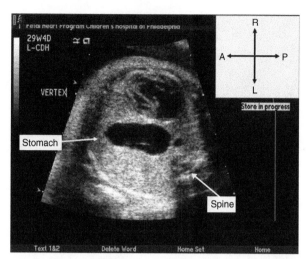

FIGURE 3-9 ■ Displaced heart into the right chest in a fetus with a left congenital diaphragmatic hernia. Left ventricular hypoplasia is also noted.

lung mass that is usually restricted to one lobe of the lung. An intrathoracic mass, such as a CCAM, has the ability to become quite large in prenatal life and may lead to cardiac compression with mediastinal shift and fetal demise.[27] When cardiac compression is significant, changes on fetal echocardiogram occur. These include hydrops, impaired filling of the heart, decreased heart size, and abnormal Doppler patterns across the mitral and tricuspid valves.[28] The natural history of a fetal CCAM is variable: Some lesions have been shown to regress, whereas others increase in size over the course of gestation.[29] Fetal resection may be performed when hydrops and significant cardiac compression are identified.[30]

Congenital Diaphragmatic Hernia

Congenital diaphragmatic hernia (CDH) is a lesion in which the diaphragm is breached and abdominal contents

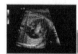

Echocardiographic Parameters in the Fetus with Sacrococcygeal Teratoma and Other Volume-Loading Conditions

▨ Evaluate for structural abnormalities
▨ Presence of hydrops (pericardial fluid, pleural effusion, ascites, scalp edema)
▨ Cardiothoracic ratio
▨ Ventricular function
▨ Combined cardiac output
▨ Atrioventricular valve regurgitation
▨ Doppler assessment of umbilical vessels, middle cerebral artery, and ductus venosus
▨ Superior and inferior vena cava dimensions

occupy the thoracic cavity. There are a number of important effects on the fetal cardiovascular system that can be seen on fetal echocardiography. The heart is often malpositioned opposite the side of the diaphragmatic hernia, most commonly into the right chest, as shown in Figure 3-9. Small branch pulmonary arteries on the side of the hernia correspond to the degree of lung hypoplasia.[31] Abnormal lung development in patients with CDH has a significant impact on morbidity and mortality and development of pulmonary hypertension.[32,33] Interestingly, there is a strong association of CDH with the presence of congenital heart disease.[34] The most common intracardiac abnormalities seen include ventricular septal defects and left-sided obstructive lesions.

Twin–Twin Transfusion Syndrome

Twin–twin transfusion syndrome (TTTS) is a disease of monochorionic twins defined sonographically by the presence of polyhydramnios of one twin (recipient twin) and oligohydramnios of the other twin (donor twin). It is reported to occur in 10% to 15% of monochorionic pregnancies.[35] Despite advances in perinatal management, TTTS still carries a high risk for significant fetal and neonatal morbidity and mortality. There is a spectrum of important cardiovascular manifestations that occurs secondary to abnormal intertwin vascular connections with a net transfusion of blood products from the donor to the recipient twin. Hypervolemia and polycythemia with subsequent polyhydramnios are seen in the recipient with cardiomyopathic changes, which follow a well-described path.[36] The cardiovascular manifestations can follow 3 typical pathways. In the first pathway, subtle cardiovascular changes (eg, right ventricular dilation and dysfunction) are observed in the recipient twin that are typically well tolerated without significant progression. In the second pathway, the recipient twin experiences progressive cardiomyopathic changes, leading to hydrops and fetal demise. The third possible pathway is an interesting manifestation in the recipient twin where there is acquired right ventricular outflow obstruction in the form of pulmonary stenosis or atresia.[37] Placental laser therapy disrupts the vascular connections between the recipient and donor and has been shown to reverse the cardiomyopathic changes in some cases.

LEFT-SIDED OBSTRUCTIVE LESIONS

Left-sided obstructive lesions (LSOLs) are a category of congenital heart defects that demonstrates inadequate development of 1 or more of the left heart structures. These include a wide variety of abnormalities that share the common features of inadequacy of the left heart to provide systemic output after birth. In this section, we will describe 3 of the more common forms of LSOLs.

Hypoplastic Left Heart Syndrome

Hypoplastic left heart syndrome (HLHS) is one of the more severe forms of congenital heart disease that the fetal cardiologist is faced with. In HLHS, there is failure of adequate development of the left heart structures, leading to stenosis or atresia of the mitral and aortic valves with varying degrees of hypoplasia of the left ventricular cavity (Figure 3-10). Fetal echocardiography is extremely sensitive in diagnosing HLHS syndrome and other single-ventricle defects. Once the diagnosis has been established, it is important to identify the presence of other intracardiac abnormalities such as

tricuspid regurgitation or right ventricular dysfunction because these significantly affect outcomes.[38] Fetuses with HLHS are followed closely throughout pregnancy with serial echocardiography to detect progression of any tricuspid regurgitation, assess ventricular function, and rule out development of a restrictive atrial septal defect. Diagnosis is commonly made at 18 to 22 weeks after an abnormal obstetrical ultrasound leads to a referral to a pediatric cardiologist. Early fetal imaging can allow for a diagnosis of HLHS as early as 12 weeks of gestation. Expecting families are counseled on the details of the anatomy and the plan for surgical palliation that includes 3 procedures leading to the Fontan procedure at the age of 2 to 3 years. Recommendations are made for delivery at a tertiary medical center with an obstetrical, neonatal, and cardiology team experienced with postnatal care of these complex patients. Prostaglandin infusion is initiated after birth, and the initial surgical procedure is typically performed within the first few days of life.

Coarctation of the Aorta

Coarctation of the aorta (CoA) describes narrowing of the lumen of the aortic arch. CoA can occur in isolation or in the setting of more complex cardiac lesions and is commonly associated with other left-sided lesions such as anomalies of the mitral and aortic valve. CoA can be challenging to diagnose in the fetus for multiple reasons. The fetal circulation is unique with 2 fetal arches, the smaller aortic arch and the larger ductal arch. Insertion of the ductal arch occurs at the point that is often narrowed in coarctation of the aorta, potentially masking the presence of an abnormality. Moreover, there are situations in which maternal acoustic windows and fetal position make it difficult to obtain definitive images

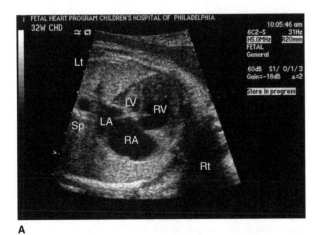
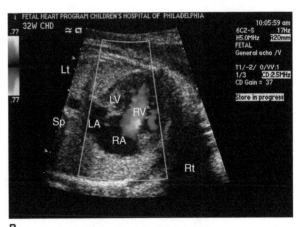

FIGURE 3-10 ■ Four-chamber view of hypoplastic left heart syndrome. Note the small left ventricle (LV) cavity on 2-dimensional imaging **(B).** There is absence of color flow filling the small left ventricle on color flow imaging **(B).** LA, left atrium; RA, right atrium; RV, right ventricle. Lt, left; Rt, right; Sp, spine.

of the aortic arch. Therefore, indirect signs of a CoA, such as discrepant ventricular and great artery size with larger right than left heart structures, are often used as a surrogate markers for LSOLs.[39] Direct measurements of the fetal aortic arch are the most specific markers for predicting postnatal obstruction when clear images can be obtained.[40] There is a known association with Turner XO syndrome, in which 35% of patients are affected, and a documented familial recurrence, suggesting a genetic substrate. Amniocentesis is often recommended to families.

The fetus tolerates narrowing of the aortic arch well as the large ductus arteriosus allows flow around any narrowed region providing unobstructed cardiac output to the body. There is usually normal growth and development with the fetus reaching term. In fetuses that are predicted to have postnatal arch obstruction, a planned delivery at a tertiary referral center with neonatal and cardiology specialists is recommended. This allows for a controlled delivery and transfer of the neonate to the intensive care unit for assessment of clinical status, initiation of prostaglandin infusion, and confirmation of the diagnosis by transthoracic echocardiography.

RIGHT-SIDED OBSTRUCTIVE LESIONS

Right-sided obstructive lesions (RSOLs) result in a spectrum of congenital heart defects that range from adequate to ductal-dependent pulmonary blood flow after birth. In many cases, the right ventricle is adequate, resulting in a 2-ventricle repair, whereas in some cases, the right ventricle is inadequate to support optimal pulmonary blood flow, resulting in single-ventricle palliation. In this section, we describe 4 of the more common forms of RSOLs.

Pulmonic Stenosis

Pulmonic stenosis (PS) typically is identified as a result of the pulmonary artery appearing smaller than the aorta. As described earlier, the pulmonary artery is approximately 20% larger than the aorta in utero. When the pulmonary artery appears smaller, it raises suspicion of right-sided disease. An important aspect of the fetal echocardiographic evaluation is whether these patients have critical PS with ductal-dependent pulmonary blood flow requiring prostaglandins at birth. The size of the pulmonary artery in relation to the aorta and the direction of the ductal flow in utero are 2 fetal parameters that are used to determine whether the patient will require prostaglandins postnatally. Prenatally, if the pulmonary artery is less than 50% of the aorta and the ductal flow is left to right (aorta to pulmonary artery),

parents are counseled that their baby will require prostaglandins at birth and will require a neonatal intervention, most likely balloon dilation of the pulmonary valve in the cardiac catheterization lab. When isolated critical PS is identified, additional ultrasound screening for extracardiac anomalies and genetic testing for Noonan syndrome are recommended. In TTTS, approximately 5% to 10% of the cases are complicated by development of RSOLs in the recipient twin. The recipient fetus may have only mild acceleration and/or narrowing of the pulmonary valve or may develop pulmonary atresia. Fetuses with a pulmonary artery size greater than 50% of the aorta and normal right to left ductal flow require cardiac evaluation after birth.

Tetralogy of Fallot

Fetal echocardiographic diagnosis of tetralogy of Fallot (TOF) involves identification of a pulmonary artery size smaller than the aorta, a ventricular septal defect (VSD), and an aorta that overrides the ventricular septum. Once TOF is diagnosed, the fetus is followed prenatally to monitor for indicators for ductal dependency after birth. As described for isolated PS, fetuses with a pulmonary artery measuring less than 50% of the size of the aorta with left-to-right flow in the duct will require prostaglandins at birth. Expectant parents are counseled that their child will likely require palliation with a Blalock-Taussig shunt or a complete TOF repair in the neonatal period. Neonatal palliation versus repair is determined after a postnatal echocardiographic evaluation for anatomic variants. Neonates identified with a coronary artery crossing the right ventricular outflow tract will require a Blalock-Taussig shunt during the neonatal period with delayed full repair due to need for placement of a right ventricle to pulmonary artery conduit. In most cases of TOF with ductal-dependent PS or pulmonary atresia, the neonate undergoes a full repair including VSD closure and a right ventricular outflow tract patch or a right ventricle to pulmonary artery conduit. In cases of mild to moderate PS that are not ductal dependent, elective repair takes place at 3 to 4 months of age. Because there is a high association of the 22q11 deletion with TOF, amniocentesis is highly recommended.[41]

Pulmonary Atresia with Intact Ventricular Septum

Pulmonary atresia with intact ventricular septum (PA/IVS) involves a spectrum of right ventricle (RV) lesions that, depending on the adequacy of the RV, lead to either single-ventricle or 2-ventricle repair (Figure 3-11). The fetal tricuspid valve (TV) z-score has been used as a predictor of RV adequacy, with a TV z-score of less than −3.5 identified as a predictor of RV hypoplasia.[42,43] In fetuses

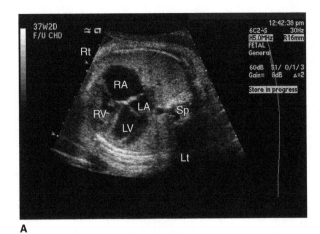
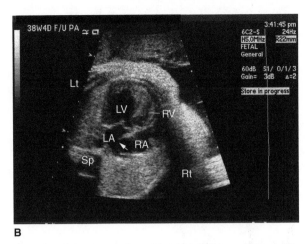

FIGURE 3-11 ■ The appearance of the ventricles in pulmonary atresia with intact ventricular septum. In panel **A**, there is a good-sized right ventricle (RV) and only mild hypoplasia of the tricuspid valve. The ventricle is hypertrophied, yet is likely suitable for a 2-ventricle repair strategy. In panel **B**, the RV is very hypoplastic. Note the bowing of the atrial septum from the right atrium (RA) into the left atrium (LA; arrow). Lt, left; LV, left ventricle; Rt, right; Sp, spine.

with TV z-score of −2.5 to −3.5, identification of tricuspid regurgitation is also important because RV coronary sinusoids and potential RV coronary cameral fistulae are not associated with borderline RVs with significant tricuspid regurgitation. Whether there is an adequate or inadequate RV, the neonate will require prostaglandins at birth. Adequacy of the RV is confirmed with a postnatal echocardiogram. Neonates with PA/IVS with an adequate RV undergo cardiac catheterization with radiofrequency perforation and balloon dilation of the pulmonary valve. After the intervention, prostaglandin is discontinued, and the neonate is observed for adequacy of pulmonary blood flow. In some patients, as a result of severe RV hypertrophy, there is inadequate antegrade pulmonary blood flow. These neonates require an additional procedure during the neonatal period to augment pulmonary blood flow either via ductal stenting or a Blalock-Taussig shunt. In cases where the RV is suspected to be inadequate or there is a suspicion of RV-dependant coronaries, expectant parents are counseled about a 3-stage palliation pathway culminating in a Fontan. As mentioned previously, the neonate would require prostaglandin with subsequent placement of a Blalock-Taussig shunt. The second stage of palliation, a bidirectional Glenn, takes place at 4 to 6 months of age, culminating with a Fontan at 2 to 3 years of age.

Tricuspid Atresia/VSD

Tricuspid atresia with a VSD is a rare lesion involving hypoplasia of the TV and RV. Assessment of the size of the branch pulmonary arteries, size of the VSD, and the direction of flow in the ductus is important in determining whether the fetus will need an intervention in the neonatal period. Fetuses with good size pulmonary arteries, an adequate size VSD, and right to left flow across the duct typically do not need prostaglandins and may or may not need a pulmonary band due to excessive pulmonary blood flow. Patients in whom the VSD appears inadequate as determined by left to right shunting at the ductus will need prostaglandins at birth and will likely need a neonatal Blalock-Taussig shunt to provide pulmonary blood flow. The second stage of palliation, a bidirectional Glenn, takes place at 4 to 6 months of age, culminating with a Fontan at 2 to 3 years of age.

DEXTRO-TRANSPOSITION OF THE GREAT ARTERIES

Dextro-transposition of the great arteries (d-TGA) is one of the most commonly missed prenatal diagnoses because the 4-chamber view will appear completely normal on a 20-week anatomic scan. Further evaluation for crossing of the outflow tracts (Figure 3-12) will result in the recognition of d-TGA. Currently, American Congress of Obstetricians and Gynecologists guidelines for ultrasonography in pregnancy state that a basic cardiac examination includes a 4-chamber view of the heart and, as part of the cardiac screening examination, an attempt should be made, if technically feasible, to view the outflow tracts.[44] As a result, it is not uncommon for neonates to be diagnosed postnatally with d-TGA.

d-TGA is a cyanotic lesion that is due to incomplete rotation of the outflow tracts during embryologic development, resulting in the aorta arising from the RV and the pulmonary artery arising from the left ventricle. In utero, the cerebral vasculature is perfused with "bluer" blood, while the oxygenated blood is pumped through the pulmonary artery, across the ductus arteriosus toward the

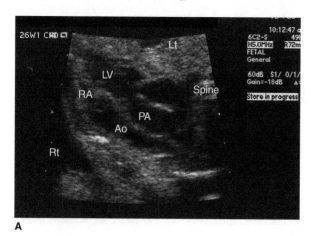
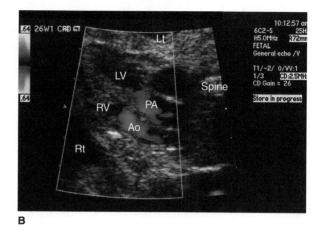

FIGURE 3-12 ■ Dextro-transposition of the great arteries. Both great vessels arise from the heart in parallel and do not cross. **(A)** Two-dimensional image. **(B)** Color flow image. Ao, aorta; Lt, left; LV, left ventricle; PA, pulmonary artery; Rt, right; RV, right ventricle.

placenta. Increasing data suggest that this aberrant circulation impacts brain development. Fetuses with d-TGA have a lower middle cerebral artery pulsatility index compared to normal fetuses, consistent with the "brain-sparing" response of cerebral autoregulation leading to increased blood flow to the brain.[18,45] Although there is a compensatory "brain-sparing" response in utero, there is likely a threshold that, once reached, results in altered brain growth and development. Delayed fetal brain maturation and development in utero is consistent with postnatal data demonstrating smaller head circumferences and structurally immature brains in term gestation neonates with d-TGA compared to normal term neonates.[20] Research is ongoing to understand the impact that altered brain development has on risk for white matter brain injury during the preoperative and postoperative period and the relation of these findings to long-term neurodevelopmental outcome.

Fetal diagnosis of d-TGA allows for planning, so if the atrial communication is deemed inadequate, the cardiac catheterization team will be ready. Inadequacy of the atrial communication can lead to profound cyanosis with severe hypoxia requiring an urgent need for balloon atrial septostomy to provide optimal mixing of deoxygenated and oxygenated blood. Lower average daily partial pressure of oxygen in arterial blood (PaO_2) and time to surgery are risk factors for white matter brain injury in neonates with d-TGA.[46] Therefore, it is important to recognize that even in neonates with a VSD who are on prostaglandin, there may not be optimal PaO_2 levels reaching the brain, and these patients may benefit from a balloon atrial septostomy while awaiting surgical repair. In either case, the neonate undergoes an arterial switch operation within a few days of age. Overall, operative mortality is low after the arterial switch operation, and these children have a relatively normal quality of life with good exercise capacity and normal IQ, although

approximately 50% of these children will have behavioral problems such as attention-deficit hyperactivity disorder and/or mild learning disabilities.

FETAL ARRHYTHMIA

Abnormalities of cardiac rhythm are quite common in the human fetus and most commonly present with an abnormally slow, fast, or irregular heart rate. These abnormalities can be detected on fetal heart tone auscultation at routine prenatal visits. Fetal arrhythmia may also present secondary to its adverse effects on the fetus that can lead to nonimmune hydrops and even fetal demise. Normal fetal heart rate ranges from approximately 120 to 180 beats per minute (bpm). Normal variations occur with fetal activity and are a sign of well-being. It is generally accepted that 1% to 3% of pregnancies manifest some disturbance of cardiac rhythm, with the majority being transient and benign and with about 10% being regarded as life threatening.

Electrocardiography is difficult in the fetus because electrical signals are weak due to the distance to the maternal abdomen surface as well as interference from maternal signals. The mainstay of diagnosis for fetal arrhythmia remains the 2-dimensional, transabdominal echocardiogram. This allows for observation of the mechanical movements caused by the electrical signals, namely contraction of the atria and ventricles and blood flow patterns within the heart. Within this modality, M-mode or pulsed wave Doppler measurements taken via a sample volume encompassing both atrial and ventricular tissue allow for accurate assessment of cardiac rhythm. Arrhythmias in the fetus can be classified as follows: atrial and ventricular extrasystoles (premature atrial contractions and premature ventricular contractions), supraventricular tachycardias, ventricular tachycardias, and disturbances of atrioventricular conduction.

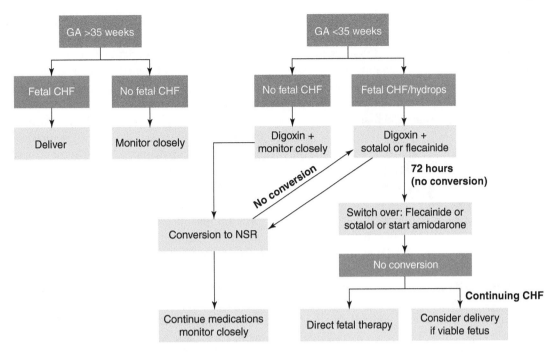

FIGURE 3-13 ■ Management algorithm for fetal supraventricular tachycardia. CHF, congestive heart failure; GA, gestational age; NSR, normal sinus rhythm.

Premature atrial contractions are the most common arrhythmia seen in the fetus. In general, premature atrial contractions are benign and in isolation are not associated with underlying disease. However, frequent premature atrial contractions may herald the development of sustained tachyarrhythmia. Supraventricular tachycardia (SVT) is the most common fetal arrhythmia having the potential for deleterious effects on fetal well-being. SVT typically presents with fetal heart rates of 220 to 280 bpm with 1:1 motion of the atria and ventricles. Close observation is warranted for fetuses with tachycardia who are near term, have intermittent (ie, less than the duration of the ultrasound scan) bouts of tachycardia, and display no signs of hydrops. Delivery of the premature infant with signs of compromise secondary to SVT is best limited to the near-term infant in a center with a multidisciplinary team approach to the critically ill premature infant.

The most commonly used drugs for fetal atrial tachycardia include digoxin, sotalol, flecainide, and amiodarone and are successful in most cases. Most antiarrhythmic drugs are well tolerated in the pregnant patient; however, closer monitoring for the proarrhythmic effects of certain drugs should be used due to the physiologic changes in cardiac output and first-pass hepatic metabolism during pregnancy. Digoxin is the most frequently used agent with the longest described experience in its use. Digoxin may be administered to the mother orally or intravenously or via direct intramuscular or intraumbilical therapy

to the fetus. A management algorithm from our institution is shown in Figure 3-13.

Congenital complete heart block (CCHB) is a rare disorder of atrioventricular conduction affecting approximately 1 in 20,000 newborns. The hallmark of CCHB is atrioventricular dissociation, in which atrial impulses are not conducted to the ventricles and have no relationship to the slower ventricular rhythm. Cardiac output is thus dependent on the intrinsic ventricular "escape" rhythm, the rate of which may be as low as 30 to 40 bpm. The bradycardia associated with CCHB is easily detected on routine auscultation and is confirmed by routine echocardiography. Fetal echocardiography can measure a mechanical PR interval (the time from atrial contraction to aortic outflow), which can provide important information about delay of conduction at the atrioventricular node. This time interval should be less than 130 ms in the fetus.

CCHB typically presents in association with either immunologic evidence of maternal connective disease or fetal structural congenital heart disease. Together, these account for approximately 90% of presentations; the remaining approximately 10% are regarded as being "idiopathic" CCHB. CCHB is a well-known manifestation of neonatal lupus, an autoimmune disease mediated by the transplacental transfer of the maternal autoantibodies anti-Ro (anti-SSA) and anti-La (anti-SSB) during gestation. The prevailing theory is that these antibodies have a particular predilection for the conduction tissue within the atrioventricular node and Purkinje fibers. The incidence of CCHB in mothers positive for anti-Ro or anti-La is quite low (approximately 1%-2%). Pharmacologic management of CCHB, once diagnosed, is based on reversal of immune-mediated damage to the atrioventricular conduction system and increasing fetal cardiac output via augmentation of the fetal heart rate. The mainstay of such therapy thus far has been maternal administration of dexamethasone and β-agonists.

CONGENITAL HEART DISEASE AND GENETIC/CHROMOSOMAL DEFECTS

Many genetic or chromosomal abnormalities have been associated with congenital heart lesions. Table 3-4 summarizes congenital heart disease (CHD) with associated syndromes or genetic defects and extracardiac manifestations.[47] When CHD is diagnosed, amniocentesis is recommended to rule out potential chromosomal and genetic abnormalities. When additional extracardiac anomalies are identified, as noted in Table 3-4, there should be a high index of suspicion for associated syndromes. Typically, amniocentesis provides karyotype screening for trisomy 13, 18, and 21 and Turner syndrome (XO). Improvement in laboratory assays has provided the ability to screen for additional genetic syndromes in utero. If a conotruncal defect such as TOF or truncus is identified, additional testing for 22q11 deletion is performed most commonly by fluorescein in situ hybridization. As cost and availability improve, DNA microarray testing will allow more sensitive

detection for microdeletions in 22q11 along with more specific gene testing for syndromes associated with CHD such as Alagille and Noonan syndromes.[47-51]

Availability of genetic testing results allows the fetal cardiologist to incorporate this information during counseling, discussing how these syndromes impact the overall outcome of infants and children with CHD. In pregnancies at less than 24 weeks of gestation, this information provides parents the ability to make an educated decision about continuing the pregnancy. In addition, knowledge of associated genetic defects/syndromes allows physicians caring for these neonates in the intensive care unit to provide optimal care. Neonates with 22q11 deletion have DiGeorge syndrome or velocardiofacial syndrome that is associated with hypocalcemia and T-cell immunologic problems. Although the immunologic issues are typically not a neonatal problem, the risk for hypocalcemia is significant, resulting in increased calcium requirements during intensive care management. These patients are at risk for neurodevelopmental abnormalities during childhood and for schizophrenia in adulthood.[41] In the case of Alagille syndrome, awareness of the associated problem of bile duct cholestasis, which requires a Kasai procedure and has a high risk of liver failure associated with it, is important information for parents to understand.[47,48] In addition, knowledge of these potential abnormalities allows for postnatal observation and evaluation. For instance, infants and children with Alagille syndrome may require numerous interventions in the cardiac catheterization lab for periperal PS.

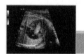

CHD Defects with Commonly Associated Genetic or Chromosomal Abnormalities

CHD Defect	Chromosome/ Genetic Defect	Syndrome	Extracardiac Findings
Conotruncal: TOF/ truncus	22q11 deletion	DiGeorge/VCF	Cleft palate, hypocalcemia, immunologic/T-cell dysfunction, feeding/speech issues, neurodevelopmental issues, schizophrenia
PPS	*JAG-1*	Alagille	Bile duct paucity, butterfly vertebrae
Coarctation/LSOL	*XO*	Turner	Cervical cystic hygroma, lymphedema/pedal edema, IUGR, horseshoe kidney, infertility, variable mental and developmental problems
PS/ cardiomyopathy	*PTPN11, KRAS, SO1*	Noonan	Posterior nuchal cystic hygroma, polyhydramnios, special facial features (low-set ears, depressed nasal bridge, large head)
AV canal defect	T21	Down	Increased NT, macroglossia, hypoplastic fifth metacarpal, duodenal atresia
VSD, PS	T18	Edward	IUGR, clinodactyly, rocker bottom feet, esophageal atresia
VSD	T13	Ptau	Holoprosencephaly, cleft lip/palate
Interrupted IVC		Heterotaxy syndrome	Biliary atresia, polysplenia, gut malrotation
ASD	*TBX5*	Holt-Oram	Upper limb abnormalities, absence of thumb, club hand

ASD, atrial septal defect; AV, atrioventricular; CHD, congenital heart disease; IUGR, intrauterine growth restriction; IVC, inferior vena cava; LSOL, left-sided obstructive lesion; NT, nuchal translucency; PPS, peripheral pulmonic stenosis; PS, pulmonic stenosis; TOF, tetralogy of Fallot; VCF, velocardiofacial syndrome; VSD, ventricular septal defect.

Clinical Pearls

■ Screening fetal echocardiograms are typically performed between 18 and 22 weeks of gestation.

■ Multiple cross-sectional tomographic views of the heart, including outflow tract views and arch views, are required for accurate diagnosis of congenital heart disease in the fetus.

■ Absence of flow or reversal of flow in the umbilical artery in diastole is abnormal, indicative of elevated placental resistance.

■ Venous pulsations in the umbilical vein and reversal of flow with atrial contraction in the ductus venosus are abnormal and correspond to elevated central venous pressure.

■ Significant constriction of the ductus arteriosus secondary to corticosteroids, high-dose aspirin, or prostaglandin synthetase inhibitors may cause right heart failure and prompt early delivery of the fetus.

■ Extracardiac anomalies, such as a sacrococcygeal teratoma, congenital cystic adenomatoid malformation, and congenital diaphragmatic hernia, may have a significant negative impact on the fetal cardiovascular system.

■ Complicating 10% to 15% of monochorionic pregnancies, the twin–twin transfusion syndrome is characterized by abnormal intertwin vascular connections, which can lead to a spectrum of cardiovascular abnormalities.

■ Serial assessment of congenital heart disease over the course of gestation is important to evaluate for progression of disease, which may impact the timing or mode of delivery.

■ In left-sided obstructive lesions, reversal of flow at the patent foramen ovale or at the transverse arch is a marker for possible inadequacy of the left-sided structures.

■ In hypoplastic left heart syndrome, right ventricular dysfunction, restriction at the atrial septal defect, severe tricuspid regurgitation, prematurity, extracardiac abnormality, and genetic abnormalities are associated with worse perinatal outcomes.

■ In right-sided obstructive lesions, reversal of flow at the ductus arteriosus and a pulmonary annulus less than 50% of the aortic annulus are prenatal markers suggestive of ductal-dependent pulmonary blood flow, which will likely require neonatal intervention.

■ In dextro-transposition of the great arteries, one of the most commonly missed diagnoses prenatally, the outflow tracts are arranged in parallel and do not cross.

■ Fetal arrhythmia is usually diagnosed with M-mode or pulsed wave Doppler measurements taken with a sample volume encompassing both the atria and the ventricles.

■ Fetal supraventricular tachycardia, which usually presents with fetal heart rates ranging from 220 to 280 beats per minute with 1:1 atrioventricular conduction, may be treated with digoxin, sotalol, flecainide, or amiodarone.

■ Congenital complete heart block secondary to maternal autoimmune disease can be treated with dexamethasone and β-agonists if the fetal heart rate is less than 55 beats per minute.

■ Amniocentesis should be offered when congenital heart disease is diagnosed, particularly if extracardiac abnormalities are also present, due to the high prevalence of genetic or chromosomal abnormalities.

Knowledge of the potential extracardiac abnormalities and/or addition of a genetic defect can greatly impact future quality of life. Therefore, it is important to incorporate this information into counseling.

In HLHS, identification of a genetic defect has been identified as a risk factor for poorer outcome.[38] Preterm delivery, extracardiac abnormalities, genetic defects, and cardiac findings of tricuspid regurgitation, impaired RV function, and atrial restriction are all factors that impact stage I survival. Therefore, having this information available is important because it has a significant influence on overall outcome.

REFERENCES

1. Mielke G, Benda N. Cardiac output and central distribution of blood flow in the human fetus. *Circulation.* 2001;103:1662-1668.

2. Friedman WF. The intrinsic physiologic properties of the developing heart. *Prog Cardiovasc Dis.* 1972;15:87-111.

3. Mahony L. Calcium homeostasis and control of contractility in the developing heart. *Semin Perinatol.* 1996;20:510-519.

4. Johnson P, Sharland G, Maxwell D, Allan L. The role of transvaginal sonography in the early detection of congenital heart disease. *Ultrasound Obstet Gynecol.* 1992;2:248-251.

5. Rychik J, Ayres N, Cuneo B, et al. American Society of Echocardiography guidelines and standards for performance of the fetal echocardiogram. *J Am Soc Echocardiogr.* 2004;17:803-810.

6. Friedberg MK, Silverman NH. Changing indications for fetal echocardiography in a University Center population. *Prenat Diagn.* 2004;24:781-786.

7. Ghi T, Huggon IC, Zosmer N, Nicolaides KH. Incidence of major structural cardiac defects associated with increased nuchal translucency but normal karyotype. *Ultrasound Obstet Gynecol.* 2001;18:610-614.

8. Hansen M, Kurinczuk JJ, Bower C, Webb S. The risk of major birth defects after intracytoplasmic sperm injection and in vitro fertilization. *N Engl J Med.* 2002;346:725-730.

9. Sharland GK, Allan LD. Normal fetal cardiac measurements derived by cross-sectional echocardiography. *Ultrasound Obstet Gynecol.* 1992;2:175-181.

10. Hofstaetter C, Hansmann M, Eik-Nes SH, Huhta JC, Luther SL. A cardiovascular profile score in the surveillance of fetal hydrops. *J Matern Fetal Neonatal Med.* 2006;19:407-413.

11. Chaoui R, Bollmann R, Goldner B, Heling KS, Tennstedt C. Fetal cardiomegaly: echocardiographic findings and outcome in 19 cases. *Fetal Diagn Ther.* 1994;9:92-104.

12. Messing B, Porat S, Imbar T, Valsky DV, Anteby EY, Yagel S. Mild tricuspid regurgitation: a benign fetal finding at various stages of pregnancy. *Ultrasound Obstet Gynecol.* 2005;26:606-609.

13. Gembruch U, Smrcek JM. The prevalence and clinical significance of tricuspid valve regurgitation in normally grown fetuses and those with intrauterine growth retardation. *Ultrasound Obstet Gynecol.* 1997;9:374-382.

14. Huggon IC, DeFigueiredo DB, Allan LD. Tricuspid regurgitation in the diagnosis of chromosomal anomalies in the fetus at 11-14 weeks of gestation. *Heart.* 2003;89:1071-1073.

15. Berning RA, Silverman NH, Villegas M, Sahn DJ, Martin GR, Rice MJ. Reversed shunting across the ductus arteriosus or atrial septum in utero heralds severe congenital heart disease. *J Am Coll Cardiol.* 1996;27:481-486.

16. Makikallio K, McElhinney DB, Levine JC, et al. Fetal aortic valve stenosis and the evolution of hypoplastic left heart syndrome: patient selection for fetal intervention. *Circulation.* 2006;113:1401-1405.

17. Prucka S, Clemens M, Craven C, McPherson E. Single umbilical artery: what does it mean for the fetus? A case-control analysis of pathologically ascertained cases. *Genet Med.* 2004;6:54-57.

18. Kaltman JR, Di H, Tian Z, Rychik J. Impact of congenital heart disease on cerebrovascular blood flow dynamics in the fetus. *Ultrasound Obstet Gynecol.* 2005;25:32-36.

19. Miller SP, McQuillen PS, Hamrick S, et al. Abnormal brain development in newborns with congenital heart disease. *N Engl J Med.* 2007;357:1928-1938.

20. Licht DJ, Shera DM, Clancy RR, et al. Brain maturation is delayed in infants with complex congenital heart defects. *J Thorac Cardiovasc Surg.* 2009;137:529-536.

21. Licht DJ, Wang J, Silvestre DW, et al. Preoperative cerebral blood flow is diminished in neonates with severe congenital heart defects. *J Thorac Cardiovasc Surg.* 2004;128: 841-849.

22. Rudolph AM. The fetal circulation and its response to stress. *J Dev Physiol.* 1984;6:11-19.

23. Flake AW, Harrison MR, Adzick NS, Laberge JM, Warsof SL. Fetal sacrococcygeal teratoma. *J Pediatr Surg.* 1986;21:563-566.

24. Silverman NH, Schmidt KG. Ventricular volume overload in the human fetus: observations from fetal echocardiography. *J Am Soc Echocardiogr.* 1990;3:20-29.

25. Schmidt KG, Silverman NH, Harison MR, Callen PW. High-output cardiac failure in fetuses with large sacrococcygeal teratoma: diagnosis by echocardiography and Doppler ultrasound. *J Pediatr.* 1989;114:1023-1028.

26. De Smedt MC, Visser GH, Meijboom EJ. Fetal cardiac output estimated by Doppler echocardiography during mid- and late gestation. *Am J Cardiol.* 1987;60:338-342.

27. Adzick NS, Flake AW, Crombleholme TM. Management of congenital lung lesions. *Semin Pediatr Surg.* 2003;12:10-16.

28. Mahle WT, Rychik J, Tian ZY, et al. Echocardiographic evaluation of the fetus with congenital cystic adenomatoid malformation. *Ultrasound Obstet Gynecol.* 2000;16:620-624.

29. Winters WD, Effmann EL, Nghiem HV, Nyberg DA. Disappearing fetal lung masses: importance of postnatal imaging studies. *Pediatr Radiol.* 1997;27:535-539.

30. Adzick NS. Open fetal surgery for life-threatening fetal anomalies. *Semin Fetal Neonatal Med.* 2009;15:1-8.

31. Sokol J, Bohn D, Lacro RV, et al. Fetal pulmonary artery diameters and their association with lung hypoplasia and postnatal outcome in congenital diaphragmatic hernia. *Am J Obstet Gynecol.* 2002;186:1085-1090.

32. Geggel RL, Murphy JD, Langleben D, Crone RK, Vacanti JP, Reid LM. Congenital diaphragmatic hernia: arterial structural changes and persistent pulmonary hypertension after surgical repair. *J Pediatr.* 1985;107:457-464.

33. Katz AL, Wiswell TE, Baumgart S. Contemporary controversies in the management of congenital diaphragmatic hernia. *Clin Perinatol.* 1998;25:219-248.

34. Cohen MS, Rychik J, Bush DM, et al. Influence of congenital heart disease on survival in children with congenital diaphragmatic hernia. *J Pediatr.* 2002;141:25-30.

35. Danskin FH, Neilson JP. Twin-to-twin transfusion syndrome: what are appropriate diagnostic criteria? *Am J Obstet Gynecol.* 1989;161:365-369.

36. Rychik J, Tian Z, Bebbington M, et al. The twin-twin transfusion syndrome: spectrum of cardiovascular abnormality and development of a cardiovascular score to assess severity of disease. *Am J Obstet Gynecol.* 2007;197:392.e1-8.

37. Lougheed J, Sinclair BG, Fung Kee Fung K, et al. Acquired right ventricular outflow tract obstruction in the recipient twin in twin-twin transfusion syndrome. *J Am Coll Cardiol.* 2001;38:1533-538.

38. Rychik J, Szwast A, Natarajan S, et al. Perinatal and early surgical outcome for the fetus with hypoplastic left heart syndrome: a 5-year single institutional experience. *Ultrasound Obstet Gynecol.* 2010;36:465-470.

39. Quartermain MD, Cohen MS, Dominguez TE, Tian Z, Donaghue DD, Rychik J. Left ventricle to right ventricle size discrepancy in the fetus: the presence of critical congenital heart disease can be reliably predicted. *J Am Soc Echocardiogr.* 2009;22:1296-1301.

40. Pasquini L, Mellander M, Seale A, et al. Z-scores of the fetal aortic isthmus and duct: an aid to assessing arch hypoplasia. *Ultrasound Obstet Gynecol.* 2007;29:628-633.

41. McDonald-McGinn DM, Sullivan KE. Chromosome 22q11.2 deletion syndrome (DiGeorge syndrome/velocardiofacial syndrome). *Medicine (Baltimore).* 2011;90:1-18.

42. Salvin JW, McElhinney DB, Colan SD, et al. Fetal tricuspid valve size and growth as predictors of outcome in pulmonary atresia with intact ventricular septum. *Pediatrics.* 2006;118:e415-e420.

43. Peterson RE, Levi DS, Williams RJ, Lai WW, Sklansky MS, Drant S. Echocardiographic predictors of outcome in fetuses with pulmonary atresia with intact ventricular septum. *J Am Soc Echocardiogr.* 2006;19:1393-1400.

44. American College of Obstetricians and Gynecologists. ACOG Practice Bulletin No. 101: ultrasonography in pregnancy. *Obstet Gynecol.* 2009;113:451-461.

45. Jouannic JM, Benachi A, Bonnet D, et al. Middle cerebral artery Doppler in fetuses with transposition of the great arteries. *Ultrasound Obstet Gynecol.* 2002;20:122-144.

46. Petit CJ, Rome JJ, Wernovsky G, et al. Preoperative brain injury in transposition of the great arteries is associated with oxygenation and time to surgery, not balloon atrial septostomy. *Circulation.* 2009;119:709-716.

47. Callen PW, ed. *Ultrasonography in Obstetrics and Gynecology.* Philadelphia, PA: Saunders Elsevier; 2008.

48. Alessandro G, Incerti M, Andreani M. Alagille syndrome: prenatal sonographic findings. *J Clin Ultrasound.* 2007;35:156-158.

49. Lee KA, Williams B, Roza K, et al. PTPN11 analysis for the prenatal diagnosis of Noonan syndrome in fetuses with abnormal ultrasound findings. *Clin Genet.* 2009;75:190-194.

50. Sahoo T, Cheung SW, Ward P, et al. Prenatal diagnosis of chromosomal abnormalities using array-based comparative genomic hybridization. *Genet Med.* 2006;8:719-727.

51. Van den Veyver IB, Patel A, Shaw CA, et al. Clinical use of array comparative genomic hybridization (aCGH) for prenatal diagnosis in 300 cases. *Prenat Diagn.* 2009;29:29-39.

CHAPTER 4

The Genetics of Abnormal Cardiac Development

Lisa C.A. D'Alessandro,
Shabnam Peyvandi*,
Susan Schachtner and
Elizabeth Goldmuntz*

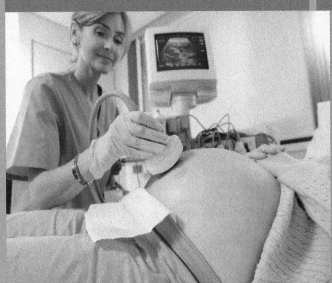

INTRODUCTION

Congenital heart disease (CHD) is the most common major birth defect, and yet its etiology remains poorly understood. It is generally accepted that both genetic and environmental factors contribute to abnormal cardiac development. With rapid advances in the field of genetics, specific gene alterations underlying named syndromes or groups of cardiac malformations continue to be identified. Our understanding of both positive and negative environmental influences also continues to evolve. Identifying the etiology of cardiac malformations is important, as environmental changes can aid normal development and information on inheritance patterns and recurrence rates aids early identification of at-risk individuals and informs future plans for individuals and families.

In this chapter, we briefly summarize the current knowledge of environmental and genetic causes of CHD.[1,2,3] A brief guide to clinical screening by history, examination, and testing for genetic causes is also presented.

EPIDEMIOLOGY

CHD is the most common major birth defect. Estimates of the birth prevalence of CHD range from 4 to 50 cases per 1000 live births depending on the epidemiologic study.[1] The variation in estimates is explained in part

by differences in study design, case ascertainment, and disease classification. In addition, the advent of ultrasound in the 1980s has resulted in identification of milder abnormalities[1] and more accurate classification and prenatal diagnosis. The latter may in fact have led to an increase in pregnancy termination and a decline in birth prevalence.

ENVIRONMENTAL FACTORS

Multiple environmental risk factors have been implicated in the development of CHD. Although unproven, some occurrences of CHD are potentially preventable through changes in the fetal environment. A select group of environmental risk factors are briefly reviewed in this section, although a growing body of epidemiologic literature is dedicated to this topic (Figure 4-1).

Diabetes

Pregestational diabetes is a known risk factor for CHD as well as abnormal development of other organ systems. Heart defects most often associated with maternal diabetes include conotruncal defects, laterality defects and, less commonly, left ventricular outflow obstructive defects (Table 4-1).[3] Hypertrophic cardiomyopathy is commonly associated with maternal diabetes but typically resolves after birth, once exposure to the hyperglycemic fetal environment ceases. The risk of birth defects secondary to diabetes can be reduced with strict glycemic control prior to conception and throughout pregnancy.[3] Identification of this risk factor is crucial

*Drs. Peyvandi and D'Alessandro contributed equally to this work.

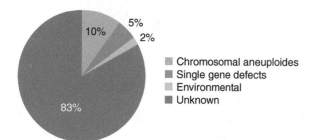

FIGURE 4-1 ■ Currently the vast majority of congenital heart disease does not have an identified underlying etiology. An as-of-yet undefined percentage is likely attributable to unknown environmental effects and single-gene defects. However, newer diagnostic techniques suggest that congenital heart disease is frequently a complex trait arising from a combination of environmental and heterogeneous genetic effects. (*Adapted with permission from van der Born et al.* Nat Rev Cardiol. *2011.*)

because the prevalence of type 2 diabetes increases in women of childbearing age.

Maternal Medications

The U.S. Food and Drug Association (FDA) classifies medications according to the risk of birth defects. Many medications have been associated with malformations of the heart, although there are no specific estimates quantifying risk of specific types of heart defects. Examples of therapeutic maternal medications associated with CHD include antiepileptic drugs (eg, phenytoin, hydantoin,

Common Maternal Conditions Associated with an Increased Risk of Congenital Heart Defects

Maternal Condition	Heart Defect
Diabetes	Conotruncal defects*
	Laterality defects
	CAVC
Febrile illness	Pulmonic stenosis
	Tricuspid atresia
	Aortic coarctation
Influenza	Outflow tract defects
	Aortic coarctation
	Tricuspid atresia
	VSD
Rubella	VSD
	PDA
	Pulmonary valve defects
	Peripheral pulmonic stenosis

*such as tetralogy of Fallot, truncus arteriosus and transposition of the great arteries
CAVC, common atrioventricular canal; PDA, patent ductus arteriosus; VSD, ventricular septal defect.

valproic acid), vitamin A, sulfa antibiotics, and lithium.[4] Examples of nontherapeutic maternal substances associated with CHD include alcohol and, in some cases, possibly tobacco.

Protective Factors

There are multiple lines of evidence suggesting that the use of multivitamins and folic acid supplementation decreases the risk of CHD. Most, but not all, studies demonstrate a reduced incidence of heart defects, such as conotruncal defects and ventricular septal defect (VSD), with prenatal use of multivitamins.[5]

Approach to Prevention of CHD

Environmental risk factors for CHD continue to be identified, providing opportunities for primary prevention. Recommendations have been published to guide prospective parents on known risk factors and emphasize proper preconceptional care.[3]

Recommendations include the following:

■ Women of childbearing age should take a multivitamin containing folic acid daily.
■ Prospective mothers should have a preconceptional evaluation of associated medical conditions such as diabetes and metabolic disorders.
■ Prospective mothers should discuss any medication use with a healthcare professional.
■ Women should avoid contact with people with febrile illnesses or the flu early in their pregnancy.
■ Women planning a pregnancy or those already pregnant should cease smoking or ingesting alcohol.

Finally, in order to properly counsel families on recurrence risk, an accurate assessment of genetic risk factors is also required. This may include referral for genetic counseling or clinical genetic evaluation and testing.

GENETIC SYNDROMES

The recognition that CHD is present in the context of a genetic syndrome has important implications for the pediatric patient, including the identification and management of multisystem involvement and development. The following provides a brief overview of common genetic syndromes and their associated heart diseases, with a summary of these conditions and their cardinal features in Table 4-2. Table 4-3 provides an overview classified by specific cardiac diseases with a list of genetic syndromes that should be considered at the time of diagnosis.

Genetic Syndromes and Associated Cardiac Disease

Syndrome	Genetic Alteration	Prevalence (per live births)	Frequency of CVS Anomalies	Cardiac Diagnosis	Dysmorphology	Systemic Involvement
Down syndrome	Trisomy 21 Translocation (3%–4%) Mosaicism (1%)	1.4:1000	40%–50%	CAVC VSD ASD PDA TOF	Upslanting palpebral fissures Epicanthal folds Brushfield spots Low nasal bridge Macroglossia Brachycephaly and third fontanelle Excess nuchal skin Low-set, small, posteriorly rotated ears Single palmar crease Clinodactyly Wide space between first and second toe	Developmental delay Hypothyroidism Strabismus, refractive errors Hearing loss Atlantoaxial instability Duodenal atresia Malrotation Hirschsprung Hip dysplasia Polycythemia Leukemia Obstructive sleep apnea
Edward syndrome	Trisomy 18 Mosaicism (5%) Partial trisomy (<1%)	1:6000	90%	VSD Polyvalvar disease TOF Complex CHD Pulmonary hypertension	Craniofacial features Overriding fingers Nail hypoplasia Short sternum	Growth deficiency Renal/GU anomalies Umbilical/inguinal hernias
Patau syndrome	Trisomy 13 Translocation (up to 20%)	1:5000 to 1:29,000	80%	ASD VSD DORV Pulmonary hypertension	Orofacial clefts Microphthalmia/anophthalmia Postaxial polydactyly Holoprosencephaly	Renal/GU anomalies
Turner syndrome	45,XO (50%) Mosaicism	1:2000–5000	17%–45%	Left-sided lesions ■ CoA ■ BAV/AS ■ HLHS (rare) ■ Mitral valve prolapse ■ Aortic root dilation/dissection	Unusual shape/rotation of ears Narrow maxilla, dental crowding Micrognathia Low posterior hairline Webbed neck Widely spaced or inverted nipples Shield chest Cubitus valgus Hyperconvex nails	Short stature Lymphedema/cystic hygroma Hypertension (essential)

(Continued)

Genetic Syndromes and Associated Cardiac Disease (Continued)

Syndrome	Genetic Alteration	Prevalence (per live births)	Frequency CVS Anomalies	Cardiac Diagnosis	Dysmorphology	Systemic Involvement
DiGeorge/velocardiofacial syndrome	22q11 microdeletion 90% sporadic 6%-10% inherited	1:5950	75%	Conotruncal defects TOF IAA Type B Truncus arteriosus Conoventricular VSD Aortic arch anomalies (right-sided aortic arch, cervical aortic arch, abnormal branching pattern)	Tubular nose Hypoplastic alae nasi Bulbous tip nose Low-set and/or dysplastic ears Myopathic facies	Immunodeficiency Hypocalcemia Cleft palate Velopharyngeal insufficiency Feeding disorders Learning and speech disabilities Behavioural and psychiatric disorders Renal anomalies
Williams-Beuren syndrome	7q11.23 microdeletion (90%)	1:10,000	80%	Supravalvar AS (75%) Supravalvar PS Peripheral pulmonary artery stenosis Arteriopathy Sudden death	Periorbital fullness Short nose with bulbous nasal tip Long philtrum Wide mouth, full lips Dental malocclusion with small, widely spaced teeth Mild micrognathia Stellate irises	Developmental delay Short stature Unique cognitive profile Hoarse voice Hernias, diverticulae, joint laxity Hypertension
CHARGE syndrome	CHD7 gene mutation (65%) Sporadic and inherited	1:10,000	70-90%	Conotruncal defects Aortic arch abnormalities VSD	Coloboma Facial asymmetry (cranial nerve weakness)	Coloboma Choanal atresia Retardation of growth and development GU anomalies (hypogonadotropic hypogonadism) Ear anomalies/deafness Cleft lip/palate
Alagille syndrome	JAG1 gene mutation (90%) 20p12 deletion (7%) NOTCH 2 gene mutation (<1%)	1:100,000	>90%	PPS or hypoplasia TOF VSD ASD AS, CoA	Triangular facies Prominent forehead and chin Hypertelorism	Paucity of interlobular bile ducts Chronic cholestasis Butterfly vertebrae Posterior embryotoxon

Syndrome	Gene	Incidence	CVS involvement	CVS defects	Extracardiac features
Holt-Oram syndrome	*TBX5* gene mutation (70%)	1:10,000	75%	ASD AV conduction delay VSD CAVC Left-sided lesions Conotruncal defects	Upper limb anomalies
Noonan/LEOPARD syndrome	*PTPN11* mutation (40%) (other genes detailed in text)	1:1000–2500	50%–90%	Pulmonic stenosis Hypertrophic cardiomyopathy ASD VSD	Epicanthal folds Downslanting palpebral fissures Ptosis Triangular facies Low-set, thickened pinnae Webbed neck with low posterior hairline Short stature Lymphatic dysplasias Cryptorchidism

AS, aortic stenosis; ASD, atrial septal defect; BAV, bicuspid aortic valve; CAVC common atrioventricular canal; CHD, congenital heart defect; CoA, coarctation of the aorta; CVS, cardiovascular system; DORV, double outlet right ventricle; GU, genitourinary; HLHS, hypoplastic left heart syndrome; IAA, interrupted aortic arch; PDA patent ductus arteriosus; PPS, peripheral pulmonary stenosis; PS, pulmonary stenosis; TOF, tetralogy of Fallot; VSD, ventricular septal defect.

Cardiac Disease and Associated Genetic Syndromes

Cardiac Lesion	Associated Syndromic and Familial Etiologies
Atrial septal defects	Trisomy 21
	Trisomy 18
	Trisomy 13
	Holt-Oram syndrome
	NKX2.5 gene mutations
	GATA4 gene mutations
	Ellis-van Creveld syndrome
	Noonan syndrome
Ventricular septal defects*	Holt-Oram syndrome
	Trisomy 21
	Trisomy 18
	Trisomy 13
	22q11.2 deletion (DiGeorge syndrome)
Common atrioventricular canal	Trisomy 21
	Trisomy 13
	Trisomy 18
Valve/arterial disease	
Polyvalvar disease	Trisomy 18
Aortic stenosis/bicuspid aortic valve/coarctation	Trisomy 13
of the aorta	Turner syndrome
	Familial aggregation of left-sided lesions
	NOTCH1 gene mutations
Supravalvar aortic stenosis	Williams syndrome
	Elastin gene mutations
Pulmonary stenosis	Noonan syndrome
	Alagille syndrome
	Costello syndrome
	LEOPARD syndrome
Branch pulmonary artery stenosis	Alagille syndrome
	Williams syndrome
Conotruncal defects	
Tetralogy of Fallot	22q11.2 deletion (DiGeorge Syndrome)
	Trisomy 21
	Alagille syndrome
	CHARGE syndrome
Truncus arteriosus	22q11.2 deletion (DiGeorge Syndrome)
Interrupted aortic arch, type B	22q11.2 deletion (DiGeorge Syndrome)
Single ventricle	
Hypoplastic left heart syndrome	Turner syndrome
Laterality defects	
Heterotaxy	*ZIC3* gene mutations
	CFC1 gene mutations
	HTX3 gene mutations

Conoventricular/Perimembranous ventricular septal defects.

Down Syndrome (Trisomy 21)

Down syndrome is the most common chromosomal aneuploidy in live births. It most often arises from maternal nondisjunction during meiosis, resulting in 3 copies of chromosome 21. Therefore, the birth prevalence increases with maternal age, from 1 in 1445 live births at age 20 years to 1 in 25 births at age 45 years.[6] Down syndrome patients have characteristic dysmorphic features, including upslanting palpebral fissure, epicanthal folds, low nasal bridge, large tongue, brachycephaly and third fontanelle, excess nuchal skin, single palmar crease, and clinodactyly. All patients with Down syndrome have an intellectual disability, although there is a wide range of abilities and functioning. Other common features are outlined in Table 4-2. Cardiac disease is an important feature of Down syndrome. Forty to 50% of patients are affected with CHD, and of those, 40% to 50% have common atrioventricular canal (CAVC), a characteristic lesion of this syndrome.[7] Many patients also have variants of CAVC, including incomplete canal with a primum atrial septal defect (ASD) and cleft mitral valve. VSDs, patent ductus arteriosus, ASD, and tetralogy of Fallot (TOF) are all associated, in decreasing order of frequency. Patients with Down syndrome are at increased risk of persistent pulmonary hypertension as neonates and also have an increased risk of developing pulmonary hypertension beyond the neonatal period. This risk is an important consideration in the timely repair of large left-to-right shunt lesions. Currently, the American Academy of Pediatrics health supervision guidelines for children with Down syndrome recommend that all children with Down syndrome undergo cardiac evaluation and echocardiogram at diagnosis.[8] Patients with Down syndrome have been shown to have equivalent outcomes for CAVC repair compared with non–Down syndrome patients.

The clinical diagnosis of Down syndrome should be confirmed by karyotype to identify cases arising from an unbalanced translocation (3%-4% of patients) rather than nondisjunction. Parents of a child with a translocation require genetic screening to assess for a balanced translocation, which has a higher recurrence risk of 10% to 15%.

Trisomy 18 (Edward) and Trisomy 13 (Patau) Syndromes

Trisomy 18 (Edward) syndrome results from 3 copies of chromosome 18 in 94% of patients, likely arising from nondisjunction. It occurs in 1 in 6000 live births.[6] Greater than 90% of patients have CHD, characteristically VSD and/or polyvalvar disease (Figure 4-2), although 10% have complex CHD. The syndrome is also characterized by intrauterine growth retardation and poor postnatal growth, small facial features, overlapping fingers, rocker bottom feet, short sternum, and renal/genitourinary anomalies.

Trisomy 13 (Patau) syndrome arises from 3 copies of chromosome 13, with translocation seen in up to 20%. The prevalence is 1 in 5000 to 29,000 live births. Patients have multiple congenital anomalies, characteristically holoprosencephaly, microphthalmia, cleft lip and palate, polydactyly, and renal/genitourinary anomalies. CHD is present in 50% to 80% of patients. ASD and VSD are the most common defects; polyvalvar disease is also seen in trisomy 13, although less commonly than in trisomy 18.

Both trisomy 18 and 13 have greater than 90% mortality in the first year of life and are associated with severe mental retardation. The high rate of mortality is postulated to be secondary to central apnea as the cardiac disease in either condition is rarely lethal. In patients who survive the neonatal period, many questions remain about the indications for cardiac surgery. All patients with multiple congenital anomalies and phenotypic features suggestive of trisomy 18 and 13 should undergo a karyotype to confirm the diagnosis and identify chromosomal translocations.

Turner Syndrome

Turner syndrome is present in 1 in 2500 to 3000 live births. The overall incidence is much higher because there is a high frequency of prenatal loss. Monosomy

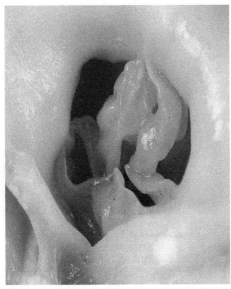 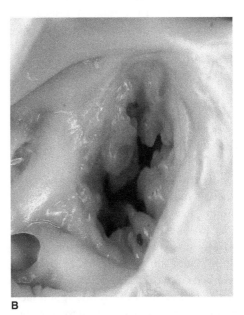

A **B**

FIGURE 4-2 ■ Cardiac pathology specimen from a patient with trisomy 18 showing polyvalvar disease with characteristic nodules on the leaflets of the pulmonary valve **(A)** and the tricuspid valve **(B)**. (*Image contributed by Dr. Paul M. Weinberg, Cardiac Registry, Children's Hospital of Philadelphia.*)

of the X chromosome (45,X) is seen in 50% of cases. Another 5% to 10% of cases have duplication of the long arm with loss of the short arm, and the remainder have mosaicism for 45,X with 1 or more other cell lines, including 46,XX, 47,XXX, and 46,XY.

Patients with Turner syndrome have characteristic physical findings, including short stature, webbed neck and low posterior hairline, narrow maxilla and dental crowding, widely spaced nipples, barrel-shaped thorax, cubitus valgus, hyperconvex nails, and lymphedema of the hands and feet. Multiple organ systems are involved, including renal, endocrine, and musculoskeletal (Table 4-2). Many patients have learning disabilities. There is a spectrum with regard to gonadal dysgenesis, the development of secondary sex characteristics and fertility, and there is some genotype–phenotype correlation, with mosaic forms having a greater incidence of spontaneous menarche. Patients with mosaic forms that include a Y chromosome (5%-6%) are at increased risk of gonadal malignancy.

CHD is present in 17% to 45% of patients with Turner syndrome.[6] Left-sided obstructive lesions are characteristic, including bicuspid aortic valve, aortic stenosis, and coarctation of the aorta. Hypoplastic left heart syndrome, mitral valve prolapse (MVP), and total anomalous pulmonary venous return are seen less commonly. Aortic root dilation and dissection are reported in older patients with Turner syndrome; however, this is typically in the context of risk factors including a history of coarctation, bicuspid aortic valve, and hypertension. There is no difference in the natural history of cardiac lesions in patients with Turner syndrome compared to those without. The American Academy of Pediatrics health supervision guidelines for girls with Turner syndrome recommend a pediatric cardiology evaluation at diagnosis. Follow-up is individualized to diagnosis; however, blood pressure should be monitored regularly.[9] The diagnosis should be confirmed with karyotype.

22q11.2 Microdeletion Syndrome

22q11.2 microdeletion syndrome encompasses DiGeorge, velocardiofacial, and conotruncal anomaly facial syndromes. With an estimated prevalence of 1 in 4000 to 6000, it is the most common microdeletion disorder yet identified. Although most microdeletions are *de novo*, they are transmitted in an autosomal dominant fashion in approximately 6% of cases. The most common deletion is large (3 Mb) and encompasses a region coding for more than 30 genes, although smaller deletions in the region have been detected. The *TBX1* gene maps into the deleted locus and encodes a transcription factor that participates in cardiovascular development. This gene is deleted in most, but not all, patients with the associated disease phenotype. Missense mutations have

also been detected in *TBX1* in patients with a DiGeorge phenotype who did not have the microdeletion on fluorescent in situ hybridization (FISH), suggesting that *TBX1* haploinsufficiency contributes to the disease phenotype.

Patients with a 22q11.2 microdeletion present with highly variable clinical phenotypes. Many have characteristic facial features, including a tubular nose with hypoplastic nasal alae and bulbous nose tip, low-set ears, and myopathic faces (Figure 4-3). Palatal anomalies are also common (70%), including velopharyngeal incompetence, submucosal clefts, and cleft palate, and contribute to the frequent feeding difficulties observed. Other characteristics include immune deficiency, hypocalcemia (parathyroid dysfunction), renal anomalies, learning difficulties, and developmental delay (70%)

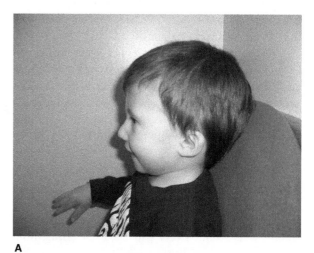

A

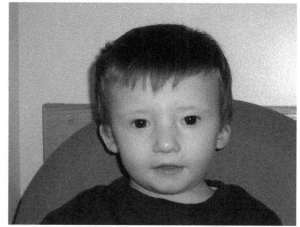

B

FIGURE 4-3 ■ Photographs of child with 22q11.2 microdeletion syndrome demonstrating typical features: narrow palpebral fissures, overfolded "hooded" eyelids, nose with squared nasal root and narrow alae giving a "bulbous" appearance, malar hypoplasia, micrognathia, and small ears with posterior rotation and an overfolded superior helix. (*Images contributed by Dr. Elizabeth Goldmuntz, Children's Hospital of Philadelphia.*)

(Table 4-2). CHD is present in approximately 74% of individuals and is the most common cause of mortality.[6] Conotruncal and arch abnormalities are characteristic including TOF (22%), truncus arteriosus (7%), interrupted aortic arch type B (15%), and vascular ring (5%). VSDs (conoventricular and posterior malalignment types) are also common (13%). Diagnosis can be confirmed with FISH, multiplex ligation-dependent probe amplification (MLPA), and genome wide array. Because patients with 22q11.2 microdeletion syndrome have widely variable phenotypes and multisystem involvement, care is often facilitated by multidisciplinary clinic visits with providers familiar with the range of problems in this population.

Williams Syndrome

Williams syndrome is a contiguous gene deletion syndrome caused by a microdeletion at 7q11.23 that disrupts the elastin gene, among others. The deletion is detectable by FISH in 99% of patients. Typically, deletions are de novo but can be inherited in an autosomal dominant fashion. The prevalence is approximately 1 in 8000 to 10,000 live births, and the syndrome occurs equally in males and females. Patients with Williams syndrome have characteristic facial features, including periorbital fullness, stellate irises, short nose with an upturned nasal tip, long philtrum, wide mouth and full lips, dental malocclusion, and small widely spaced teeth (Figure 4-4). Genotype-phenotype analyses demonstrate that deletion of the elastin gene is associated with the following features: cardiovascular disease, voice hoarseness, diverticula, rectal prolapse, inguinal and umbilical hernias, joint hypermobility and contractures,

and soft, lax skin. Children with Williams syndrome have developmental delay (95%), difficulties with visuospatial cognition, and a characteristic personality. Hypercalcemia is a characteristic feature of Williams syndrome, although relatively uncommon (15%), and may manifest with irritability, constipation, vomiting, and muscle cramps. Altered calcium metabolism can persist to adulthood, and therefore, multivitamins and vitamin D should be avoided.

Approximately 80% of children with Williams syndrome have CHD and vasculopathy, which is the greatest cause of morbidity and mortality.[6] The characteristic lesions are supravalvar aortic stenosis (SVAS) and peripheral pulmonary artery stenosis (PPAS). In a recent retrospective review of 270 patients with Williams syndrome, 45% had SVAS, 37% had PPAS, and 20% had both. Other common lesions included MVP and mitral regurgitation in 15%, VSD in 13%, and supravalvar pulmonary stenosis in 12%. Mild and moderate SVAS and PPAS are seen to improve over time without intervention. Overall, mortality and sudden death are rare.[10] Sudden death in Williams syndrome has been estimated to occur in approximately 1 in 1000 patients[11] and is thought to be secondary to bilateral outflow tract obstruction and coronary ostial stenosis. Recognition of outflow tract obstruction is of critical importance when considering sedation and general anesthesia in this population, as is the awareness that coronary ostial stenosis may be underappreciated in the asymptomatic patient. Currently the American Academy of Pediatrics health supervision guidelines for children with Williams syndrome recommend a cardiac evaluation at diagnosis, followed by annual assessments until age 5 years (or as dictated by clinical findings). If results of previous evaluations are

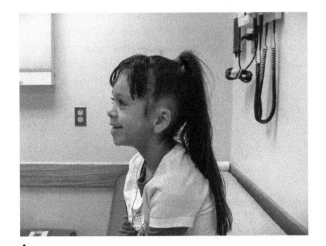
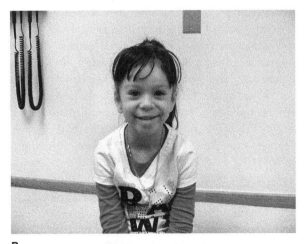

A   **B**

FIGURE 4-4 ■ Photographs of an affected child demonstrating typical features of Williams syndrome: eyes with periorbital fullness, short palpebral fissures, broad eyebrows, slightly short nose, full lips with a wide mouth, full cheeks, and ears with prominent lobes. (*Images contributed by Dr. Elizabeth Goldmuntz, Children's Hospital of Philadelphia.*)

negative, re-evaluation at puberty is recommended to assess for arterial stenosis and hypertension.[12]

CHARGE Syndrome (Hall-Hittner Syndrome)

Previously known as the CHARGE association, CHARGE is actually a genetically heterogeneous syndrome. Sixty-five percent of patients who are clinically diagnosed with CHARGE have a mutation in the gene *CHD7* on chromosome 8q12.1. The birth prevalence of CHARGE syndrome is 1 per 10,000 to 1 per 15,000 live births. Most cases are sporadic; however, autosomal dominant inheritance and germline mosaicism are possible as well.[13] The diagnostic criteria are as follows:

C–coloboma (retinal or choroid)
H–heart defects
A–choanal atresia
R–retardation of growth and development
G–genitourinary anomalies
E–external ear anomalies/deafness

Other clinical features include cranial nerve weakness and facial palsy/asymmetry, hypoplasia of the cochlea and semicircular canals, oral clefts, and neurogenic swallowing problems.

CHD is present in the majority of patients, independent of mutation status. A wide range of CHDs have been associated with CHARGE, including conotruncal and aortic arch anomalies.

Alagille Syndrome

Alagille syndrome is an autosomal dominant disorder whose diagnosis originally required the presence of bile duct paucity in conjunction with 3 of the following 5 characteristics: cholestasis, CHD, skeletal anomalies, ocular anomalies, or facial features. Subsequent studies demonstrated a highly variable clinical phenotype, including some cases with minimal hepatic findings or only a subset of classic features. Alagille syndrome is a genetically heterogeneous disorder. *JAG1* was the first disease gene identified for this syndrome and remains the most common, with mutations identified in approximately 95% of patients with clinical features of the disease. Frameshift mutations are the most common. Mutations in *NOTCH2* have also been detected in *JAG1* mutation–negative patients with features of Alagille syndrome.

Characteristic dysmorphic features include a broad forehead, deep-set eyes, rounded tip of the nose, and a pointed chin. These features typically give the face an inverted triangle shape. Nearly 90% of patients have some cardiac involvement, and peripheral pulmonary stenosis is the most common. Pulmonary valve stenosis and TOF are also associated. Other anomalies include

noncardiac vascular anomalies and skeletal (butterfly vertebrae), ocular, hepatic, hematologic (bleeding tendency), and renal anomalies.[14] Ocular anomalies usually consist of anterior chamber defects, pigmentary retinal anomalies, and posterior embryotoxon.[13]

Patients suspected of having Alagille syndrome should undergo testing for a *JAG1* mutation. Obtaining a detailed family history in a patient with isolated right-sided CHD can reveal a family history of right-sided defects, such as mild valvar pulmonary stenosis or peripheral pulmonary stenosis, which should also prompt testing for *JAG1* mutations. This will allow the clinician to provide proper genetic counseling to a family regarding recurrence risk.[2]

Holt-Oram Syndrome

Holt-Oram syndrome is an autosomal dominant "heart-hand" syndrome characterized by upper limb anomalies and CHD. This syndrome is estimated to occur in 1 per 10,000 individuals.[13] Skeletal anomalies are fully penetrant; therefore, all patients with this diagnosis have preaxial radial ray malformations. The severity of the skeletal anomaly varies, ranging from severe defects such as phocomelia to defects only appreciated radiographically. Common upper limb anomalies include triphalangeal, hypoplastic, or absent thumb and radial dysplasia.[2]

In contrast, CHD is not fully penetrant and is seen in approximately 75% of patients. ASDs are the most common, occurring in 60% of the patients, followed by VSD and AV conduction delay. Additional heart defects are reported, including atrioventricular septal defects, conotruncal anomalies, and left-sided defects, but are much less common.

Patients with Holt-Oram syndrome have a mutation in the gene *TBX5*. Mutations are found in approximately 70% of the patients and include nonsense, frameshift, and missense mutations. Because this syndrome is not thought to be genetically heterogeneous, patients without gene mutations are posited to have mutations in the regulatory region that is not routinely tested.[2]

The diagnosis of Holt-Oram syndrome should be considered in patients with CHD and upper limb anomalies. Because the phenotype is variable, the syndrome should also be considered in patients with septal defects and a family history of septal or upper limb anomalies. The evaluation of a patient with suspected Holt-Oram syndrome should include a radiograph for radial ray abnormalities and testing for cardiac and conduction abnormalities.

Noonan, LEOPARD, and Costello Syndrome

Noonan, LEOPARD, Costello, and cardio-facio-cutaneous syndromes and neurofibromatosis type 1 all arise from defects in various proteins involved in the Ras/MAPK signaling pathway.[7] Many of the phenotypic features of these disorders overlap; therefore, accurate diagnosis relies on identification of a subset of pathognomonic features or identifying a mutation in a disease-related gene.

Noonan syndrome is the most common of this group of disorders, occurring in 1 in 1000 to 2500 patients. Noonan syndrome is inherited in an autosomal dominant manner, and an affected parent is identified in 30% to 75% of families. It is a genetically heterogeneous disorder with 4 disease-related genes identified. Approximately 50% of patients have gain-of-function mutations in *PTPN11*, 13% have *SOS1* mutations, 3% to 17% have *RAF1* mutations, and less than 5% have *KRAS* mutations.[7] Clinical features include dysmorphic features (epicanthal folds, downslanting palpebral fissures, ptosis, low-set ears), webbed neck, pectus carinatum superiorly and pectus excavatum inferiorly, short stature, and lymphatic dysplasias. Cardiovascular disease is present in 50% to 90% of patients. A dysplastic, stenotic pulmonary valve is characteristic and present in 20% to 50%. Hypertrophic cardiomyopathy is also commonly seen (20%-30%). Other cardiac disease includes ASD, VSD, branch pulmonary artery stenosis, coarctation of the aorta, and incomplete CAVC. In addition to the overlap with genetically related syndromes, Noonan syndrome in a female can overlap with the phenotype of Turner syndrome, which should be considered in the differential diagnosis.

LEOPARD syndrome is genetically related to Noonan syndrome, with gain-of-function mutations in *PTPN11* in 90% of patients. Mutations in *RAF1* and *BRAF* have also been identified in less than 5% of patients with LEOPARD syndrome. It is also inherited in an autosomal dominant fashion. LEOPARD is an acronym for the phenotype of lentigines, electrocardiogram (ECG) abnormalities, ocular hypertelorism, pulmonary stenosis, abnormalities of genitalia, retardation of growth, and deafness. Approximately 80% of patients have CHD, most commonly hypertrophic cardiomyopathy (70%) and pulmonary stenosis (25%). ECG abnormalities include findings related to hypertrophic cardiomyopathy, as well as conduction defects. Skin findings include multiple lentigines on the face, neck, and trunk and cafe-au-lait spots.

Costello syndrome is a rare pediatric disorder; the incidence is unknown.[6] Patients with Costello syndrome have distinctive coarse facies, perinasal papillomata, loose skin of the hands and feet with deep creases, joint laxity, and ulnar deviation of the wrist. Poor growth, short stature, and intellectual disability are common. There is also an increased lifetime risk of solid tumors. Approximately 30% to 75% of patients have cardiovascular disease, including pulmonary stenosis (25%-50%),

hypertrophic cardiomyopathy (30%-47%), and mitral valve prolpase (MVP). Approximately 42% to 74% of patients have atrial tachycardia, most commonly multifocal chaotic atrial tachycardia, which can be very difficult to treat. Eighty to 90% of patients with Costello syndrome will have detectable mutations in the *HRAS* oncogene, and common mutations are postulated to be activating mutations affecting the Ras/MAPK pathway.[7]

Marfan Syndrome

Marfan syndrome (MFS) is an autosomal dominant connective tissue disorder that affects the cardiovascular, skeletal, ocular, and neural systems. The prevalence of MFS ranges from 1 in 5000 to 10,000 live newborns. There is equal prevalence in males and females.

The majority of cases are caused by a mutation in the gene *FBN1* located on chromosome 15q21.1. Over 1000 mutations have been described in this gene, leading to abnormalities in the protein product fibrillin-1. The disease is highly penetrant and exhibits phenotypic heterogeneity. Fibrillin-1 is a glycoprotein responsible for the formation of microfibrils, which make up elastic fibers in the extracellular matrix. The mutation in *FBN1* is thought to cause reduced or mutated forms of fibrillin-1, which in turn leads to alterations in the mechanical properties of tissues, increased transforming growth factor-beta (TGF-β) activity and signaling, and loss of cell-matrix interactions causing connective tissue weakness. Recent mouse models and studies have demonstrated that the increased TGF-β activity is the cause of aortic root aneurysms.[15]

The organ systems typically involved include skeletal, ocular, cardiovascular, and pulmonary. Features within the skeletal system include pectus carinatum or excavatum, scoliosis, and increased arm span-to-height ratio. Common dysmorphic features include dolichocephaly, downslanting palpebral fissures, malar hypoplasia, and retrognathia. Ectopia lentis, dislocation of the lens upward and temporally, is the characteristic ocular abnormality seen in approximately 60% of patients with MFS. The cardiovascular manifestations, particularly aortic pathology, are the main cause of morbidity and mortality in these patients, although the most common form of heart disease is MVP. Aortic dilation typically occurs in the sinuses of Valsalva and is found in 60% to 80% of patients with MFS. Aortic dissection is a life-threatening complication of aortic root dilation. Rarely, pulmonary artery dilation is seen in MFS but is not specific to this diagnosis and is not included in the diagnostic criteria.

The diagnosis of MFS is predominantly clinical. The original diagnostic guidelines separated organ involvement into major and minor criteria; however, the revised Ghent criteria give more weight to the 2 cardinal features of MFS—aortic root dilation and ectopia lentis.[16] Family history remains a crucial component of the diagnosis. Other organ system involvement is organized into a scoring system. These criteria also emphasize the importance of genetic testing because most patients carry a mutation in *FBN1*. Patients who are found to have a mutation and at least one of aortic root dilation or ectopia lentis are deemed to have the diagnosis. The updated Ghent criteria are depicted in Table 4-4.

MFS shares many features with other connective tissue disorders such as Ehlers-Danlos syndrome and Loeys-Dietz syndrome. In Loeys-Dietz syndrome, patients have tortuosity and dilation of the abdominal aorta, pelvic vessels, and intracranial vessels.[17] Aortic dilation and dissection can occur at a significantly younger age (eg, 6 months) in these patients. Also patients typically have a bifid uvula or cleft palate and hypertelorism. The genes involved in this syndrome are TGFBR1 and TGFBR2. Ehlers-Danlos syndrome is characterized by hypermobility, easy bruising, and thin, translucent skin in addition to aortic root dilation in medium-sized arteries. The genes involved in this syndrome include *COL3A1*, *COL1A2*, and *PLOD1*. These syndromes should always be considered in the differential diagnoses of MFS because each of these conditions has unique management, risks, and prognosis.

With the involvement of so many organ systems in MFS, a multidisciplinary assessment is recommended. This includes referral to a cardiologist for a transthoracic echocardiogram, referral to an ophthalmologist for a slit-lamp examination, and referral to an orthopedist for evaluation of possible skeletal abnormalities. Skeletal abnormalities are usually investigated radiographically including computed tomography or magnetic resonance imaging of the lumbar spine to rule out dural ectasia. A pediatric cardiologist should follow patients with aortic root dilation to monitor for progression, initiate medication, and refer to surgery if necessary. Those pediatric patients with a family history of MFS without clinical findings should be evaluated periodically because many issues do not manifest until adulthood.

VATER Association

VATER is a nonrandom association first described in 1973.[18] The acronym describes the associated malformations of vertebral defects, atresia, tracheoesophageal fistula, esophageal atresia, radial limb anomalies and renal defects. The acronym has sometimes been expanded to VACTERL to include cardiac malformations and limb defects. Diagnosis is made when three of the defining malformations are present. It is usually sporadic and occurs in 0.4 to 5.1 per 100,000 births.[19] There is some indirect evidence for an underlying genetic etiology, including findings that 9% of probands have a first-degree relative with at least 1 feature of the association, which is higher than would be expected to occur by chance.[20] Additionally, some subgroups have been defined, such as VACTERL with hydrocephalus (particularly aqueductal stenosis) that is inherited in a Mendelian fashion. Autosomal dominant, recessive, and X-linked patterns have been described. The VATER/VACTERL association overlaps considerably with other nonrandom associations, including oculoauriculovertebral spectrum (Goldenhar), Klippel-Feil syndrome, MURCS (mullerian duct aplasia or hypoplasia, renal aplasia, cervicothoracic somite dysplasia), and the caudal regression spectrum. It has been suggested that these associations are on a spectrum of axial mesodermal dysplasia resulting from failure of mesodermal cell migration during early blastogenesis.[21]

The inclusion of cardiac defects as a criterion in this association is a matter of ongoing debate. In 2001, Kallen et al.[22] identified 5260 infants with multiple malformations and used pair-wise associations between malformations to determine which associations were in fact nonrandom (ie, not attributable to confounding variables). These authors advocate for restricting

Ghent Criteria for Diagnosis of Marfan Syndrome – Updated (2011)*

Absence of Family History	Positive Family History
Aortic root dilation + ectopia lentis	Ectopia lentis alone
Aortic root dilation + *FBN1* mutation	Systemic findings (score >7)
Aortic root dilation + systemic findings (score >7)	Aortic root dilation
Ectopia lentis + *FBN1* mutation	

*NOTE. Updated Ghent criteria for the diagnosis of Marfan syndrome based on recommendations from an expert panel. Aortic root dilation is defined as a z-score >2 by echocardiography. Systemic findings include involvement in other organ systems such as skeletal malformations and facial features. A scoring system has been created to define significant systemic findings (score >7). The diagnosis of Marfan syndrome is made depending on the presence or absence of family history.
Adapted with permission from Loeys B, Dietz H, Braverman A, et al. The revised Ghent nosology for the Marfan syndrome. J Med Genet. 2010;47:476-485.*

the inclusion criteria for VATER association to vertebral malformations, anal atresia, esophageal atresia, and preaxial upper limb reduction defects. Cardiac malformations were not found to occur more often in infants with VATER compared with other infants with multiple malformations; however, they were primarily associated with esophageal atresia.[22] The types of cardiac defects are wide ranging and not well delineated.[19,22]

HERITABLE HEART DISEASE

NKX2.5/GATA4 (Nonsyndromic Single-Gene Disorders)

NKX2.5 and GATA4 have been identified as disease genes for a subset of patients with specific types of nonsyndromic CHD. In 1998, using linkage analysis and positional cloning techniques, Schott et al.[23] identified 3 mutations within the gene encoding the homeobox transcription factor NKX2.5 in 4 families with ASD and atrioventricular (AV) conduction disorders with no other syndromic features. Animal models had already demonstrated that NKX2.5 participates in cardiovascular development, but these finding in humans led to the novel discovery that NKX2.5 is critical to AV nodal development and long-term function. These and other studies demonstrate that patients with ASD and AV conduction abnormalities may have underlying NKX2.5 mutations and that patients with an NKX2.5 mutation are at risk of progressive AV block. As such, patients with ASD should be screened for AV conduction delay, and those with NKX2.5 mutations should be followed for progressive degrees of AV block even after surgical repair of their cardiac defect. Other investigations have identified mutations in NKX2.5 that are associated with AV block alone[24] and rarely additional different cardiac lesions such as TOF without conduction defects.[25]

Similar to NKX2.5, investigators identified mutations in GATA4 in families with septal defects and no syndromic features. Studies are currently ongoing to discover other phenotypes associated with genetic alterations in these transcription factors and their interactions with each other.

Left-Sided Lesions

Bicuspid aortic valve (BAV) is the most common congenital heart lesion and occurs in approximately 1% of the general population. It frequently underlies aortic stenosis in children (up to 70%)[26] and adults (up to 50%)[27] and is associated with other left-sided lesions, including coarctation of the aorta (50%-80%), interrupted aortic arch, and VSD.[26,28] Aortic stenosis (with or without BAV) in the fetus can progress to hypoplastic

left heart syndrome (HLHS) during gestation,[29] indicating a mechanistic link between these conditions. In family-based studies of HLHS, the recurrence risk in first-degree relatives is 3.5%, but up to 18.3% for all cardiovascular malformations.[30] Both BAV and HLHS can be familial conditions, and family-based genome-wide linkage studies have shown an overlap in loci, confirming that the 2 conditions are genetically related.[31,32] Multiple associated loci were demonstrated; however, even within families, indicating that left-sided lesions are a complex trait and, in most cases, cannot be attributed to a classical Mendelian mode of inheritance.[30,32,33] It remains to be determined how associated loci contribute to the development of left-sided lesions. One autosomal dominant cause of aortic valve disease has been identified. Mutations in the transcription factor–encoding gene NOTCH1 result in various lesions including BAV and calcific aortic stenosis.[34]

APPROACH TO THE SYNDROMIC PATIENT WITH HEART DISEASE

History

In addition to a thorough cardiac history (covered elsewhere; see Chapter 1), an assessment of multisystem involvement and family history is the key to identifying syndromic and heritable heart disease. The underlying etiology of the cardiac disease may affect prognosis and will alter how recurrence counseling is conducted.

Inquiring about the pregnancy and birth history is an opportunity to elicit potential harmful environmental exposures during fetal life such as gestational diabetes, medications, alcohol and drug use, and infections, as well as potential protective effects such as folate and prenatal vitamin use. Children with chromosomal and genetic problems typically have poor growth and may have a history of intrauterine growth retardation. Growth problems are likely to be multifactorial in a syndromic child with heart disease; therefore, a careful history can help differentiate altered growth potential (eg, chromosomal abnormality) from inadequate intake (eg, feeding intolerance) and increased caloric requirements (eg, heart failure). Calorie counts and serial growth measurements may be helpful.

To elicit information about dysmorphology, parents can be asked whom the child most resembles or if they have had any concerns about unusual features or appearance. A thorough review of systems is important to elicit a history of other birth defects and problems with vision and hearing, impaired growth and development, other systemic disease (eg, endocrine, renal, gastrointestinal), skeletal malformations, birthmarks and skin changes, and frequent infections. One should also ask if other specialists or consultants are following the child, if other investigations have been conducted, and if any therapies are ongoing (eg, physiotherapy, speech therapy).

Family History

The goal of a thorough family history is to elicit information that will help characterize the phenotype and provide clues to diagnosis, identify family members who have subtle manifestations of disease that may have not been previously appreciated, identify a pattern of inheritance, and assist with recurrence risk counseling. Constructing a pedigree can be a useful tool (Figure 4-5) and requires inquiry about every member of each generation (Does your sister/brother have a heart problem, palpitations, or a pacemaker? Did he/she have surgery as a child?) rather than asking overly general questions (Does anyone in the family have a heart problem?).

The following are important features to review when detailing the family history:

■ Consanguinity (Are the parents related in any way other than by marriage?)
■ Other family members with CHD or acquired heart disease (eg, aortic stenosis, pacemaker/implantable cardioverter-defibrillator)
■ Other family members with birth defects/congenital anomalies

■ Familial short or tall stature or growth problems
■ Problems with hearing or vision
■ Other family members with developmental delay/mental retardation, learning problems, psychiatric problems, or genetic or chromosomal problems
■ Sudden unexpected death at any age (sudden infant death syndrome or beyond)
■ Pregnancy loss or termination

Because the medical histories of family members may not be known, it can be helpful to ask about the presence of symptoms (Does anyone else complain about palpitations? Does anyone else in the family pass out?), ongoing medication use, hospitalizations, or follow-up with a cardiologist. It is important to clarify biologic relationships (Do all of the children have the same mother and father?) and to identify consanguinity, family members who have died, miscarriages, and pregnancy terminations. Additional information about family members and new diagnoses may become available over time.

Examination

In addition to a thorough cardiovascular examination (covered elsewhere; see Chapter 1) and signs of cardiac compromise (eg, heart failure symptoms, cyanosis), there are many readily assessed physical findings that may suggest an underlying genetic defect. Documenting growth over time is essential. From head to toe, a rapid survey can

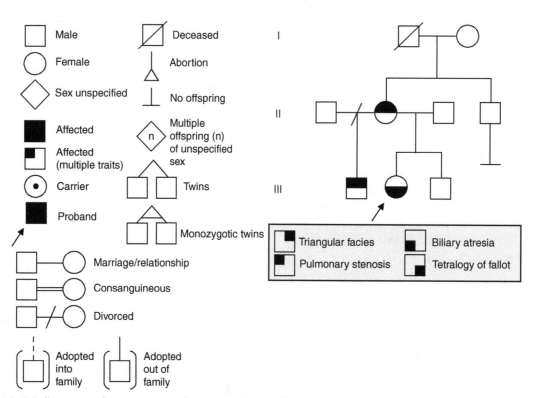

FIGURE 4-5 ■ Pedigree nomenclature. Common pedigree nomenclature is illustrated. A sample 3-generation pedigree of a family with Alagille syndrome is shown. Each generation is numbered in Roman numerals. An arrow indicates individual III-2, the proband. The various phenotypes are designated in the legend.

reveal a vast number of abnormalities. Examination of the head and neck includes facial shape (eg, long, narrow, triangular), skull shape (eg, frontal bossing, brachycephaly), eye spacing and shape, orientation of the palpebral fissures, flattening or hypoplasia of the midface, nasal shape, philtrum, ear shape (eg, malformed pinnae) and position/rotation (eg, low set, posteriorly rotated), palate (eg, cleft, narrow, high arching), nuchal webbing or excess skin, and hairline (eg, low set). Inspection of the chest may reveal the presence of pectus excavatum, pectus carinatum, or widely spaced nipples. Palpation of the abdomen should include assessment of liver position (right, left, or midline). Examination of the back should note scoliosis and sacral dimples. Limb abnormalities including ulnar deviation and increased joint laxity can be quickly assessed. Examination of the hands should be performed; long tapered or short digits, wide palms, single palmar creases, clinodactyly, polydactyly, absent thumbs, and webbing between the digits are easily noted. Additional items to note include birth marks, skin elasticity, scars, and stigmata of organ disease (eg, jaundice). Syndromic phenotypic features may become more or less characteristic with increasing age.

DIAGNOSTIC APPROACHES

There are a number of genetic tests that can assist clinicians in diagnosing genetic alterations in children with CHD. Significant advances have occurred in the field of genetic testing with increasingly sensitive methods to detect genetic alterations (Figure 4-6).

Chromosomal Analysis/Karyotype

The chromosome karyotype displays the 23 pairs of human chromosomes in metaphase and can detect changes in chromosome number such as trisomies or monosomies. It can also detect large changes in chromosome architecture such as translocations and is the best method of detecting balanced translocations. It has been estimated that standard chromosome analysis reveals a chromosomal aberration in 8% to 13% of neonates with CHD.[2] Common syndromes that can be identified by a karyotype include trisomy 21, trisomy 18, trisomy 13, and Turner syndrome (45,XO).

In prenatal life, amniocentesis is the primary means of prenatal chromosomal diagnosis. This test can be performed at 15 to 16 weeks of gestation.

Fluorescence In Situ Hybridization

Fluorescent in situ hybridization (FISH) can be used to detect submicroscopic deletions of chromosome segments. These small deletions cannot be seen on standard or even high-resolution karyotype. Control and test DNA probes are hybridized with metaphase chromosomes to determine whether the test region is normal or deleted. FISH technology was paramount in the detection of the 22q11 microdeletion. It has also been useful with other deletion syndromes such as Williams syndrome.

The disadvantage of FISH is that it is targeted to a particular locus and therefore is unable to detect unsuspected genetic alterations elsewhere in the genome. Although FISH technology has been extremely useful in the diagnosis of deletion syndromes, there are more advanced techniques that allow for the diagnosis of smaller defects within the genome. MLPA is another method of identifying deletions within the genome. MLPA is similar to a polymerase chain reaction (PCR); however, it can detect and amplify multiple targets (up to 40 sequences) with a single primer. The advantage of MLPA over FISH is that smaller deletions as well as duplications can be detected.

Genome-Wide Microarray

Microarray technology permits wide-scale scanning across the whole genome to detect areas of structural variation including deletions and duplications. Oligonucleotides (short fragments of DNA) of known sequence are embedded on the microarray chip, testing up to 1 million single-nucleotide polymorphisms. Patient DNA is labeled with fluorescent probes and then hybridized to the chip. The degree of fluorescence at each location on the chip correlates with the degree of correspondence between the patient DNA and the chip DNA. Areas of structural variation can be compared to known reference DNA sequences to determine if known genes are disrupted by the alteration. The advantage of genome-wide array technology is that the entire genome can be assessed simultaneously and areas of alteration can be detected without prior knowledge of where a disruption may have occurred. Interpretation can be complicated if areas of structural variation do not correspond to known genes or if multiple regions are detected, and it may not be clear if and how the change has contributed to the observed phenotype. Additionally, the technique is not sensitive enough to detect small deletions, insertions, or single-nucleotide mutations within genes. Therefore, if a phenotype corresponding to a known single-gene disorder is suspected, then specific mutation screening must still be conducted. Arrays can also be constructed with dense probe coverage for regions of interest to increase the likelihood of detecting potential disease-causing alterations.

Targeted Mutation Screening and Sequencing

Mutation analysis identifies changes in the coding sequence of a gene of interest, including base pair

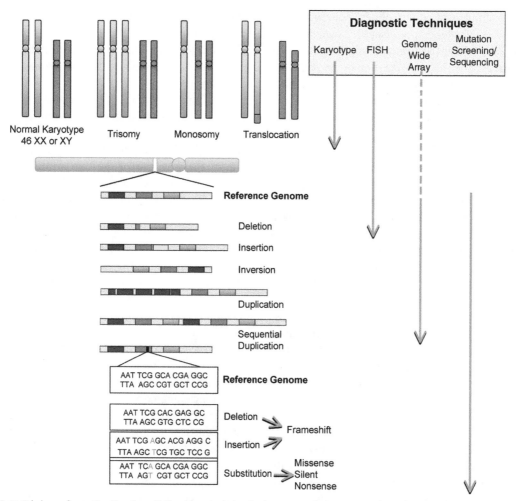

FIGURE 4-6 ■ Echelons of genetic alteration. At the microscopic level, chromosome karyotype can detect large alterations in genetic information including chromosomal aneuploidy and large translocations. Fluorescent in situ hybridization (FISH) can detect chromosomal aneuploidy and large translocations, as well as targeted submicroscopic structural variation (deletions and some noncontiguous duplications). Genome-wide array technology can detect structural variation at a genome-wide level without necessitating probes for targeting screening; arrays cannot detect balanced translocations. Mutation and sequencing will detect down to single base pair alterations in genetic information within targeted genes.

deletions and insertions resulting in frameshift mutations or missense mutations. Nucleotide changes can result in altered amino acid sequences, consequently affecting protein structure. The most common method of detecting mutations is to amplify the gene of interest with PCR and perform sequencing. The sequence is then compared to a reference sequence to detect alterations. Newer methods use array technology to test groups of genes at once. This technique is most helpful when a patient has a phenotype that corresponds to a known single-gene disorder, such as Alagille or Holt-Oram syndrome. Table 4-3 lists some of the common single-gene disorders that cause CHD.

Recurrence Risk

There are a growing number of adults with CHD and families with affected children who wish to reproduce.

Healthcare providers are commonly asked about the risk of having a child or second child with CHD. The recurrence risk of CHD varies based on the type of lesion, the presence of additional affected family members, and the presence of known genetic or syndromic risk factors.

Certain types of CHD exhibit familial recurrence such as left-sided lesions, which can be seen in multiple members of 1 family. In general, in families with 1 affected child, the risk of recurrence in a sibling is estimated to be 3% to 4%. When 2 siblings are affected, this risk increases to 10%. When 1 parent is affected, the risk of having a child with CHD is slightly higher at 4%.[1] These percentages can be higher based on the type of cardiac lesion. For example, recurrence of cardiovascular malformations in a sibling of a child with HLHS has been reported to be as high as 22%.[30] The genetic etiology of CHD is complex: Mendelian transmission is evident with autosomal dominant, autosomal recessive, and X-linked inheritance, but complex traits with non-Mendelian patterns of inheritance are also suspected.

CONCLUSIONS

An increasing body of research demonstrates that genetic and environmental factors contribute to the etiology of CHD in both the syndromic and nonsyndromic child. It is of increasing importance to identify these causes to define, and perhaps decrease, the risk of recurrence in a young family or recurrence in offspring of an affected adult. In addition, identifying the genetic basis will not only answer an important question for the family (Why was my child born with a heart defect?), but may also help identify comorbidities (such as AV block in cases with *NKX2.5* mutations or feeding disorders in patients with 22q11.2 deletion) and assist with risk stratification. Identification of the associated environmental and genetic risks begins with a careful family history and physical examination and requires diligent thought and collaboration with colleagues in clinical genetics. With the increasing complexity of available genetic testing, referral to and/or collaboration with a clinical genetics service becomes of increasing importance. To that end, several centers have started multidisciplinary clinics that combine cardiovascular assessment and genetic testing. The future promises to further define the genetic contribution to these disorders and provide additional insight into etiology, prevention, and variability in clinical outcome.

Clinical Pearls

- CHD is the most common major birth defect, occurring in 1 in 200 live births. Both genetic and environmental risk factors have been identified.
- A thorough examination for commonly associated-dysmorphic features, other congenital anomalies, and genetic syndromes is imperative. The presence of any such findings should prompt referral to a clinical geneticist or cardiovascular genetics clinic for evaluation and genetic testing.
- The etiology of CHD is markedly heterogeneous and not well understood, but an increasing number of genetic tests, including microarray analyses and gene mutation studies, can help pinpoint a genetic basis, the results of which may markedly influence recurrence risk assessments and future management.
- Environmental risk factors for CHD continue to be identified, providing opportunities for primary prevention.

REFERENCES

1. van der Born T, Zomer A, Zwinderman A, Meijboom F, Bouma B, Mulder B. The changing epidemiology of congenital heart disease. *Nat Rev Cardiol.* 2011;8:50-60.
2. Pierpont ME, Basson CT, Benson DW, et al. Genetic basis for congenital heart defects: current knowledge: a scientific statement from the American Heart Association Congenital Cardiac Defects Committee, Council on the Cardiovascular Disease in the Young: endorsed by the American Academy of Pediatrics. *Circulation.* 2007;115:3015-3038.
3. Jenkins K, Correa A, Feinstein J, et al. Noninherited risk factors and congenital cardiovascular defects: current knowledge: a scientific statement from the American Heart Association Council on Cardiovascular Disease in the Young: endorsed by the American Academy of Pediatrics. *Circulation.* 2007;115;2995-3014.
4. Hernandez-Diaz S, Werler M, Walker A, Mitchell A. Folic acid antagonists during pregnancy and the risk of birth defects. *N Engl J Med.* 2000;343:1608-1614.
5. Botto L, Mulinare J, Erickson D. Do multivitamin or folic acid supplements reduce the risk for congenital heart defects? Evidence of gaps. *Am J Med Genet.* 2003;121A: 95-101.
6. Cassidy SB, Allanson JE, eds. *Management of Genetic Syndromes.* 2nd ed. Hoboken, NJ: Wiley; 2005.
7. Pagon RA, Bird TD, Dolan CR, Stephens K, eds. *GeneReviews.* Seattle, WA: University of Washington; 1993.
8. American Academy of Pediatrics. Health supervision for children with Down syndrome. American Academy of Pediatrics. Committee on Genetics. *Pediatrics.* 2001;107:42-49.
9. American Academy of Pediatrics. Health supervision for children with Turner syndrome. American Academy of Pediatrics. Committee on Genetics. *Pediatrics.* 2003;111:692-702.
10. Collins RT, Kaplan P, Somes GW, Rome JJ. Long-term outcomes of patients with cardiovascular abnormalities and Williams syndrome. *Am J Cardiol.* 2010;105:874-878.
11. Wessel A, Gravenhorst V, Buchhorn R, Gosch A, Partsch CJ, Pankau R. Risk of sudden death in the Williams-Beuren syndrome. *Am J Med Genet A.* 2004;127A:234-237.
12. American Academy of Pediatrics. Health supervision for children with Williams syndrome. American Academy of Pediatrics. Committee on Genetics. *Pediatrics.* 2001;107:1192-1204.
13. Goldmuntz E, Lin A. Genetics of congenital heart defects. In: Allen H, Driscoll D, Shaddy R, Feltes T, eds. Moss and Adams' Heart Disease in Infants, *Children and Adolescents.* Philadelphia, PA: Lippincott Williams & Wilkins; 2008:545-572.
14. Kamath B, Spinner N, Emerick K, et al. Vascular anomalies in Alagille syndrome. *Circulation.* 2004;109:1354-1358.
15. Canadas V, Villacosta I, Bruna I, Fuster V. Marfan syndrome. Part 1: pathophysiology and diagnosis. *Nat Rev Cardiol.* 2010;7:256-265.
16. Loeys B, Dietz H, Braverman A, et al. The revised Ghent nosology for the Marfan syndrome. *J Med Genet.* 2010;47:476-485.

17. Hemelrijk C, Renard M, Loeys B. The Loeys-Dietz syndrome: an update for the clinician. *Curr Opin Cardiol.* 2010;25:546-551.

18. Quan L, Smith DW. The VATER association. Vertebral defects, anal atresia, T-E fistula with esophageal atresia, radial and renal dysplasia: a spectrum of associated defects. *J Pediatr.* 1973;82:104-107.

19. Botto LD, Khoury MJ, Mastroiacovo P, et al. The spectrum of congenital anomalies of the VATER association: an international study. *Am J Med Genet.* 1997;71:8-15.

20. Solomon BD, Pineda-Alvarez DE, Raam MS, Cummings DAT. Evidence for inheritance in patients with VACTERL association. *Hum Genet.* 2010;127:731-733.

21. Bergman C, Zerres K, Peschgens T, Senderek J, Hornchen H, Rudnik-Schoneborn S. Overlap between VACTERL and hemifacial microsomia illustrating a spectrum of malformations seen in axial mesodermal dysplasia complex (AMDC). *Am J Med Genet.* 2003;121A:151-155.

22. Kallen K, Mastroiacovo P, Castilla EE, Robert E, Kallen B. VATER non-random association of congenital malformations: study based on data from four malformation registers. *Am J Med Genet.* 2001;101:26-32.

23. Schott J, Benson W, Basson C, et al. Congenital heart disease caused by mutations in the transcription factor NKX2.5. *Science.* 1998;281:108-111.

24. Benson W, Silberbach M, Kavanaugh-McHugh A, et al. Mutations in the cardiac transcription factor NKX2.5 affect diverse cardiac developmental pathways. *J Clin Invest.* 1999;104:1567-1573.

25. Goldmuntz E, Geiger E, Benson W. NKX2.5 mutations in patients with tetralogy of Fallot. *Circulation.* 2001;104:2565-2568.

26. Mack G, Silberbach M. Aortic and pulmonary stenosis. *Pediatr Rev.* 2000;21:79-85.

27. Ward C. Clinical significance of the bicuspid aortic valve. *Heart.* 2000;83:81-85.

28. Duran AC, Frescura C, Sans-Coma V, Angelini A, Basso C, Thiene G. Bicuspid aortic valves in heart with other congenital heart disease. *J Heart Valve Dis.* 1995;4:581-590.

29. Hornberger LK, Sanders SP, Rein A, Spevak PF, Parness IA, Colan SD. Left heart obstructive lesions and left ventricular growth in the midtrimester fetus. A longitudinal study. *Circulation.* 1995;92:1531-1538.

30. Hinton RB, Martin LJ, Tabangin ME, et al. Hypoplastic left heart syndrome is heritable. *J Am Coll Cardiol.* 2007;50:1590-1595.

31. Hinton RB, Maartin LJ, Rame-Gowda S, Tabangin ME, Cripe LH, Benson DW. Hypoplastic left heart syndrome links to chromosomes 10q and 6q and is genetically related to bicuspid aortic valve. *J Am Coll Cardiol.* 2009;53:1065-1071.

32. McBride KL, Zender GA, Fitzgerald-Butt SM, et al. Linkage analysis of left ventricular outflow tract malformations (aortic valve stenosis, coarctation of the aorta, and hypoplastic left heart syndrome). *Eur J Hum Genet.* 2009;17:811-819.

33. Cripe L, Andelfinger G, Martin LJ, Shooner K, Benson DW. Bicuspid aortic valve is heritable. *J Am Coll Cardiol.* 2004;44:138-143.

34. Garg V, Muth AN, Ransom JF, et al. Mutations in NOTCH1 cause aortic valve disease. *Nature.* 2005;437:270-274.

Evaluation and Therapy: Neonatal Critical Heart Disease

Shyam K. Sathanandam,
Stephanie Fuller and
Matthew J. Gillespie

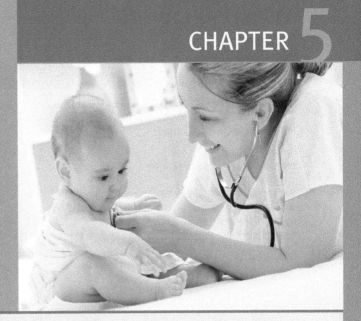

INTRODUCTION

Critical heart disease in the newborn includes all congenital heart lesions that would result in neonatal demise unless immediate intervention is undertaken. It is estimated that congenital heart disease occurs in about 8 per 1000 live births.[1] Not all congenital heart disease (CHD) presents in the newborn period. However, there are a handful of conditions that need immediate management in a newborn infant, the failure of which precludes survival. Roughly 3.5 in 1000 live births have critical CHD.[1] Neonatal critical heart diseases can be broadly described as those that present as severe cyanosis (right heart obstruction) and those that present as shock (left heart obstruction). Table 5-1 lists common conditions in both categories. The common denominator to all critical heart diseases presenting in the neonatal period is that they need a patent ductus arteriosus for survival until further palliative procedures can be undertaken. To understand the physiology of these lesions, it is important to have knowledge of the circulatory changes that happen right after birth.

Fetal Circulation

Blood oxygenated in the placenta is returned by way of the umbilical veins. Most of the umbilical venous blood shunts through the ductus venosus to the inferior vena cava (IVC), which provides a low-resistance bypass.[2] The IVC blood is composed of streams of hepatic venous blood, umbilical venous blood, and blood from lower extremities. The stream of umbilical venous blood selectively enters the left atrium, though the foramen ovale guided by the eustachian valve. The left ventricle (LV) pumps out this blood into the ascending aorta for distribution to the coronaries, head, and upper extremities.[2] The superior vena caval stream and rest of the IVC blood pass into the right ventricle (RV). The RV pumps out this blood into the pulmonary trunk. A small amount of this blood enters the pulmonary circulation, and the rest passes through the ductus arteriosus into the descending aorta and finally reaches the placenta via the umbilical arteries. Figure 5-1 shows the key elements of fetal circulation. The main differences between fetal circulation and postnatal circulation consist of the following:

- Placental circulation provides gas exchange for the fetus
- Absence of gas exchange in the collapsed lungs; this results in very little flow of blood to the lungs
- Presence of a ductus venosus providing a low-resistance bypass for umbilical venous blood to reach the IVC
- Widely open foramen ovale to provide a route to the oxygenated blood to reach the left atrium
- Widely open ductus arteriosus to allow RV blood to reach descending aorta

Circulatory Changes After Birth

After birth, the lungs expand and provide oxygenation of blood. The increased flow of blood to the pulmonary artery passing though the lungs and reaching the left atrium increases the left atrial pressure. The effect of this is that the septum primum approximates with the septum secundum and the foramen ovale closes functionally. Clamping of the cord increases the systemic vascular resistance (SVR). Thus, the systemic pressure increases, while the pulmonary artery pressure falls due to lowering of the pulmonary vascular resistance.[2] As a result, flow of blood though the ductus arteriosus reverses. Instead of blood flowing from the pulmonary artery to the aorta, as in the fetus, the blood flows from aorta to pulmonary

Common Neonatal Critical Congenital Heart Diseases (CHD)

CHD Presenting with Cyanosis	CHD Presenting with Shock
Tetralogy of Fallot (TOF)	Critical aortic stenosis
Dextro-transposition of great arteries (d-TGA)	Coarctation of aorta
Tricuspid atresia	Interrupted aortic arch
Total anomalous pulmonary venous connection (TAPVC)	Hypoplastic left heart syndrome (HLHS)
Pulmonary atresia with intact ventricular septum (PAIVS)	
Critical pulmonary stenosis	

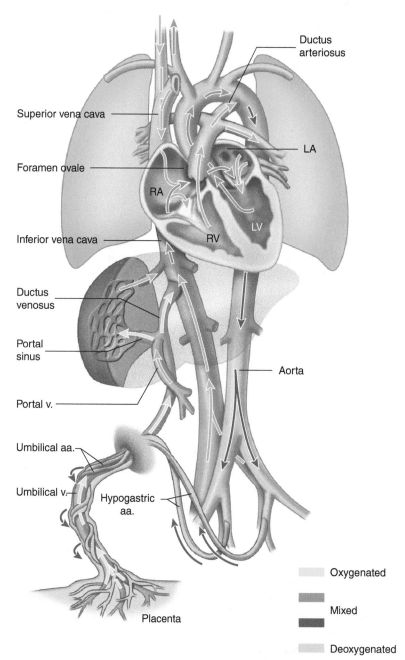

FIGURE 5-1 ■ Diagram of fetal circulation showing 4 sites of shunt: placenta, ductus venosus, foramen ovale, and ductus arteriosus. aa, artery; LA, left atrium; LV, left ventricle; RA, right atrium; RV, right ventricle; v, vein. (*Reproduced, with permission, from Cunningham FG, Leveno KJ, Bloom SL, Hauth JC, Rouse DJ, Spong CY. Williams Obstetrics. 23rd ed. New York, NY: McGraw-Hill; 2010.*)

artery. The ductus arteriosus constricts and closes off. The pulmonary and systemic circulations thus separate from each other soon after birth.

GENERAL PRINCIPLES OF MANAGEMENT OF NEWBORN WITH CRITICAL HEART DISEASE

Outcome of a newborn with critical CHD ultimately depends on the timely assessment and accurate diagnosis of the underlying defect, as well as the prompt evaluation of potential secondary end-organ damage. Fetal ultrasound has become a vital tool in prenatal diagnosis of critical CHD. Prenatal diagnosis avoids hemodynamic compromise that is frequently seen following postnatal diagnosis.[3,4]

In general, lesions that mandate delivery near a pediatric tertiary cardiac care center include (1) those that require immediate surgery or cardiac catheterization, (2) those that require ductal patency for cardiac output, and (3) those that require ductal patency for pulmonary blood flow.

Spontaneous delivery close to full term is generally recommended. Delivery room resuscitation should follow general guidelines for neonatal resuscitation. Airway should be stabilized. Vascular access should be obtained by placement of umbilical venous and arterial catheterization. Metabolic abnormalities and hypovolemia should be corrected. Inotropic agents and prostaglandin should be available and administered when indicated. Oxygen should be used with caution, particularly in those with single-ventricle physiology. Oxygen is a potent pulmonary vasodilator and will cause pulmonary overcirculation at the expense of systemic circulation. Conversely, oxygen should be administered when a cyanotic right-sided obstructive lesion is suspected or when there is concurrent lung disease. In general, arterial oxygen saturations should be maintained between 80% and 85%, which in a neonate with single-ventricle physiology and good cardiac output translates to a balanced circulation.

Once the neonate is resuscitated and stabilized, a thorough evaluation is warranted. Although there are numerous cardiac lesions, there are many similarities in their clinical presentation. Signs and symptoms include cyanosis, discrepant pulses, signs of congestive heart failure, and cardiogenic shock. The initial evaluation of a newborn with suspected critical CHD includes a thorough physical examination, 4-extremity blood pressure, preductal and postductal saturation, a chest radiograph (Figure 5-2), electrocardiogram, hyperoxia test, and an echocardiogram. Features particular to individual lesions will be discussed in detail later in this chapter.

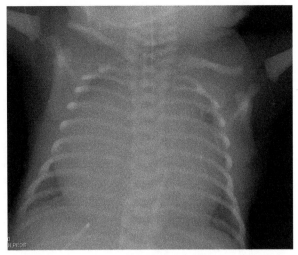

FIGURE 5-2 ■ Chest radiograph of a newborn who developed cyanosis soon after birth. The radiograph demonstrates severe cardiomegaly, which is seen with Ebstein anomaly. Sometimes a chest radiograph gives clues to the diagnosis.

Once the diagnosis is made, attention should continue to focus on the basic principles of neonatal life support and maintenance of a patent ductus arteriosus. Airway must be stabilized, vascular access must be secured, volume status and inotropic support must be maintained, and systemic and pulmonary circulations must be balanced. Prostaglandin E_1 (PGE_1) is administered in nearly all cases of critical CHD. When administration of PGE_1 does not improve the clinical condition, total anomalous pulmonary venous return with obstruction, hypoplastic left heart syndrome with an intact atrial septum, or transposition of great arteries with restrictive atrial communication should be suspected, and urgent catheterization or surgical intervention is indicated.

For most neonates with critical CHD whose ductal patency is maintained with PGE_1, attention to balancing pulmonary (Qp) and systemic circulation (Qs) is essential.[5] This is particularly important for patients with single-ventricle physiology and complete intracardiac mixing of systemic and pulmonary venous return. In this situation, the relative resistances to flow govern the ratio of distribution of flow between the systemic and pulmonary circuits. Resistance to Qp is encountered by subvalvar or valvar pulmonary stenosis, pulmonary vascular resistance (PVR), and elevated pulmonary venous and left atrial pressures. Resistance to Qs likewise occurs by subvalvar or valvar aortic stenosis, aortic arch hypoplasia or coarctation, and SVR. The management goal of patients with single-ventricle physiology is to provide adequate pulmonary blood flow without compromising systemic oxygen delivery and tissue perfusion.

Using the Fick equation:

$$Qp : Qs = \frac{SaO_2 - SvO_2}{SpvO_2 - SpaO_2}$$

Strategies to Balance Qp:Qs

Qp:Qs			
Increased Qp:Qs		Decreased Qp:Qs	
Increased SVR	Decreased SVR	Increased PVR	Decreased PVR
Epinephrine, high-dose dopamine	Oxygen, hyperventilation, alkalosis, nitric oxide	Hypoxia, hypercarbia, hypoventilation, acidosis	Milrinone, dobutamine
Unrestrictive interatrial communication		Restrictive interatrial communication	

NOTE. The balance between pulmonary and systemic circulation (Qp:Qs) is dependent on the relative resistances between systemic (SVR) and pulmonary vasculature (PVR).

Ideally in patients with good cardiac output, with a mixed venous oxygen saturation (SvO_2) of 60% and no lung pathology and thus a pulmonary vein oxygen saturation ($SpvO_2$) of 100%, a systemic arterial oxygen saturation (SaO_2) of 80% would represent a Qp:Qs ratio of 1:1, because pulmonary artery saturation ($SpaO_2$) is the same as SaO_2 because of complete mixing. An SaO_2 of 90% may lead to an SvO_2 of 70% and a Qp:Qs of 2:1. An SaO_2 of 70% and SvO_2 of 50% will result in a Qp:QS of 0.66:1.

Neonates with unbalanced physiology can be broadly categorized as (1) those with inadequate Qp resulting in hypoxemia and (2) those with excessive Qp resulting in systemic hypoperfusion. Inadequate Qp results from increased PVR. Hence, to increase Qp, the underlying cause of diminished Qp should be identified. For example, patients with hypoplastic left heart spectrum hypoxemia because of restrictive interatrial communication should undergo transcatheter or surgical septostomy. Excessive Qp leads to hypotension, acidosis, and decreased tissue perfusion. It can result from either increased SVR or diminished PVR. Elevated SVR can be a result of increased exogenous catecholamines or secondary to exogenous vasoactive agents. Table 5-2 summarizes strategies to balance Qp:Qs.

NEONATES PRESENTING WITH CYANOSIS

Cyanosis results from right-to-left shunting of blood. It is invariably due to some degree of right heart obstruction. Consequently, the venous blood has no outlet and has to mix with the arterial blood across either an interatrial communication (atrial septal defect [ASD]) or interventricular communication (ventricular septal defect [VSD]). In the fetal life, the venous blood shunts across an ASD or a VSD to get to the aorta. Depending on the degree of right heart obstruction, there may be little flow from the pulmonary artery to the aorta across a patent ductus arteriosus (PDA) to even reversal of flow from the aorta to the pulmonary artery. This may be the first clue on a fetal ultrasound for suspicion of a cyanotic heart disease. Soon after birth, the lung is the organ where gas exchange takes place. Hence, the entire cardiac output needs to go to the lungs. However, with right heart obstruction, this is not feasible unless there is a PDA. If not diagnosed prenatally or early after birth, these infants could develop severe cyanosis due to decreased, effective pulmonary blood flow. Hence, they require prostaglandin infusion to keep ductal patency. The common cyanotic heart diseases are listed in Table 5-1. We will now discuss each heart disease in detail.

Tetralogy of Fallot

The classic example of cyanotic patients with pulmonic stenosis is tetralogy of Fallot (TOF). It is the most common cyanotic CHD. TOF occurs in 7% of all CHDs.[6] Anatomically, TOF consists of:

■ VSD
■ Pulmonic stenosis or pulmonary atresia
■ Overriding aorta
■ Right ventricular hypertrophy

Hemodynamics

Physiologically, pulmonic stenosis causes concentric right ventricular hypertrophy without cardiac enlargement. Once the right and left ventricular pressures have become identical, increasing severity of pulmonic stenosis reduces the flow of blood into the pulmonary artery and increases the right-to-left shunt. The VSD is silent, but the pulmonic stenosis produces a systolic ejection murmur. The severity of cyanosis is directly proportional to the severity of pulmonic stenosis, but the intensity of the systolic murmur is inversely related to the severity of pulmonic stenosis. The P_2 component of S_2 is soft and generally inaudible.

Neonates and infants with TOF may develop hypoxic spells. Hypoxic or hypercyanotic spells are also commonly referred to as "Tet spells." Tet spells occur predominantly after waking up or following exertion.[7] They are characterized by a period of uncontrollable crying, rapid and deep breathing (hyperpnea), deepening of cyanosis, limpness or convulsions, and occasionally death. Events such as crying lower the SVR, increase the right-to-left shunt, and initiate the spell by establishing a vicious cycle of hypoxic spells. The fall in arterial PO_2, in addition to an increase in PCO_2 and a fall in pH, stimulates the respiratory center and produces hyperpnea, which increases the negative intrathoracic pressure and increases the systemic venous return to the RV.

Clinical features

Patients with TOF may become symptomatic anytime after birth. The degree of obstruction determines the severity of cyanosis. Electrocardiogram (ECG) in TOF shows a right axis deviation with RV hypertrophy. The chest radiograph shows a normal-sized heart with upturned apex suggestive of RV hypertrophy (Figure 5-3). The absence of main pulmonary artery segment gives it the shape described as "coeur-en-sabot" or boot-shaped heart. The pulmonary fields are oligemic.

Critical care management

Neonates with TOF should be monitored in the neonatal intensive care unit. The degree of cyanosis is determined by the degree of pulmonary blood flow. PGE_1 infusion is generally not required. However, as the duct starts occluding, the extent of RV outflow obstruction becomes apparent. Severely cyanotic infants need to be started on PGE_1 infusion to maintain ductal patency for adequate pulmonary blood flow.

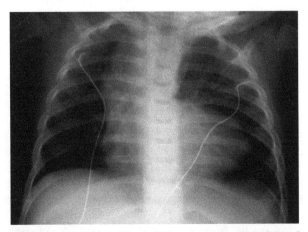

FIGURE 5-3 ■ Chest radiograph from a newborn with tetralogy of Fallot. It shows a normal-sized heart with upturned apex suggestive of right ventricular hypertrophy. The absence of main pulmonary artery segment gives it the shape described as "coeur-en-sabot" or boot-shaped heart. The pulmonary fields are oligemic.

Hypoxic spells of TOF require immediate recognition and appropriate treatment, because they can cause serious central nervous system complications. Treatment of hypoxic spell strives to break the vicious cycle. The infant should be picked up and held in a knee–chest position. Morphine sulfate 0.2 mg/kg subcutaneously or intramuscularly suppresses the respiratory center and abolishes hyperpnea. Alternatively, ketamine 2 mg/kg intravenously (IV) works by increasing the SVR and sedates the infant. Oxygen can be administered, but it has little demonstrable effect on arterial oxygen saturation. Acidosis stimulates the respiratory center causing hyperpnea. Hence, it should be aggressively corrected. Vasoconstrictors, such as phenylephrine 0.02 mg/kg IV, increase SVR and may break the spell. β-Blockers such as propranolol (0.1 mg/kg) or esmolol administered IV reduce the heart rate and may reverse the spell.

Neonatal interventions

Neonates with TOF who are duct dependent or having hypercyanotic spells require some form of intervention before full repair. Balloon dilatation/stent implantation of the RV outflow tract and pulmonary valve, although not widely practiced, has been attempted to delay repair for several months.[8,9] Stent implantation of the ductus arteriosus has also been attempted to allow adequate pulmonary blood flow. Stenting of the ductus arteriosus allows for discontinuation of PGE_1 and discharge from the intensive care unit (ICU). This will buy time for nutrition and growth and ultimately a complete repair.

Surgical palliative shunt procedures may be warranted in the neonate for similar indications (eg, TOF with pulmonary atresia, TOF with severely hypoplastic pulmonary artery, severely cyanotic neonate, or medically unmanageable hypoxic spells). Typically a Gore-Tex interposition shunt is placed between the subclavian artery and the ipsilateral pulmonary artery via a lateral thoracotomy (Figure 5-4A). The operative mortality rate is 1% or less.

Neonatal surgical repair

Total repair of TOF is carried out under cardiopulmonary bypass and circulatory arrest. The procedure includes patch closure of the VSD, resection of infundibular tissue, and placement of a transannular patch (Figure 5-4B). The mortality rate is 2% to 3%.[10-12]

Postoperative critical care management

Most patients can be extubated in the operating room or soon after surgery. Bleeding could be a problem during the postoperative period especially in polycythemic patients. Right bundle-branch block caused by the right ventriculotomy occurs in over 90% of patients and is well tolerated. Complete heart block occurs in less than 1% of patients.[10-12] Junctional ectopic tachycardia and

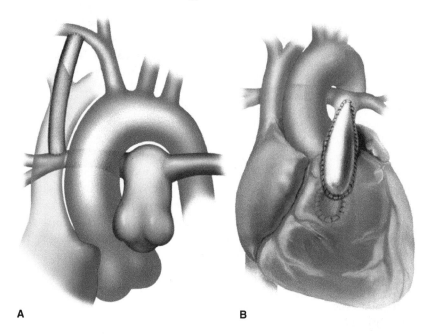

A   **B**

FIGURE 5-4 ■ **A.** Picture illustrating a modified right Blalock-Taussig shunt. It involves placement of an extended polytetrafluoroethylene shunt between the innominate artery and the right pulmonary artery. **B.** Picture illustrating a complete repair of tetralogy of Fallot with ventricular septal defect patch closure, resection of right ventricle muscle bundle, and a transannular patch. (*Reproduced, with permission, from McDonald RW.* Ped US Today. *2008;13:161-228. Copyright © Chrestomathis Press Inc., All rights reserved.*)

ventricular arrhythmia occur in 2% to 5% of postoperative patients.[10-12]

Pulmonary Atresia with Intact Ventricular Septum

Pulmonary atresia with intact ventricular septum (PAIVS) is a rare CHD, accounting for 1% of all CHDs. The pulmonary valve is atretic and is replaced by a membrane. However, the pulmonary artery trunk and branch pulmonary arteries are usually well developed. The size of the tricuspid valve and the RV varies and relates to survival.[13,14] When all 3 portions of the RV are present, the tricuspid valve and the RV are almost of normal size. This is called the tripartite type of pulmonary atresia, because all portions of the RV (the inlet, tubercular, and infundibular portions) are present. In this chapter, we discuss only this variant of PAIVS. Because there is no outlet to the right heart, an interatrial communication (ASD or patent foramen ovale [PFO]) is obligatory. The mixed blood from the left heart is pumped out to the aorta, and a PDA is necessary for survival after birth.

Clinical features

The neonate is severely cyanotic and may have mild respiratory distress. The physical examination reveals a single second heart sound with a faint pansystolic murmur caused by tricuspid valve regurgitation. The chest radiograph demonstrates mild cardiomegaly with decreased pulmonary vascular markings. The ECG demonstrates a normal axis with decreased right-sided forces. Echocardiography is diagnostic. It will reveal the atretic, nonmobile pulmonary valve, with no flow of blood across it. The RV cavity is usually smaller than

normal and hypertrophied. There is right-to-left shunt across the interatrial communication and left-to-right shunt across the PDA.

Critical care management

Neonates with PAIVS are dependent on a PDA for pulmonary circulation. Hence, PGE_1 infusion should be started right after birth if there was a prenatal diagnosis or immediately after the diagnosis is suspected or confirmed. Neonates with PAIVS usually require a catheter or surgical intervention soon after birth. Hence, they are typically not fed until then.

Neonatal catheter intervention

Routine cardiac catheterization and angiocardiography are undertaken in almost all neonates born with PAIVS. Angiocardiography will demonstrate the presence or absence of coronary sinusoids[15] from the RV and whether the coronary flow is dependent on the RV (Figure 5-5).

The determination of either the presence or absence of RV-dependent coronary sinusoids[15] is critical in the management of these patients. If the RV, pulmonary artery, and tricuspid valve are determined to be of adequate size that will allow a future biventricular repair and if there are no RV-dependent coronary sinusoids, then radiofrequency-assisted valvotomy and balloon dilatation can be performed (Figure 5-6).

There is usually a plate-like membrane that separates the RV from the pulmonary artery.[16] A radiofrequency tipped wire is used to perforate through this membrane followed by balloon dilatation of this valvotomy site to establish patency between the RV outflow tract to the pulmonary artery. After this procedure, the

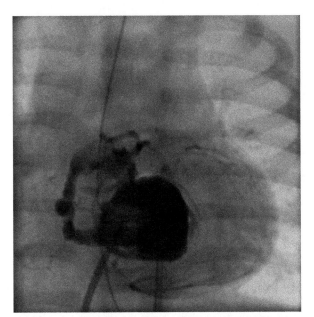

FIGURE 5-5 ■ Right ventriculogram in a patient with pulmonary atresia with intact ventricular septum showing multiple dilated fistulous connections from the right ventricle to the coronary arteries.

baby is taken back to the ICU and PGE₁ is discontinued. In approximately 50% of those who undergo this procedure, there is no need for further palliation at this point.[17,18] The other 50% of patients still do not have adequate pulmonary blood flow and need further palliation to establish pulmonary blood flow. One such palliation could be stenting of the PDA in the catheterization lab.

Surgical palliation in the neonatal period

There are several surgical palliative procedures that are available for neonates with an adequately sized tricuspid valve and RV. One approach would be to perform a closed surgical valvotomy without cardiopulmonary bypass plus a modified Blalock-Taussig shunt (Figure 5-4A).

Another approach involves placement of a transannular RV outflow patch (Figure 5-4B) and a Blalock-Taussig shunt under cardiopulmonary bypass. These procedures are palliative, allowing the neonate to grow after being discharged from the hospital. They will require a definitive biventricular repair in the future.[17,18]

When the RV or tricuspid valve is small and will not allow for a future biventricular repair, then a Blalock-Taussig shunt without the RV outflow patch is performed. A Fontan operation is performed at a later time. Postoperative critical care management of neonates after a palliative surgical procedure is similar to that described for TOF.

Dextro-Transposition of Great Arteries

Dextro-transposition of the great arteries (d-TGA) is defined as the aorta arising from the RV and the pulmonary artery arising from the LV. It account for about 5% of all CHD. It is more prevalent in males than females (3:1).[19]

Hemodynamics

In complete d-TGA, the aorta lays anterior and to the right of the pulmonary artery and carries desaturated blood from the RV to the body, and the pulmonary artery arises posteriorly from the LV and carries oxygenated blood to the lungs (Figure 5-7).

Because the systemic and pulmonary circulations are separate, survival depends on the presence of atrial, ventricular, or aortopulmonary (PDA) communications. Complete d-TGA is classified as (1) with intact ventricular septum or (2) with VSD. The latter group is further subdivided into cases with or without pulmonic stenosis. The physiology of d-TGA with VSD and pulmonic stenosis is similar to TOF.[20] In this section, we will only discuss patients with TGA with intact ventricular septum.

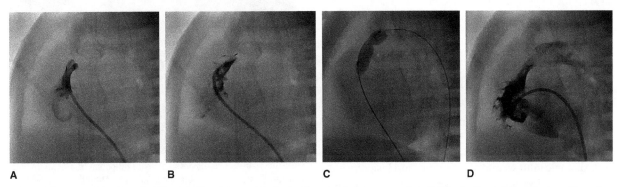

A B C D

FIGURE 5-6 ■ A. Injection of contrast in the right ventricular outflow tract shows no communication to the pulmonary artery. There is a plate-like atresia of the pulmonary valve. B. Radiofrequency (RF) perforation of the pulmonary valve. The tip of the RF wire can be seen to cross through the atretic pulmonary valve into the main pulmonary artery. C. Balloon valvuloplasty of the pulmonary valve over a wire that has now been passed across the perforation made in the pulmonary valve. D. Right ventriculogram after intervention shows contrast to fill the main pulmonary artery through the pulmonary valve.

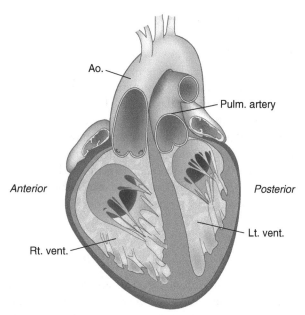

FIGURE 5-7 ■ Diagram representing dextro-transposition of the great arteries showing the aorta arising from the right ventricle and the pulmonary artery arising from the left ventricle. (*Reproduced, with permission, from Fyler DC, ed. Nadas' Pediatric Cardiology. Philadelphia, PA: Hanley & Belfus; 1992.*)

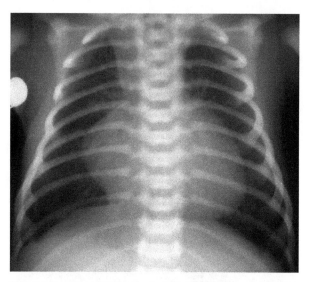

FIGURE 5-8 ■ Chest radiograph of a newborn with dextro-transposition of the great arteries shows a narrow superior mediastinum because of the anteroposterior relationship of the aorta and the pulmonary artery giving an "egg on string" appearance.

In patients with d-TGA, the oxygenated pulmonary venous blood recirculates in the lungs, whereas the systemic venous blood recirculates in the systemic circulation.[19] Survival depends on the mixing available between the 2 circulations. In patients with intact ventricular septum, the mixing site is the atrial communication. Generally, the atrial communication is the PFO, and being small, the mixing is poor. The neonates will become symptomatic due to severe hypoxemia and systemic acidosis. As the PVR falls, the PDA shunts from aorta to pulmonary artery and does not serve as a site for mixing. The extra pulmonary blood flow across the PDA returns to the left atrium and shunts across the PFO to mix at the atrial level provided the atrial communication is unrestrictive.[19] Hence, it is generally a good idea to keep the PDA open with infusion of PGE$_1$.

Clinical features

Neonates with d-TGA are cyanotic at birth. If undiagnosed, the neonate presents with rapid breathing and congestive heart failure within the first week of life. If the interatrial communication results in poor mixing, the neonate continues to remain severely cyanotic. Physical examination shows severe cyanosis with or without signs of congestive heart failure, normal first heart sound, single loud second heart sound, and insignificant grade 1 to 2 ejection systolic murmur. The ECG shows right axis deviation and RV hypertrophy. The chest radiograph shows cardiomegaly with a narrow base and plethoric lung fields. The cardiac silhouette has an "egg on side" appearance (Figure 5-8).

Two-dimensional echocardiography and color flow Doppler studies usually are diagnostic (Figure 5-9). Careful assessment of the size of the interatrial communication will help in the management of neonates with severe cyanosis. Coronary artery anatomy is quite variable and can usually be sorted out by echocardiography. Associated defects such as a VSD, LV outflow tract obstruction, or pulmonary valve stenosis can be evaluated. Rarely, a coarctation of aorta (COA) occurs with d-TGA.

Progressive hypoxia and acidosis could lead to death unless the mixing of systemic and pulmonary

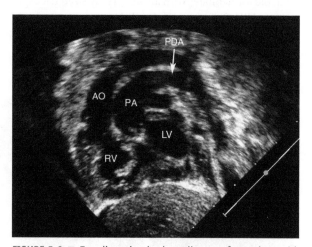

FIGURE 5-9 ■ Two-dimensional echocardiogram of a newborn with dextro-transposition of the great arteries. The aorta can be seen arising from the right ventricle and the pulmonary artery from the left ventricle. AO, aorta; LV, left ventricle; PA, pulmonary artery; PDA, patent ductus arteriosus; RV, right ventricle. (*Reproduced, with permission, from Fuster V, Walsh RA, Harrington RA. Hurst's the Heart'. 13th ed. New York, NY: McGraw-Hill; 2011.*)

blood improves. There is a higher tendency to develop pulmonary vascular obstructive disease at an earlier age especially with associated VSD or PDA than with acyanotic heart defects with left-to-right shunt, making surgical repair necessary during early infancy. Cerebrovascular accidents have been reported in neonates with d-TGA before repair with or without balloon atrial septostomy.[21]

Critical care management

Metabolic acidosis, hypoglycemia, and hypocalcemia should be treated. PGE$_1$ infusion may improve oxygen saturation slightly until preparation for a balloon atrial septostomy is made in severely cyanotic infants. Oxygen administration may lower PVR and increase pulmonary blood flow and may improve oxygenation. Congestive heart failure can be treated with diuretics and digoxin.

Neonatal intervention

Balloon atrial septostomy, called the Rashkind procedure, is often needed for severely cyanotic neonates to improve atrial-level mixing. The procedure could be carried out on the bedside under echocardiography guidance or in the catheterization laboratory under fluoroscopic and echocardiographic monitoring. A balloon-tipped catheter is advanced into the left atrium through the PFO. The balloon is inflated with diluted radiopaque dye and rapidly withdrawn to the right atrium (Figure 5-10). This can be repeated again to create a large defect in the atrial septum. Rarely in older infants, the balloon atrial septostomy may not be successful, and a blade atrial septostomy may be preferred.

Neonatal surgical repair

The arterial switch operation performed shortly after birth (before 2 weeks of age) has become the standard surgical procedure for d-TGA with intact ventricular septum. The aorta is transected slightly above the coronary ostia, and the pulmonary artery is also transected at about the same level. Both coronary arteries are removed from the aorta with triangular buttons. Triangular buttons of similar size are made at the proper position in the pulmonary artery trunk. The coronary arteries are transplanted to the pulmonary artery trunk. The ascending aorta is brought behind the pulmonary artery and connected to the proximal pulmonary artery to form a neo-aorta (Figure 5-11).

Postoperative critical care management

The mortality rate for the arterial switch operation ranges between 1% and 2%. The success of the procedure depends on the timing of the procedure and presence of associated lesions. Common complications in the immediate postoperative period include ventricular dysfunction[22,23] and dysrhythmias. Neonates who develop ventricular dysfunction require careful evaluation for coronary artery stenosis including sometimes a coronary angiography. Most children could be extubated the same day or the following day after the operation. The usual postoperative recovery period is about 1 week.

Total Anomalous Pulmonary Venous Connection

Total anomalous pulmonary venous connection (TAPVC) is an uncommon cyanotic congenital anomaly constituting less than 1% of CHD, with a 4:1 male preponderance.[24] All of the pulmonary veins, instead of joining the left atrium, are connected anomalously to result in the total pulmonary venous blood reaching the right atrium. TAPVC is classified anatomically as supracardiac, cardiac, infracardiac, and mixed varieties. In supracardiac TAPVC, the pulmonary veins join together to form a common pulmonary vein, which may drain into the innominate vein or the right superior vena cava. In cardiac TAPVC, the veins join the coronary sinus or

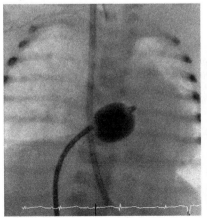
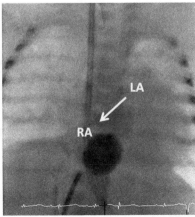

A   B

FIGURE 5-10 ■ Balloon atrial septostomy in a newborn with dextro-transposition of the great arteries and restrictive interatrial communication. The balloon is inflated in the left atrium and rapidly pulled across the septum to create an adequate-size communication. LA, left atrium; RA, right atrium.

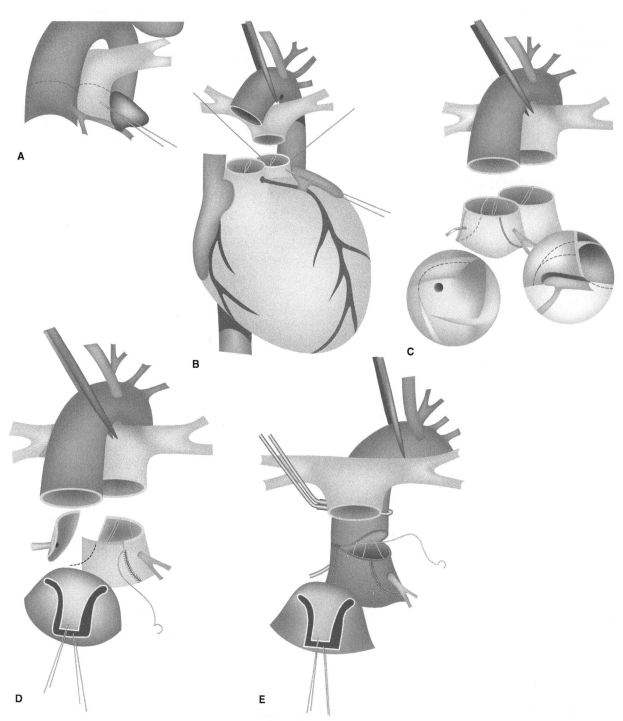

FIGURE 5-11 ■ Arterial switch operation. **A.** The dotted lines indicate the incision sites on the aorta and the pulmonary artery. **B.** The aorta and the pulmonary arteries are incised and switched positions. **C.** The dotted lines indicate the sites of harvesting the coronary buttons from the native aortic root. **D.** The coronary buttons are transferred to the neoaortic root (native pulmonary root) posteriorly and sutured. **E.** The aorta and pulmonary arteries are switched and sutured. (*Modified, with permission, from Castaneda AR. Anatomic correction of transposition of the great arteries at the arterial level. In: Sabiston DC Jr, Spencer FC, eds. Surgery of the Chest. 5th ed. Philadelphia, PA: WB Saunders; 1990.*)

enter the right atrium directly. In infracardiac TAPVC, the common pulmonary vein drains into the ductus venosus or the portal or hepatic veins.

Hemodynamics

TAPVC results in the pulmonary venous blood reaching the right atrium, which also receives systemic venous blood. This results in almost complete mixing of the 2 venous returns. The blood flow to the left atrium is the right-to-left shunt through a PFO or ASD. The oxygen saturation of the blood in the pulmonary artery is higher or identical to that in the aorta because of mixing of the blood in the right atrium. Physiologically TAPVC can be divided into (1) patients with pulmonary venous obstruction, which results in pulmonary arterial hypertension as well as restriction to pulmonary blood flow; and (2) patients without pulmonary venous obstruction, where there is increased pulmonary blood flow and consequently congestive heart failure. TAPVC of the infracardiac type is nearly always obstructive, whereas the cardiac and supracardiac types may or may not have pulmonary venous obstruction. Generally the left atrium and ventricle are of normal size or can be small. In this section, we discuss TAPVC with obstruction because it presents in the newborn period.

Clinical features

Patients with obstructive type of TAPVC present with marked cyanosis, respiratory distress, and shock. Because there is obstruction to pulmonary venous return, the lungs are congested, which causes difficulty in oxygenation and ventilation.

The physical findings consist of a normal-sized heart with parasternal heave, normal first heart sound, normally or widely split second sound with accentuated pulmonic component, and insignificant murmurs. Right-sided fourth heart sound is audible. Tricuspid regurgitation occurs and results in cardiomegaly.

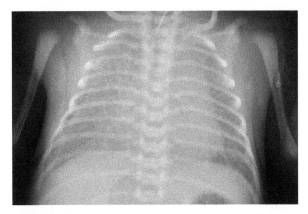

FIGURE 5-12 ■ Chest radiograph of a newborn with obstructed total anomalous pulmonary venous connection showing "ground glass" appearance secondary to pulmonary venous congestion.

The ECG in TAPVC shows right axis deviation and RV hypertrophy. The characteristic chest radiograph of obstructive TAPVC consists of a normal-sized heart with severe pulmonary venous congestion resulting in a "ground glass" appearance of the lungs (Figure 5-12). Two-dimensional echocardiography with color Doppler could demonstrate the abnormal course of the pulmonary veins. However, it may be difficult to confirm the diagnosis by echocardiography alone, and cardiac catheterization with angiography may be necessary to determine the correct diagnosis (Figure 5-13).

Critical care management

It is crucial to have a high level suspicion to diagnose this entity. Once the diagnosis is made, every effort should be taken to stabilize the critically ill neonate. It is not uncommon for these neonates to require mechanical ventilation, oxygen, and inhaled nitric oxide.

Acidosis should be corrected. Rarely, in extreme cases that do not respond to conventional therapy, the

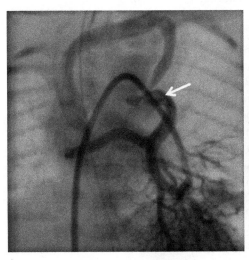
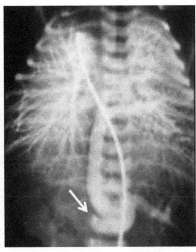

A   B

FIGURE 5-13 ■ Angiography of newborn with obstructed total anomalous pulmonary venous connection (TAPVC). **A.** Obstructed supracardiac type of TAPVC. The arrow points to the level of obstruction. **B.** Obstructed infracardiac type of TAPVC. The arrow points to the level of obstruction.

neonate may require extracorporeal membrane oxygenation support. The congenital heart surgeon should be contacted for early operative intervention. PGE$_1$ infusion may sometimes be used to keep the ductus arteriosus open in order to allow for decompression of the pulmonary circulation and provide for systemic cardiac output because the PDA shunts from right to left.

Neonatal surgical repair

For obstructive TAPVC, surgical management is superior to medical management. There are no palliative procedures for this condition. All neonates with pulmonary venous obstruction should be operated upon as soon as the diagnosis is confirmed. There are several different operations available for this condition. All procedures are intended to redirect the pulmonary venous return to the left atrium.

Postoperative critical care management

The surgical mortality rate is between 5% and 10%. The rate can be as high as 20% for infants who go into surgery in a state of shock.[25] The 2 common causes of death are postoperative paroxysms of pulmonary hypertension and the development of pulmonary vein stenosis. Paroxysms of pulmonary hypertension, which relate to a small and poorly compliant left heart with resultant heart failure and pulmonary edema, may require prolonged respiratory support postoperatively.

Atrial arrhythmias are not uncommon in the immediate postoperative state. Obstruction at the site of anastomosis or pulmonary vein stenosis is usually not seen in the immediate postoperative period but can sometimes happen quite early after the operation.

Tricuspid Atresia

Congenital absence of the tricuspid valve is called tricuspid atresia. The RV is hypoplastic. It constitutes approximately 3% of all CHDs.[26]

Hemodynamics

Atresia of the tricuspid value results in the absence of a communication between the right atrium and the RV. The RV is underdeveloped, the inflow portion being absent. The only exit for the systemic venous blood coming to the right atrium is by way of the PFO or an ASD. There is complete mixing of the systemic venous and pulmonary venous blood in the left atrium from where the blood passes to the LV. A VSD provides communication between the LV and the outflow portion of the RV. The great vessels are normally related in 70% of cases, whereas in 30% of patients, the vessels are transposed. Therefore, the LV maintains both the systemic and the pulmonary circulation. The physiology is that of any other single ventricle, wherein the saturation of blood

in the pulmonary artery and the aorta is identical. The size of the VSD and the presence of subpulmonic stenosis determine the amount of pulmonary blood flow and the type of initial palliation.

Clinical features

The clinical presentation depends on the state of pulmonary flow, which may be increased or decreased. Clinically, patients with diminished pulmonary blood flow have symptoms and physical signs more or less identical to Fallot's tetralogy. The ECG is characterized by left axis deviation and LV hypertrophy. The mean QRS axis is approximately −45 degrees. The P waves may show both right and left atrial enlargement (Figure 5-14). The chest radiograph suggests LV configuration of the cardiac silhouette. Prominent superior vena cava shadow is present. The lungs are oligemic. Echocardiogram identified a large LV cavity. The atretic tricuspid valve can be recognized in the 4-chamber view. The size of the VSD, presence of subpulmonic stenosis, and the great vessel relationship can also be established by echocardiography.

Critical care management

Neonates with decreased pulmonary blood flow either because of a restrictive VSD or pulmonic stenosis are severely cyanotic. PGE$_1$ infusion should be started to maintain the patency of the ductus arteriosus before planned surgical shunt placement or cardiac catheterization and stenting of the ductus. A balloon atrial septostomy is rarely needed to improve right atrium–left atrium shunt, because the interatrial communication is usually adequate. Neonates with adequate pulmonary blood flow rarely develop congestive heart failure. When the great arteries are normally related and there is adequate pulmonary blood flow through a VSD, no palliative procedure is required in the newborn period. Patients need to be closely watched for decreased oxygen saturation resulting from reduction in the size of the VSD.

Neonatal surgical palliation

Neonates with decreased pulmonary blood flow need a systemic to pulmonary artery shunt as the initial palliation. Rarely, older infants with cyanosis could have a bidirectional superior cavopulmonary anastomosis. This procedure helps to increase the oxygen saturation without adding volume load to the LV. Pulmonary artery banding is rarely necessary for infants with congestive heart failure. The Damus-Kaye-Stansel procedure and shunt operation are performed for neonates with d-TGA and restrictive VSD. In this operation, the main pulmonary artery is transected, and the pulmonary artery stump is sewn over. The proximal pulmonary artery is connected end to side to the ascending aorta, and a systemic–pulmonary artery shunt is created

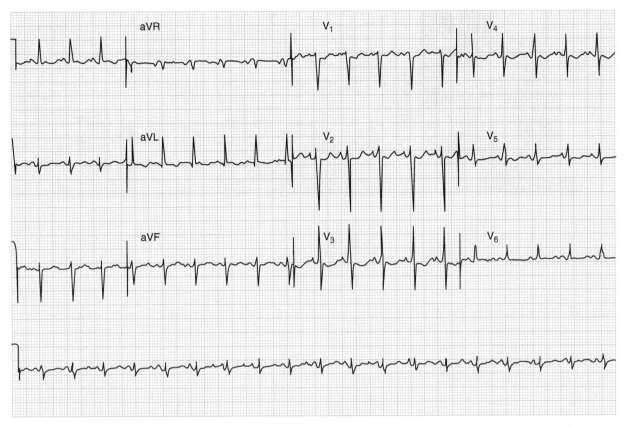

FIGURE 5-14 ■ Electrocardiogram from a newborn with tricuspid atresia characterized by left axis deviation. The QRS axis is −45 degrees.

to supply blood flow to the lungs. The mortality rate for this procedure is between 5% and 10%.

Critical Pulmonary Stenosis

Pulmonary stenosis is a relatively common CHD, accounting for 8% to 10% of all defects.[27] Anatomically, pulmonary stenosis is located at the valvular, subvalvar, supravalvar, or peripheral branches. Subvalvar pulmonary stenosis is called infundibular pulmonary stenosis. In valvular pulmonary stenosis, the pulmonary valve is thickened, with fused or absent commissures. Patients with Noonan syndrome have dysplastic valves that are thick and irregular and a variably small pulmonary valve annulus. The term critical pulmonary stenosis is used for severe pulmonary stenosis presenting in the newborn period with cyanosis, decreased pulmonary blood flow, and signs of right heart failure.[28] Neonates with critical pulmonary stenosis have a nearly atretic valve. The RV is usually normal in size but may be hypoplastic in those with critical pulmonary stenosis.

Hemodynamics

To keep the flow normal across the pulmonary valve, the RV increases its systolic pressure and develops concentric RV hypertrophy. The pulmonary artery beyond the obstruction shows poststenotic dilatation. Because of the obstruction, the RV systole is prolonged, resulting in delayed closure of the pulmonary valve. This results in a widely split second heart sound that is variable, becoming wider during inspiration. The width of the splitting during expiration is directly related to the severity of pulmonary valvar obstruction. The flow across the narrow pulmonary valve results in a pulmonary ejection systolic murmur. The duration of the systolic murmur is also related to the severity of obstruction. The more severe the pulmonary stenosis is, the longer the systolic murmur and the wider the splitting of the second sound. A pulmonary ejection click is audible during expiration but disappears or becomes softer during inspiration. The more severe the pulmonary stenosis, the closer the click is to the first heart sound. In severe pulmonary stenosis, with marked RV hypertrophy, the RV diastolic pressure also increases. The right atrium pressure increases to be able to fill the RV, which results in a fourth heart sound (S₄) as well as a prominent a wave in the jugular venous pulse.

Clinical features

With severe pulmonary stenosis, if the foramen ovale is patent, a right-to-left shunt at the atrial level may result in cyanosis. The hypertrophied RV results in a left

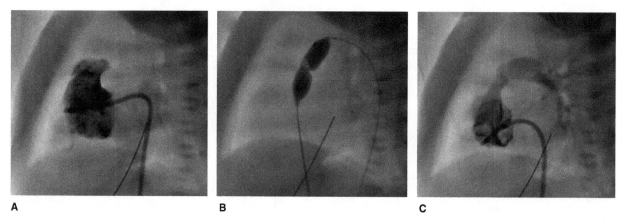

A   **B**   **C**

FIGURE 5-15 ■ Balloon valvuloplasty in critical pulmonary stenosis. **A.** Right ventriculogram demonstrating a thin jet of contrast through the stenotic pulmonary valve. **B.** Balloon dilation of the pulmonary valve shows a waist on the balloon. **C.** Right ventriculogram after balloon valvuloplasty demonstrates contrast opacification of the main pulmonary artery through the pulmonary valve.

parasternal heave. A systolic thrill is palpable at the second and third left interspace. The P_2 is widely split and varies with respiration. In critical pulmonary stenosis, the P_2 is diminished in intensity and may be so widely split in expiration that further widening during inspiration may not be appreciated on auscultation, suggesting a fixed split second sound. A pulmonary ejection click varying with respiration follows the first heart sound. S_4 is audible in critical pulmonary stenosis. Newborns with critical pulmonary stenosis show signs of RV failure with hepatomegaly.

With increasing severity of pulmonary stenosis, the duration and intensity of the murmur increase and the peak gets delayed. In critical pulmonary stenosis, the murmur goes through the aortic component of the second heart sound, partially or completely masking it. The ECG shows right axis deviation and RV hypertrophy. The systolic overload of the RV is suggested by a pure R or a qR type of complex in leads V_4R and V_1. Thoracic roentgenogram shows a normal-sized heart with pulmonary oligemia seen only in critical pulmonary stenosis. Echocardiogram is used to assess the site and severity of pulmonic obstruction.

Critical care management

Neonates with critical pulmonary stenosis who present with cyanosis have a high mortality rate without emergent and appropriate management. PGE_1 infusion may temporarily improve pulmonary blood flow by reopening the ductus arteriosus. Other supportive measures must be taken to stabilize the baby before sending for cardiac catheterization.

Neonatal catheter intervention

Balloon pulmonary valvuloplasty is the initial treatment of choice for critical pulmonary stenosis. A balloon catheter introduced through the femoral vein is inflated across the pulmonary valve to separate the fused valves (Figure 5-15). The mortality rate is less than 1%, and the major complication rate is less than 3%. Hence, balloon valvuloplasty is the first-line therapy, and surgical treatment of valvular pulmonary stenosis is indicated only if balloon valvuloplasty is unsuccessful. Excellent results have been obtained with balloon valvuloplasty.[29,30]

Neonatal surgical repair

Surgical pulmonary valvotomy is performed only if balloon valvuloplasty is unsuccessful. Neonates with critical pulmonary stenosis may require a transventricular valvotomy and/or the insertion of a transannular patch. Alternatively, it can be done through an incision on the pulmonary artery. If severe infundibular hypoplasia is present, a systemic to pulmonary artery shunt is also performed. Dysplastic valves often require complete excision of the valves.

NEONATES PRESENTING WITH SHOCK

Critical Aortic Stenosis

The term critical aortic stenosis is used to describe congenital aortic valve stenosis presenting in the newborn period with signs and symptoms of congestive heart failure. The valve may be bicuspid or unicuspid, with thickening and myxoid dysplasia. Sometimes, there may be no identifiable cusps or commissures.

Hemodynamics

The hemodynamic consequences of critical aortic valve stenosis start in utero. It leads to LV hypertrophy. LV hypertrophy is initially well tolerated in utero. But over time, the LV compliance may decrease, and this results in decreased LV filling, which ultimately could lead to hypoplasia of the LV, mitral valve, aortic valve annulus, and LV outflow tract. COA can also develop with or without aortic arch hypoplasia. Endomyocardial fibroelastosis with or without infarction of papillary muscle may occur due to oxygen supply demand mismatch. Fetal aortic stenosis could evolve into hypoplastic left heart syndrome.[31]

Clinical features

The fetus usually tolerates severe aortic stenosis, even in the presence of severe LV hypoplasia, because the RV is capable of handling the entire cardiac output. Soon after birth, symptoms develop rapidly. If the LV size and function are adequate to handle the entire cardiac output, signs and symptoms may be mild even after closure of the ductus arteriosus. However, if the LV does not have the capacity to handle the entire cardiac output, closure of the ductus arteriosus may result in circulatory collapse. Shock ensues quickly. The newborn becomes pale with poor peripheral perfusion, weak pulses, hepatomegaly, hyperdynamic precordium, and respiratory distress. The prolongation of LV ejection causes delayed closure of the aortic valve, resulting in a delayed A_2. The delay results in closely split, single, or paradoxically split second sound according to the severity of obstruction. With immobile valves, the A_2 diminishes in intensity and may become inaudible. Turbulent flow across the obstruction results in aortic ejection systolic murmur. A thrill may be palpable at the second right interspace. With increase in LV diastolic pressure, a forceful left atrial contraction results in a palpable and audible fourth heart sound (S_4). With LV failure, a third heart sound (S_3) also becomes audible. In valvar aortic stenosis, there is poststenotic dilatation of the ascending aorta. A dilated ascending aorta is associated with an ejection click that follows the first sound and precedes the start of the murmur. The aortic ejection click is best heard at the apex. The pulse pressure gets narrower as the stenosis becomes severe.

ECG in aortic stenosis reveals LVH. Presence of ST-T wave changes suggests severe aortic stenosis. However, a normal ECG does not exclude aortic stenosis. The thoracic roentgenogram exhibits a normal-sized heart with dilated ascending aorta. Echocardiogram and Doppler evaluations confirm the diagnosis and delineate anatomic details. The aortic valve is frequently thickened with reduced mobility and a small orifice. The LV is frequently hypertrophic, but it may be dilated and poorly contractile.

Critical care management

For critically ill neonates with congestive heart failure, rapidly acting inotropic agents such as dopamine and diuretics should be started. PGE_1 infusion may be necessary to reopen the ductus arteriosus. Intubation and positive pressure ventilation are frequently required. Patient must be stabilized before balloon valvuloplasty or surgery.

Neonatal catheter intervention

Percutaneous balloon valvuloplasty to relieve the stenosis is now regarded as the first step in management of symptomatic neonates.[32] A balloon catheter introduced through the femoral artery can be placed at the level of the aortic valve and inflated to tear the valve along the commissure (Figure 5-16). Sometimes during cardiac catheterization, there may be no demonstrable gradient across the valve because of poor LV function, and after valvuloplasty, there may be recovery of LV function and a higher gradient can be obtained. Although the results of balloon valvuloplasty are promising, they are not as good as those for pulmonary stenosis. Serious complications such as avulsion of part of the aortic valve leaflet leading to aortic insufficiency and perforation of mitral valve or LV have been reported. Other complications include loss of femoral artery pulse and major hemorrhage.

Neonatal surgical repair

Closed aortic valvotomy, using calibrated dilators or balloon catheters without cardiopulmonary bypass, may be performed in sick neonates. Newborns with a small aortic annulus, small mitral annulus, small LV cavity, and mitral regurgitation from papillary muscle infarction have a poor prognosis. These neonates may require a Norwood procedure and future single-ventricle palliation.[33]

Alternatively, aortic valve replacement using pulmonary root autografts (the neonatal Ross procedure) can be performed.[34] In this procedure, the autologous pulmonary valve is used to replace the aortic valve, and an allograft conduit is used to replace the pulmonary valve. The coronary arteries have to be reimplanted. The pulmonary valve autograft has the advantage of long-term durability and possibility of autograft growth; it does not require anticoagulation and remains uncompromised by host reactions.

When aortic stenosis is associated with complex LV outflow tract obstruction, an annular enlargement with or without aortoventriculoplasty called the Konno operation can be done along with the Ross procedure.

Coarctation of Aorta

Congenital COA is located at the junction of the arch with the descending aorta. It is a sharp indentation involving the posterior wall of the aorta. It is neither distal nor proximal to the ductus arteriosus; hence, it is described as being juxtaductal in position. Just like other left-sided obstructive lesions, it is more common in males than females (2:1).[35] Other left heart lesions such

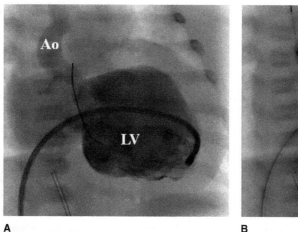 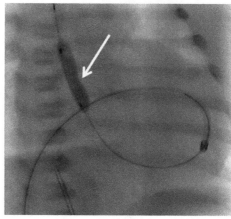

FIGURE 5-16 ■ Balloon valvuloplasty in critical aortic stenosis. **A.** Left ventriculogram demonstrating a very dilated and poorly functioning left ventricle (LV) because of critical aortic valve stenosis. **B.** Balloon dilation of the aortic valve shows a waist on the balloon. The arrow points to the waist on the balloon. Ao, aorta.

as aortic annular hypoplasia, bicuspid aortic valve, VSD, and mitral valve anomalies are frequently associated.[36,37]

Hemodynamics

In newborns with significant coarctation of aorta, the RV via the ductus arteriosus supplies the descending aorta, similar to fetal life. With the closure of the ductus soon after birth, the neonate becomes symptomatic, because good collaterals have not developed. The neonate develops shock secondary to severe LV failure. In extreme situations, renal failure and gut ischemia can occur because of poor perfusion to these organs.

Clinical features

The newborn with COA may be asymptomatic. As the ductus arteriosus constricts, the neonate becomes pale and tachypneic. As the LV fails and the ductus completely closes, oliguria, severe acidemia, and circulatory shock ensue. The neonate can become extremely sick without re-establishing ductal patency. Differential cyanosis may be present, as the lower extremity gets ductal blood flow from the right heart. Peripheral pulses may be weak and thready as a result of LV dysfunction. A blood pressure differential may become apparent only after improvement of cardiac function with administration of inotropes. The S_2 is loud and single, and an S_3 gallop is usually present. An aortic ejection systolic murmur may be present because of bicuspid aortic valve. The ECG shows LV hypertrophy. Presence of ST and T-wave changes suggests additional aortic stenosis or endocardial fibroelastosis. Thoracic roentgenogram shows a normal-sized heart with prominent ascending aorta and the aortic knuckle. From the suprasternal notch view, a wedge-shaped "shelf" of tissue in the posterior aspect of the isthmus can be visualized and the gradient across the narrowing obtained with Doppler. Other associated defects can also be imaged.

Critical care management

The extremely sick neonate should be stabilized appropriately with correction of acidosis. PGE_1 infusion should be started as soon as possible to reopen the ductus arteriosus and establish flow to the descending aorta and the kidneys. Short-acting inotropes such as dopamine, diuretics, and oxygen should be started. Intubation and mechanical positive pressure ventilation may be necessary.[38]

Balloon angioplasty of the COA is usually not very helpful and is associated with a high rate of complications and a higher rate of recoarctation. Balloon angioplasty can be attempted for very sick neonates in whom standard surgical management carries a high risk.

Neonatal surgical repair

Resection of the coarctation segment and end-to-end anastomosis is the common approach. Subclavian flap aortoplasty is another procedure that involves dividing the distal subclavian artery and inserting a flap of the proximal portion of this vessel between the 2 sides of the longitudinally split aorta through the narrow segment. Alternatively, a Dacron patch can be inserted instead of the subclavian artery flap. If there is a long segment coarctation, a conduit may be inserted between the ascending and descending aorta. In sick patients with a large VSD associated with coarctation of aorta, a pulmonary artery band is applied to limit pulmonary blood flow. The VSD can be repaired at a later date. In experienced centers, the mortality rate for surgical repair of isolated coarctation in infancy is extremely low.[39] However, the surgical risks are higher for infants who present with congestive heart failure.[40]

Interrupted Aortic Arch

This is an extreme form of COA in which the aortic arch is atretic or a segment of the arch is absent. Depending on the location of the interruption, the defect is divided into 3 types (Figure 5-17).

■ Type A: The interruption is distal to the left subclavian artery.
■ Type B: The interruption is between the left carotid and left subclavian arteries. This is the most common type, and 50% of these patients have DiGeorge syndrome.
■ Type C: The interruption is between the innominate and left carotid arteries.

There may be associated lesions such as VSD, bicuspid aortic valve, mitral valve deformity, persistent truncus arteriosus, or subaortic stenosis.

Hemodynamics

During fetal life, the descending aorta and the portion of the arch distal to the interruption are supplied by the ductus arteriosus. After birth, the neonate becomes symptomatic just as the ductus begins to constrict. The hemodynamics are similar to those of a neonate with severe coarctation of aorta.

Clinical features

The clinical picture is similar to that of a neonate with severe coarctation of aorta. The neonate becomes progressively tachypneic, with poor peripheral pulses, and signs of left heart failure and/or circulatory shock develop. Differential cyanosis can be seen after re-establishing ductal patency. If there is an associated VSD, the neonate could be cyanotic in the upper extremity as well because of some right-to-left shunt across the VSD. Thoracic roentgenogram shows cardiomegaly, increased pulmonary vascular markings, and pulmonary venous congestion and edema. There may be absence of a thymic shadow in the upper mediastinum if there is associated DiGeorge syndrome. The ECG may show RV hypertrophy. Echocardiography is useful in diagnosis of the interruption and associated defects. However, sometimes computerized tomographic angiography, magnetic resonance imaging, or angiocardiography may be needed for accurate diagnosis of the interruption and defects.

Critical care management

PGE₁ infusion is necessary to keep the ductus arteriosus patent. Occasionally in sick neonates, intubation and oxygen administration may be needed. These neonates should be worked up to rule out DiGeorge syndrome. If the neonate has DiGeorge syndrome, transfusion of citrated blood causes chelation of calcium, leading to severe hypocalcemia. Blood should be irradiated before transfusion. Cardiac catheterization and stenting of the ductus arteriosus may be performed in extremely sick neonates who are not ideal surgical candidates.

Neonatal surgical repair

Complete repair of the interruption is needed for all neonates. A primary anastomosis can be done if the interrupted segment is short. Dacron vascular graft or homograft may be used to repair long-segment interruption. Simple VSDs can be repaired as well. However, if the VSD is complex and multiple, pulmonary artery banding can be performed and the VSD repaired later.

Hypoplastic Left Heart Syndrome

Hypoplastic left heart spectrum (HLHS) is a spectrum of abnormalities in which the LV and other left-sided structures are poorly formed.[41] The LV is of inadequate size and cannot provide sufficient cardiac output. It could grossly be classified into 3 anatomic subtypes: (1) atresia of mitral and aortic valves; (2) stenosis of

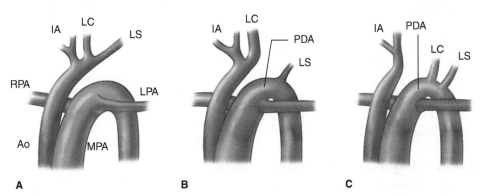

FIGURE 5-17 ■ Diagram showing the various types of aortic arch interruption. **A.** Type A: The interruption is distal to the left subclavian artery (LS). **B.** Type B: The interruption is between the left carotid (LC) and left subclavian arteries (LS). **C.** Type C: The interruption is between the innominate (IA) and left carotid arteries (LC). AO, aorta; LPA, left pulmonary artery; MPA, main pulmonary artery; PDA, patent ductus arteriosus; RPA, right pulmonary artery. (*Reproduced, with permission, from Jonas RA. Interrupted aortic arch. In: Marvoudis C, Backer CL, eds.* Pediatric Cardiac Surgery. *2nd ed. St. Louis, MO: Mosby; 1994:184. Copyright Elsevier.*)

mitral valve with aortic valve atresia; and (3) stenosis of mitral and aortic valves. Hypoplasia of the ascending aorta is usually associated, unless there is a VSD, in which case the aorta may be normal in size. Until the early 1980s, infants born with this anomaly had no treatment options. Today, neonates are expected to survive via staged reconstruction or heart transplantation.[42] Because this is an extensive topic, we will discuss only some of the challenges faced during the newborn period before staged palliation.

Hemodynamics

During fetal life, oxygenated blood is not shunted across the foramen ovale to the left atrium because of the underdevelopment of left heart structures. In the right atrium, the oxygen-rich umbilical venous blood and the systemic venous return mix with the pulmonary venous return from the left atrium. This admixture of venous blood passes through the tricuspid valve into the RV. The RV pumps a portion of this into the pulmonary circulation and the rest to the aorta by way of the ductus arteriosus. The cerebral and myocardial circulations are derived via retrograde flow from the ductus into the transverse arch and ascending aorta. The fetus tolerates this circulation quite well throughout gestation. After birth, systemic and pulmonary venous blood mix in the atrium. Thus, an adequate-sized interatrial communication is essential. The RV handles the entire systemic and pulmonary circulations. As the PVR falls, the pulmonary circulation (Qp) increases. The systemic circulation (Qs) is entirely dependent on the ductus arteriosus. Hence, an adequate size ductus arteriosus is essential for systemic circulation.

Neonatal critical care management

Most neonates with HLHS are prenatally diagnosed via fetal ultrasound. When diagnosis is available before delivery, management is easier and safer. Soon after delivery, the neonate should be examined thoroughly after standard care. Umbilical venous and arterial catheters are useful in preoperative management. Vascular access and PGE infusion can be started prior to transport to the ICU. PGE_1 dose of 0.01 to 0.025 µg/kg/min is usually sufficient for stabilization. Arterial blood gas, electrolytes, ionized calcium, and glucose should be measured. Blood should be sent to the blood bank for cross-matching. Neonates with apnea secondary to PGE_1 may require endotracheal intubation. Acidosis should be corrected. A chest radiograph is necessary to determine proper placement of endotracheal tube, nasogastric tube, and central venous access. Mild cardiomegaly and increased pulmonary vascular markings are usually seen. In the absence of an infection risk, no antibiotics are necessary. After assurance of stability from the initial assessment, a complete echocardiogram

should be obtained. Besides confirming the diagnosis, helpful information to obtain from the initial echocardiogram includes myocardial function, ductal patency, and restriction to pulmonary venous return.

Management of the undiagnosed newborn

When there is no fetal diagnosis, diagnosis may be challenging and often late. The newborn usually appears well and is transported to the newborn nursery. Symptoms appear several hours to 48 hours after birth, as the ductus arteriosus begins to close. The neonate becomes tachypneic due to excess pulmonary blood flow. The neonate feeds poorly. As the duct starts constricting, the perfusion to organs declines. The pulses are often weak, and extremities are cool. The neonate becomes shocky and acidotic. Without timely diagnosis and intervention, this can be rapidly fatal. Once diagnosis is suspected, vascular access and PGE_1 infusion should be commenced right away. Patients presenting with significant restriction to ductal flow often require higher doses of PGE_1 (0.1 µg/kg/min) to reopen the ductus. However, at high doses, PGE_1 causes hypotension in the already compromised infant. The prognosis of the "shocky" infant who is successfully resuscitated is generally not as good as the prenatally diagnosed infant. Fluid resuscitation (10-20 mL/kg) and low-dose dopamine (3-5 µg/kg/min) will counter the vasodilatory effects of PGE_1. Endotracheal intubation and mechanical ventilation are helpful to control pulmonary overcirculation. In general, supplemental oxygen should be avoided because oxygen acts as a pulmonary vasodilator, decreasing PVR and increasing Qp:Qs.

Once stabilized, an echocardiogram will help to confirm the diagnosis. Most infants tend to have a low-grade base deficit, lactic acidosis, and mild hypotension. They often benefit from low-dose dopamine. Dopamine at low doses has minimal effect on Qp:Qs but increases total cardiac output and may increase oxygen delivery and improve systemic hypotension.

Balancing pulmonary and systemic blood flow

Too little pulmonary blood flow (low Qp) results in hypoxemia, whereas too much pulmonary blood flow (high Qp) can result in systemic hypoperfusion, hypotension, metabolic acidosis, acute renal failure, necrotizing enterocolitis, and cerebral ischemia.[43] Qp:Qs can be easily calculated using the modified Fick equation.

$$Qp : Qs = \frac{SaO_2 - SvO_2}{SpvO_2 - SaO_2}$$

Assuming that the newborn has normal cardiac output, with a mixed venous oxygen saturation (SvO_2) of 60%, and no lung pathology, and thus a pulmonary vein oxygen saturation (Spvo$_2$) of 100%, then a systemic arterial oxygen saturation (Sao$_2$) of 80% would represent a Qp:Qs of 1:1. An Sao$_2$ of 90% may lead to an Svo$_2$ of 70% in the presence of normal cardiac output and Qp:Qs of 2:1. An Sao$_2$ of 70% and Svo$_2$ of 50% will result in a Qp:QS of 0.66:1. The clinically stable infant may tolerate pulmonary overcirculation without significant intervention. However, those who are diagnosed late can develop shock. The use of inspired gas mixtures to balance Qp:QS is a topic of interest and controversy. Hypoxia (10% Fio$_2$),[44] hypercarbia (5% Fioc$_2$),[45] and increased inspired nitrogen (17% Fio$_2$)[46] have been tried in intubated infants with pulmonary overcirculation to limit Qp.

HLHS with restrictive or intact atrial septum

An adequate interatrial communication, either a PFO or a secundum ASD, is essential for mixing of oxygenated pulmonary venous return. The atrial septum primum is abnormally deviated posterosuperiorly and leftward, leading to several degrees of interatrial restriction.[47] Rarely the interatrial septum is intact. Neonates born with an intact or highly restrictive atrial septum are severely hypoxemic and exhibit signs of pulmonary venous obstruction.

Newborns with HLHS and an intact atrial septum are difficult to manage following birth. If the restriction of the atrial communication is diagnosed prenatally, the infant can be delivered electively and immediately stabilized with endotracheal intubation and umbilical venous and arterial access and transported to the catheterization laboratory as soon as possible. Alternatively, some centers deliver these infants by elective cesarean section close to the catheterization lab to prevent delay in transport. After quick stabilization, catheter intervention should be attempted with surgical backup for possible

extracorporeal membrane oxygenation or surgical atrial septectomy.[48] The atrial septum is thicker than normal, and balloon septostomy is usually ineffective. An alternate strategy is transseptal puncture followed by static balloon dilation of the atrial septum. The most reliable catheterization strategy for achieving an adequate atrial communication is radiofrequency wire perforation followed by stent implantation across the atrial septum (Figure 5-18).

Approach of high-risk neonates with HLHS

Most neonates with HLHS undergo staged palliation. However several preoperative factors have been found to lead to adverse outcome following stage I palliation. The presence of restrictive interatrial communication, prematurity, small for gestational age, chromosomal anomaly, presence of severe tricuspid valve regurgitation, and associated anomalous pulmonary venous connections are some factors that result in poor outcomes.[49] Presence of shock, need for cardiopulmonary resuscitation, end-organ injury (renal dysfunction), size of the ascending aorta, and intracranial hemorrhage are other factors that may considerably affect outcome following stage I palliation. Also, the presence of congenital malformation of other organs may preclude operative palliation. For these high-risk infants, there is a combined surgical-catheterization hybrid option that is available. The 2 most important factors for survival beyond the neonatal period are maintaining an adequate size ductus arteriosus to provide systemic cardiac output and limiting pulmonary blood flow and balancing Qp:Qs. These can be adequately achieved by the hybrid strategy. This involves median sternotomy, bilateral branch pulmonary artery banding, and stent implantation in the ductus arteriosus (Figure 5-19). This is a relatively low-risk procedure[50] and effectively allows the infant to

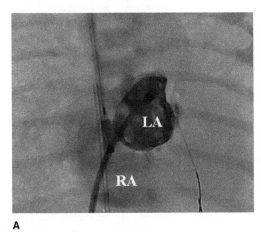
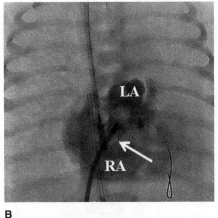

A **B**

FIGURE 5-18 ■ Hypoplastic left heart syndrome with intact atrial septum. **A.** A sheath is inserted into the left atrium (LA) through a hole created in the interatrial septum by radiofrequency perforation. Contrast injection through the sheath in the LA shows that the LA is dilated, globular, and hypertensive because of LA outflow obstruction. **B.** The arrow points to the stent that has been inserted in the interatrial septum between the LA and right atrium (RA). The LA appears decompressed after stent insertion.

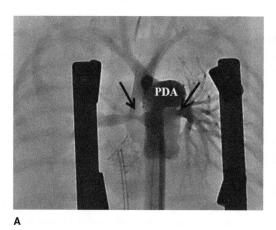
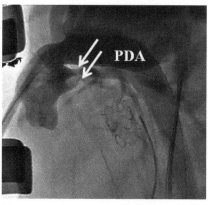

A   B

FIGURE 5-19 ■ Hypoplastic left heart syndrome: hybrid procedure. **A.** Median sternotomy and bilateral branch pulmonary artery banding (arrows) and stenting of the patent ductus arteriosus (PDA) through a sheath inserted directly in the main pulmonary artery. **B.** Lateral projection of the same angiogram demonstrates the bilateral branch pulmonary artery banding (arrows) and stenting of the PDA through a sheath inserted directly in the main pulmonary artery.

be weaned off PGE_1. The Qp:Qs is usually well balanced for 2 to 3 months. When the infant becomes more cyanotic around that time, a comprehensive stage II palliation (integrating stage I and II) can be performed. The hybrid procedure can also be used as a bridge to heart transplantation in neonates who are not candidates for staged palliation.

MISCELLANEOUS NEONATAL HEART DISEASES

Ectopia Cordis

Ectopia cordis is characterized by a partial or complete displacement of the heart outside the thorax (Figure 5-20). It is a form of pericardial defect. In the classic form, it is associated with a sternal cleft and an omphalocele. It is associated with CHD, especially TOF, d-TGA, or double

outlet right ventricle. Although it is not a critical CHD, care must be taken to cover the heart carefully and properly and avoid compression and kinking of the heart. General principles to avoid sepsis must be followed. Most advocate some form of prosthetic reconstruction of the chest wall and covering the heart with skin along with surgical repair of the CHD.

Clinical Pearls

- Critical heart disease in the newborn includes all congenital heart lesions that would result in neonatal demise unless immediate intervention is undertaken.
- Neonatal critical heart disease can be broadly described as those that present as severe cyanosis and those, which present as shock (approximately 3.5/1000 live births).
- Critical cyanosis occurs when effective pulmonary blood flow is limited following the transition from fetal to postnatal circulation. Cyanotic structural heart diseases include: pulmonary stenosis, tetralogy of Fallot, tricuspid atresia, pulmonary atresia with intact ventricular septum, transposition of the great arteries and total anomalous pulmonary venous connection.
- Cardiogenic shock occurs once the ductus arteriosus begins to close in infants born with severe left-sided heart abnormalities. Left-sided defects include: aortic stenosis, coarctation of the aorta, interrupted aortic arch, and hypoplastic left heart syndrome.
- Outcome of a newborn with critical congenital heart disease ultimately depends on the timely assessment and accurate diagnosis of the underlying defect.
- Once the diagnosis is made, attention should continue to focus on the basic principles of neonatal life support and maintenance of a patent ductus arteriosus via prostaglandin (PGE_1) infusion.
- Definitive therapy to repair or palliate the underlying structural heart defect is ideally performed once the patient is stabilized. Invasive procedures are performed in the operating room and/or cardiac catheterization laboratory.

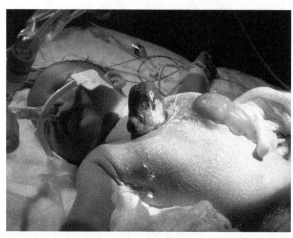

FIGURE 5-20 ■ Ectopia cordis: a newborn baby with ectopia cordis arising through a cleft in the sternum. An omphalocele is also present.

REFERENCES

1. Zeltser I, Tabbutt S. Critical heart disease in the newborn. In: Bell LM, Vetter VL, eds. *Pediatric Cardiology: The Requisites in Pediatrics*. New York, NY: Mosby Elsevier; 2006:31-50.

2. Rudolph AM. The fetal circulation. In: Rudolph AM, ed. *Congenital Diseases of the Heart: Clinical-Physiological Considerations*. 3rd ed. New York, NY: Wiley-Blackwell; 2009:3-10.

3. Cohen MS. Fetal diagnosis and management of congenital heart disease. *Clin Perinatol*. 2001;28:11-29.

4. Verheijen PM, Lisowski LA, Stoutenbeek P, et al. Prenatal diagnosis of congenital heart disease affects preoperative acidosis in the newborn patient. *J Thorac Cardiovasc Surg*. 2001;121:798-803.

5. Park MK. Invasive procedures. In: *Pediatric Cardiology for Practitioners*. 4th ed. New York, NY: Mosby Inc.; 2002:83-87.

6. Perry LW, Neill CA, Ferencz C, et al. Infants with congenital heart disease: the cases. In: Ferencz C, Rubin JD, Loffredo CA, eds. *Perspectives in Pediatric Cardiology. Epidemiology of Congenital Heart Disease, the Baltimore-Washington Infant Study 1981-1989*. Armonk, NY: Futura Publishing; 1993:33-62.

7. Kothari SS. Mechanism of cyanotic spell in tetralogy of Fallot: the missing link? *Int J Cardiol*. 1992;37:1-5.

8. Sluysmans T, Nevan B, Rubay J, et al. Early balloon dilation of the pulmonary valve in infants with tetralogy of Fallot. Risks and benefits. *Circulation*. 1995;91:1506-1511.

9. Kreutzer J, Perry SB, Jonas RA, et al. Tetralogy of Fallot with diminutive pulmonary arteries: preoperative pulmonary valve dilation and transcatheter rehabilitation of pulmonary arteries. *J Am Coll Cardiol*. 1996;27: 1741-1747.

10. Reddy VM, Liddicoat JR, McElhinney DB, et al. Routine primary repair of tetralogy of Fallot in neonates and infants less than three months of age. *Ann Thorac Surg*. 1995;60(Suppl):592-596.

11. Hennein HA, Mosca RS, Urcelay G, et al. Intermediate results after complete repair of tetralogy of Fallot in neonates. *J Thorac Cardiovasc Surg*. 1995;109:332-342.

12. Sousa Uva M, Lacour-Gayet F, Komiya E, et al. Surgery for tetralogy of Fallot at less than six months of age. *J Thorac Cardiovasc Surg*. 1994;107:1291-1300.

13. Hanley FL, Sade RM, Blackstone EH, et al. Outcomes in neonatal pulmonary atresia with intact ventricular septum. A multi-institutional study. *J Thorac Cardiovasc Surg*. 1993;105:406-407.

14. Humpl T, Soderberg B, McCrindle BW, et al. Percutaneous balloon valvotomy in patients with pulmonary atresia with intact ventricular septum: impact on patient care. *Circulation*. 2003;108:826-832.

15. Satou GM, Perry SB, Gauvreau K, et al. Echocardiographic predictors of coronary artery pathology in pulmonary atresia with intact ventricular septum. *Am J Cardiol*. 2000;85:1319-1324.

16. Walsh KP, Abdulhamed JM, Tometzki JP. Importance of right ventricular outflow tract angiography in distinguishing critical pulmonary stenosis from pulmonary atresia. *Heart*. 1997;77:456-460.

17. Ashburn DA, Blackstone EH, Wells WJ, et al. Determinants of mortality and type of repair in neonates with pulmonary atresia with intact ventricular septum. *J Thorac Cardiovasc Surg*. 2004;127:1000-1007.

18. Rychik J, Levy H, Gaynor JW, et al. Outcome after operations for pulmonary atresia with intact ventricular septum. *J Thorac Cardiovasc Surg*. 1998;116:924-931.

19. Wernovsky G. Abnormalities of the origin of the great arteries. In: Allen HD, Driscoll DJ, Shaddy RE, et al., eds. *Moss and Adams' Heart Disease in Infants, Children, and Adolescents*. 7th ed. Philadelphia, PA: Lippincott Williams & Wilkins; 2008:1038-1099.

20. Kirklin JW, Barratt-Boyes BG. Complete transposition of great arteries. In: Kirklin JW, Barratt-Boyes BG, eds. *Cardiac Surgery*. New York, NY: Churchill Livingston; 1993:1383-1467.

21. McQuillen PS, Hamrick SE, Miller SP, et al. Balloon atrial septostomy is associated with preoperative stroke in neonates with transposition of the great arteries. *Circulation*. 2006;113:280-285.

22. Daebritz SH, Tiete AR, Sachweh JS, et al. Systemic right ventricular failure after arterial switch operation. *Ann Thorac Surg*. 2001;71:1255-1259.

23. Wernovsky G, Mayer JE, Jonas RA, et al. Factors influencing early and late outcome of the arterial switch operation for transposition of great arteries. *J Thorac Cardiovasc Surg*. 2000;109:289-302.

24. Abbott ME. *Atlas of Congenital Heart Disease*. New York, NY: American Heart Association; 1936.

25. Cobanoglu A, Menashe VD. Total anomalous pulmonary venous connection in neonates and young infants: repair in the current era. *Ann Thorac Surg*. 1993;55:43-49.

26. Report of the New England Regional Infant Cardiac Program. *Pediatrics*. 1980;65(Suppl 2):388-461.

27. Driscoll DJ, Michels VV, Gersony WM, et al. Occurrence risk for congenital heart defects in relatives of patients with aortic stenosis, pulmonary stenosis and ventricular septal defect. *Circulation*. 1993;87(Suppl 2):1114-1120.

28. Freed MD, Rosenthal AR, Bernhard WF, et al. Critical pulmonary stenosis with diminutive right ventricle in neonates. *Circulation*. 1973;48:875-882.

29. Stanger P, Cassidy SC, Girod DA, et al. Balloon pulmonary valvuloplasty: results of the valvuloplasty and angioplasty of congenital anomalies registry. *Am J Cardiol*. 1990;65:775-783.

30. McCrindle BW, Kan JS. Long term results after neonatal balloon pulmonary valvuloplasty. *Circulation*. 1991;83:1915-1922.

31. Wessels MW, Berger RM, Frohn-Mulder IM, et al. Autosomal dominant inheritance of left ventricular outflow tract obstruction. *Am J Med Genet A*. 2005;134:171-179.

32. Gatzoulis MA, Rigby ML, Shinebourne EA, et al. Contemporary results of balloon valvuloplasty and surgical valvotomy for congenital aortic stenosis. *Arch Dis Child*. 1995;73:66-69.

33. Lofland GK, McCrindle BW, Williams WG, et al. Critical aortic stenosis in the neonate: a multi-institutional study of management, outcomes, and risk factors. *J Thorac Cardiovasc Surg*. 2001;121:10-27.

34. Ohye RG, Gomez CA, Ohye BJ, et al. The Ross/Konno procedure in neonates and infants: intermediate term

results and autograft function. *Ann Thorac Surg.* 2001;72: 823-830.

35. Report of the New England Regional Infant Cardiac Program. *Pediatrics.* 1980;65:375-461.

36. Anderson RH, Lenox CC, Zuberbuhler JR. Morphology of ventricular septal defect associated with coarctation of aorta. *Br Heart J.* 1983;50:176-181.

37. Shone JD, Sellers RD, Anderson RC, et al. The development complex of "parachute mitral valve," supravalvar ring of left atrium, sub-aortic stenosis and coarctation of aorta. *Am J Cardiol.* 1963;11:714-725.

38. Kilman JW, Williams TE, Breza TS, et al. Reversal of infant mortality by early surgical correction of coarctation of aorta. *Arch Surg.* 1972;105:865-868.

39. Zehr KJ, Gillinov AM, Redmond JM, et al. Repair of coarctation of the aorta in neonates and infants: a thirty year experience. *Ann Thorac Surg.* 1995;59:33-41.

40. Quaegebeur JM, Jonas RA, Weinberg AD, et al. Outcomes in seriously ill neonates with coarctation of the aorta: a multi-institutional study. *J Thorac Cardiovasc Surg.* 1994;108:841-851.

41. Abu-Harb M, Wyllie J, Hey E, et al. Presentation of obstructive left heart malformations in infancy. *Arch Dis Child Fetal Neonatal Ed.* 1994;71:F179-F183.

42. Mahle WT, Spray TL, Wernovsky G, et al. Survival after reconstructive surgery for hypoplastic left heart syndrome: a 15 year experience from a single institution. *Circulation.* 2000;102:136-141.

43. Tweddell JS, Hoffman GM, Berger S, et al. Hypoplastic left heart syndrome. In: Allen HD, Driscoll DJ, Shaddy RE, et al., eds. *Moss and Adams' Heart Disease in Infants, Children, and Adolescents.* 7th ed. Philadelphia, PA: Lippincott Williams & Wilkins; 2008:1005-1038.

44. Tabbutt S, Ramamoorthy C, Montenegro LM, et al. Impact of inspired gas mixtures on the pre-operative infants with hypoplastic left heart syndrome during controlled ventilation. *Circulation.* 2001;104:159-164.

45. Jobes DR, Nicolson SC, Steven JM, et al. Carbon dioxide prevents pulmonary overcirculation in hypoplastic left heart syndrome. *Ann Thorac Surg.* 1992;54:150-151.

46. Shime N, Nashimoto S, Hiramatsu N, et al. Hypoxic gas therapy using nitrogen in the preoperative management of neonate with hypoplastic left heart syndrome. *Pediatr Crit Care Med.* 2000;1:38-44.

47. Rychik J. Echocardiographic imaging. In: Rychik J, Wernovsky G, eds. *Hypoplastic Left Heart Syndrome.* Philadelphia, PA: Springer; 2002:39-68.

48. Kreutzer J, Rome J. Cardiac catheterization. In: Rychik J, Wernovsky G, eds. *Hypoplastic Left Heart Syndrome.* Philadelphia, PA: Springer; 2002:193-228.

49. Tabbutt S, Dominguez TE, Ravishankar C, et al. Outcomes after the stage I reconstruction comparing the right ventricular to pulmonary artery conduit with the modified Blalock-Taussig shunt. *Ann Thorac Surg.* 2005;80: 1582-1590.

50. Holzer RJ, Chisolm JL, Hill SL, et al. "Hybrid" stent delivery in the pulmonary circulation. *J Invasive Cardiol.* 2008;20:592-598.

CHAPTER 6

Care of the Postprocedural Patient

Javier J. Lasa,
Roxanne Kirsch,
Stephanie Fuller and
Jonathan J. Rome

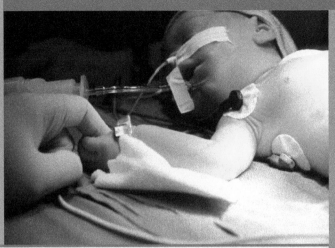

INTRODUCTION

The care of infants, children, and adults with congenital heart disease (CHD) can be complex and challenging. In particular, the inpatient periprocedural setting can pose unique management challenges and represents one of the highest risk periods for the patient with CHD. Successful congenital heart surgery and interventional cardiac catheterization require a comprehensive, well-coordinated, team-based mode of care delivery that incorporates a solid knowledge base with sound clinical judgment. Management of the postprocedural patient should reflect a firm understanding of common congenital heart defects and surgical interventions, cardiopulmonary anatomy and physiology, advanced technical skills, pharmacology, and common complications. Patient and family-centered anticipatory guidance should be effective and confident with similarly comprehensive communication with primary care providers throughout the hospitalization and discharge process. This chapter provides an informative overview in the approach to the care of the postoperative and postcatheterization patient with CHD, specifically focusing on the immediate postprocedure and post–hospital discharge time periods.

CARE OF THE POSTSURGICAL PATIENT

Preoperative Stabilization

The goals of preoperative intensive care unit (ICU) care are focused on stabilizing the patient (often with a ductal-dependent cardiac lesion), maintaining stable hemodynamics, and accurately identifying abnormal cardiac anatomy for appropriate procedural planning. In the current era, many neonates with CHD are diagnosed prenatally. Families should be encouraged to seek obstetrical care at a tertiary center with specialized pediatric cardiac services that allow for safe delivery of the infant while avoiding potentially life-threatening complications related to transfer and delays in care. However, a significant percentage of neonates with CHD continue to present in the postnatal period[1] (Table 6-1). Immediate stabilization with initiation of prostaglandins, where appropriate, and transfer to a surgical and interventional cardiac center should be initiated promptly.

Once in the ICU setting, preoperative stabilization of the neonate consists of maintaining hemodynamic stability while avoiding preoperative morbidity that may impact the timing or effectiveness of definitive therapies such as surgery or interventional catheterization. Intravenous prostaglandin may be required for the neonate to maintain ductal patency prior to surgery. Hemodynamic support in the form of inotropes and/or mechanical ventilation may be required in the setting of severe cardiorespiratory compromise. Prostaglandin therapy and its associated side effects, including apnea, require close monitoring, although effective administration with low-dose infusions (0.01 μg/kg/min) have been successful without the need for tracheal intubation (Table 6-2).

Cardiopulmonary Bypass in Neonates, Infants, and Children

Surgical techniques and intraoperative care advancements have extended the limits of patients being exposed to cardiopulmonary bypass (CPB). Technology

Presenting Symptoms of Patients Diagnosed Postnatally with Critical Congenital Heart Disease

	Diagnosis in Nursery, n = 73 (%)	Diagnosis After Discharge, n = 16 (%)
Murmur	38	25
Cyanosis	32	0
Respiratory distress	7	19
Shock	4	38
Arrhythmia	3	0
Other	3	6
Multiple symptoms	14	13

Modified with permission from Dorfman AT, Marino BS, Wernovsky G, et al. Critical heart disease in the neonate: presentation and outcome at a tertiary care center. Pediatr Crit Care Med. 20089:193-202.

has allowed for the relative miniaturization of elements of the CPB circuit, thereby minimizing the volume load and inflammatory responses observed after CPB. Yet there are several important considerations with regard to managing the infant and child after undergoing CPB. The challenges of balancing this vulnerable time period with essential life-sustaining interventions are not trivial and require a comprehensive understanding of perioperative factors, including oxygen-carrying capacity (eg, maintaining optimal hematocrit),[2] temperature regulation, acid-base balance, and timing of intervention.

Ultrafiltration is a commonly used technique at the end of CPB that removes plasma water and inflammatory mediators from CPB circuit blood volume. This step is performed after separation from the bypass circuit in

Common Versus Uncommon Side Effects of Prostaglandin E$_1$ Therapy in the Neonatal Population

	Side Effect
Common	Apnea
	Hypotension
	Peripheral vasodilation
	Tachycardia
	Temperature elevation
	Hypoventilation
Uncommon	Hypoglycemia
	Hypocalcemia
	Diarrhea
	Thrombocytopenia
	Rash

an effort to further minimize the inflammatory response after CPB. However, it is impossible to completely mitigate the inflammatory response from CPB. Furthermore, the resulting hemodilution from the bypass circuit yields a significantly decreased hematocrit, level of circulating clotting factors, and plasma protein, leading to dysfunction in the prothrombotic and anticoagulation balance of the coagulation system.[3] In addition, the relative immaturity of the liver in neonates further exacerbates the dilutional coagulopathy due to diminished production of vitamin K–dependent clotting factors. Impaired thermoregulation requires intensive monitoring of core temperatures after CPB, especially when hypothermia is used as the primary strategy for surgical repair (deep hypothermic circulatory arrest [DHCA]). The immature lung of the neonate and infant predisposes the pulmonary vascular bed and surrounding parenchyma to increased reactivity, potential pulmonary edema, and pulmonary hypertension. The diminished fat and carbohydrate reserves and the higher metabolic rate and oxygen consumption observed in the neonate account for rapid hypoxia in the setting of apnea. The presence of intracardiac or extracardiac shunting can exacerbate the relative flow distribution between systemic and pulmonary vascular beds. Additional immature organ systems include the renal, central nervous, and immune systems. Renal vascular resistance is elevated in the neonate and infant, resulting in limited acid-base balance control, sodium reabsorption, excretion, and dilutional capabilities. Brain maturation is significantly delayed in infants with complex CHD compared with similarly gestational age–matched neonates.[4] Additionally, immature neonatal and infant immune defenses result in poor antibody and complement generation as well as dysfunctional mononuclear cells.

Low Cardiac Output States and Hemodynamic Monitoring

Significant surgical and CPB stressors can lead to low cardiac output syndrome (LCOS) after cardiac surgery, predominately affecting neonates and infants but also affecting older children and adults who undergo complex operations with long myocardial ischemic times or in any patient with pre-existing ventricular dysfunction, atrioventricular valve regurgitation, or arrhythmias. To maintain adequate systemic perfusion, an age-appropriate heart rate for the patient's clinical condition, adequate preload and intravascular volume, normal myocardial function, and appropriate afterload are ideal.

The interplay between diminished cardiac output, increased metabolic demand, inflammatory responses to CPB, and maladaptive responses to stress contributes to a predictable period of low cardiac output approximately 8 to 12 hours after separation from CPB circuit. This condition, often described as LCOS, is reflective of the transient myocardial ischemia and related myocyte swelling and noncompliance observed after CPB. Exposure of circulating blood volumes to the bypass circuit leads to the release of inflammatory factors that induces capillary leak and subsequent alterations in pulmonary compliance, vascular resistances, and loading conditions of the heart. Inadequate cardiac output leads to a period of relative oliguria, decreased skin perfusion, and systemic blood pressure and ultimately results in the requirement of fluid resuscitation, escalation of inotropic support, and vigilance. This transient depression in cardiac output generally improves after the first 24 hours as increased urine output is matched by decreasing inotropic support.[5,6] Table 6-3 highlights the hemodynamic profile of conditions that can lead to cardiovascular instability in the postoperative period and should be differentiated from LCOS.

Residual postoperative lesions will contribute greatly to the degree of LCOS postoperatively. For this reason, intraoperative transesophageal echocardiography is often used to identify significant residual lesions (intracardiac shunts, obstruction to inflow or outflow, valve regurgitation) prior to separation from CPB, thus allowing for repeat correction if indicated prior to discontinuation of support.

Postoperative ICU management should evaluate for significant contributors to decreased intravascular volume as measured by intracardiac lines (right and/or left atrial pressure) and systemic blood pressure monitoring. Systemic arterial catheters can aid in real-time blood pressure measurements while providing ready access for frequent phlebotomy and arterial blood gas sampling.

Contributors to postoperative intravascular volume depletion include hemorrhage, excessive diuresis or inadequate fluid administration, and excessive capillary leak after CPB. Blood products including packed red blood cells, platelets, and fresh frozen plasma should be administered when postoperative bleeding is prolonged or when abnormal coagulation laboratory values are observed. Recombinant factor VII should be administered in cases of significant postoperative hemorrhage resistant to routine blood product administration and repletion of fibrinogen with cryoprecipitate.[7] Sudden cessation of bloody output from a previously draining chest tube in conjunction with tachycardia, rising intracardiac pressures, hypotension, and narrowing pulse pressure herald the clinical diagnosis of cardiac tamponade. Simple maneuvers to clear occluded chest tubes are required regularly to prevent fluid accumulation in the mediastinum and pericardial space. Ultimately, re-exploration of the mediastinum is required to restore hemodynamic stability when there is suspicion of tamponade. Complicated surgical procedures associated with long CPB times may result in myocardial swelling and/or excess bleeding. Both sequelae prohibit immediate sternal closure. Hemodynamic instability or ongoing bleeding can be managed more efficiently with delayed sternal closure, although mechanical ventilatory strategies must reflect the changes in functional residual capacity and respiratory compliance that occur with sternal closure. Delayed sternal closure can be associated with transient respiratory deterioration and a similar decrease in cardiac output often requiring a temporary escalation of ventilatory support and increase in inotropic support.[8]

Pharmacologic therapies are often used for additional hemodynamic support in the postoperative period and can include adrenergic-based therapies, phosphodiesterase inhibitors, and afterload-reducing agents such as α-blockers or direct vasodilators. The mechanism of action and side effect profile of each vasoactive agent should be weighed on an individual basis for each lesion and/or condition in the postoperative period (Table 6-4). Catecholaminergic medications such as dopamine, dobutamine, epinephrine, and isoproterenol can lead to excessive chronotropy and increased inotropic demands, thereby increasing myocardial oxygen

Hemodynamic Profile of Conditions That Lead to Cardiovascular Instability in the Postoperative Period

	HR	CVP	Pulse Pressure	MAP	Urine Output	Capillary Refill Time
Hypovolemia	↑	↓	Normal	↓	↓	↑
Tamponade	↑	↓	Narrow	↓	↓	Normal/↓
LCOS	↑	↓/↑	Normal	↓	↓	↑

CVP, central venous pressure; HR, heart rate; LCOS, low cardiac output syndrome; MAP, mean arterial blood pressure.

Inotropic and Vasopressor Classification, Standard Dose Range, Receptor Binding (Catecholamines), and Major Clinical Side Effects

Drug	Dose Range	Receptor Binding				Major Side Effects
		α_1	β_1	β_2	DA	
Dopamine	2-20 μg/kg/min	+++	++++	++	+++++	Hypertension, ventricular arrhythmias, cardiac ischemia
Dobutamine	2-20 μg/kg/min	+	+++++	+++	N/A	Tachycardia, hypertension, ventricular arrhythmias, cardiac ischemia, hypotension
Norepinephrine	0.01-3 μg/kg/min	+++++	+++	++	N/A	Arrhythmias, bradycardia, peripheral ischemia, hypertension
Epinephrine	0.01-0.1 μg/kg/min; mg IV every 3-5 minutes (max, 0.2 mg/kg)	+++++	++++	+++	N/A	Ventricular arrhythmias, severe hypertension, cardiac ischemia, cerebrovascular hemorrhage
Isoproterenol	0.01-2 μg/kg/min	0	+++++	+++++	N/A	Ventricular arrhythmias, cardiac ischemia, hypertension, hypotension
Phenylephrine	0.4-9 μg/kg/min; 0.1-0.5 mg IV every 10-15 minutes	+++++	0	0	N/A	Reflex bradycardia, hypertension, severe peripheral and visceral vasoconstriction, tissue necrosis with extravasation

Adapted with permission from Overgaard C, Dzavik V. Inotropes and vasopressors: review of physiology and clinical use in cardiovascular disease. Circulation. 2008;118;1047-1056. DA, dopamine; IV, intravenous.

consumption. Atrial and ventricular dysrhythmias can be seen with higher frequency when using chronotropic and inotropic agents. Additionally, activation of peripheral α-receptors may lead to increased peripheral vascular resistance with a concomitant decrease in cardiac output. Because of the many undesirable adverse effects associated with the use of high-dose endogenous or synthetic adrenergic therapies, afterload-reducing agents such as phosphodiesterase type III inhibitors (eg, milrinone) are being increasingly used in the postoperative period. Demonstrating both vasodilatory and lusitropic (myocardial relaxation) properties, these agents also act synergistically with β-agonists and have fewer side effects. Vasodilator therapy with afterload-reducing agents such as sodium nitroprusside or phenoxybenzamine can also improve cardiac output in select patient populations who experience elevated systemic vascular resistance in the postoperative period.

Mechanical support in the form of extracorporeal membrane oxygenation (ECMO) has been used increasingly as an adjuvant therapy when conventional measures such as fluid resuscitation, inotropic support, and afterload reduction fail. Indications include ventricular dysfunction resistant to inotropic support, inability to wean off CPB, severe pulmonary hypertension with resultant right ventricular failure, intractable arrhythmias with compromised cardiac output, and palliations with catastrophic shunt occlusion. ECMO support has become the most widely used mode of mechanical cardiopulmonary support for children with CHD, both before and after heart surgery.[9] Prior to initiation of ECMO support, one must consider the need for a dedicated team of ECMO specialists, immobilization of the patient, use of intensive and invasive monitoring, and the risks of coagulopathy, thrombosis, stroke, infection, and multiorgan failure. In addition, patients should be perceived as having a potentially reversible cardiac or pulmonary disease to be considered candidates for ECMO.

Mechanical assist devices, such as pulsatile and axial flow ventricular assist devices, are also being used increasingly as bridges to transplantation (in the case of CHD or cardiomyopathy) or recovery (in select cases of myocarditis/cardiomyopathy). These devices have several advantages including their ease of use, chronic support capabilities, mobility for cardiac rehabilitation, need for low-level anticoagulation, capability for biventricular support without oxygenation, and higher rate of extubation. Risks include thromboembolic complications, increased risk of presensitization in the pretransplant population, infection, and size limitations.

Cardiopulmonary Interactions and Respiratory Distress in the Postoperative Period

Respiratory mechanics and cardiovascular function are linked primarily through the changes in intrathoracic pressure that alter systemic venous return to the heart, as well as through alterations in pulmonary vascular resistance and left ventricular afterload. Positive pressure ventilation increases intrathoracic pressure during inspiration, thus decreasing venous return to the right atrium and reducing right ventricular preload. This decrease in venous return is mirrored by the left ventricle and leads to decreased stroke volume with a subsequent decrease in cardiac output. Additional alterations in lung recruitment may exacerbate changes in pulmonary vascular resistance. Although pulmonary vascular resistance will reach a nadir at function residual capacity, alveolar overrecruitment above function residual capacity or underrecruitment at residual volume can lead to subsequent increases in pulmonary vascular resistance.

The predominant effect of increased intrathoracic pressure during inspiration with positive pressure ventilation is likely to be decreased systemic venous return with a subsequent decrease in cardiac output. Ventilatory strategies should be chosen carefully to avoid adverse effects on the cardiovascular system. Patients most affected by ventilatory changes are those with significant right ventricular diastolic dysfunction, those at risk for pulmonary hypertension, and those with cavopulmonary anastomoses. Although corrective surgeries may improve pulmonary compliance in cardiac lesions with significantly elevated pulmonary blood flow, pulmonary mechanics and anatomy are also affected by CPB, trauma, and/or intercurrent infection. Changes such as prominent swelling of the mucosa due to hyperemia or edema, excessive or highly viscous secretions, hyperactive bronchial smooth muscle, and/or extrinsic compression by neighboring structures can all contribute to decreased myocardial compliance. In addition, pulmonary edema, pneumonia, and atelectasis most commonly lead to lower airway and alveolar abnormalities.

Respiratory failure may also result from diaphragmatic paresis or outright paralysis, particularly in neonates and infants, who rely on diaphragmatic contraction for chest wall expansion more than older children. Intraoperative injury to the phrenic nerve (usually left-sided) is most commonly caused by direct trauma, although thermal injuries have also been reported.[10] Diagnosis is confirmed by fluoroscopy or by bedside ultrasonography demonstrating paradoxical or paretic motion of a raised hemidiaphragm in conjunction with paradoxical abdominal motion. In such cases, surgical diaphragmatic plication is recommended should the patient demonstrate increased work of breathing and/or failure to wean from mechanical ventilation.

Pleural effusions may also interfere with postoperative recovery and can lead to reintubation and prolonged length of stay in hospital. Patients undergoing specific procedures such as right ventriculotomies with subsequent transient right ventricular dysfunction and total cavopulmonary anastomoses (Fontan operation) are more likely to accumulate pleural effusions due to elevated central venous pressures and impaired lymphatic drainage. Evacuation of the pleural space with chest tubes subsequently allows for improved ventilation and less intrathoracic airspace competition.

Although many postoperative CHD patients remain intubated and mechanically ventilated after surgery, specific patient populations may benefit from early extubation. Older children, those without pulmonary hypertension, and those with less complex lesions requiring shorter CPB or DHCA times have been shown to be extubated successfully in the operating room or within hours of arrival to the ICU.[11] Several criteria should be evaluated in order to promote a higher likelihood of success of extubation in the postoperative or postprocedural cardiac patient. The patient's hemodynamic status should be evaluated with the goal of maintaining the patient with a normal heart rate and rhythm as well as adequate systemic perfusion. Higher inotropic support may require delayed extubation in order to decrease the work of breathing and improve oxygen delivery to the myocardium and other vital organs. Hemostasis should also be achieved. Lastly, the patient's neurologic status should be fully evaluated after the appropriate titration of sedative and analgesic regimens to allow for spontaneous breaths without the presence of respiratory depression or seizure activity.

Pulmonary Hypertension

Pulmonary hypertension is a major cause of morbidity and mortality following cardiac surgery in the pediatric population, especially after repair of CHD with large left-to-right shunts such as unrestrictive ventricular septal defects, complete atrioventricular (AV) canal defects, total anomalous pulmonary venous connection (TAPVC), large patent ductus arteriosus, truncus arteriosus, and dextro-transposition of the great arteries. Triggers of postoperative pulmonary hypertensive crises include hypoxia, hypercarbia, hypothermia, and hypoglycemia. Recent advances in the investigation of the pathophysiology of pulmonary hypertension, including the role of vascular endothelium in the production of vasodilators and vasoconstrictors such as endothelin, have advanced our understanding of pulmonary vascular biology and how pulmonary vascular resistance can be altered following CPB.[12] Early surgical repair in younger patients may also have contributed to the lower incidence of pulmonary hypertension in the CHD population over the past decades and should be considered in the current management of patients with early signs of pulmonary hypertension. In addition to avoiding known triggers, analgesia and sedation in the ICU play a large role in avoiding or treating postoperative pulmonary hypertensive crises. Inhaled nitric oxide (NO) is a specific pulmonary vascular smooth muscle relaxant that can lower pulmonary artery pressure in a number of diseases without the unwanted effect of systemic hypotension. Prophylactic and therapeutic use of inhaled NO has been reported after repair of obstructed TAPVC, Fontan operation, complete AV canal repair, and a variety of other anatomic lesions. Possible toxicities of inhaled NO include methemoglobinemia, production of excess nitrogen dioxide, and injury to the pulmonary surfactant system. Additionally, abrupt withdrawal of NO can lead to rebound pulmonary hypertension, thus requiring a slow wean from support. Additional therapies that may attenuate the withdrawal response to inhaled NO that may also treat active pulmonary hypertension include oxygen and the use of sildenafil, a phosphodiesterase type 5 inhibitor.[13] Pretreatment with sildenafil, which is well tolerated and available as an oral preparation, produces acute and relatively selective pulmonary vasodilatation while acting synergistically with NO. Hyperventilation was previously proposed as a strategy for the management of pulmonary hypertension but is no longer used due to the compensatory increase in systemic vascular resistance, decrease in cardiac output, reduction of both coronary and cerebral blood flow, and potential for worsening outcome of acute lung injury if large tidal volumes are used. However, adequate ventilation and avoidance of hypercarbia remains important.

Arrhythmias

Up to 25% of pediatric patients undergoing congenital heart surgery experience an arrhythmia after undergoing CPB.[14] Dysrhythmias may impact the patient's hemodynamic stability due to loss of AV synchrony, inadequate filling time, or inadequate ventricular output. Most arrhythmias occur within the first 48 hours and include both bradyarrhythmias (sinus bradycardia and varying degrees of AV block) and tachyarrhythmias (supraventricular tachycardia, atrial flutter, atrial fibrillation, junctional ectopic tachycardia, and ventricular tachycardia). Risk factors for arrhythmia include myocardial ischemia, right ventricular noncompliance, ventriculotomy, multiple intracardiac suture lines near the conducting tissue, electrolyte imbalances, irritation of the endocardium from intracardiac monitoring lines, longstanding volume overload, and direct surgical trauma to the conduction system.

Up to 3% of postoperative cardiac surgical neonates and infants will experience surgically induced permanent complete AV block. The majority requires transient pacing via temporary pacing wires that are placed and tested in the operating room. Consensus recommendations for postoperative advanced second- or third-degree AV block in the pediatric population suggest permanent pacemaker implantation if heart block is not expected to resolve or persists for more than 7 days after cardiac surgery[15] (Figure 6-1).

For life-threatening, acute tachyarrhythmias accompanied by an acute change in level of consciousness, hypotension, or impaired systemic perfusion, electrical cardioversion may take precedence over pharmacotherapy. Treatment for all arrhythmias should aim to improve the hemodynamic profile of each patient while maximizing adequate oxygenation and correcting electrolyte imbalances. Junctional ectopic tachycardia (JET) is common after pediatric cardiac surgery, especially after repair of tetralogy of Fallot in young infants and after closure of ventricular septal defects and common AV canal defects. The diagnosis of JET is made in the presence of a narrow complex tachycardia with accompanying AV dissociation observed by shorter R-R intervals compared to measured P-P intervals. Often, retrograde p waves can be seen immediately after the QRS complex, suggesting retrograde conduction via the AV node (Figure 6-2). Effective treatment strategies for this automatic tachycardia must include adequate sedation and analgesia, reduction of catecholaminergic stimulation, and avoidance of hyperthermia through the use of antipyretics or institution of mild hypothermia (35°C). Temporary overdrive AV pacing may also be instituted once the JET rate has been reduced by medical therapies in order to re-establish AV synchrony to improve cardiac output. Antiarrhythmic medications such as amiodarone (class III) are particularly effective in treatment of hemodynamically significant JET as well as other automatic and ventricular arrhythmias in the postoperative period. Amiodarone acts as a negative inotrope and decreases conductivity of nodal tissues, potentially producing significant sinus bradycardia, sinus arrest, or variable AV block, especially if pre-existing disease exists. Therefore, the medical team should be prepared to initiate temporary pacing when administering amiodarone in the early postoperative period. Permanent pacing may also be needed. Long-term systemic side effects of amiodarone use should be considered including phototoxicity, corneal deposits, altered thyroid function, and depressed liver function. Coexisting medications must also be considered when treating cardiac arrhythmias, especially adrenergic agents,

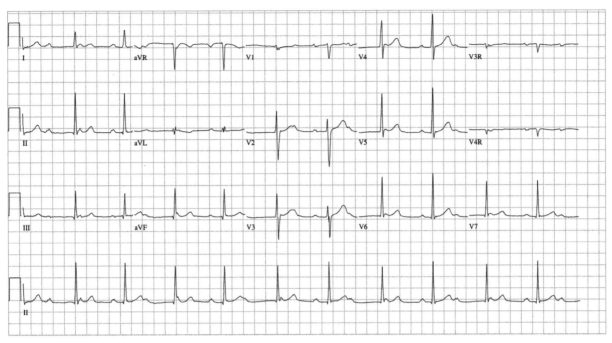

FIGURE 6-1 ■ Fifteen-lead surface electrocardiogram demonstrating complete atrioventricular block.

digoxin (dose adjustment is required when given with amiodarone), and drugs known to alter electrolyte levels. Therefore, the treatment of arrhythmias in the postoperative period should consider the presence of pre-existing rhythm disturbances, each patient's hemodynamic status, and any potential interactions with other drugs (ie, QT prolongation).

Altered Mental Status and Central Nervous System Injuries

The central nervous system (CNS) may be particularly susceptible to injury following CPB and may be further exacerbated during periods of low cardiac output. Seizures, embolic stroke, intracerebral hemorrhage,

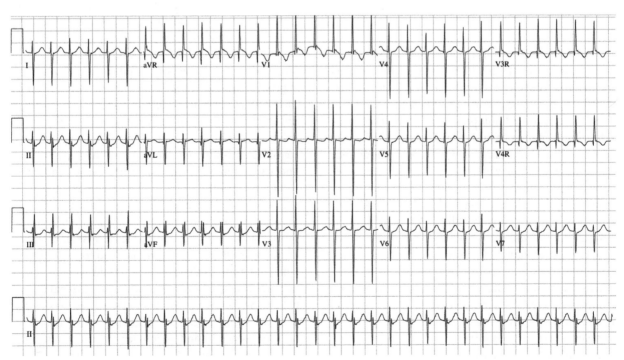

FIGURE 6-2 ■ Fifteen-lead surface electrocardiogram demonstrating junctional ectopic tachycardia with notable retrograde p waves in a 3-month-old infant after undergoing congenital heart surgery.

choreoathetosis, and long-term cognitive delay (academic difficulties, behavioral abnormalities, fine and gross motor delay, visual–motor integration, and executive planning) are all complications that may result from cardiac surgery and CPB with or without DHCA. Although usually transient, clinically detectable seizures can occur in up to 20% of neonates in the immediate postoperative period and should be investigated rapidly and treated with anticonvulsant therapy.[16] Risk factors for seizures include younger age at the time of surgery, longer periods of DHCA, and presence of coexisting abnormalities of the CNS. Perioperative seizures are a marker for early CNS injury and have been reported to be associated with worse scores on developmental testing of children several years after undergoing CPB and complex congenital heart surgery.[17] Long-term developmental sequelae of surgery for congenital heart defects continue to be the subject of ongoing research into optimal perioperative neuroprotective strategies. Preoperative risk, postoperative course, and operative variables likely play a role in the development of persistent developmental delays, in varying degrees as yet to be determined. Additional considerations during the postoperative period include the use of invasive monitoring lines, which may increase the risk of paradoxical embolus, as well as complications from prolonged hospital course such as fever, infections, hyper-/hypoglycemia, and acute swings in cerebral blood flow brought on by mechanical ventilation changes.

Acute Renal Failure and Electrolyte Abnormalities

Acute kidney injury occurs in up to 30% to 40% of adult and pediatric patients after CPB, with neonates, younger infants, and adults with comorbidities especially vulnerable to the period of planned renal ischemia. CPB with hypothermia, nonpulsatile perfusion, and reduced mean arterial pressure has been shown to cause the release of angiotensin, renin, catecholamines, and antidiuretic hormone. Acute kidney injury after CPB has been shown to be independently associated with increased mortality, longer hospital lengths of stay, increased hospital costs, and lower long-term quality of life.[18] Although multiple definitions exist for acute kidney injury, nearly all are based on an absolute or percentage change in serum creatinine levels, with relative increases of 1.5 to 3 times baseline levels indicating injury, progressing to outright failure with anuria. Impaired renal function results in decreased urine output, increased water weight gain, and elevated serum creatinine, blood urea nitrogen, and potassium values. Management varies depending on the need for volume replacement in patients with low filling pressures and diuretic administration in patients with

elevated filling pressures. Although rare in the pediatric population after CHD surgery, severe renal failure with anuria, life-threatening hyperkalemia, intractable metabolic acidosis, and fluid overload that compromises gas exchange can occur and is associated with increased mortality rates. Excessive fluid retention with renal failure delays extubation, increases risks of infection, and prolongs ICU recovery time. Additional aggressive forms of support may need to be employed including peritoneal dialysis, hemodialysis, and/or continuous venovenous hemofiltration. Peritoneal dialysis is generally technically easier to accomplish in the neonate and infant population, as there is no requirement for large intravascular catheters or anticoagulation, although control over fluid balance may be less precise when compared with continuous renal replacement therapy.

Particular vigilance must also be paid to electrolyte abnormalities during the period of active diuresis within the first 24 hours after CPB. Attention should be devoted to aggressive monitoring and supplementation of potassium, calcium, and magnesium levels. Metabolic derangements secondary to renal failure such as metabolic acidosis, hyponatremia, hyperkalemia, and hypocalcemia should be avoided because they can exacerbate underlying myocardial dysfunction. Accurate records of intake and output should be recorded and tabulated daily to assess total body fluid balance.

Pain Management and Sedation

Significant stressors associated with CHD surgery including CPB, aortic cross-clamping, deep hypothermia, myocardial ischemia, and elevations in stress hormone levels contribute to altered hemodynamics in the postoperative period. In addition, pain, agitation, and anxiety are also expected and therefore require an aggressive multidisciplinary approach with therapies including continuous or intermittent infusions of opioid and benzodiazepine agents, regional techniques (eg, epidural anesthesia), patient-controlled analgesia, nonsteroidal anti-inflammatory agents, child life therapy, and active family participation. The neonatal and infant response to painful or stressful stimuli may manifest as tachycardia and hypertension in the patient with normal cardiovascular reserve. Hemodynamically compromising tachycardia and intolerable increases in afterload associated with hypertension may lead to rapid hypoxemia and even sudden death in certain patients. These untoward complications are particularly evident among patients with labile pulmonary artery pressures and in palliated single-ventricle patients in whom the balance between systemic and pulmonary vascular resistance plays an important role in hemodynamic stability. Continuous infusions of fentanyl or morphine following intraoperative anesthetic dosing have been used traditionally for pain management in patients with unstable hemodynamics and for neonates after undergoing palliation for single-ventricle disease. The goal is to minimize hemodynamic lability in the first postoperative night when cardiac output reaches its nadir and myocardial reserve is diminished. Less labile patients who are awakened in the immediate postoperative period may receive analgesia on an as-needed basis with intermittent dosing of narcotics. In addition, analgesics are usually required to gain cooperation and alleviate pain and discomfort associated with chest tube, intracardiac monitoring lines, and pacemaker wire removal.

Infants and children who require prolonged use of opioids and benzodiazepines are more susceptible to the effects of withdrawal and require a slow wean over at least 7 to 14 days. Signs and symptoms include jitteriness, insomnia, seizures, diarrhea, diaphoresis, agitation, nausea and vomiting, tachycardia, and hypertension. Long-term pain management after transfer from the ICU to the general ward and eventual discharge home can include transition to oral acetaminophen or ibuprofen with intermittent dosing of narcotics (oxycodone). Older children and adolescents often require an additional 5 to 7 days of oral narcotics such as oxycodone or codeine.

Postoperative Infection

Perioperative use of antibiotics, initiated intraoperatively within 1 hour prior to skin incision, reduces the incidence of postoperative wound infections. Antibiotics are given during the immediate recovery phase for at least 24 hours after surgery or until sternal closure if the sternum is open for the immediate postoperative course. Low-grade fever (<38.5°C) during the early postoperative period is commonly observed after CPB and is rarely associated with an infectious cause. Early removal of indwelling catheters in the postoperative patient may reduce the incidence of mediastinitis and sepsis. Mediastinitis occurs in ≤2% of patients undergoing cardiac surgery and is characterized by persistent fever, purulent drainage from the sternotomy wound, sternal instability, and leukocytosis. *Staphylococcus* species are the most common offending pathogens, and risk factors include delayed sternal closure, early re-exploration for bleeding, diabetes, obesity, and reoperation. As with sepsis after cardiac surgery in adults, delayed diagnosis of mediastinitis can lead to mortality rates as high as 25%. Treatment is primarily surgical with debridement, irrigation, use of negative pressure wound therapy (eg, vacuum-assisted closure), and aggressive parenteral antibiotic therapy.

Wound care in the home environment is often a source of anxiety for parents and should also be addressed in preparation for discharge. Most incisions require little care if no drainage or wound separation is observed. However, more frequent cleaning with sterile saline solution and covering with a dry sterile gauze dressing are required should mild dehiscence or serosanguinous drainage be present after initial healing. Oral antibiotics are also considered for significant wound dehiscence or superficial infection demonstrated by expanding erythema without prominent edema, purulent discharge, or induration. Hospitalization with initiation of intravenous antibiotics and possible surgical debridement, as discussed earlier, is warranted in the presence of extensive wound infections. As most incisional suture material is absorbable, the only stitches that require delayed removal are those from drainage tubes and from invasive vascular monitoring line placement (arterial lines, central venous catheters), which are removed 5 to 7 days after initial catheter removal.

Transfer to the General Care Ward

The transition of care from ICU to general care ward or intermediate care unit is an important step in the recovery of patients after undergoing cardiac surgery. While the acuity of patient care and intensity of management become less complex, the goal of successful transition to life at home should remain the focus. Hemodynamic stability and precautions against hospital-associated comorbidities such as infections, malnutrition, and poor psychosocial adjustment are mainstays of care.

Initial considerations for transfer require satisfactory surgical results with hemodynamic stability, absence of inotropic support, independence from mechanical ventilatory support, and removal of most invasive vascular monitoring lines and drainage tubes. Supplemental oxygen use and enteral tube feeding are not contraindications to transfer to the general care ward or to discharge home. Neonates and infants with specialized dietary needs or preoperative caloric supplementation often require tube-feeding support throughout the entire hospitalization. Furthermore, an infrequent complication from open-heart surgery that parallels injury to the phrenic nerve is trauma to the recurrent laryngeal nerve. Injury of this nerve results in unilateral vocal cord paralysis, leading to hoarse voice or weak cry. As airway protection is potentially compromised, previously normal feeding neonates can demonstrate signs of aspiration (coughing, gagging, respiratory distress, or oxygen desaturation) when bottle-fed in recovery. Vocal cord dysfunction is transient in the majority of patients, yet consultation with an otorhinolaryngologist or speech language therapist may help determine whether the child will require thickened oral feeds or will be completely dependent on nasogastric feeds.

A late complication from cardiac surgery that may not manifest for up to 7 to 21 days after surgery is postpericardiotomy syndrome. The appearance or persistence of a pericardial effusion with associated fever, chest pain/discomfort, irritability, nausea, poor appetite, and intolerance of feeds in the infant may be diagnostic of this condition. Physical examination reveals a pleural or pericardial rub, and chest radiography confirms a widened mediastinum with occasional accompanying pleural effusions. Mild cases require observation with serial examinations and echocardiograms. However, moderate effusions with symptoms usually require treatment with nonsteroidal anti-inflammatory agents (ibuprofen, indomethacin) and close follow-up. Corticosteroids are usually reserved for cases not responding to anti-inflammatory medications. Larger pericardial effusions may require pericardiocentesis to prevent cardiac tamponade, and chronic effusions may require a surgically created pericardial window.

Preparation for Discharge

The coordination of discharge plans should reflect the age of the patient, the congenital heart lesion and corresponding surgical repair, any coexisting medical issues, and the family dynamic and environment to which the patient is entering upon discharge. A family-centered approach can help in this care delivery and has been shown to improve outcomes as well as patient, family, and provider satisfaction. Patient and family education is therefore the cornerstone of effective anticipatory guidance after hospital discharge.

Routine discharge instructions should include information about medications, suture line care, activity, diet, and bathing restrictions. Children can usually resume their usual bathing or showering routine after removal of all drains and tubes 48 hours after surgery, whereas newborn skin care is dependent on the disappearance of the umbilical cord stump. Impaired or delayed wound healing will require sponge bathing until the wound is completely healed. Infants and young children generally do not require formal activity restrictions as they move around freely and self-limit when tired or in pain. In the setting of median sternotomy healing, providing support from under the buttocks and the back of the infant's head when lifting is a preferred approach when compared to picking up the child under the arms. Usual return to school or daycare occurs about 1 to 2 weeks after discharge from the hospital. In older children and adolescents, median sternotomy incisions require 6 to 8 weeks for complete bone healing. These patients are instructed to avoid strenuous activities including contact sports, swimming, climbing, skateboarding/snowboarding, bike riding, and/or any activity that can result in chest wall trauma. They should not participate in sports or physical education classes for 6 to 8 weeks after return to school and specifically avoid lifting objects weighing greater than 10 lb. Primary care physicians are therefore the strongest advocates for these

patients, often recommending home schooling or tutoring to keep children current with school activities.

Patients demonstrating adequate intake of fluids and tolerance of oral medications can be prepared for discharge with the understanding that most children do not regain their usual appetite for 1 to 2 weeks after discharge. Nutritional counseling should begin with an assessment of home routines and preferences; families are encouraged to bring in food and treats from home, as most children do not have dietary restrictions. Narcotics are known to slow gastrointestinal motility; therefore, an adequate balance between pain control and bowel movement regularity and comfort is essential. The addition of stool softeners or prokinetic agents should also be strongly considered in all older children and adolescents.

The critically ill newborn and neonatal population often experiences difficulty with oral feeding postoperatively. Prolonged or complex hospitalizations as well as recurrent laryngeal nerve injury pose a risk to development of oral feeding intolerance and possible aversion. Newborns denied oral feeds for weeks after birth require time to relearn the oral–motor coordination required for successful oral feeding. These infants may need temporary supplemental or total nasogastric tube feeding with high-calorie formulas. As the infant recovers at home with continued help from oral and speech therapists, nasogastric feeds are eventually weaned until feeding support is no longer needed.

A comprehensive medication reconciliation process will assist the providers, nursing staff, patient, and family with a better understanding of each medication, its dosing regimen, and its side effect profile. By the time of discharge, many children have transitioned to acetaminophen or ibuprofen for pain control with intermittent dosing of a narcotic (oxycodone or codeine). Diuretics are also used aggressively in the postoperative period and are also frequently prescribed on discharge. Diuretics are preferably dosed during the day to avoid enuresis and frequent nighttime voiding. This attention to medication scheduling should also reflect the transition to home care, which is not based on 24-hour-per-day nursing availability. When appropriate, once- or twice-daily medication dosing should be prescribed to allow for uninterrupted periods of sleep and minimal disruption to school routines.

Lastly, general care guidelines also help to prepare the patient and family for other problems that may arise at home. Families are instructed to monitor their child for temperature instability, with low-grade fevers (<38°C) treated at home with antipyretics and recurring low-grade fevers or high-grade fever (>38.5°C) necessitating physician evaluation. Additional reasons to seek physician screening include wound changes, such as expanding erythema, swelling, drainage, or opening, and persistent nausea, vomiting, feeding intolerance, abdominal pain, difficulty breathing, tachypnea, or irritability. Routine immunizations may be deferred for 4 to 6 weeks after surgery to allow for immune reconstitution and appropriate antibody response after undergoing CPB. As a special patient population, heart transplantation patients are counseled to avoid live vaccines for at least 6 months after transplantation.

Follow-up appointments should include early visits to the primary care physician's office 2 to 3 days after discharge and a follow-up with the pediatric cardiologist at 1 to 2 weeks, depending on the individual needs and complexity of medical care.

CARE OF THE POSTCATHETERIZATION PATIENT

Basics of Cardiac Catheterization in the Pediatric Patient

Cardiac catheterization in the CHD population shares few common elements with routine cardiac catheterization in the adult with isolated coronary or valvular heart disease. Although the equipment and tools may be similar, the indications, techniques, and interventions performed are substantially different. A complete precatheterization assessment will ensure that appropriate indications for the procedure are reviewed, sedation strategies are considered, vascular access plans are outlined, and potential interventions are discussed among the catheterization team and with the patient and family.

Planning for sedation requires knowledge of the patient's cardiac and noncardiac medical history, with particular attention paid to the age of the patient, airway status, and prior responses to sedation and medication reactions. General anesthesia is often the optimal strategy, particularly for complex interventions and catheter procedures in unstable infants. Common intravenous regimens used for nonanesthesia cases include combinations of midazolam and ketamine, pentobarbital and morphine, or fentanyl and midazolam in older children.

Vascular access is most commonly obtained through the femoral artery and vein using the modified Seldinger technique (catheter over a wire). Beyond femoral access, many other sites may be used either because of vascular occlusion or for other directed procedures. Alternative sites for arterial access include umbilical, axillary, radial, and even carotid (via cut-down) arteries. Alterative sites for venous access include jugular, subclavian, and transhepatic. Heparin is routinely administered when arterial access is obtained both to decrease risk of arterial occlusion and to minimize the potential for thromboembolism and stroke.

Interventional Procedures and Complications

It is helpful for the practitioner caring for children with CHD to have a general understanding of the wide range of therapeutic procedures performed in the catheterization lab. Common interventions include device closure of septal defects (atrial and ventricular), balloon angioplasty for stenotic lesions (coarctation of the aorta, pulmonary arterial stenoses), stenting for vascular stenosis (coarctation of the aorta, pulmonary artery branch stenosis), percutaneous pulmonary valve implantation, balloon valvuloplasty (pulmonary and aortic stenosis), and embolization procedures (patent ductus arteriosus, collateral vessels). Some knowledge of the basic technique and the potential case-specific complications will help the practitioner in the management of patients both immediately after procedures as well as on subsequent follow-up.

Only 2 devices are currently approved in the United States for atrial septal defect (ASD) closure: the Amplatzer Septal Occluder and the Helex device. The Amplatzer device is composed of a Nitinol wire mesh external frame with polyester fiber forming occlusive material within this frame. When appropriately deployed, the device takes the shape of 2 counter occluders, 1 on each side of the atrial septum (Figure 6-3), with a connecting waist between (Figure 6-4). The Helex device consists of a long Nitinol wire over which has been sewn a continuous strip of polytetrafluoroethylene (Gore-Tex) fabric (Figure 6-5). When appropriately deployed, the device forms 2 occlusive disks, 1 on each side of the atrial septum (Figure 6-6). Upon release, these disks lock together, occluding the defect. The transcatheter closure of an ASD involves maneuvering large-bore delivery catheters from the femoral vein antegrade across the atrial defect. Device deployment is guided by a combination of fluoroscopy and echocardiography (transesophageal in younger patients or intracardiac in older ones). Apart from the general risks of hemodynamic catheterization, there are several procedure-specific risks. These include device embolization, atrial arrhythmias, heart block, and device erosion. Embolization of an ASD device is uncommon; when it occurs, it is usually within the first 12 hours and diagnosed before patient discharge. However, late embolizations have been reported. Embolization is almost never symptomatic. It is often treated in the catheterization laboratory, although surgical retrieval may be necessary. Although quite rare (approximately 1 in 1000), device erosion is perhaps the most severe complication that may occur after ASD closure. Erosion may result in aortic injury or tamponade.

Standard postprocedure care after ASD device closure includes daily aspirin and bacterial endocarditis prophylaxis for 6 months.

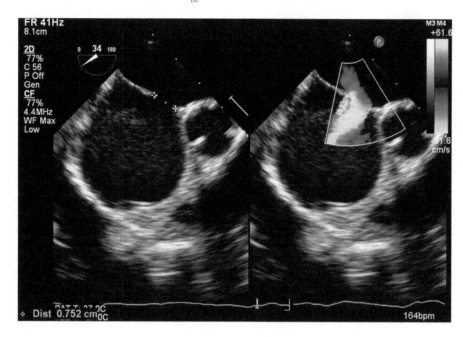

FIGURE 6-3 ■ Transesophageal echocardiogram with 2-dimensional and color spectral Doppler imaging demonstrating moderate-sized secundum atrial septal defect prior to device closure.

Patent ductus arteriosus (PDA) is treated by catheter occlusion in most patients other than the premature infant. A small PDA is usually occluded with embolization coils. Using either an antegrade or retrograde approach, spring wire coils enmeshed with polyester fibers are introduced into a delivery catheter and delivered by extrusion out of the distal catheter port with a straight metal wire serving as a loading and delivery tool. The coil then occludes the vessel by creation of a mass of fabric and wire in which a thrombus forms. Larger PDAs are usually closed with an Amplatzer Duct Occluder or Amplatzer Vascular Plug. These devices are similar in concept to the Amplatzer Septal Occluder

device described earlier but of different configurations. The devices are positioned such that a retention disk is positioned in the aortic ampulla with the remaining portion of the device deployed across the ductus, and angiograms are performed to document device position and efficacy (Figure 6-7). After the procedure, patients are observed in hospital for 6 hours. A chest x-ray is performed to confirm device position. Complications are rare after PDA occlusion. In rare instances, if occlusion is incomplete, patients may be at risk for intravascular hemolysis, embolization, or infection.

Balloon angioplasty is used to treat recurrent or native coarctation of the aorta, branch pulmonary artery

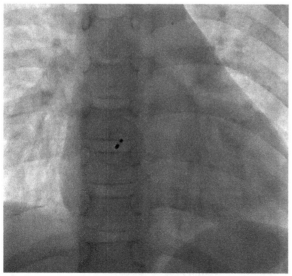

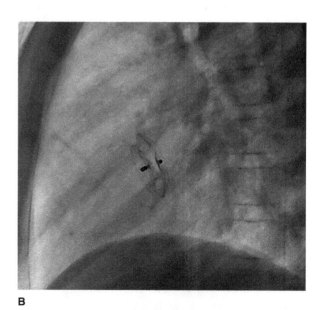

A

B

FIGURE 6-4 ■ **A.** Fluoroscopic still image (anterior-posterior camera angle) of atrial septal defect device closure with Amplatzer Septal Occluder. **B.** Fluoroscopic still image (lateral camera angle) of atrial septal defect device closure with Amplatzer Septal Occluder.

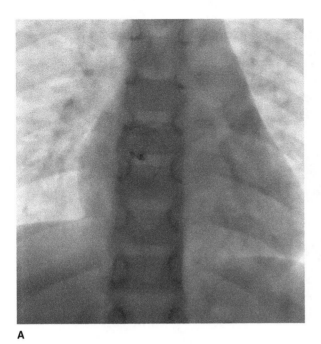

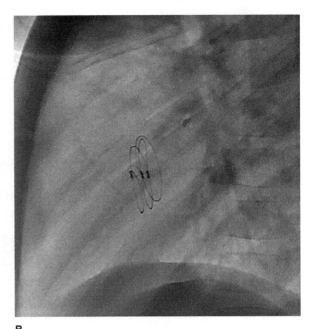

FIGURE 6-5 ■ A. Fluoroscopic still image (anterior-posterior camera angle) of atrial septal defect device closure with Helex device. **B.** Fluoroscopic still image (lateral camera angle) of atrial septal defect device closure with Helex device.

stenosis, and a variety of systemic or pulmonary venous obstructions. Dilating balloons are advanced over a guide-wire positioned through the stenotic lesion. Balloons are typically inflated to high pressures (up to 25 atmospheres). The mechanism of stenosis relief usually involves varying degrees of intimal and medial disruption. Although angioplasty can be very effective, incomplete relief of obstruction and/or restenosis may occur. In addition, angioplasty may not be safe in early postoperative stenotic lesions. In these situations, balloon expandable stents are often the treatment of choice.

Surgery is the best treatment for native coarctation of the aorta in the neonate and infant. In older children, either catheter or surgical treatment may be offered, as there is disagreement about which treatment modality is optimal. In infants through school-aged children, balloon dilation is generally recognized as the preferred method of treating recurrent coarctation. In adolescents and older patients, both native and recurrent coarctations are effectively treated with stents. Angioplasty or stenting is performed via a retrograde femoral arterial approach. Balloon dilation and/or stent implantation are successful in achieving immediate relief of the obstruction in over 90% of cases. Aortic aneurysms and dissections are potential complications of dilation and stenting. Although these events are rare, patients require follow-up imaging of the aorta to rule out late development of aneurysms after catheter treatment of coarctation. Patients are usually observed overnight after catheter treatment.

Balloon pulmonary arterioplasty has also gained wide acceptance as standard management of branch pulmonary artery stenoses particularly in distal lesions not amenable to surgical repair. Treatment modalities include the use of standard balloon angioplasty, cutting balloons, or endovascular stents. Routine in-hospital postcatheterization care includes follow-up complete blood count testing, chest radiograph, and observation overnight. Procedure-specific complications include vessel perforation or rupture, aneurysm formation, and transient pulmonary edema. Serious complications occur in approximately 1% of procedures; cutting balloon angioplasty is highest in risk. So-called reperfusion pulmonary edema is most likely to occur in patients with multiple-branch pulmonary artery obstructions after angioplasty has resulted in relief of obstruction to only some areas of lung. These areas are subjected to sudden-onset excess pulmonary flow and pressure. Clinically, these patients may manifest profound hypoxia. If this occurs, patients require immediate intubation and positive pressure ventilation. Repeat emergency catheter treatment may be necessary to redistribute pulmonary blood flow.

First reported in 1982, balloon dilation of valvar pulmonary stenosis was among the first interventions for CHD. Balloon dilation of pulmonary stenosis is usually curative except in patients with dysplastic pulmonary valve leaflets (most common in Noonan syndrome). Complications after this procedure are rare.

In contrast to pulmonary stenosis, balloon aortic valvuloplasty must be considered palliative rather than curative treatment. The goal of therapy is the reduction in aortic valve gradient without creating significant aortic insufficiency. Although the procedure achieves this goal in most patients, virtually all will require additional treatment later in life for stenosis, regurgitation, or both.

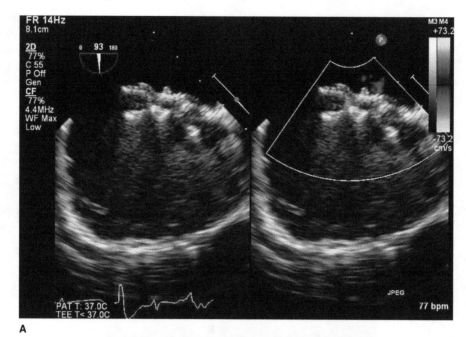

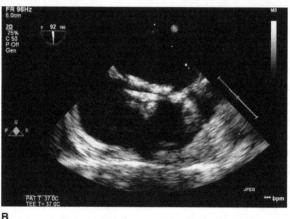

FIGURE 6-6 ■ **A.** Transesophageal echocardiogram 2-dimensional imaging of secundum atrial septal defect after device closure with Amplatzer Septal Occluder. **B.** Transesophageal echocardiogram 2-dimensional imaging of secundum atrial septal defect after device closure with Helix device.

Beyond the newborn period, aortic valve dilation is performed via a retrograde femoral artery approach. The neonatal population with critical aortic stenosis undergoing balloon valvuloplasty represents an especially high-risk population; they frequently have significant left ventricular dysfunction and mitral insufficiency. Intraprocedure events such as ventricular fibrillation are not uncommon. Even after successful valvuloplasty, these infants may require a significant period of intensive care with inotropic support. When retrograde transfemoral access is used in the neonate, loss of pulse is common after the procedure due to femoral artery thrombosis. Generally, treatment with anticoagulants or thrombolytics successfully re-establishes femoral arterial patency. Typically, a postcatheterization echocardiogram is performed to document residual gradients and insufficiency and evaluate ventricular function.

Complications

Additional complications associated with both diagnostic and interventional cardiac catheterizations in the pediatric population can be observed, although overall rates of serious complications and mortality have declined over the past 30 years. An increased risk of periprocedural mortality continues to remain significantly associated with cardiac catheterization in children with elevated pulmonary vascular resistance. The use of newer pharmacologic advancements and the advent of nonionic contrast media have helped to reduce overall mortality. Postcatheterization monitoring in an ICU setting for all patients with pulmonary hypertension has been adopted by many centers in an effort to provide ready access to needed pharmacologic rescue therapies should pulmonary hypertensive crises occur during recovery.

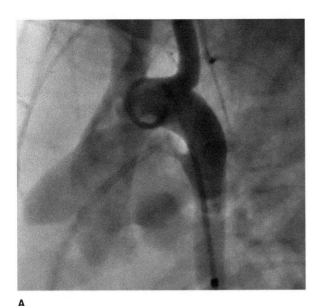 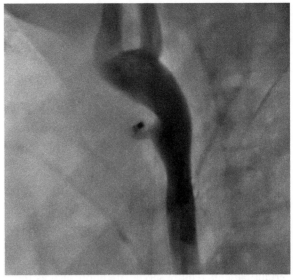

A   B

FIGURE 6-7 ■ A. Fluoroscopic still image (lateral camera angle) of an aortogram showing a patent ductus arteriosus prior to device closure. B. Fluoroscopic still image (lateral camera angle) of patent ductus arteriosus after closure with an Amplatzer ductal occluder device. Note absence of contrast in the pulmonary artery compared to prior to closure.

Additionally, improved catheter technology and better noninvasive description of cardiac anatomy have resulted in fewer catheter-related complications. Adverse events are twice as likely to occur during interventional cases as compared to diagnostic cases. Severe or catastrophic adverse events occur in approximately 9% of all interventional cases and only 5% of diagnostic cases, as reported by the participants of the Congenital Cardiac Catheterization Outcomes Project (C3PO) recently. Death occurred in only 0.3% of all cases and was associated with severity of disease prior to undergoing catheterization.

MEDICAL MANAGEMENT AFTER DISCHARGE

Goals of the Postprocedural Outpatient Evaluation

The management of pediatric patients with CHD presents challenges through the lifespan. Although the most critical aspect of care occurs in the immediate periprocedural period, continued observation and management in the outpatient setting are crucial to the growth and development of the child. The heterogeneity of CHD presents a wide spectrum of management complexities, thus requiring the general practitioner to understand each patient's individualized management strategy. Children may initially undergo palliation and subsequent repair or may receive primary repairs. After hospital discharge, management decisions revolve around

short-term postprocedural management, medication use, monitoring of growth, nutrition, development, family impact, and immunization status.

The majority of children require continued pharmacologic support after discharge from surgery. Although most postcatheterization patients will continue their precatheterization medical management, several will require adjustments or initiation of new medications to affect loading conditions of their heart or to decrease pulmonary arterial pressures. Pain management after catheterization is typically accomplished with simple nonsteroidal anti-inflammatory agents, acetaminophen, and rarely opioids. Postsurgical patients often require a variety of preload, contractility, and afterload-altering medications, including diuretics (loop and thiazide agents), digoxin, and angiotensin-converting enzyme inhibitors. Antiarrhythmics are also commonly prescribed to treat persistent atrial or ventricular tachycardias in the postoperative period. These medications may include digoxin in addition to β-blockers and amiodarone. Side effect profiles and potential drug–drug interactions need to be evaluated for each patient and reconciled with discharge instructions and the discharge summary of hospital course.

Long-term growth and development continue to remain a substantial challenge for all patients with CHD, including those who undergo "definitive repair." Up to 30% of children with CHD will be below the third percentile on weight-for-age growth curves. Preoperative management often focuses on the high metabolic state associated with congestive heart failure by increasing caloric intake. Therefore, high-calorie supplementation should continue postoperatively until the child's weight has stabilized and no additional complications are observed. Children not responding to nutritional supplementation or who have a genetic syndrome associated with poor growth may require a more comprehensive evaluation of endocrine function and gastrointestinal health. Once wound healing has occurred and postoperative pain is better controlled, stressing a healthy lifestyle and diet will help to avoid the establishment of sedentary habits in this particularly obesity-prone population.

Every effort should be made to ensure that all children with CHD receive all immunizations according to the American Academy of Pediatrics immunization schedule recommendations. This can be challenging for this population due to the frequency of associated illnesses, hospitalizations, and procedures. Additionally, certain patients require special attention such as those who have undergone orthotopic heart transplantation, those with asplenia syndromes, and those with DiGeorge syndrome. Intensive immunosuppressive regimens require that all live vaccines be delayed by 6 months in all heart transplantation patients. Asplenia syndrome patients should receive pneumococcal and *Haemophilus influenzae* type B vaccines starting at 2 months and should also receive amoxicillin prophylaxis (20 mg/kg/day). Children with document T-cell immunodeficiency from 22q11 deletion syndrome (DiGeorge syndrome) should receive inactivated vaccines. Close consultation with an immunologist can help determine the extent of response to each vaccine. Additionally, infants undergoing CPB with ultrafiltration shortly after receiving immunizations should consider repeat vaccination because exposure to blood products and ultrafiltration may affect immune responses to vaccines. Respiratory syncytial virus infections are non–immunity-conferring lower respiratory tract infections that have been shown to lead to higher hospitalization and mortality rates in the CHD population when compared to noncardiac pediatric patients. Respiratory syncytial virus prophylaxis is thus warranted in any patient less than 2 years of age with cyanotic CHD, patients with pulmonary hypertension, and patients with hemodynamically significant lesions (unrepaired or palliated) requiring cardiac medications such as digoxin, diuretics, and/or angiotensin-converting enzyme inhibitors.

Dental care in children with CHD is another important consideration due to the risk of bacterial endocarditis. Transient bacteremia occurs frequently with routine dental hygiene and can increase substantially with dental procedures associated with instrumentation and preventive care. Updated American Heart Association and American Dental Association guidelines have been published recently.[19] These recommendations have simplified and reduced the need for antibiotic prophylaxis in this population, limiting the use of antibiotics to the following patients: those with artificial heart valves, prior history of infective endocarditis, unrepaired or incompletely repaired cyanotic CHD (including those with palliative shunts or conduits), completely repaired CHD with prosthetic material or device within first 6 months after procedure, any repaired CHD with residual defect, and cardiac transplantation with any valve abnormality (stenosis, regurgitation).

Lastly, postprocedural care should seek to engage family and care providers. Education about medications and nutritional needs should be delivered with reciprocal feedback of understanding demonstrated. Follow-up of the postoperative child is a lifelong process that requires active participation between cardiologist, surgeon, primary care physician, and family to ensure a successful, healthy, and meaningful life.

Clinical Pearls

- Management of the postprocedural patient should reflect a firm understanding of common congenital heart defects and surgical interventions, cardiopulmonary anatomy and physiology, advanced technical skills, pharmacology, and common complications.
- The primary care provider should understand that the use of mechanical support in the form of extracorporeal membrane oxygenation (ECMO) has become widely used and should be considered when assessing cardiopulmonary and developmental status of growing children.
- Pulmonary hypertension is a major cause of morbidity and mortality following cardiac surgery in the pediatric population, especially after repair of congenital heart disease with large left-to-right shunts, truncus arteriosus, dextro-transposition of the great arteries, and total anomalous pulmonary venous connection.
- Up to 25% of pediatric patients undergoing congenital heart surgery experience an arrhythmia after cardiopulmonary bypass, with most arrhythmias occurring within the first 48 hours. These include both bradyarrhythmias (sinus bradycardia and varying degrees of atrioventricular block) and tachyarrhythmias (supraventricular tachycardia, atrial flutter, atrial fibrillation, junctional ectopic tachycardia, and ventricular tachycardia).
- Perioperative seizures are an early marker for central nervous system (CNS) injury with risk factors including younger age at the time of surgery, longer periods of deep hypothermic circulatory arrest, and presence of coexisting abnormalities of the CNS.
- Although rates of serious complications and mortality have declined over the past 30 years, an increased risk of periprocedural mortality remains for patients with elevated pulmonary vascular resistance.
- After hospital discharge, the primary care provider must be aware of short-term postprocedural management plans; medication use; monitoring of growth, nutrition, and development; family stress; and immunization implications.

REFERENCES

1. Dorfman AT, Marino BS, Wernovsky G, et al. Critical heart disease in the neonate: presentation and outcome at a tertiary care center. *Pediatr Crit Care Med.* 2008;9:193-202.

2. Wypij D, Jonas RA, Bellinger DC, et al. The effect of hematocrit during hypothermic cardiopulmonary bypass in infant heart surgery: results from the combined Boston hematocrit trials. *J Thorac Cardiovasc Surg.* 2008;135:355-360.

3. Naik SK, Knight A, Elliott M. A prospective randomized study of a modified technique of ultrafiltration during pediatric open-heart surgery. *Circulation.* 1991;84(5 Suppl):422-431.

4. Licht DJ, Shera DM, Clancy RR, et al. Brain maturation is delayed in infants with complex congenital heart defects. *J Thorac Cardiovasc Surg.* 2009;137:529-536.

5. Wernovsky G, Wypij D, Jonas RA, et al. Postoperative course and hemodynamic profile after the arterial switch operation in neonates and infants: a comparison of low-flow cardiopulmonary bypass and circulatory arrest. *Circulation.* 1995;92:2226-2235.

6. Tweddell JS, Hoffman GM. Postoperative management in patients with complex congenital heart disease. *Semin Thorac Cardiovasc Surg Pediatr Card Surg Annu.* 2002;5:187-205.

7. Razon Y, Erez E, Vidne B, et al. Recombinant factor VIIa (Novoseven) as a hemostatic agent after surgery for congenital heart disease. *Paediatr Anaesth.* 2005;15:235-240.

8. Tabbutt S, Duncan BW, McLaughlin D, et al. Delayed sternal closure after cardiac operations in a pediatric population. *J Thorac Cardiovasc Surg.* 1997;113:886-893.

9. Duncan BW, Hraska V, Jonas RA, et al. Mechanical circulatory support in children with cardiac disease. *J Thorac Cardiovasc Surg.* 1999;117:529-542.

10. Joho-Arreola AL, Bauersfeld U, Stauffer UG, et al. Incidence and treatment of diaphragmatic paralysis after cardiac surgery in children. *Eur J Cardiothorac Surg.* 2005;27:53-57.

11. Alghamdi AA, Singh SK, Hamilton BC, et al. Early extubation after pediatric cardiac surgery: systematic review, meta-analysis, and evidence-based recommendations. *J Card Surg.* 2010;25:586-595.

12. Suesaowalak M, Cleary JP, Chang AC. Advances in diagnosis and treatment of pulmonary arterial hypertension in neonates and children with congenital heart disease. *World J Pediatr.* 2010;6:13-31.

13. Steinhorn RH, Kinsella JP, Pierce C. Intravenous sildenafil in the treatment of neonates with persistent pulmonary hypertension. *J Pediatr.* 2009;155:841-847.

14. Delaney JW, Moltedo JM, Dziura JD, et al. Early postoperative arrhythmias after pediatric cardiac surgery. *J Thorac Cardiovasc Surg.* 2006;131:1296-1300.

15. Villain E. Indications for pacing in patients with congenital heart disease. *Pacing Clin Electrophysiol.* 2008;31(Suppl 1):S17-S20.

16. Gaynor JW, Jarvik GP, Bernbaum J, et al. The relationship of postoperative electrographic seizures to neurodevelopmental outcome at 1 year of age after neonatal and infant cardiac surgery. *J Thorac Cardiovasc Surg.* 2006;131:181-189.

17. Rappaport LA, Wypij D, Bellinger DC, et al. Relation of seizures after cardiac surgery in early infancy to neurodevelopmental outcome. *Circulation.* 1998;97:773-779.

18. Li S, Krawczeski CD, Zappitelli M, et al. Incidence, risk factors, and outcomes of acute kidney injury after pediatric cardiac surgery: a prospective multicenter study. *Crit Care Med.* 2011;39:1493-1499.

19. Wilson W, Taubert KA, Gewitz M, et al. Prevention of infective endocarditis: guidelines from the American Heart Association: a guideline from the American Heart Association Rheumatic Fever, Endocarditis, and Kawasaki Disease Committee, Council on Cardiovascular Disease in the Young, and the Council on Clinical Cardiology, Council on Cardiovascular Surgery and Anesthesia, and the Quality of Care and Outcomes Research Interdisciplinary Working Group. *Circulation.* 2007;116:1736-1754.

CHAPTER 7

Acyanotic Shunt Lesions

Shari Wellen,
Andrew C. Glatz and
Shobha Natarajan

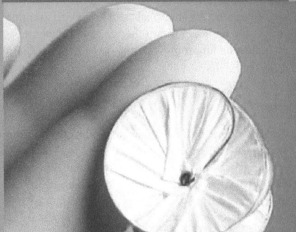

INTRODUCTION

Acyanotic cardiac defects are a group of diverse cardiac malformations that share a common physiology of increased pulmonary blood flow in the setting of normal systemic perfusion and oxygen saturation. Most of these defects produce varying degrees of shunting of blood from the left side of the heart to the right side. Patients with shunt lesions often present initially to the general pediatrician with problems ranging from failure to thrive and poor weight gain to respiratory distress and exercise intolerance. Alternatively, the patient may be asymptomatic but have an abnormal cardiovascular physical examination. Some of these defects, when left untreated, can affect long-term cardiovascular health. Therefore, this chapter will address the pathophysiology of shunt lesions, modes of presentation, indications for referral, and general treatment algorithms of shunt lesions.

Pathophysiology of Shunt Lesions: General Principles

Although specific defects within the group of shunt lesions present at different ages depending on the location and degree of shunting, the common pathophysiology involves increased pulmonary blood flow.

In utero, the placenta provides oxygenated blood to the fetus. The pulmonary vasculature is constricted, and blood flow is largely shunted away from the lungs across the patent foramen ovale and the patent ductus arteriosus. The first breaths of life initiate a sharp decline in pulmonary vascular resistance that then continues for the first few months of life.[1] The degree of shunting through some of the shunt lesions, such as

patent ductus arteriosus and ventricular septal defect, depend on the relative resistances between the pulmonary and systemic vascular beds. Therefore, infants with these types of shunt lesions present beyond the neonatal period but within the first few months of life when pulmonary vascular resistance is low, promoting more pulmonary blood flow.

In contrast, the degree of shunting in other defects, such as atrial septal defects, depends on right ventricular compliance. The right ventricle is relatively stiff and noncompliant in utero. Unlike the relatively brisk drop in pulmonary vascular resistance after birth, the right ventricle can take months to remodel. Therefore, patients with these types of defects present in late childhood or early adulthood.

Clinical Manifestations: General Principles

Excessive pulmonary blood flow leads to respiratory symptoms of tachypnea and increased work of breathing. The exact mechanism of these symptoms is unknown, but it likely is explained by increased lymphatic flow. As pulmonary blood flow continues to increase, lymphatic channels in the lungs are overwhelmed and interstitial fluid accumulates, leading to peribronchial edema and inflammation.[2] Tachypnea and retractions ensue. This increased work of breathing, in turn, makes it difficult to feed well and increases oxygen and caloric demands, leading to poor weight gain and failure to thrive. Unlike adults with low-output heart failure, infants and children with shunt lesions have high-output heart failure. Increased metabolic demand stimulates neurohormonal mechanisms and increases cardiac output. Hepatic veins dilate to accommodate the increased blood volume, and hepatomegaly results. Adrenergic drive is also increased and accounts for the tachycardia and diaphoresis that are often seen.[3] An abnormal cardiac physical examination in the setting of these other signs and symptoms is an indication for prompt referral to a pediatric cardiologist (Table 7-1).

General Treatment Principles

The goals of medical therapy are to minimize respiratory symptoms and optimize growth. Fortified feeds with additional calories and supplemental enteral nutrition with nasogastric feeds can improve weight gain. Close monitoring during these therapies is critical.

Diuretic medications reduce the interstitial fluid that has accumulated in the lungs and can ameliorate the respiratory symptoms. Furosemide is a loop diuretic that acts by inhibiting the sodium-potassium-chloride channel in the thick ascending limb of the loop of Henle. It can be prescribed at an initial dose of 1 mg/kg/dose twice daily and increased as needed, in conjunction with a pediatric cardiologist. Possible side effects of furosemide include dehydration, hypokalemia, and mild hypocalcemia.[4] Additional diuretics can be used if this is inadequate therapy or not tolerated by the patient. Chlorothiazide is a thiazide diuretic that inhibits sodium and chloride reabsorption from the distal convoluted tubules. Side effects include dehydration and hypokalemia.[4] Spironolactone is a mild diuretic that acts by inhibiting the effect of aldosterone. It is a potassium-sparing diuretic and, thus, can be used in conjunction with other diuretics to prevent hypokalemia. Spironolactone is considered to help with myocardial remodeling in patients with heart failure. Some pediatric cardiologists prescribe digoxin for patients with evidence of ventricular dysfunction and congestive heart failure. There are limited data supporting its use for ventricular remodeling. In some patients, enalapril may be used to decrease systemic afterload, particularly with ventricular septal defects and patent

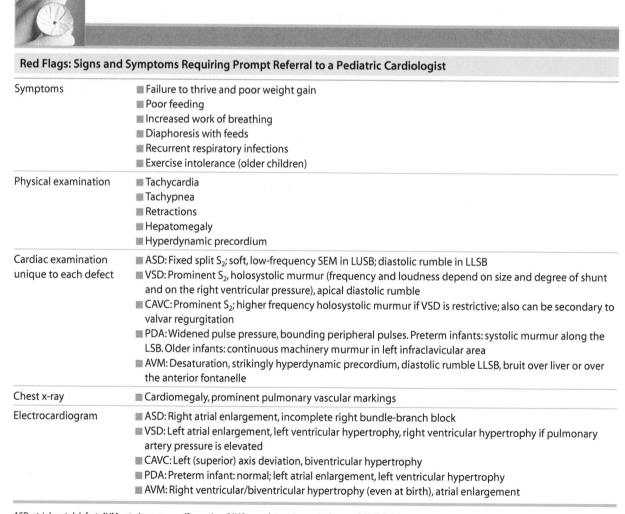

Red Flags: Signs and Symptoms Requiring Prompt Referral to a Pediatric Cardiologist

Symptoms	■ Failure to thrive and poor weight gain ■ Poor feeding ■ Increased work of breathing ■ Diaphoresis with feeds ■ Recurrent respiratory infections ■ Exercise intolerance (older children)
Physical examination	■ Tachycardia ■ Tachypnea ■ Retractions ■ Hepatomegaly ■ Hyperdynamic precordium
Cardiac examination unique to each defect	■ ASD: Fixed split S_2; soft, low-frequency SEM in LUSB; diastolic rumble in LLSB ■ VSD: Prominent S_2, holosystolic murmur (frequency and loudness depend on size and degree of shunt and on the right ventricular pressure), apical diastolic rumble ■ CAVC: Prominent S_2; higher frequency holosystolic murmur if VSD is restrictive; also can be secondary to valvar regurgitation ■ PDA: Widened pulse pressure, bounding peripheral pulses. Preterm infants: systolic murmur along the LSB. Older infants: continuous machinery murmur in left infraclavicular area ■ AVM: Desaturation, strikingly hyperdynamic precordium, diastolic rumble LLSB, bruit over liver or over the anterior fontanelle
Chest x-ray	■ Cardiomegaly, prominent pulmonary vascular markings
Electrocardiogram	■ ASD: Right atrial enlargement, incomplete right bundle-branch block ■ VSD: Left atrial enlargement, left ventricular hypertrophy, right ventricular hypertrophy if pulmonary artery pressure is elevated ■ CAVC: Left (superior) axis deviation, biventricular hypertrophy ■ PDA: Preterm infant: normal; left atrial enlargement, left ventricular hypertrophy ■ AVM: Right ventricular/biventricular hypertrophy (even at birth), atrial enlargement

ASD, atrial septal defect; AVM, arteriovenous malformation; CAVC, complete atrioventricular canal; LLSB, left lower sternal border; LSB, lower sternal border; LUSB, left upper sternal border; PDA, patent ductus arteriosus; SEM, systolic ejection murmur; VSD, ventricular septal defect.

Medications Frequently Used for Symptoms of Congestive Heart Failure

Medication	Usage	Mechanism of Action	Dosage	Side Effects
Furosemide	Diuresis	Loop diuretic (inhibits Na-K-Cl channel in thick ascending loop of Henle)	Neonates: 1-4 mg/kg/dose once or twice daily; children: 1-6 mg/kg/d divided twice daily	Hypokalemia, hypocalcemia, nephrocalcinosis, hyponatremia, dehydration, ototoxicity
Chlorothiazide	Diuresis	Thiazide diuretic (inhibition of sodium and chloride reabsorption from distal convoluted tubule)	20 mg/kg/d divided twice daily	Hypokalemia, hypochloremic metabolic alkalosis, hyperglycemia, dehydration
Spironolactone	Potassium-sparing diuretic; cardiac remodeling	Potassium-sparing diuretic (aldosterone inhibition to increase excretion of sodium, chloride, and water)	1-3 mg/kg/d every 12-24 hours	Hyperkalemia, hypernatremia, hyperchloremic metabolic alkalosis, gynecomastia
Digoxin	Congestive heart failure; antiarrhythmic	Inhibits ATPase to inhibit conduction through the sinus and atrioventricular nodes; increases influx of calcium into the cellular cytoplasm; increases cardiac parasympathetic activity and arterial baroreceptor activity, which decreases central sympathetic outflow	PO neonates: Load 20-30 μg/kg; maintenance 5-10 μg/kg/d; PO 1 month-2 years: Load 40-60 μg/kg; maintenance 10-12 μg/kg/d; PO 2-5 years: Load 30-40 μg/kg, maintenance 7.5-10 μg/kg/d; PO 5-10 years: Load 20-30 μg/kg, maintenance 5-10 μg/kg/d; PO >10 years: Load 10-15 μg/kg, maintenance 2.5-5 μg/kg/d	Tachyarrhythmia, bradycardia, confusion; diplopia, yellow vision
Enalapril	Systemic afterload reduction; ventricular remodeling	ACE inhibitor (blocks conversion of angiotensin I to angiotensin II)	Initial: 0.1 mg/kg/d divided twice daily Maintenance: titrate up to 0.5 mg/kg/d	Hypotension, syncope, cough, hyperkalemia, loss of taste reception
Indomethacin	Closure of a patent ductus arteriosus	Cyclooxygenase inhibitor	<48 hours (all weights) or 2-7 days (<1250 g): time 0, 0.2 mg/kg/dose; 12 hours, 0.1 mg/kg/dose; 24-36 hours, 0.1 mg/kg/dose 2-7 days (>1250 g) or >7 days (all weights): time 0, 12 hours, 24-36 hours, 0.2 mg/kg/dose	Necrotizing enterocolitis, renal failure, thrombocytopenia, oliguria
Caloric fortification	Failure to thrive		As needed	

ACE, angiotensin-converting enzyme; PO, oral.

arterial ducts. Enalapril decreases the systemic vascular resistance, resulting in decreased left-to-right shunting in these lesions. This medication is also used to reduce significant left-sided atrioventricular (AV) valve regurgitation (Table 7-2).

Although it may seem counterintuitive, oxygen therapy can be harmful in these conditions. Oxygen acts as a pulmonary vasodilator, causing a decrease in the pulmonary vascular resistance and leading to increased pulmonary blood flow and worsening of symptoms in the setting of isolated shunt lesions.

If there are enough symptoms to warrant medical management with medication and nutrition, the patient should be followed closely by the primary physician and cardiologist. In cases where the patient does not adequately respond to medical therapy, surgical or catheter-based interventions should be considered as discussed later for individual defects.

ATRIAL SEPTAL DEFECT

Embryology

The atrial septum develops from a series of invaginations beginning in the fifth week of gestation.[5] The septum primum forms during the fifth week of gestation as tissue that grows toward the endocardial cushions.[5,6] The space between is called the ostium primum. Small perforations develop in the superior portion of the septum primum, forming the ostium secundum, which allows for flow across the atrial septum in the fetus.[5] The septum secundum forms during the seventh week of gestation as tissue that evaginates from the posterior wall of the atrium, leaving a space between the septum primum and secundum called the fossa ovalis[5,7] (Figure 7-1). In utero, there is right-to-left shunting through this patent foramen ovale (PFO). Following birth, the increase in pulmonary blood flow results in increased pulmonary venous return to the left atrium. The resultant increased left atrial pressure closes the flap valve of the PFO, eliminating the shunt.[5,7]

Definitions and Epidemiology

Atrial septal defects (ASDs) are among the more common congenital heart defects, occurring in 1 per 1500 births, with a female preponderance of 2:1 and accounting for 6% to 10% of all cardiac lesions.[6,8,9] The classification of ASDs refers to their location within the atrial septum (Figure 7-2). Ostium secundum ASDs are the most common, comprising 80% to 90% of all ASDs. These defects are located in the septum primum. There are a few rare genetic defects associated with these defects. Holt-Oram syndrome is caused by a mutation in the *TBX5* gene and is associated with anomalies of the upper extremities and the presence of an ASD.[6] An association has also been found between AV conduction delay, noted by PR prolongation on electrocardiogram, and the presence of an ASD that is localized to the *NKX2.5* gene. [6]

Ostium primum defects are less common, representing 2% to 3% of ASDs.[5] Primum defects are located anterior to the fossa ovalis between septum primum and endocardial cushions.[6] These defects are along the spectrum of endocardial cushion defects and can be found with an isolated cleft mitral valve or as part of an AV septal defect (see below), where they are often associated with trisomy 21.[5,6,10]

Sinus venosus ASDs result from incomplete septation between the pulmonary veins, the vena cavae, and the right atrium.[5,6] These defects are posterior and superior to the fossa ovalis and are often associated with anomalous pulmonary venous drainage of the right pulmonary veins. They collectively account for 5% to 10% of ASDs.[8,11]

The rarest type of ASD is the coronary sinus septal defect. This defect results from a lack of septation of the

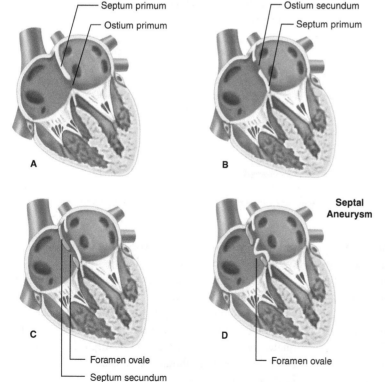

FIGURE 7-1 ■ Atrial septal anatomy. **A.** Embryologically, the septum primum (first septum) divides the atrium by migrating to the ventricles. The gap preceding the septal migration is the ostium primum. **B.** Once the septum primum completes its journey, fenestrations (holes) appear and generally coalesce into a single ostium secundum. **C.** A second septum (septum secundum) grows down on the right atrial side of the septum primum and covers the entire septal area except for a large oval hole that forms in its distal portion (the foramen ovale). **D.** If there is redundancy of either the septum primum (as shown) or both septae, then that defines a septal aneurysm. (*Reproduced, with permission, from McPhee SJ, Papadakis MA.* Current Medical Diagnosis and Treatment 2011. *50th ed. New York, NY: McGraw-Hill; 2011.*)

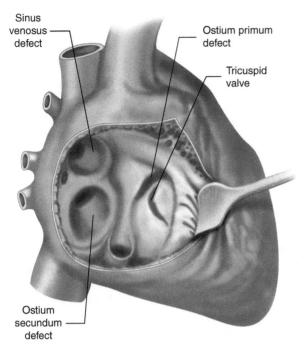

Sinus venosus defect

Ostium primum defect

Tricuspid valve

Ostium secundum defect

FIGURE 7-2 ■ Anatomic features of atrial septal defect. (*Reproduced, with permission, from Cheitlin MD, Sokolow M, McIlroy MB. Clinical Cardiology. 6th ed. Originally published by Appleton & Lange. Copyright © 1993 by The McGraw-Hill Companies, Inc.*)

coronary sinus from the left atrium (unroofed coronary sinus), allowing for a communication between the left and right atria via the coronary sinus.[5] It is often seen in conjunction with a persistent left superior vena cava.

As previously discussed, the foramen ovale is a normal fetal structure that typically closes after birth. However, autopsy studies have shown that as many as 17% to 35% of adults may have an open or probe-patent foramen ovale.[5] These small residual communications may be noted on echocardiograms performed for other reasons. They are not felt to be of any hemodynamic significance and typically do not cause symptoms or changes in the physical examination.[6,7] However, patients with a history of an embolic stroke may be evaluated for the presence of a PFO. It is possible that during an episode of transiently increased right atrial pressure, an embolus in the systemic veins could shunt right to left through a PFO (a "paradoxical shunt"), resulting in an embolic event.[6]

Pathogenesis

The direction of blood flow across an ASD is determined by the relative ventricular compliances. In the immediate newborn period, the right and left ventricles are both stiff, resulting in little shunting across the defect. As the newborn grows, the right ventricle becomes more compliant than the left ventricle and pulmonary vascular resistance decreases, resulting in increasing left-to-right flow across the ASD.[7,12] The increased blood flow across the ASD results in a volume load to the right side of the heart, including the right atrium, right ventricle, and pulmonary arteries.

Clinical Presentation

Symptoms

Most infants with ASDs are asymptomatic, because the left-to-right shunt is not very significant early in life. Infants with genetic syndromes or chronic lung disease of prematurity are 2 groups of patients who are more likely to be symptomatic from an ASD in the first months of life.[7] Some infants or young children with an ASD may have frequent respiratory tract infections. But even in childhood, most ASDs do not cause symptoms because the right ventricle tolerates the volume load well.[6] Instead, children typically present to the cardiologist because of an abnormal cardiac physical examination.

Physical examination

In infancy, the physical examination is often normal. Children can have a hyperdynamic cardiac impulse and a prominent RV heave, secondary to the volume load on the right side of the heart and right ventricular dilation.[6] Auscultation reveals a fixed, widely split S_2 and/or a low-frequency systolic ejection murmur at the left upper sternal border from augmented flow across the pulmonary valve. With large shunt volumes, a diastolic rumble may be audible at the left lower sternal border, secondary to the increased volume across the tricuspid valve.[6]

Diagnosis

Chest x-ray may reveal an enlarged cardiac silhouette, a dilated pulmonary artery, and increased pulmonary vascular markings.[6,12] These findings are more prominent with a larger left-to-right shunt and increase with age. An electrocardiogram may show evidence of right atrial enlargement with tall, peaked p waves. In addition, an incomplete right bundle-branch block pattern may be seen as an rSR' pattern in lead V_1.[6] Most often, patients remain in normal sinus rhythm in the presence of an ASD, although older untreated patients may have significant right atrial dilation from chronic left-to-right shunting with resultant supraventricular tachyarrythmias.[6]

The mainstay for diagnosis of an ASD is echocardiography. Transthoracic echocardiographic images can demonstrate the size and location of the defect within the atrial septum, as well as the direction of shunt through the defect.[13] Transthoracic echocardiography also allows for definition of the pulmonary vein and mitral valve anatomy and assessment of right atrial and right ventricular dilation.[6,7,13] Echocardiography serves an important role in determining which ASDs are amenable to catheter-based intervention versus surgical intervention.

Treatment

Medical management

ASDs rarely cause symptoms of heart failure in childhood in the absence of other pulmonary or genetic abnormalities. However, if a patient demonstrates poor growth or symptoms of tachypnea and respiratory distress with activity or feeds, diuretics may be warranted[6] (see Table 7-2). Subacute bacterial endocarditis (SBE) prophylaxis is not indicated in the setting of an ASD.[14]

Surgical/catheter-based intervention

Secundum ASDs can often close spontaneously. Previously published studies report that 92% of defects diagnosed in infancy close before 1 year of age. Defects are most likely to close if they are less than 7 mm in diameter.[6,13] Newly diagnosed infants and toddlers are usually followed. If the secundum ASD persists and echocardiography demonstrates volume load to the right side, these patients are usually referred for closure around the age of 3 to 4 years.[6] In older children, an ASD is often closed soon after diagnosis if there is evidence for significant right ventricular dilation. The defect should be closed sooner if a patient develops symptoms of congestive heart failure refractory to the medical interventions outlined earlier.[6,11] If left untreated, patients are at risk for increasing pulmonary arterial pressures and the development of pulmonary hypertension in the third or fourth decade of life. Pulmonary vascular disease occurs in 5% to 10% of untreated ASDs and is more commonly seen in females.[6] There is also a risk of supraventricular tachyarrhythmias secondary to the dilation of the right atrium as the patient ages.[6]

Transcatheter closure of ostium secundum ASDs has been used with increasing frequency and is now the most commonly used therapy for the appropriate defect. There are multiple catheter devices available, whose description is beyond the scope of this chapter (Figure 7-3). Some ostium secundum ASDs are not amenable to transcatheter closure because of the size of the patient, the size of the defect, or the location of the defect within the atrial septum.[9] In these patients, surgical closure is recommended.

Ostium primum defects, sinus venosus defects, and unroofing of the coronary sinus will not spontaneously close and ultimately require elective surgical intervention. These defects are not amenable to catheter-based intervention.

A PFO rarely causes symptoms or significant right heart dilation and, thus, does not typically require intervention unless it is diagnosed in the context of a cryptogenic stroke.

Postoperative concerns and follow-up

Both catheter-based and surgical techniques can successfully close nearly all ASDs with a very low rate of serious complications. Nevertheless, there are a few considerations that require attention during the follow-up period after ASD closure. After surgical ASD closure, there is a risk for postpericardiotomy syndrome consisting of accumulation of pericardial fluid and inflammation. Symptoms of respiratory distress, fever, fatigue, or emesis within the first weeks after intervention should prompt an evaluation for pericardial effusion.[9,12] Typically, this complication is treated with anti-inflammatory medication or steroids. In rare cases, pericardial fluid drainage is required. Patients who undergo repair of sinus venosus ASDs are at increased risk of sinus node dysfunction, superior vena cava obstruction, and pulmonary venous obstruction.[11] In addition, patients are at risk of developing supraventricular tachyarrhythmias, including atrial fibrillation, a risk that increases with age at closure.[9,15]

After catheter-based intervention, there is a risk of device embolization, which usually occurs in the first 24 hours after the procedure.[6,9] There is also a risk of thrombus formation on the device, with an incidence of 1.2%.[9] Commonly, anticoagulation with aspirin therapy is recommended for at least 6 months after device placement. Some patients develop AV conduction delay or atrial ectopy that typically resolves in the days to weeks after device placement.[9] Finally, there have been rare isolated reports of late device embolization and device erosion through the atrial or aortic wall.[9] Patients require 6 months of SBE prophylaxis after device placement (Table 7-3).

VENTRICULAR SEPTAL DEFECT

Embryology

The ventricular septum is a complex structure that forms through a sequence of events in the fetus between 4 and 7 weeks of gestation and involves fusion of several tissues including endocardial cushion–derived mesenchyme, primary atrial septum, and muscular components of atrial and ventricular septae.[16] The muscular intraventricular septum forms by infolding of the ventricular muscle within the primitive cardiac tube. This muscular septum aligns with the conal septum, which is positioned between the 2 outflow tracts.[16] Lastly, the membranous septum closes, which is adjacent to the anteroseptal commissure of the tricuspid valve.[17] Ventricular septal defects (VSDs) can occur anywhere in the septum.

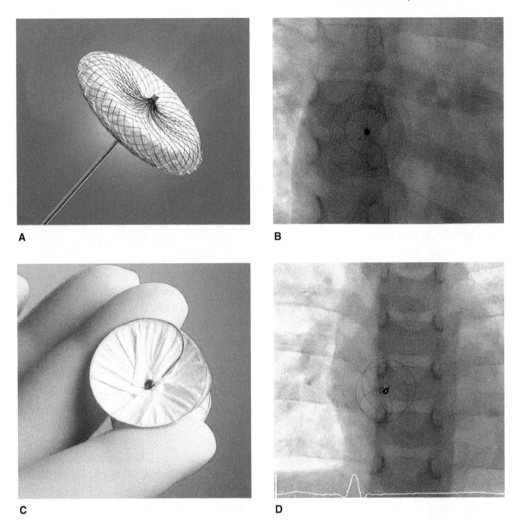

FIGURE 7-3 ■ Two commonly used devices for percutaneous closure of secundum atrial septal defects (ASDs). **A.** The Amplatzer Septal Occluder attached to its delivery cable. The device is made of an alloy, nitinol, shaped into 2 flat discs and a middle "waist," with polyester fabric inserts designed to help close the hole and provide a foundation for growth of tissue over the device. **B.** A frontal fluoroscopic image of the Amplatzer Septal Occluder after deployment. **C.** The GORE HELEX Septal Occluder is composed of expanded polytetrafluoroethylene patch material supported by a single nitinol wire frame shaped to bridge the ASD. **D.** A frontal fluoroscopic image of the GORE HELEX Septal Occluder after deployment.

Summary of ASD

Medical management	Asymptomatic: None Symptomatic: Diuretics, caloric fortification	
Indications for intervention	Elective ASD closure in childhood (after age 3-4 years) if asymptomatic with evidence of right-sided volume load by examination or echocardiogram; earlier intervention if symptomatic	
Treatment options	Surgical closure via midline sternotomy	Catheter-based device closure (depends on location of defect and size of patient)
Postintervention issues	Pericardial effusion, arrhythmias, residual ASD	Residual ASD; small risk of device embolization, atrial arrhythmias, disruption of adjacent structures (SVC/pulmonary vein obstruction, etc), and thrombus
Follow-up	Frequent assessments after surgery and continued cardiology follow-up if there is a residual defect or if there are associated defects	Aspirin and endocarditis prophylaxis for first 6 months after procedure; yearly follow-up with cardiologist

ASD, atrial septal defect; SVC, superior vena cava.

Definitions and Epidemiology

VSD accounts for 20% of congenital heart disease, making it the most common form of congenital heart disease after bicuspid aortic valve.[18] The incidence of isolated VSDs has increased over time, but this increase may be related to improved ultrasound technology and increased diagnosis in the prenatal and antenatal periods. There is a slight female predominance of 56%.[18] More than 75% of small defects close within the first 2 years of life.[17,19] VSDs are the most common heart defect in many chromosomal anomalies, including patients with trisomies 13, 18, and 21.[18] VSDs are also associated with Holt-Oram syndrome.

VSDs are classified according to their location within the ventricular septum (Figure 7-4). Spontaneous closure rate and the presence of associated defects depend on the defect type. Conoventricular defects account for 80% of all VSDs.[18,19] Other terms include membranous or perimembranous defects. These VSDs lie between the outlet and inlet portion of the right ventricle, adjacent to the tricuspid valve and the aortic valve. These defects can be restricted by overlapping tricuspid valve tissue or by prolapse of the aortic valve cusp into the defect.[19] Some smaller defects can close spontaneously.

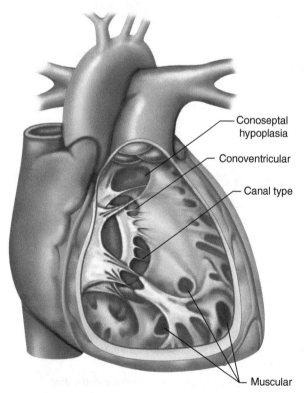

FIGURE 7-4 ■ Different types of ventricular septal defects when viewed from the right ventricle. (*Adapted with permission, from Fyler DC, ed. Nadas' Pediatric Cardiology. Philadelphia, PA: Hanleuy and Belfus; 1992.*)

Muscular defects account for 5% to 20% of all VSDs.[18,19] They can occur anywhere along the muscular septum and are further classified according to their location within the muscular septum (midmuscular, anterior muscular, or posterior muscular). These defects often close spontaneously.[19]

Malalignment VSDs occur when the conal septum, the septum between the right and left ventricular outflow tracts, is malaligned with the inlet septum. A posterior malalignment VSD results from posterior deviation of the conal septum.[16] This type of VSD can be associated with subaortic obstruction, aortic valve hypoplasia, and arch obstruction. Anterior malalignment VSD results from anterior deviation of the conal septum and is associated with subpulmonary obstruction (eg, tetralogy of Fallot).[16,18] These defects do not close spontaneously.

Conoseptal hypoplasia defects result from underdevelopment of the conal septum. The deficiency in the subvalvar area can result in prolapse of the right coronary cusp of the aortic valve into the defect with the subsequent development of aortic insufficiency.[19] This type of defect will not close spontaneously, but a prolapsed aortic cusp may restrict flow partially or fully. These defects account for only 5% to 7% of VSDs in Western populations but up to 30% in Asian populations.[18,19]

Canal-type VSDs are located at the level of the AV valves. The tricuspid valve may straddle across the defect with attachments into the left ventricle. These defects account for 5% to 7% of all VSDs.[18,19] This type of defect will not close spontaneously.

Pathogenesis

The relative pulmonary and systemic vascular resistances and the size of the defect determine the hemodynamic effect of the VSD.[3,19] In the early newborn period, the pulmonary and systemic vascular resistances are relatively equal, resulting in little or no shunting of blood across the defect. As the pulmonary vascular resistance declines in the first weeks of life, the degree of shunting across the defect increases.[3,17,19] Shunting occurs largely in systole and is directed to the lungs and the left side of the heart. In infants with a hemodynamically significant VSD, increased pulmonary blood flow from a moderate to large defect leads to symptoms and signs of heart failure and to left atrial and left ventricular dilation.

Left undetected or untreated, this chronic elevation in pulmonary blood flow can alter the pulmonary vascular bed, initiating intimal proliferation and muscularization of the arterioles. This process can eventually lead to Eisenmenger syndrome, a condition where the increased pulmonary vascular resistance leads to right-to-left shunting across the VSD, pulmonary hypertension, and cyanosis.[17–19]

Labels: Conoseptal hypoplasia, Conoventricular, Canal type, Muscular

Clinical Presentation

Symptoms

Infants and children with small VSDs may not develop symptoms early in life. In infants with moderate to large defects, symptoms only begin to develop after the first few weeks of life when the pulmonary vascular resistance is low enough to promote left-to-right shunt through the defect.[3,19] Affected infants will develop tachycardia with tachypnea and increased work of breathing. They may have recurrent respiratory infections. They may experience difficulty feeding, diaphoresis, poor weight gain, and failure to thrive.[17–19] Older infants and children with large shunts that go unrecognized can eventually develop symptoms of pulmonary hypertension and Eisenmenger syndrome including shortness of breath, dyspnea on exertion, and cyanosis.[18,19]

Physical examination

Often there are no obvious abnormalities on the cardiovascular physical examination in the immediate newborn period. Both a drop in the pulmonary vascular resistance and the physiologic nadir of hemoglobin at 6 to 8 weeks of age may produce positive examination findings. For the smaller, pressure-restrictive defects, the only abnormal finding may be a murmur—a grade 2-3/6 medium- to high-frequency, holosystolic murmur heard at the left lower sternal border or toward the apex (depending on VSD location).[18,19]

In infants with hemodynamically significant defects, vital signs often demonstrate tachycardia and tachypnea. Blood pressure and saturation are not affected in isolated defects. The infant may have retractions or flaring. Pulses and perfusion are usually normal. The abdominal examination is extremely important and demonstrates hepatomegaly secondary to a high-output state. Lungs are usually clear to auscultation. The precordium may be hyperactive, and there may be a palpable thrill produced by a pressure-restrictive defect with a high-velocity jet directed anteriorly across the septum.[18,19] S_1 is usually normal, and it is often difficult to evaluate the S_2 in the setting of a loud holosystolic murmur from the VSD.[18,19] The higher the frequency of the holosystolic murmur, the more pressure restrictive the defect is. Keep in mind that even the most restrictive defects can produce a large-volume shunt. A middiastolic rumble may be audible at the apex because of increased blood flow across the mitral valve and signifies a larger magnitude shunt.[18,19] In patients with Eisenmenger physiology, the oxygen saturation is low, there may be clubbing of the hands and feet, the precordium is hyperdynamic, the P_2 component of the S_2 is loud, and there may not be a significant murmur because systemic right ventricular pressure will limit the shunt across the defect.[17–19]

Diagnosis

If there are any concerns on history or physical examination for a hemodynamically significant VSD, a prompt cardiology referral is recommended. When there is suspicion of a VSD, additional studies can be performed to confirm the diagnosis.

The electrocardiogram in infants with small VSDs is normal. Patients with larger defects will have findings consistent with left atrial dilation and left ventricular hypertrophy, particularly a wide, biphasic p wave and increased left-sided forces, respectively.[17–19] As the right ventricular pressure increases from exposure to the pressures of the systemic left ventricle, right ventricular hypertrophy may also become evident.[17] Chest x-ray is normal in infants with a small VSD. Patients with moderate-sized VSDs have an enlarged cardiac silhouette with evidence of pulmonary vascular congestion.[17–19]

Transthoracic echocardiography identifies the type and size of the VSD and determines the hemodynamic significance of the defect. Two-dimensional imaging in various planes is used to localize the defect.[16,19] Depending on the type of defect, involvement of tricuspid valve tissue and prolapse of the aortic cusp can also be evaluated. Both color and spectral Doppler assessments determine the direction of the shunt, the peak velocity, and the peak pressure gradient across the defect. In addition to assessing the anatomy and physiology of the VSD, echocardiography can also assess the impact of the shunt on the heart.[16,19] Tricuspid regurgitation peak velocity allows for calculation of a right ventricle pressure estimate. Two-dimensional and M-mode assessment enables accurate assessment of left atrium and left ventricle enlargement and left ventricle dimensions and function. Ventricular septal curvature assessed by 2-dimensional imaging in short axis also gives a rough estimate of right ventricle pressure elevation. Associated abnormalities such as aortic insufficiency and right ventricular outflow tract obstruction can be demonstrated.[16,19] All of these parameters can be followed serially on follow-up studies.

Cardiac catheterization is no longer routinely performed to diagnose the presence of a VSD.[18] However, it may be useful in determining the degree of left-to-right shunt across the defect in patients in whom the indication for surgery is not clear. It also allows for identification of additional defects and determination of the pulmonary vascular resistance.[18] In patients with significantly elevated pulmonary vascular resistance, closure of the VSD may not be tolerated.[18,19]

Treatment

Medical management

Children with small VSDs rarely develop symptoms of heart failure and require neither medical nor surgical intervention.[17] However, in infants with symptoms of failure to thrive and heart failure, medical management with diuretics and fortified nutrition is often the first line of therapy[18] (see Table 7-2). Medical therapy is often conducted with close collaborative efforts between the cardiologist and pediatrician. During respiratory season, infants with significant hemodynamic shunts should receive proper vaccines and monthly respiratory syncytial virus immunoprophylaxis with palivizumab.

Surgical intervention

Surgery is indicated for (1) infants who continue to have failure to thrive and heart failure symptoms despite maximal medical management; (2) asymptomatic children with increasing left ventricular dilation and/or progressive aortic insufficiency; and (3) asymptomatic older infants and children who have defects (eg, malalignment defects, canal defects, conoseptal hypoplasia defects) that will not likely close on their own.[17-19] Surgery is performed via a median sternotomy. Depending on the location of the VSD, the repair may be approached through the tricuspid valve or through either the pulmonary or aortic valve.[17]

Some VSDs are amenable to catheter-based device occlusion of the defect. Typically, catheter-based interventions are considered for hemodynamically significant muscular defects or in critically ill patients.

Postoperative complications and follow-up

Surgery for an isolated VSD is generally tolerated well with minimal complications. Early on, some patients may have a small residual VSD that will likely not be hemodynamically significant. Postoperative electrocardiogram may demonstrate a right bundle-branch block due to manipulation of the conduction system during the repair.[18] These patients can sometimes develop pericardial or pleural effusions that often only need medication and resolve over time. Patients should be followed closely in the first few weeks after discharge by their pediatrician and cardiologist.

Patients with unrepaired, isolated VSDs do not require prophylaxis for infective endocarditis under the new guidelines. All patients who have had surgery to close their VSD should receive endocarditis prophylaxis for 6 months after surgery if patch material is used. If a residual peri-patch VSD persists after 6 months, endocarditis prophylaxis should continue.[14]

Long-term outcomes are quite good in patients with isolated VSDs who undergo intervention prior to the development of pulmonary hypertension or in those who are being followed for a hemodynamically insignificant defect. In patients with conoventricular and conoseptal hypoplasia VSDs, there is a risk of developing progressive aortic regurgitation from prolapse of the aortic

---

Summary of VSD

Medical management	■ Small, pressure-restrictive defects with no symptoms: none ■ Symptomatic: Diuretics, caloric fortification, and nasogastric feeds ± digoxin and ACE inhibition
Indications for intervention	■ Symptomatic infants who fail medical management should be referred for surgical closure. ■ Infants whose symptoms are well controlled with medical management should be referred for elective closure if VSD continues to be significant in the first year of life. ■ Elective closure in childhood should be considered for asymptomatic children with continued left atrial/ventricular enlargement. ■ Children with large defects and evidence of Eisenmenger physiology should have a thorough evaluation with catheterization to determine eligibility for surgical closure. ■ Asymptomatic children with small, pressure-restrictive defects without left-sided volume load or evidence of pulmonary hypertension should be followed only.
Treatment options	■ Surgical closure via midline sternotomy; catheter-based device closure considered for critically ill patients in most centers
Postoperative issues	■ Pericardial effusion, arrhythmias, residual VSD, RBBB pattern on ECG
Follow-up	■ Frequent assessments after surgery ■ Endocarditis prophylaxis for first 6 months after procedure; continued prophylaxis if there is a residual defect adjacent to patch material from the repair ■ Continued cardiology follow-up to follow residual VSD and to assess for the development of associated defects (double-chambered right ventricle, subaortic stenosis, arrhythmias, etc)

ACE, angiotensin-converting enzyme; ECG, electrocardiogram; RBBB, right bundle branch block; VSD, ventricular septal defect.

valve cusp.[16] There is also a risk of the development of a subaortic membrane and double-chambered right ventricle with right ventricular outflow tract obstruction in patients with conoventricular septal defects.[16] This risk persists even after operative intervention or after spontaneous closure of the VSD. Therefore, these patients should receive lifelong follow-up with a cardiologist (Table 7-4).

COMMON ATRIOVENTRICULAR CANAL DEFECTS

Embryology

The common AV canal defects are a group of congenital heart defects that develop from abnormal development of the endocardial cushions and subsequent septation of the heart. These defects can range from ostium primum ASDs (see section on ASDs) to inlet VSDs (see section on VSDs). These defects also involve a common AV valve.[20,21] It is the size of the atrial and/or ventricular defects that dictates the clinical presentation and timing of intervention (Figure 7-5).

Epidemiology

AV septal defects (AVSDs) account for 3% to 5% of all congenital heart disease, with an incidence of 0.24 to 0.31 per 1000 births.[21,22] There is a slight predominance of AVSD in females, with a 1.3:1 female-to-male ratio.[21,22] Most notably, patients with trisomy 21 have a 40% to 45% incidence of congenital heart disease, of which 40% have an AVSD.[21,23] In fact, any infant diagnosed with trisomy 21 should undergo a cardiology evaluation at diagnosis to assess for congenital heart disease. In addition, heterotaxy syndrome is associated with AVSD, particularly the asplenia form.[20] There is also an autosomal dominant form of AVSD.[20] When an AVSD is not balanced equally over both ventricles, ventricular hypoplasia may develop and single ventricle palliation may be required. These defects will not be addressed here.

Physiology

The degree of left-to-right shunting depends on the presence of atrial level (ostium primum) and ventricular level communications.[20,21,23] The physiology associated with this lesion is similar to that of an ASD and VSD. The degree of left-to-right shunting across the defect increases as the pulmonary vascular resistance falls. Children often present in infancy because of the large ASD and the VSD with failure to thrive, tachypnea, hepatomegaly, and recurrent respiratory infections. In addition, the common AV valve may be regurgitant, exacerbating these clinical findings.[20,21]

Clinical Presentation

Symptoms

As with other types of shunt lesions, the timing and severity of symptoms depend on the relative vascular resistances and ventricular compliances. Complete AV canal defects have a large atrial and ventricular defect. These infants present with failure to thrive, diaphoresis, and tachypnea in the first several weeks of life.[20,21,23] Infants with transitional AV canal defects where the VSD component is small and restrictive or those with incomplete AV canal defects where there is no VSD may have minimal symptoms and grow fairly well in infancy. These patients will more likely present with a murmur on physical examination.[21] Infants with trisomy 21 are at risk for pulmonary hypertension regardless of whether or not they have congenital heart disease.[21] Therefore, these infants may have minimal symptoms even with a complete AV canal defect because the pulmonary vascular

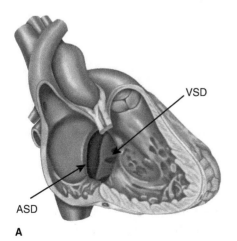

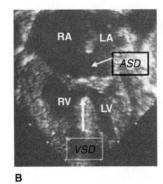

FIGURE 7-5 ■ **A.** Image of a complete atrioventricular canal defect with a common atrioventricular valve, an atrial septal defect (ASD), and a ventricular septal defect (VSD). **B.** Two-dimensional echocardiography of a complete atrioventricular canal defect. LA, left atrium; LV, left ventricle; RA, right atrium; RV, right ventricle.

A

B

resistance is elevated, limiting the left-to-right shunt and pulmonary blood flow.

Physical examination

The physical examination findings are dependent on the size and/or shunting across the VSD, the pulmonary artery pressure, and the degree of AV valve regurgitation. In symptomatic patients, vital signs may demonstrate low weight percentile, tachypnea with retractions, and tachycardia.[20,21] Unless the defect is unbalanced or there is elevated pulmonary vascular resistance, patients are not typically desaturated. Their pulses and perfusion are adequate. In patients with increased pulmonary blood flow and symptoms, the liver will be enlarged. On cardiovascular examination, the precordium is hyperdynamic, and S_2 may be prominent if there is elevated pulmonary vascular resistance. Splitting of S_2 may not be appreciated in the setting of tachycardia. A restrictive or small VSD may produce a higher frequency holosystolic murmur along the left sternal border.[20,21] If the VSD is large or the pulmonary resistance is high, there may not be an appreciable murmur even in the setting of a common AV canal defect. There may be a higher frequency holosystolic murmur at the apex signifying left-sided regurgitation through a cleft in the left AV valve.[20,21] Extra heart sounds are rare. A diastolic rumble may be heard due to the large amount of blood flow crossing the AV valve in large shunts.

Diagnostic Studies

The electrocardiogram in infants with a common AV canal defect typically shows left axis deviation (QRS axis between 0 and −120 degrees). Biventricular hypertrophy can also be seen.[20,23] Chest x-ray typically demonstrates cardiomegaly with a prominent right atrial border due to right atrial enlargement and prominent lung markings.[20,23] Transthoracic echocardiography demonstrates the anatomy of the common AV valve and the atrial and/or ventricular level defects.[20] Color Doppler can be used to show the direction of shunting across these defects and the degree of common AV valve regurgitation.[20,24] Echocardiography is also important to assess the relative balance of AV valve inflow into each ventricle and to identify associated defects such as subaortic obstruction, coarctation of the aorta, additional septal defects, and patent ductus arteriosus.[20,24] Evaluation of right-sided pressure and pulmonary artery pressure can also be performed.

Treatment

Medical management

As with ASDs and VSDs, medical management is targeted toward optimizing weight gain and minimizing symptoms of heart failure with medications and caloric fortification (see Table 7-2). In addition, systemic afterload reduction, typically with an angiotensin-converting enzyme inhibitor, may be necessary in patients with significant AV valve regurgitation.[20]

Surgical repair

For complete common AV canal defects, elective repair is scheduled in the first few months of life regardless of whether the baby is symptomatic. Early surgical repair minimizes the risk of early pulmonary vascular disease due to the large ventricular level shunt.[20] For patients with incomplete or transitional AV canal defects, surgery is often performed electively around 2 to 3 years of age unless symptoms or significant AV valve regurgitation prompt earlier surgical referral.

There are many surgical techniques to repair AV canal defects, but they all involve closure of the septal defects and repair of the common AV valve.[20]

Postoperative concerns and follow-up

Surgical results for complete intracardiac repair of AVSD are quite good, with an overall mortality of 5% to 10% and a freedom from reoperation of 80% to 95%.[20,22] In the immediate postoperative period, the risks are the same as those for closure of an ASD or VSD, as described earlier. During the first 6 postoperative months, patients should receive SBE prophylaxis. Patients who undergo surgical repair of an AVSD are at risk for residual ASDs or VSDs and should continue to receive prophylaxis if a peri-patch ASD or VSD remains after 6 month. Probably the most notable postoperative issue is left AV valve regurgitation.[20] Typically, this issue, even with significant regurgitation, can be managed for many months to years with close cardiology follow-up and medication. Although the data are limited in this population, angiotensin-converting enzyme inhibition therapy is usually initiated in the setting of significant left AV valve regurgitation. Patients also need to be monitored long term for AV valve stenosis and arrhythmias. Due to the anatomy of the left ventricular outflow tract in the setting of a common AV canal defect, monitoring for the development of subaortic obstruction is also warranted.[20] Although these issues can develop over time, patients with repaired common AV canal defects have a favorable prognosis and do well (Table 7-5).

PATENT DUCTUS ARTERIOSUS

Definitions and Epidemiology

Patent ductus arteriosus (PDA) is defined as persistence of the ductus arteriosus beyond 3 months of life. PDA occurs in 2 to 4 per 1000 live, full-term births with a female predominance of 2:1.[25,26] PDA accounts for approximately 5% to 10% of all forms of congenital

Summary of CAVC Defect

Medical management	■ Symptomatic infants (typically with complete CAVC defect): Diuretics, caloric fortification and nasogastric feeds; ACE inhibition in the setting of significant AV valve regurgitation ■ Asymptomatic: None ■ Asymptomatic with significant AV valve regurgitation: ACE inhibition ■ Endocarditis prophylaxis for complete, transitional, or incomplete CAVC defects
Indications for intervention	■ Infants with trisomy 21 and complete CAVC defect who are either asymptomatic or whose symptoms are well controlled with medical management should be scheduled for elective surgical repair in the first 3-6 months of life to prevent onset of pulmonary vascular disease. ■ Symptomatic infants who fail medical management should be referred for surgical closure Asymptomatic children with transitional or incomplete CAVC and a pressure-restrictive ventricular septal defect with normal pulmonary artery pressure can have elective closure in the first 2 years of life.
Treatment options	■ Surgical closure via midline sternotomy
Postoperative issues	■ Pericardial effusion, arrhythmias, residual defects, residual AV valve regurgitation or stenosis
Follow-up	■ Frequent assessments after surgery ■ Endocarditis prophylaxis for first 6 months after procedure; continued prophylaxis if there is a residual defect adjacent to patch material from the repair ■ Lifelong cardiology follow-up to monitor residual defects and to assess for the development of associated issues (subaortic stenosis, arrhythmias, etc) ■ Children with significant residual AV valve regurgitation may need continued ACE inhibition and further intervention on the valve.

ACE, angiotensin-converting enzyme; AV, atrioventricular; CAVC, complete atrioventricular canal.

heart disease.[25–27] It is seen more frequently in preterm infants, with an incidence of 8 per 1000 live births. PDA is associated with prematurity and low birth weight, congenital rubella, chromosomal anomalies, birth at high altitudes, and birth asphyxia.[25]

Siblings of patients with an isolated PDA have a recurrence rate of 1% to 5%.[25] There are also genetic syndromes associated with patency of the ductus arteriosus. Patients with trisomies 21 and 18, CHARGE syndrome, and Rubinstein-Taybi syndrome have a higher incidence of PDA.[25] In addition, there are case reports of increased recurrence rates of PDA within families. Char syndrome (chromosome 6p12-p21) is an autosomal dominant syndrome with a constellation of physical features, including low-set ears, ptosis, short philtrum, "duck-bill" lips, mild learning impairment, pharyngeal anomalies, and a PDA. The syndrome has been mapped to *TFAP2B*, which is a gene involved in neural crest development.[25] Familial thoracic aortic aneurysm/dissection with PDA has been described and attributed to a locus at chromosome 16, p12.2-p13.3.[25]

Pathogenesis

The ductus arteriosus is a normal fetal structure formed from the embryonic sixth aortic arch.[25,28] In utero, because the lungs are collapsed and the pulmonary resistance is high, the shunt across the ductus arteriosus is from the pulmonary artery to the aorta. The PDA connection to the aorta can vary depending on the arch sidedness and branching pattern. The duct directs blood flow to the lower body. Postnatally, through various changes in the neonatal transitional circulation, the duct normally closes in the first 1 to 2 weeks of life.[23,25,29] Premature infants have immature ductal tissue that exhibits an abnormal response to these mechanisms and the duct can persist.[25,29]

The physiologic consequences of a PDA are similar to those of a VSD. As the pulmonary vascular resistance decreases, the direction of the shunt becomes increasingly left to right from the aorta to the pulmonary artery.[27] In fact, the shunt through a PDA occurs in systole and diastole. Therefore, patients with significant PDAs often become symptomatic sooner (often in the first several weeks of life) than infants with a significant VSD, whose shunt only occurs in systole.

If left untreated, there is a risk of pulmonary vascular disease. As the lungs continue to be exposed to systemic pressures transmitted through a large PDA, irreversible changes within the pulmonary vascular bed, including intimal proliferation, arteriolar medial hypertrophy, and fibrosis, ensue, ultimately resulting in pulmonary hypertension.[25,27] As the pulmonary vascular resistance rises, the direction of blood flow may reverse from left to right to right to left at the ductus arteriosus.[25,28]

Clinical Presentation

Symptoms

The degree of symptoms from a PDA depends on its size and degree of shunt. Premature infants may have difficulty weaning from the ventilator and require high ventilatory settings.[25,28] These infants may experience pulmonary hemorrhage and be at risk for necrotizing enterocolitis.[28]

Full-term infants and children with small PDAs may not develop symptoms early in life. In infants with moderate to large defects, symptoms may begin to develop in the first few weeks of life when the pulmonary vascular resistance is low enough to promote left-to-right shunt through the defect both in systole and diastole. Affected infants will develop tachycardia with tachypnea and increased work of breathing.[25,28] They may have recurrent respiratory infections. They may experience difficulty feeding, diaphoresis, poor weight gain, and failure to thrive.[28] Older infants and children with large shunts that go unrecognized can eventually develop symptoms of pulmonary hypertension and pulmonary vascular disease, including shortness of breath, dyspnea on exertion, hemoptysis, and cyanosis.[25,28]

Physical examination

In term newborns, the only finding may be a nonspecific, systolic murmur. In fact, 50% of infants in the newborn nursery typically have murmurs, and the majority are just closing PDAs. The presence of a continuous murmur audible at the left upper chest and back is often the reason for referral to a pediatric cardiologist.[23,25,28] In the setting of a hemodynamically significant PDA, the precordium may be hyperactive. The peripheral pulses are often bounding because the diastolic PDA run-off of blood from the aorta to the pulmonary artery causes a widened pulse pressure.[23,25,28] In conjunction with this examination finding, the diastolic pressure may be low. Silent PDAs are aptly termed by the absence of an audible murmur or other abnormality on physical examination. These PDAs are usually hemodynamically insignificant and are an incidental finding.[25]

Patients with untreated moderate to large PDAs develop pulmonary hypertension. These patients present with differential cyanosis or lower oxygen saturation of the lower extremities secondary to the right-to-left shunting of desaturated pulmonary arterial blood flow across the ductus arteriosus and into the descending aorta. They also may develop clubbing of the hands and feet.[25,28] The precordium is hyperdynamic, and the P_2 component of the S_2 is loud.

Evaluation

The electrocardiogram in patients with a PDA is typically normal in infancy and early childhood. If left untreated, left atrial enlargement may be evident with broad, notched p waves secondary to the increased volume of blood shunted to the left atrium. The electrocardiogram usually does not show evidence of ventricular hypertrophy in childhood, although right ventricular hypertrophy may become evident as the pulmonary vascular bed remodels and pulmonary hypertension develops.[25,28] Chest x-ray in patients with a moderate-to large-sized PDA demonstrates an enlarged cardiac silhouette and pulmonary vascular congestion.

Transthoracic echocardiography is performed to confirm the presence of a PDA.[25,28,29] The size of the PDA can be measured with 2-dimensional imaging. The direction of the shunt can be determined by Doppler echocardiography.[25,28,29] Echocardiography can also show the degree of left atrial and left ventricular enlargement. Imaging can calculate the right ventricular pressure with the peak tricuspid regurgitation velocity and evaluate the degree of septal curvature as well as the degree of right ventricular enlargement and hypertrophy to assess the degree of pulmonary hypertension.[29]

Treatment

Medical management

Infants and children with symptomatic PDAs can be supported with caloric fortification with supplemental feeds and diuretic therapy (see Table 7-2).[25] In preterm infants, in particular those with extreme prematurity below 30 weeks, fluid restriction to decrease the interstitial lung fluid and optimization of hemoglobin levels are also considered. For the preterm infant, medical therapy for closure is often considered.[30] Indomethacin is a cyclooxygenase-1 (COX-1) receptor inhibitor and causes vasoconstriction of the PDA. Ibuprofen may be used as well, but it is a less potent inhibitor of the COX-1 receptors.[25] Indomethacin is given as 3 doses: 0.2 mg/kg/dose followed by 0.1 mg/kg/dose at 12 and 24 hours. Prophylactic treatment with indomethacin is recommended in infants born at less than 27 weeks of gestation. These medications have significant side effects themselves, including renal dysfunction, necrotizing enterocolitis, and impaired cerebral blood flow. Infants may also develop a rise in free bilirubin.[25] The most recent guidelines do not recommend the use of SBE prophylaxis for patients with an unrepaired PDA.[14]

Surgical and catheter-based therapy

Methods of ductal closure have improved significantly over the years. The goals of closure are to prevent the development of pulmonary vascular disease in those with

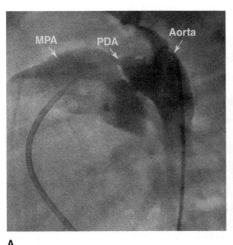
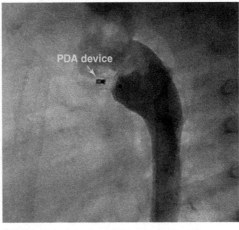

FIGURE 7-6 ■ Patent ductus arteriosus (PDA). **A.** Lateral projection of an angiogram taken at catheterization through a catheter in the descending aorta. Contrast fills the aorta as well as a PDA, with left-to-right flow of contrast into a dilated main pulmonary artery (MPA) segment. This is a "typical" conical PDA, with a larger aortic ampulla tapering to a smaller opening on the MPA side. A second catheter is positioned in the MPA, passed antegrade from venous access. **B.** Similar angiogram from the aortic catheter after deployment of a PDA occlusive device. In this example, an Amplatzer Duct Occluder device was used with complete occlusion of flow through the PDA.

large, unrestrictive PDAs and to minimize the lifetime risk of infective endarteritis.[30] Intervention, either surgical or catheter-based, is considered in (1) premature infants who do not respond to indomethacin or ibuprofen therapy or in whom medical therapy is contraindicated; (2) premature infants who fail to wean ventilator settings, develop signs of necrotizing enterocolitis or pulmonary hemorrhage, or have other evidence of hemodynamic instability or end-organ damage; (3) older infants or children with persistence of heart failure symptoms; and (4) asymptomatic patients with an audible murmur or cardiomegaly by chest x-ray or echocardiogram (Table 7-6). Cardiopulmonary bypass is not required for surgical intervention, which is performed via a lateral thoracotomy. In addition, the surgeon may use video-assisted thoracoscopy to close the PDA.[30] In some centers, surgical ductal closure is performed at the bedside.

Transcatheter closure of PDAs has been used with increasing frequency and is now the most commonly used therapy for the appropriate defect in older infants, children, and adults. Hemodynamic data are also acquired during the catheterization procedure.[30] There are multiple coils and devices available for PDA closure, whose description is beyond the scope of this chapter.[30] Some PDAs are not amenable to transcatheter closure because of the size of the patient or the size of the PDA (Figure 7-6). In these patients, surgical closure is recommended.

Postoperative complications and follow-up

Surgical and catheter-based closure techniques are generally well tolerated with minimal complications. Postoperative issues can include pleural effusions, infection, and hemothorax. There is a risk of interfering with the recurrent laryngeal nerve during the procedure.[27]

Patients may present with difficulty swallowing and a hoarse voice. After an initial postoperative follow-up clinic visit by a pediatric cardiologist, patients who undergo closure of the patent arterial duct often do not need further follow-up with cardiology. There is a small long-term risk of scoliosis and restrictive lung disease secondary to the thoracotomy.[27] The latter may present as asthmatic symptoms, exercise intolerance, or recurrent respiratory infections. The use of SBE prophylaxis is not required after surgical ligation of a patent arterial duct unless there is a residual shunt.[14]

Catheter-based device closure of a PDA is associated with few risks. Patients are routinely discharged the same day of the procedure. Embolization of the coil or device can occur.[26,27] Close monitoring of the patient after the procedure and assessment of device position by chest x-ray are performed. The device or coil can obstruct aortic or pulmonary artery flow and can be assessed by examination and echocardiography.[30] Lastly, infection can occur. Patients with fever or other generalized symptoms after device placement should be evaluated. For the first 6 months after the procedure, the patient should receive endocarditis prophylaxis. There are no significant long-term risks of the procedure (Table 7-6).

ARTERIOVENOUS MALFORMATION

Embryology

Embryonic vascular endothelium is derived from primitive mesenchymal cells during the third to tenth week of gestation. These cells form masses and cords and develop into the capillary bed. Separate venous and arterial

Summary of PDA	
Medical management	■ No medical treatment for hemodynamically insignificant or silent PDA
	■ Preterm infant: Diuresis, caloric fortification, optimize hemoglobin and ventilator management; indomethacin or ibuprofen to promote PDA closure
	■ Older infants and children with symptoms: Diuresis, caloric fortification
Indications for intervention	■ Premature infants who do not respond to indomethacin or ibuprofen therapy or in whom medical therapy is contraindicated
	■ Premature infants who fail to wean ventilator settings, develop signs of necrotizing enterocolitis or pulmonary hemorrhage, or have other evidence of hemodynamic instability or end-organ damage
	■ Older infants or children with persistence of heart failure symptoms
	■ Asymptomatic patients with an audible murmur or cardiomegaly by chest x-ray or left atrial/left ventricular enlargement on echocardiogram
Treatment options	■ Surgical PDA ligation via lateral thoracotomy
	■ Catheter-based coil or device closure
Postoperative issues	■ s/p surgical ligation: Pleural effusion, hemothorax, infection, disruption of recurrent laryngeal nerve function (often transient); small long-term risk of scoliosis and restrictive lung disease
	■ s/p catheter-based closure: Groin hematoma, loss of femoral artery pulse, device embolization, pulmonary artery or aortic obstruction from the device/coil, infection
Follow-up	■ Endocarditis prophylaxis for 6 months after procedure, or longer if there is residual defect

PDA, patent ductus arteriosus; s/p, status post

vessels form on either side of the capillary bed. Arteriovenous malformations (AVMs) result from abnormal morphogenesis of these structures, although the exact molecular mechanisms and timing of the developmental abnormalities are still unclear.[31] AVMs can occur in the pulmonary or systemic circulations.

Definitions and Epidemiology

AVMs are typically congenital; however, acquired forms can result from trauma, arterial dysplasia, and vascular puncture. There are no known teratogenic or toxic causes. Hereditary hemorrhagic telangiectasia (Osler-Weber syndrome) is an autosomal dominant syndrome where there is normal vascular morphogenesis; however, the walls of the small arteries are weak, and vascular malformations can develop later in life.[31]

The most common cerebral AVM is the vein of Galen malformation, located deep in the brain parenchyma. Hepatic AVMs are also seen. Pulmonary AVMs are seen in hereditary hemorrhagic telangiectasia, significant liver disease, and patients with single-ventricle congenital heart disease palliated with a cavopulmonary anastomosis. This "acquired" pulmonary AVM is thought to be due to lack of hepatic flow to the lungs. Pulmonary AVMs will not be discussed further here.

Pathogenesis

Large systemic AVMs can produce significant hemodynamic effects with a left-to-right shunt and volume load to the right side of the heart. There is also a concomitant decrease in systemic vascular resistance resulting in a compensatory widened pulse pressure and increase in heart rate, stroke volume, and plasma volume.[32] Increase in the myocardial oxygen demand and decreased coronary perfusion due to decreased diastolic blood pressure can develop, and patients can often present with high-output failure and progress to low-output failure if left untreated.[31,32] Unlike other shunt defects such as ASDs or VSDs, AVMs are obligatory shunts, meaning that the degree of shunting does not depend on relative vascular resistance or ventricular compliance. Therefore, symptoms and signs can manifest as early as fetal life in the larger malformations.

Clinical Presentation

Symptoms

The presentation of an AVM is determined by the size of the defect and its location. As stated earlier, shunting through an AVM is independent of vascular resistance. Therefore, patients with large AVMs can present in utero with hydrops fetalis. Newborns can present with profound congestive heart failure and cyanosis due to the large left-to-right shunt through the AVM and right-to-left shunting across the PFO and PDA. AVMs that present in the newborn period are usually cerebral, hepatic, or intrathoracic.

Children with small AVMs may by relatively asymptomatic due to a relatively small shunt. These patients may first present with a murmur. Other symptoms relate to the location of the AVM. Smaller vein of Galen AVMs, for example, can present with hydrocephalus in infancy and with headaches in older patients.[33]

Physical examination

Neonates who present with a large AVM may appear cyanotic and in respiratory distress. They will have notable tachycardia, tachypnea, and widened pulse pressure. Oxygen saturation may be lower in the lower extremities due to right-to-left ductal shunt. Extremities may be warm and well perfused, and bounding pulses may accompany the widened pulse pressure. Alternatively, if the patient is in a low-output state, extremities may be cool and capillary refill may be sluggish. Patients with hepatic AVMs may have hepatomegaly and a bruit auscultated over the liver. In neonates with large AVMs, the precordium will be strikingly hyperdynamic to palpation. S_2 may be prominent. A mid-diastolic rumble due to increased flow across the tricuspid valve or a holosystolic murmur of AV valve regurgitation may be heard. Auscultation of the anterior fontanel may reveal an audible bruit, which is reported in 30% of vein of Galen malformations.[31]

Children with smaller AVMs often do not manifest many signs on cardiac physical examination. A mid-diastolic murmur may be audible due to increased flow across the tricuspid valve. If the AVM is superficial, a thrill may be palpable. Upon compression of the AVM, the mid-diastolic murmur may resolve due to disruption of the increased venous return to the right side of the heart (Nicoladoni-Branham sign).[31]

Diagnosis

The electrocardiogram is often normal. In neonates with large AVMs, there may be evidence of right axis deviation, right atrial enlargement, and right ventricular hypertrophy. Chest roentgenograms may show cardiomegaly, increased pulmonary vascular markings and pulmonary edema due to the increased left-to-right shunting across the defect.

Echocardiography can assess the hemodynamic impact of the AVM.[34] The superior vena cava may appear dilated in patients with a cerebral AVM, whereas the inferior vena cava and hepatic veins are dilated in patients with a hepatic AVM. Large AVMs lead to right atrial and right ventricular enlargement, and right ventricular function may be hyperdynamic. Valvar regurgitation may be noted. A general anatomic survey will ensure there are no associated cardiac defects. Doppler assessment is important in the evaluation of a significant AVM. Retrograde diastolic flow in the aorta is noted in arterial vessels proximal to the AVM.

Ultimately, diagnosis is achieved by direct assessment of the region of the AVM, via a variety of imaging modalities including ultrasound, angiography, computed tomography, or magnetic resonance imaging.[32]

Treatment

Once neonates are stabilized with ventilation and supportive measures to maintain systemic output and decrease oxygen consumption, intervention to eliminate or limit flow through the AVM must be pursued. Systemic AVMs can be excised with surgery only if the lesion is accessible and localized. Often, however, the

Summary of AVM	
Medical management (cardiac)	■ Neonates: Mechanical ventilation, diuretics, inotropic medications ■ Infants/children: Diuresis, caloric fortification
Cardiac indications for intervention	■ Failed medical management and persistence of heart failure in the neonate ■ Symptomatic infants whose symptoms are responsive to medical management can defer intervention until 5-6 months of age
Treatment options	■ Endovascular treatment with percutaneous embolization of the AVM ■ Surgical excision ■ Microsurgery, radiosurgery
Postoperative issues	■ Heart failure symptoms may persist with partial embolization. ■ Other issues relate to the location of the AVM and interventional techniques.
Follow-up	■ Once AVM is treated and cardiac manifestations have resolved, no further follow-up is necessary.

AVM, arteriovenous malformation.

malformation recurs. Transcatheter embolization is a newer strategy to disrupt the arteriovenous connections. This technique is limited by the ability to access all of the small, tortuous vessels and the ability of new arterial supply to develop.[31,32] Depending on the size and location of the AVM, embolization may only partially occlude the shunt and may require multiple procedures. Large cerebral malformations have a very poor prognosis and are associated with significant neurologic consequences. Patients often suffer from hydrocephalus, seizures, intracranial hemorrhage, and mental retardation.[31] These patients should be managed in conjunction with appropriate specialists, depending on the location of the malformation (Table 7-7).

Clinical Pearls

- Increased pulmonary blood flow occurs in shunt lesions from shunting of blood from the left side of the heart to the right side of the heart.
- Patients with ASDs and small VSDs are typically asymptomatic at birth and in infancy, although premature infants or those with chromosomal abnormalities may manifest symptoms earlier.
- Typical symptoms range from failure to thrive, recurrent respiratory infections, and poor weight gain in infants to respiratory distress and exercise intolerance in older children.
- Clinical examination may be normal. When it is abnormal, there may be tachypnea, hepatomegaly, hyperdynamic precordium, rales, and/or an audible murmur consistent with the specific lesion.
- Children with the described symptoms and concerning physical examination findings should be referred to a pediatric cardiologist for further evaluation.
- Echocardiography is used to confirm the diagnosis of acyanotic shunt lesions.
- Medical management includes optimization of caloric intake and symptomatic management with diuretics, afterload reduction, and digoxin.
- Acyanotic shunt lesions can be closed by surgical or catheter-based intervention with excellent outcomes and minimal long-term complications. The timing of intervention varies by lesion and presentation.

REFERENCES

1. Abraham R. Perinatal and postnatal changes in the circulation. In: Abraham R, ed. *Congenital Diseases of the Heart: Clinical-Physiological Considerations.* 3rd ed. West Sussex, United Kingdom: Wiley-Blackwell; 2009:25-36.

2. Artman M, Mahony L, Teitel DF. *Neonatal Cardiology.* New York, NY: McGraw-Hill; 2002.

3. Rudolph AM. Ventricular septal defect. In: Rudolph AM, ed. *Congenital Diseases of the Heart: Clinical-Physiological Considerations.* 3rd ed. West Sussex, United Kingdom: Wiley-Blackwell; 2004:148-178.

4. Munoz R, Schmitt CG, Roth SJ, Cruz ED. *Handbook of Pediatric Cardiovascular Drugs.* London, United Kingdom: Springer; 2008.

5. Rojas CA, El-Sherief A, Medina HM, et al. Embryology and developmental defects of the interatrial septum. *AJR Am J Roentgenol.* 2010;195:1100-1104.

6. Coburn J, Porter WDE. Atrial septal defects. In: Hugh D, Allen DJD, Shaddy RE, Feltes TF, eds. *Moss and Adams' Heart Disease in Infants, Children, and Adolescents Including the Fetus and Young Adult.* 7th ed. Philadelphia, PA: Lippincott Williams & Wilkins; 2008:632-645.

7. Abraham R. Atrial septal defect and partial anomalous drainage of the pulmonary veins. In: Abraham R, ed. *Congenital Diseases of the Heart: Clinical-Physiological Considerations.* 3rd ed. West Sussex, United Kingdom: Wiley-Blackwell; 2009:179-202.

8. Kharouf R, Luxenberg DM, Khalid O, Abdulla R. Atrial septal defect: spectrum of care. *Pediatr Cardiol.* 2008;29:271-280.

9. Gervasi L, Basu S. Atrial septal defect devices used in the cardiac catheterization laboratory. *Prog Cardiovasc Nurs.* 2009;24:86-89.

10. Najm HK, Williams WG, Chuaratanaphong S, Watzka SB, Coles JG, Freedom RM. Primum atrial septal defect in children: early results, risk factors, and freedom from reoperation. *Ann Thorac Surg.* 1998;66:829-835.

11. Attenhofer Jost CH, Connolly HM, Danielson GK, et al. Sinus venosus atrial septal defect: long-term postoperative outcome for 115 patients. *Circulation.* 2005;112: 1953-1958.

12. Jonas R. Atrial septal defect. In: Jonas R, ed. *Comprehensive Surgical Management of Congenital Heart Disease.* London, United Kingdom: Hodder Arnold; 2004:225-241.

13. Geva T. Anomalies of the atrial septum. In: Wyman W, Lai LLM, Cohen MS, Geva T, eds. *Echocardiography in Pediatric and Congenital Heart Disease.* West Sussex, United Kingdom: Wiley-Blackwell; 2009:158-174.

14. Wilson W, Taubert KA, Gewitz M, et al. Prevention of infective endocarditis: guidelines from the American Heart Association: a guideline from the American Heart Association Rheumatic Fever, Endocarditis, and Kawasaki Disease Committee, Council on Cardiovascular Disease in the Young, and the Council on Clinical Cardiology, Council on Cardiovascular Surgery and Anesthesia, and the Quality of Care and Outcomes Research Interdisciplinary Working Group. *Circulation.* 2007;116:1736-1754.

15. Glatz AC, McBride MG, Paridon SM, et al. Long-term noninvasive arrhythmia assessment after surgical repair of sinus venosus atrial septal defect. *Congenit Heart Dis.* 2010;5:141-148.

16. Forbus GA, Shirali GS. Anomalies of the ventricular septum. In: Lai W, Mertens L, Cohen MS, Geva T, eds. *Echocardiography in Pediatric and Congenital Heart Disease from Fetus to Adult.* West Sussex, United Kingdom: Wiley-Blackwell; 2009:175-187.

17. Jonas RA. Ventricular septal defect. In: Jonas R, ed. *Comprehensive Surgical Management of Congenital Heart Disease.* London, United Kingdom: Hodder Arnold; 2004:243-255.

18. McDaniel NL, Gutgesell HP. Ventricular septal defects. In: Allen HD, Shaddy RE, Feltes TF, eds. *Moss and Adams' Heart Disease in Infants, Children, and Adolescents Including the Fetus and Young Adult.* 7th ed. West Sussex, United Kingdom: Lippincott Williams & Wilkins; 2008:667-682.

19. Aguilar N, Eugenio Lopez J. Ventricular septal defects. *J Bol Assoc Med P R*. 2009;101:23-29.

20. Craig B. Atrioventricular septal defect: from fetus to adult. *Heart*. 2006;92:1879-1885.

21. Cetta F, Edwards WD, Dearani JA, Puga FJ. Atrioventricular septal defects. In: Allen HD, Shaddy RE, Feltes TF, eds. *Moss and Adams' Heart Disease in Infants, Children and Adolescents Including the Fetus and Young Adult.* Philadelphia, PA: Lippincott Williams & Wilkins; 2008:646-667.

22. Calabro R, Limongelli G. Complete atrioventricular canal. *Orphanet J Rare Dis*. 2006;1:8.

23. Rudolph AM. The ductus arteriosus and persistent patency of the ductus arteriosus. In: Rudolph AM, ed. *Congenital Disease of the Heart: Clinical-Physiological Considerations*. West Sussex, United Kingdom: Wiley-Blackwell; 2004:115-147.

24. Cohen MS. Common atrioventricular canal defects. In: Lai W, Mertens L, Cohen MS, Geva T, eds. *Echocardiography in Pediatric and Congenital Heart Disease from Fetus to Adult*. West Sussex, United Kingdom: Wiley-Blackwell; 2009:230-248.

25. Forsey JT, Elmasry OA, Martin RP. Patent arterial duct. *Orphanet J Rare Dis*. 2009;4:17.

26. Fortescue EB, Lock JE, Galvin T, McElhinney DB. To close or not to close: the very small patent ductus arteriosus. *Congenit Heart Dis*. 2010;5:354-365.

27. Radtke WA. Current therapy of the patent ductus arteriosus. *Curr Opin Cardiol*. 1998;13:59-65.

28. Tacy TA. Abnormalities of the ductus arteriosus and pulmonary arteries. In: Lai W, Mertens L, Cohen MS, Geva T, eds. *Echocardiography in Pediatric and Congenital Heart Disease from Fetus to Adult*. West Sussex, United Kingdom: Wiley-Blackwell; 2009:283-296.

29. Moore P, Heymann MA. Patent ductus arteriosus and aortopulmonary window. In: Lai W, Mertens L, Cohen MS, Geva T, eds. *Moss and Adams' Heart Disease in Infants, Children, and Adolescents Including the Fetus and Young Adult*. 7th ed. West Sussex, United Kingdom: Lippincott Williams & Wilkins; 2008:683-702.

30. Giroud JM, Jacobs JP. Evolution of strategies for management of the patent arterial duct. *Cardiol Young*. 2007;17(Suppl 2):68-74.

31. Grifka RG, Preminger TJ. Vascular anomalies. In: Allen HD, Shaddy RE, Feltes TF, eds. *Moss and Adams' Heart Disease in Infants, Children, and Adolescents Including the Fetus and Young Adult*. 7th ed. Philadelphia, PA: Lippincott Williams & Wilkins; 2008:715-729.

32. Konez O, Burrows PE. An appropriate diagnostic workup for suspected vascular birthmarks. *Cleve Clin J Med*. 2004;71:505-510.

33. Khullar D, Andeejani AM, Bulsara KR. Evolution of treatment options for vein of Galen malformations. *J Neurosurg Pediatr*. 2010;6:444-451.

34. Starc TJ, Krongrad E, Bierman FZ. Two-dimensional echocardiography and Doppler findings in cerebral arteriovenous malformation. *Am J Cardiol*. 1989;64:252-254.

CHAPTER 8

Acyanotic Heart Disease: Valves, Outflow Tracts, and Vasculature

Matthew C. Schwartz,

Joseph W. Turek, Therese M. Giglia,

Stephanie Fuller and Andrew C. Glatz

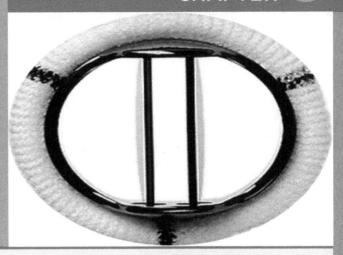

INTRODUCTION

Acyanotic cardiac lesions represent a significant portion of all congenital heart disease. Although acyanotic shunt lesions are discussed in Chapter 7, this chapter focuses on acyanotic valve and ventricular outflow tract lesions as well as common vascular abnormalities. The chapter begins with a discussion of the semilunar valves (aortic valve and pulmonary valve) and their associated ventricular outflow tracts. Next, lesions of the atrioventricular valves (mitral valve and tricuspid valve) are addressed. Finally, the chapter concludes with a discussion of aortic arch anomalies and peripheral pulmonary stenosis. Each section begins with a description of the normal cardiac structures prior to describing the lesions that affect them. Tables 8-1 and 8-2 summarize the salient points from each section. Endocarditis prophylaxis for various lesions is discussed in Chapters 14 and 16.

SEMILUNAR VALVES

Aortic Valve

The aortic valve connects the left ventricle to the aorta. The normal aortic valve is made up of 3 cusps and does not have a tensor apparatus. Aortic stenosis (AS) results from obstruction at any point between the left ventricle and the aorta. It can occur below the valve in the left ventricular outflow tract (subvalvar AS), at the level of the valve itself (valvar AS), or above the valve in the proximal aorta (supravalvar AS). AS in some form accounts for 3% to 8% of all congenital heart disease.[1]

Valvar aortic stenosis

Definitions and epidemiology. Congenital valvar AS is a malformation of the aortic valve that occurs before birth and results in varying degrees of obstruction to blood flow. Valvar AS accounts for 75% of congenital AS. Although not always stenotic, the most common congenital lesion of the aortic valve is a bicuspid aortic valve, which occurs in 1% of the population.[1] A bicuspid aortic valve occurs when 2 cusps fuse to form a valve that functionally has 2 cusps instead of 3. Unicuspid aortic valves have a slit-like opening and are associated with critical AS. Less commonly, stenosis results from a hypoplastic valve annulus with normal cusps. Valvar AS occurs more often in males than females. Additional congenital heart defects are present in 20% of patients including patent ductus arteriosus (PDA), aortic coarctation, and ventricular septal defect (VSD).[1]

Pathogenesis. The congenital aortic valve abnormality decreases the size of the orifice through which blood flows from the left ventricle to the aorta causing left ventricular outflow obstruction. A unicuspid valve typically results in "critical AS" in which severe obstruction prevents adequate antegrade blood flow across the aortic valve and systemic perfusion is dependent on right-to-left flow across the PDA. In patients with a bicuspid aortic valve, the orifice size can be relatively preserved during life. If the orifice size does not increase normally with growth, then obstruction develops later in childhood or adolescence. The left ventricle hypertrophies over time to maintain normal wall stress in the setting of the increased afterload, which predisposes the myocardium to chronic ischemia and can lead to left ventricular dilatation and systolic dysfunction.

A Summary of Common Acyanotic Congenital Cardiac Lesions and Associated Findings

Lesion	Common Etiologies	Classic Murmur	Other Examination Findings	Common Presentation	ECG	CXR
Valvar aortic stenosis	Infant: unicuspid valve Children: bicuspid aortic valve	SEM loudest at RUSB with radiation to neck	Systolic ejection click if bicuspid valve present	Neonates: critical AS presents with low cardiac output/shock Children: asymptomatic murmur	LVH may be present	Infants: pulmonary edema, cardiomegaly Children: usually normal
Aortic regurgitation	Bicuspid aortic valve	Medium- to high-frequency diastolic murmur at left sternal border	Wide pulse pressure Bounding pulses	Asymptomatic murmur	LVH may be present	Cardiomegaly may be present
Valvar pulmonary stenosis	Conical valve or unicuspid valve Often associated with Noonan syndrome	SEM loudest at LUSB with radiation to back	Systolic ejection click may be present	Neonates: critical PS presents with cyanosis Children: asymptomatic murmur	RVH RAE may be present	Infants: decreased pulmonary vascular markings Children: usually normal
Mitral stenosis	Leaflet, chordae, or papillary muscle abnormalities	Low-frequency, mid-diastolic murmur at apex	Second heart sound can be narrowly split if pulmonary HTN present	Usually presents in infancy with tachypnea, frequent pneumonia, FTT	LAE	May show pulmonary edema
Mitral regurgitation	Leaflet, chordae, or papillary muscle abnormalities	Holosystolic, blowing murmur at apex	MS murmur if significant MR exists	Neonates: tachypnea, FTT Children: exercise intolerance	LAE LVH	Cardiomegaly may be present
Ebstein anomaly	Tethered septal and posterior tricuspid valve leaflets	Holosystolic murmur at LLSB	PS murmur if significant TR exists	Mild: murmur, arrhythmias, fatigue with exertion Severe: cyanosis in infancy	RAE	Cardiomegaly
Aortic coarctation	Associated with left-sided obstructive lesions and Turner syndrome	SEM loudest at LUSB with radiation to back Murmur can be absent	Upper extremity HTN Blood pressure gradient between RUE and LE and diminished femoral pulses	Neonates: may present with low cardiac output/shock Children: upper extremity HTN	LVH may be present	Infants: pulmonary edema, cardiomegaly Children: 3 sign, rib notching

AS, aortic stenosis; CXR, chest radiograph; ECG, electrocardiogram; FTT, failure to thrive; HTN, hypertension; LAE, left atrial enlargement; LE, left extremity; LLSB, left lower sternal border; LUSB, left upper sternal border; LVH, left ventricular hypertrophy; MR, mitral regurgitation; MS, mitral stenosis; PS, pulmonary stenosis; RAE, right atrial enlargement; RUE, right upper extremity; RUSB, right upper sternal border; RVH, right ventricular hypertrophy; SEM, systolic ejection murmur; TR, tricuspid regurgitation.

Concerning Signs or Symptoms in Children or Adolescents with Congenital Cardiac Lesions

Lesion	Signs/Symptoms That Should Prompt Concern
LVOT obstructive lesion	■ Chest pain or syncope with exercise
RVOT obstructive lesion	■ Chest pain or syncope with exercise ■ Dyspnea on exertion
Mitral stenosis	■ Dyspnea on exertion ■ Syncope ■ Recurrent pneumonia
Mitral regurgitation	■ Dyspnea on exertion ■ Recurrent pneumonia
Ebstein anomaly	■ Dyspnea on exertion ■ Palpitations ■ Syncope
Aortic coarctation	■ Severe upper extremity hypertension ■ Dyspnea on exertion

LVOT, left ventricular outflow tract; RVOT, right ventricular outflow tract.

Clinical presentation. Newborns with severe aortic obstruction may have ductal-dependent systemic circulation after birth. If perfusion to the head and neck and upper extremity vessels as well as the descending aorta is dependent on flow from the pulmonary artery through a PDA, this is termed "critical AS." If not identified either prenatally or before ductal closure, infants with critical AS will present in shock in the first week of life as the ductus arteriosus closes and systemic perfusion is compromised. Such patients often appear well immediately after birth, although frequently they are "comfortably tachypneic." They usually do not have differential saturations between the upper and lower body since the ductus supplies the ascending as well as descending aorta. Following ductal constriction, these infants appear pale and often have a systolic ejection murmur at the right upper sternal border as well as a gallop. Peripheral pulses will be diminished. Laboratory testing will reveal a significant metabolic acidosis. Some neonates with significant (although not critical) valvar AS may tolerate ductal closure. These patients often present within the first few months of life with severe congestive heart failure due to left ventricular failure. They present with poor feeding, tachypnea, and growth failure, and physical examination shows a systolic ejection murmur, gallop, and decreased peripheral pulses.

Only 10% of patients with congenital valvar AS present during infancy. Instead, most patients with a bicuspid valve are diagnosed later. Some are referred to a pediatric cardiologist to evaluate a cardiac murmur. Dyspnea, chest pain, or syncope with exercise may be present if the stenosis and resultant left ventricular hypertrophy are substantial. On physical examination, a thrill may be present in the suprasternal notch. The first heart sound will be normal, and splitting of the second sound may not be present in severe AS due to prolonged left ventricular ejection. Patients with a bicuspid aortic valve may have a systolic ejection click that shortly follows S$_1$; the click is best heard at the left lower sternal border or apex. The characteristic murmur of AS is a systolic ejection murmur that begins shortly after S$_1$ and is crescendo–decrescendo in shape (Figure 8-1). The murmur is best heard at the right upper sternal border and can radiate to the carotid arteries. As the stenosis worsens, the murmur becomes louder and harsher and peaks later in systole.

Diagnostic tests. Chest radiograph (CXR) is usually normal in isolated AS unless left ventricular failure is present, in which case cardiomegaly can be observed. Patients with significant obstruction may show signs of left ventricular hypertrophy on electrocardiogram (ECG), but typically the tracing is normal. Clinical symptoms and physical examination can suggest AS, but the test of choice to confirm the diagnosis is echocardiography. The echocardiogram can demonstrate the morphology of the aortic valve (Figure 8-2) and can characterize the degree of obstruction using Doppler

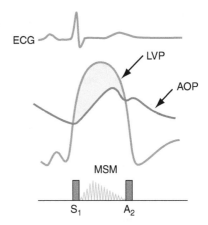

FIGURE 8-1 ■ Left ventricle pressure (LVP) and aortic pressure (AOP) tracings shown with simultaneous electrocardiogram (ECG) and auscultatory characteristics in a patient with left ventricular outflow tract obstruction. Due to the obstruction, left ventricular pressure exceeds aortic pressure during systolic ejection. The midsystolic murmur (MSM) begins after the first heart sound (S$_1$) and is crescendo–decrescendo in character. The murmur is loudest at the peak of left ventricular ejection when the pressure difference between ventricle and aorta is the greatest. During late systole, the pressure difference diminishes and the murmur ends prior to aortic valve closure (A$_2$). (*Reproduced, with permission, from Fauci AS, Kasper DL, Braunwald E, et al. Harrison's Principles of Internal Medicine. 17th ed. New York, NY: McGraw-Hill; 2008.*)

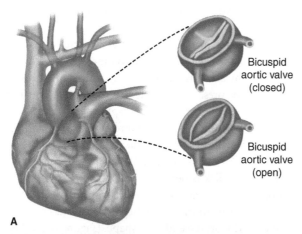

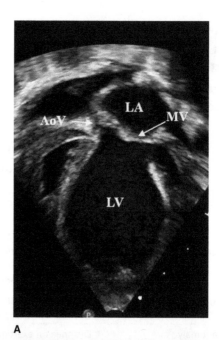

A

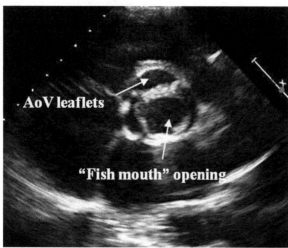

B

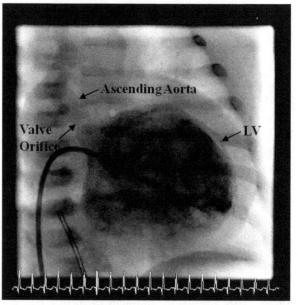

B

FIGURE 8-2 ■ **A.** Picture illustrating a bicuspid aortic valve when open and closed. (*Reproduced, with permission, from Siu SC, Silversides CK. Bicuspid aortic valve disease. J Am Coll Cardiol. 2010;55:2789-2800. Copyright © Elsevier Inc., All rights reserved.*) **B.** Echocardiogram showing parasternal short axis view of an open bicuspid aortic valve in an adolescent. The aortic valve (AoV) is shown in cross-section with the characteristic "fish mouth" appearance.

FIGURE 8-3 ■ **A.** Echocardiogram showing the apical 4-chamber view in a neonate with severe valvar aortic stenosis. The left ventricle (LV) is severely dilated and the aortic valve (AoV) is unicuspid and hypoplastic. LA, left atrium; MV, mitral valve. **B.** Left ventricular angiography in the same patient highlighting the dilated LV and the small orifice through which contrast flows from LV to aorta.

to estimate the pressure gradient between left ventricle and aorta during systole. The echocardiogram can also determine left ventricular size (hypertrophy, dilatation) and systolic function (Figure 8-3A). In neonates with critical AS, the echocardiogram is crucial in determining if the aortic valve and left ventricle are large enough to support a biventricular circulation. Cardiac catheterization can be diagnostic and therapeutic in patients with AS and is considered the gold standard for measuring the pressure gradient from left ventricle to ascending aorta. Angiography can also differentiate left ventricular size and function and the effective aortic valve orifice (Figure 8-3B).

Treatment. Patients who present in infancy with ductal-dependent circulation or heart failure require

intervention. If the left ventricle, mitral valve annulus, and aortic valve annulus are of adequate size, a 2-ventricle circulation is viable. In these patients, transcatheter balloon dilation of the aortic valve is preferred over open surgical valvotomy in most centers. Balloon dilation is effective, but many patients will develop aortic insufficiency after dilation. Patients with significant aortic regurgitation or refractory stenosis will require a surgical intervention. Patients who require transcatheter intervention in infancy often require repeat balloon dilation in childhood and many ultimately require surgical intervention.

Patients who present in childhood or adolescence with congenital AS usually can be managed expectantly as most are asymptomatic with mild obstruction. Medical management of these patients includes appropriate exercise restrictions and serial evaluations of the aortic valve obstruction with echocardiogram. Guidelines for exercise restriction in congenital AS exist; patients with mild AS and no symptoms can participate in all competitive sports.[2] Of note, patients with a bicuspid aortic valve can also develop valve regurgitation and dilatation of the ascending aorta that must also be considered when determining exercise restrictions. Exercise guidelines for patients who have undergone prosthetic aortic valve replacement are discussed in the aortic regurgitation section.

In children or adolescents who do require valve intervention, balloon valvuloplasty is generally preferred to surgery as the initial intervention. Typically, balloon valvuloplasty is performed if the catheter-derived gradient across the valve is ≥50 mm Hg and there is no significant aortic insufficiency. Children or adolescents with progressive aortic regurgitation or stenosis that is refractory to balloon dilation typically require surgery.

Surgical options in infants and small children include replacement of the diseased aortic valve with an aortic homograft or with a pulmonary autograft (Ross procedure). In the Ross procedure, the aortic valve is completely removed and the patient's pulmonary valve is transferred into the aortic position. A conduit is then placed from right ventricle to pulmonary artery. In larger children and adolescents, mechanical or bioprosthetic valves can also be used. Mechanical valves are durable but require anticoagulation with warfarin. Bioprosthetic valves may not require anticoagulation but have limited longevity and durability compared to mechanical valves.

Subvalvar aortic stenosis

Definitions and epidemiology. Subvalvar AS results when obstruction to left ventricular outflow exists below the aortic valve. It represents 10% to 20% of AS in children and, like valvar AS, is more common in males. Subvalvar AS is most often caused by a subaortic membrane, a ridge of membranous or fibromuscular tissue that encircles the left ventricular outflow tract. Subaortic obstruction can also occur in hypertrophic obstructive cardiomyopathy, but this is discussed in Chapter 13. Other congenital cardiac anomalies such as VSD, aortic coarctation, atrioventricular septal defect, valvar AS, and mitral valve abnormalities are often found in association with a subaortic membrane.[1]

Pathogenesis. The pathophysiology of subvalvar AS is similar to that of valvar AS: Afterload is increased on the left ventricle, and over time, this results in left ventricular hypertrophy. As in valvar disease, severe subaortic obstruction and ventricular hypertrophy can result in endocardial ischemia and fibrosis. In patients with subaortic disease, the aortic valve can be trileaflet or bicuspid. The valve leaflets thicken due to the damage from the turbulent flow below the valve that may lead to valvar stenosis as well as aortic regurgitation.

Clinical presentation. Patients with subvalvar AS usually present with a heart murmur in the absence of symptoms. In other patients with accompanying cardiac lesions such as aortic coarctation, the subaortic obstruction will be diagnosed incidentally at the time of echocardiogram. If obstruction is severe, symptoms can mimic valvar AS. Physical examination will show a systolic ejection murmur loudest at the left midsternal border that radiates to the suprasternal notch and neck. The murmur will resemble that of valvar AS, but patients with subvalvar obstruction will not have a systolic click, an important finding that can help differentiate between valvar and subvalvar obstruction.

Diagnostic tests. The ECG can be normal, but may also show left ventricular hypertrophy. Echocardiography is needed to establish the diagnosis and to determine the severity of the obstruction (Figure 8-4). The echocardiogram will define associated cardiac lesions and determine if the aortic valve has incurred damage from the turbulent subaortic flow. Cardiac catheterization can be used to determine the gradient from left ventricle to aorta. However, catheterization is used less often in the evaluation of subaortic obstruction because transcatheter interventions are not used for treatment.

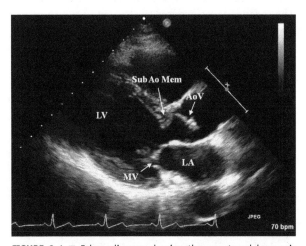

FIGURE 8-4 ■ Echocardiogram showing the parasternal long axis view in a child with left ventricular outflow tract obstruction due to a subaortic membrane. AoV, aortic valve; LA, left atrium; LV, left ventricle; MV, mitral valve; Sub Ao Mem, subaortic membrane.

Treatment. The treatment of choice for subaortic obstruction is surgical resection of the obstructive left ventricular outflow tract tissue. Although often successful, complications include surgically created VSDs and complete heart block.

Mild subaortic obstruction can remain stable for years but may progress. Indications for surgery are not universally agreed upon, but patients with progressive obstruction should undergo operation. Likewise, patients with progressive left ventricular hypertrophy, left ventricular systolic dysfunction, or symptoms (eg, chest pain, exercise intolerance, syncope) should have resection. Progressive aortic regurgitation is also an indication for membrane resection. The valvar AS guidelines for exercise restriction can be applied to those with subvalvar obstruction.[2]

Supravalvar aortic stenosis

Definitions and epidemiology. Supravalvar AS is obstruction to left ventricular outflow above the aortic valve and is the least common form of congenital AS. Roughly 30% to 50% of patients with supravalvar AS have Williams syndrome.[1] The lesion can be familial in patients who do not have other features of Williams syndrome. In half of the patients, the lesion is sporadic. In those with the familial form, abnormal elastin gene expression is thought to cause the supravalvar narrowing. The stenosis is typically localized to the sinotubular junction, but some can have narrowing of the entire ascending aorta. Other lesions associated with supravalvar AS can include branch pulmonary artery stenosis, aortic coarctation, VSD, and bicuspid aortic valve.[1]

Pathogenesis. The physiology of supravalvar AS is similar to subvalvar and valvar stenosis. However, in supravalvar AS, the coronary arteries are uniquely affected because they arise proximal to the obstruction. The coronaries are exposed to elevated systolic pressure that can lead to abnormal remodeling. Also, the coronary ostia may be compromised due to the supravalvar stenosis. As a result, patients with supravalvar AS are at risk for ischemia and endocardial fibrosis. In addition, because the sinotubular junction does not expand normally, shear stress is placed on aortic valve leaflets, leading to thickening and damage in many patients.

Clinical presentation. Most patients are diagnosed when referred for an asymptomatic murmur. Similar to valvar and subvalvar stenosis, patients with supravalvar AS can experience chest pain or syncope with exercise if severe obstruction exists. The quality and location of the murmur are similar to valvar AS, but a systolic click is uncommon.

Diagnostic tests. ECG can show left ventricular hypertrophy but is typically normal. Echocardiography

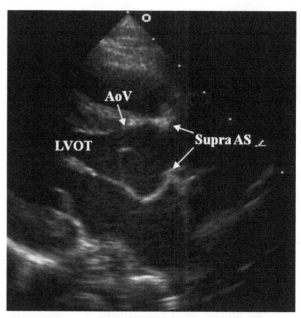

FIGURE 8-5 ■ Echocardiogram showing the parasternal long axis view in a 5-year-old female with Williams syndrome and supravalvar aortic stenosis. AoV, aortic valve; LVOT, left ventricular outflow tract; Supra AS, supravalvar aortic stenosis.

is necessary to make the diagnosis and to evaluate the severity of obstruction (Figure 8-5). Cardiac catheterization can determine the degree of obstruction, and angiography defines the anatomy of the ascending aorta and coronary arteries. However, at catheterization, patients with supravalvar AS are at increased risk of cardiac arrest, likely due to impairment of coronary flow during catheter manipulation. It is important to use noninvasive methods to evaluate other arteries that can be affected by the elastin abnormality including the aortic arch branches, pulmonary arteries, and renal arteries.

Treatment. Like subvalvar AS, surgery is the treatment of choice for supravalvar obstruction. Criteria for intervention are similar to those used for valvar AS. Surgical repair consists of patch plasty of 1, 2, or all 3 aortic sinuses. Exercise restrictions for patients with valvar AS can also be applied to patients with supravalvar AS.[2]

Aortic regurgitation

Definitions and epidemiology. Aortic valve regurgitation (AR) is uncommon in the pediatric population and can be congenital or acquired. Congenital causes include primary valve abnormality, VSDs, subaortic membranes, and aortic root dilation associated with connective tissue disorders. The most common primary valve abnormality is a bicuspid aortic valve. Some VSDs that are located close to the aortic valve (ie, conoventricular or conal septal hypoplasia types) lead to valve insufficiency via leaflet prolapse into the defect. Sub-aortic membranes cause turbulence below the aortic valve that can damage the valve cusps and lead to regurgitation. Aortic root dilation in the setting of Marfan syndrome or Ehlers-Danlos syndrome can lead to root dilation that ultimately compromises coaptation of the aortic valve leaflets. Acquired causes of AR also exist and include endocarditis, rheumatic heart disease, infectious aortitis, and valve dysfunction after transcatheter balloon dilation for AS.[3]

Pathogenesis. In the presence of AR, blood flows backward from the aorta to the ventricle during diastole. This regurgitant volume must be ejected again during the next cardiac cycle and, thus, acts as a volume load for the left ventricle, leading to ventricular dilation. As the left ventricle dilates, the myocardium hypertrophies to maintain wall stress. Forward flow is maintained, but over time, systolic dysfunction can result, eventually leading to symptoms of heart failure. Aortic diastolic pressure will be lower due to the valve regurgitation and, if severe, coronary perfusion can be reduced, further compromising left ventricular performance.

Clinical presentation. Mild to moderate AR can be tolerated very well for years. As discussed in the section on valvar AS, patients with a bicuspid valve rarely present with symptoms in childhood or adolescence. The onset of severe regurgitation will often be associated with clinical signs of congestive heart failure including shortness of breath and failure to thrive. Chest pain with exercise and syncope can also occur but are less common. Patients with severe AR may have tachypnea, tachycardia, and a low diastolic blood pressure on examination. The diastolic leakage of blood from the aorta to the ventricle and the increased volume of blood ejected during systole will lead to increased systolic pressure, a wide pulse pressure, and bounding or "water hammer" pulses on palpation (Corrigan pulse). Even patients with mild AR will have a medium- to high-frequency early diastolic murmur (Figure 8-6). It is heard best at the left sternal border in those with valvular disease and at the right upper sternal border in patients with aortic root dilation. Due to an increased stroke volume, a systolic ejection murmur can also be present that resembles the murmur in valvar AS. Also, true valvar AS can accompany AR, particularly in patients with a bicuspid aortic valve.

A second diastolic murmur can also be present called an Austin Flint murmur. It results from turbulent inflow of blood from the left atrium into the left ventricle. The aortic regurgitant flow impedes the opening of the anterior mitral valve leaflet during left ventricular filling, leading to a relative mitral stenosis murmur. The Austin Flint murmur is low pitched, occurs in late diastole, and is appreciated near the apex.

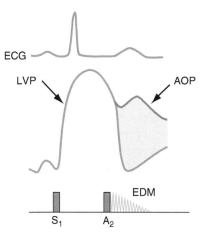

FIGURE 8-6 ■ Left ventricle pressure (LVP) and aortic pressue (AOP) tracings shown with simultaneous electrocardiogram (ECG) and auscultatory characteristics in a patient with aortic regurgitation. During diastole, AOP always exceeds LVP. The regurgitant orifice at the aortic valve allows blood to flow from aorta to left ventricle during diastole, creating an early diastolic murmur (EDM) that starts soon after aortic valve closure (A₂). (*Reproduced, with permission, from Fauci AS, Kasper DL, Braunwald E, et al.* Harrison's Principles of Internal Medicine. *17th ed. New York, NY: McGraw-Hill Companies; 2008.*)

Diagnostic tests. Patients with significant regurgitation will often have cardiomegaly on CXR due to left ventricular dilatation. The ECG may show left ventricular hypertrophy. Echocardiography is essential in evaluating AR because it outlines aortic valve morphology and aortic root size as well as left ventricular size and function (Figure 8-7). Using color Doppler echocardiography, one can qualitatively describe the severity of the regurgitation. Cardiac magnetic resonance imaging (MRI) can be used to determine left ventricular volume and ejection fraction and can quantify the aortic valve regurgitant fraction.

Treatment. Although data in children are limited, angiotensin-converting enzyme (ACE) inhibitors can

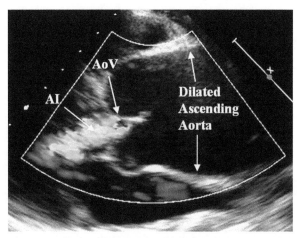

FIGURE 8-7 ■ Echocardiogram with color Doppler showing the parasternal long axis view in a 12-year-old male with Marfan syndrome. Aortic insufficiency (AI) is seen due to severe ascending aorta dilation. AoV, aortic valve.

be used to treat AR; decreasing afterload and diastolic pressure can decrease the pressure gradient between the aorta and the left ventricle, thus decreasing the volume of regurgitated blood. The presence of severe AR with any symptoms is an indication for surgical intervention. Patients with severe insufficiency who are asymptomatic should be referred for surgery if left ventricular systolic dysfunction is present or if there is progressive left ventricular enlargement.[3] Currently, no transcatheter strategies are available in children.

The primary surgical principle in managing AR in the pediatric population is to avoid valve replacement when possible. In infants and young children, replacement would require aortic homografts, which are known to have accelerated calcification and failure. Although most children with significant AR will eventually require valve replacement, delay into adolescence or early adulthood makes both bioprosthetic and mechanical valves viable options. Valve choice is dictated not only by size, but also by the need for anticoagulation that is required for all mechanical valves and some prosthetic valves. Aortic valve repair can involve commissurotomies and leaflet extensions with pericardial patches as well as other strategies.

Asymptomatic patients with mild or moderate regurgitation but normal left ventricular end-diastolic size do not require exercise restriction. Patients with mild or moderate regurgitation and any symptoms should refrain from competitive sports. Patients with mechanical or bioprosthetic aortic valves with normal valve function and normal left ventricular function may participate in moderate static and moderate dynamic competitive sports. Patients taking anticoagulation, however, should refrain from participation in any sports that risk body contact or trauma.[4]

Pulmonary Valve

Like the aortic valve, the normal pulmonary valve is made up of 3 cusps and has no tensor apparatus. Obstruction to right ventricular outflow can occur below the pulmonary valve within the outflow tract itself (subvalvar pulmonary stenosis), at the level of the valve (valvar pulmonary stenosis), or above the pulmonary valve within the proximal main pulmonary artery (supravalvar pulmonary stenosis). All forms of pulmonary stenosis and pulmonary regurgitation are addressed in this section.

Valvar pulmonary stenosis
Definitions and epidemiology. In 80% to 90% of cases, right ventricular outflow obstruction is due to congenital valvar pulmonary stenosis (PS). The diagnosis makes up 8% to 10% of all cases of congenital heart disease.[5] In severe cases, the valve is conical with no

separation into valve leaflets, with a hypoplastic valve annulus. There can be fusion of leaflets, resulting in a unicuspid or bicuspid valve. Other patients have a "dysplastic valve" defined as a trileaflet valve with thickened cusps and a hypoplastic annulus. Dysplastic valves are typical of Noonan syndrome.[5]

Pathogenesis. The valve abnormality decreases the orifice through which blood flows from the right ventricle. Similar to the effect that AS has on the left ventricle, PS increases afterload on the right ventricle. The obstruction causes right ventricular pressure to rise. The right ventricle hypertrophies to normalize wall stress. Over time, the ventricle can dilate and ultimately show systolic failure. Severe ventricular hypertrophy causes abnormal right ventricular compliance and can lead to elevated right atrial pressure. In these patients, right atrial pressure can exceed left atrial pressure during exercise, and cyanosis may be appreciated due to right-to-left shunting at a patent foramen ovale.

Neonates with severe pulmonary valve obstruction can have right ventricular hypoplasia, a significant right-to-left shunt across the patent foramen ovale, and inadequate antegrade flow across the pulmonary valve. These patients will be cyanotic after birth with ductal dependent pulmonary blood flow. This condition is referred to as "critical PS."

Clinical presentation. Most patients with PS are diagnosed after referral for an asymptomatic murmur as symptoms are rarely present in childhood. If severe obstruction is present, the patient may have symptoms of exertional fatigue due to the inability of the right ventricle to increase its output. Rarely, patients with significant stenosis may have chest pain or syncope with exercise. Neonates with critical PS will be cyanotic after birth. Typically, cardiac output is preserved because the right-to-left flow across the patent foramen ovale is unobstructed.

On auscultation, the characteristic murmur of valvar PS is ejection type (crescendo–decrescendo) and is loudest at the left upper sternal border with radiation to the back. The intensity of the murmur increases with the degree of obstruction. The first heart sound is normal. Splitting of the second heart sound increases with the degree of obstruction as right ventricular ejection is prolonged. Many patients with mild or moderate stenosis will have a systolic ejection click heard after S_1. Those with significant obstruction may have a palpable systolic thrill along the left sternal border. In critical PS, the systolic murmur may be soft because of decreased flow across the pulmonary valve in setting of right-to-left flow across the patent foramen ovale. The murmur of a PDA is likely to be present in the left upper chest in these patients.

Diagnostic tests. Patients with mild pulmonary valve obstruction will often have a normal ECG. Those with moderate or severe stenosis may show right axis deviation with signs of right ventricular hypertrophy or right atrial enlargement. CXR can show a prominent main pulmonary artery due to poststenotic dilatation. Cardiomegaly is uncommon unless right ventricular failure or other structural cardiac defects are present. In contrast, infants with critical PS will have cardiomegaly and significantly diminished pulmonary vascular markings.

Echocardiography is crucial in making the diagnosis of PS. The severity of obstruction can also be estimated using Doppler measurements. When needed, the gradient can be precisely measured at cardiac catheterization.

Treatment. In children and adolescents with mild stenosis, the obstruction rarely progresses, and only serial observation is required. The obstruction in those with moderate stenosis is more likely to progress, particularly during early periods of rapid growth. Patients with severe stenosis will often exhibit progression of obstruction and should be followed closely. Patients who are symptomatic or those with significant obstruction and elevated right ventricular pressure should undergo pulmonary valve intervention.[5]

Transcatheter balloon valvuloplasty is typically the initial intervention in patients with valvar PS (Figure 8-8). Balloon valvuloplasty is safe and effective in patients with typical valvar PS. Pulmonary regurgitation of varying degrees often results from dilation and warrants serial follow-up. Balloon dilation is typically less effective in patients with a dysplastic valve (ie, Noonan syndrome).

With the success of transcatheter balloon valvuloplasty, valvar PS rarely necessitates surgical intervention. However, the infrequent patient with inadequate relief of obstruction by balloon dilation, a dysplastic valve, severe annular hypoplasia, severe pulmonary regurgitation, or accompanying subvalvar and/or supravalvar obstruction may require surgery. The valve can largely be managed with open valvotomy and/or an anterior right ventricular outflow tract patch. Valve replacement remains an option in older children.

Neonates with critical PS require prostaglandin infusion after birth to maintain pulmonary blood flow via the PDA. Transcatheter balloon dilation is also first-line treatment in these patients. Even with successful balloon dilation, cyanosis can often persist because abnormal right ventricular compliance causes a right-to-left shunt across the patent foramen ovale. The cyanosis typically improves as the right ventricle remodels after relief of the stenosis, but this may take several weeks. Therefore, some patients will require prostaglandin infusion after balloon dilation while the right ventricular hypertrophy and diastolic dysfunction improve.

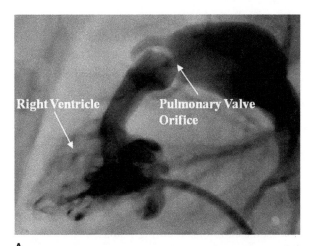

A

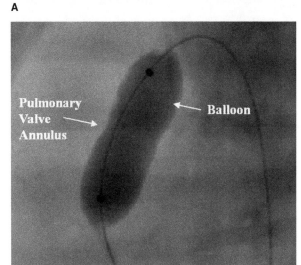

B

FIGURE 8-8 ■ **A.** Angiogram showing right ventricular injection in a 3-day-old infant with valvar pulmonary stenosis. The small pulmonary valve orifice is highlighted with the arrow. **B.** Balloon valvuloplasty of the same patient showing a "waist" in the balloon at the level of the valve annulus.

Asymptomatic patients with a peak gradient across the pulmonary valve by echocardiogram of less than 40 mm Hg and normal right ventricular function can participate in all competitive sports. Patients with a gradient of greater than 40 mm Hg can participate in low-intensity competitive sports and are often referred for pulmonary valve intervention before competitive sports participation. Following pulmonary valve intervention, those with a gradient of less than 40 mm Hg can participate in all competitive sports.[2]

Subvalvar pulmonary stenosis

Definitions and epidemiology. Isolated obstruction below the level of the pulmonary valve is rare and accounts for about 5% of right ventricular outflow lesions. The obstruction can be due to a fibrous or muscular band. An entity called double-chambered right ventricle can also be considered a form of subvalvar PS in which anomalous hypertrophied muscular bands course through the cavity of the right ventricle. The ventricle is divided into 2 chambers, a high-pressure chamber proximal to the muscle bands and a low-pressure chamber distal to the bands.[5] It has been implicated that some double-chambered right ventricles develop as a result of turbulent flow left to right from a small VSD.

Pathogenesis. The right ventricular outflow obstruction of subvalvar PS is similar to that described for valvar disease. In cases of outflow tract muscular hypertrophy or of double-chambered right ventricle, the obstruction is dynamic and worsens during systole.

Clinical presentation. Similar to patients with valvar stenosis, patients with subvalvar PS are typically asymptomatic and referred for murmur evaluation. The cardiac murmur is similar to the murmur of valvar PS and is an ejection-type (crescendo–decrescendo) systolic murmur heard at the left sternal border. Patients with subvalvar obstruction will not have a systolic ejection click.

Diagnostic tests. The CXR and ECG are similar to those seen in patients with valvar obstruction. Two-dimensional and Doppler echocardiography are used to diagnose and characterize the subvalvar anatomy and to quantify the degree of obstruction. Catheterization may be used to confirm echocardiographic pressure gradients, and angiography is useful in establishing the diagnosis of double-chambered right ventricle. Grading of subvalvar obstruction is similar to that used in valvar PS.

Treatment. Many cases of subvalvar PS are associated with tetralogy of Fallot. Cases of isolated subvalvar PS are much less frequent but also constitute a surgical disease. Through a right ventricular incision, subvalvar muscle is aggressively divided to relieve the obstruction. The right ventriculotomy is then augmented with pericardium, homograft, or a synthetic patch to provide unimpeded flow through the right ventricular outflow tract. The subvalvar PS noted with double-chambered right ventricle often progresses. In light of this observation, aggressive resection of the muscle bundles in this variant is warranted.

Exercise restrictions for patients with valvar PS can be applied to those with subvalvar obstruction.[2]

Supravalvar pulmonary stenosis

Definitions and epidemiology. Supravalvar PS is the rarest form of right ventricular outflow tract obstruction. Typically, this is due to hypertrophic tissue located at the sinotubular junction of the main pulmonary

artery. Sometimes, the pulmonary valve cusps can be tethered to the supravalvar narrowing as well, creating a valvar level of obstruction. Like supravalvar AS, supravalvar PS is associated with Williams syndrome.

Pathogenesis. The hemodynamic effect of supravalvar PS is identical to that seen in valvar or subvalvar PS.

Clinical presentation. Most patients are asymptomatic at diagnosis. Similar to valvar and subvalvar PS, the murmur is ejection type and heard loudest at the left upper sternal border. A systolic click is not present and, thus, helps differentiate supravalvar from valvar obstruction.

Diagnostic tests. ECG is typically normal but may show right ventricular hypertrophy if obstruction is moderate or severe. Echocardiography should be used to delineate the right ventricular outflow tract, pulmonary valve, and supravalvar areas. Doppler is used to quantify the degree of obstruction. Cardiac catheterization can be used to measure the pressure gradient across the supravalvar area but is uncommonly used because transcatheter therapies do not exist for supravalvar obstruction.

Treatment. There are no effective medical or transcatheter options for management. In patients with progressive or severe obstruction, surgery is recommended. Patients with mild obstruction can be followed expectantly. Operative repair consists of enlarging the pulmonary artery distal to the valve with an anterior patch. Ideally, the valve can be left unaltered.

Guidelines for exercise restriction are similar to those for valvar PS.[2] If other characteristic features are present, a diagnosis of Williams syndrome should be considered.

Pulmonary regurgitation

Definitions and epidemiology. Pulmonary regurgitation (PR) is a rare isolated congenital lesion and occurs due to idiopathic dilation of the pulmonary artery or in the setting of connective tissue disorders. In children, PR more commonly is seen following balloon valvuloplasty in patients with valvar PS. Rheumatic heart disease and endocarditis can also lead to PR. PR invariably occurs in patients with tetralogy of Fallot whose surgical repair includes a transannular patch, and this population is discussed in Chapter 9.

Pathogenesis. Similar to aortic insufficiency, leakage of blood from the main pulmonary artery to the right ventricle during diastole leads to increased end-diastolic ventricular volume. Over time, this can lead to right ventricular dilation and, ultimately, right ventricular systolic failure.

Clinical presentation. Even with severe PR, most patients are clinically asymptomatic. Over time, if right ventricular dilatation and systolic dysfunction result, patients can develop symptoms of exercise intolerance, dyspnea on exertion, and lower extremity edema. Patients with significant right ventricular dilatation are at risk for ventricular arrhythmias.

On physical examination, patients may have a parasternal lift if right ventricular dilatation is present. The murmur of PR is a soft diastolic, decrescendo murmur heard at the left upper sternal border; this is best heard in the supine position, unlike AR, which is best heard with the patient erect. Patients who have regurgitation following balloon valvuloplasty for valvar stenosis may also have a murmur of residual stenosis. If significant PR is present, then a systolic ejection murmur due to increased stroke volume from the right ventricle across the pulmonary valve may also be heard.

Diagnostic tests. The CXR may show cardiomegaly if the right ventricle is dilated. ECG can show QRS prolongation in the setting of ventricular dilatation. Echocardiogram is needed to characterize the pulmonary valve morphology and the degree of regurgitation using color and pulsed wave Doppler. Cardiac MRI has become a useful tool for quantifying the amount of PR as well as the volume and ejection fraction of the right ventricle. Cardiac catheterization is not used to evaluate PR.

Treatment. Medical management of PR is limited. Guidelines for exercise participation exist for repaired tetralogy of Fallot, and these can be applied to patients with congenital PR. Patients with significant PR and right ventricular dilatation, right ventricular systolic pressure greater than 50% systemic, or tachyarrhythmias should only participate in low-intensity sports.[2] Patients with mild PR typically have a benign clinical course and may never require intervention. Even chronic severe PR can be tolerated for many years, but eventual right ventricular dilatation may be associated with exercise intolerance and even ventricular arrhythmias.

Surgical pulmonary valve replacement is recommended in patients with severe regurgitation in association with right ventricular dilatation and symptoms of right heart failure. Right ventricular dilatation and arrhythmias are also an indication for valve replacement. Indications for pulmonary valve replacement in patients with asymptomatic right ventricular dilatation are not clearly established.[6] Bioprosthetic valves are used in the surgical replacement of the pulmonary valve. Recently, transcatheter options for restoration of pulmonary valve competency in certain patients have been introduced including the Edwards SAPIEN and Medtronic Melody Valves. These devices are valved stents that function as pulmonary valves when placed in the right ventricular outflow tract.

ATRIOVENTRICULAR VALVES

Mitral Valve

The atrioventricular valves separate the atria from the ventricles. Unlike semilunar valves, the atrioventricular valve mechanisms consist of the valve leaflets themselves as well as chordae and papillary muscles. The normal mitral valve is composed of 2 leaflets, the anterior leaflet and the posterior leaflet. The leaflets are supported by chordae tendineae that in turn attach to 2 left ventricular papillary muscles. During systole, the papillary muscles pull the 2 leaflets together and facilitate coaptation. The chordae prevent excessive valve excursion and/or prolapse into the left atrium. Abnormalities of the leaflets and/or the subvalvar apparatus can result in changes in valve function (ie, stenosis and/or regurgitation).

Mitral stenosis

Definitions and epidemiology. Obstruction to mitral inflow may result from congenital abnormalities of the annulus (hypoplasia), leaflets (thickened, commissural fusion), chordae (shortened, thickened, abnormal attachments), and/or papillary muscles (thickened, fused) with a combination of lesions not uncommon. Limited valve leaflet excursion and obstruction may result from a mitral arcade (a distinct anomaly in which the chordae are severely shortened or absent and the leaflets insert directly into the papillary muscle) or a parachute valve (anomaly characterized by chordal attachments from both leaflets to a single papillary muscle). "Typical" congenital mitral stenosis (MS) is used to describe patients with stenosis from annular or leaflet hypoplasia with symmetrical chordal distribution and attachments.[7] Mitral valve anomalies are associated with other left-sided obstructive lesions including bicuspid aortic valve, AS, and coarctation of the aorta.

Pathogenesis. The main physiologic consequences of MS are pulmonary edema and pulmonary arterial hypertension. With obstruction to mitral inflow, the left atrial and pulmonary venous pressures increase, potentially leading to pulmonary edema and pleural effusions. In some patients, the venous congestion in bronchial veins can cause bronchospasm, called "cardiac asthma." The increase in pulmonary venous pressure is also reflected to the pulmonary arteries and may lead to pulmonary hypertension. The pulmonary vascular resistance, however, may be normal, and the pulmonary artery pressures may normalize when the MS is relieved. If the MS is severe, right ventricular failure can result. In some patients with chronic mitral obstruction, an increase in pulmonary vasomotor tone and/or pulmonary vascular remodeling occurs that may lead to irreversible pulmonary vascular changes.

Clinical presentation. Infants with severe mitral obstruction will present in the newborn period with tachypnea and cyanosis. If the mitral valve and left ventricle are inadequate to handle an entire cardiac output, then the right ventricle must supply blood to both the lungs and to the body via a PDA (ductal-dependent systemic blood flow). Most of these patients are characterized as having hypoplastic left heart syndrome, which is discussed in further detail in Chapter 10. Patients with less severe obstruction will present beyond the neonatal period with tachypnea, cough, and failure to thrive. Pulmonary venous congestion makes them prone to pneumonia, either bacterial or viral.

Physical examination will show a soft S_1. A snap is not heard during mitral valve opening because the valve leaflets are relatively immobile. The second heart sound can be normally split. If pulmonary hypertension is present, however, the second heart sound may be narrowly split or loud and single (best heard at the left upper sternal border). The murmur of MS is low frequency and heard during mid-diastole at the apex (Figure 8-9). If other lesions are present, such as AS or coarctation, additional findings will be present on physical examination.

Diagnostic tests. In the setting of significant mitral obstruction, CXR may show left atrial enlargement and pulmonary vascular prominence or pulmonary edema. ECG may show left atrial enlargement. Echocardiography is essential in the evaluation of MS. The mitral valve apparatus should be evaluated for abnormalities in structure and valve mobility. Doppler interrogation of

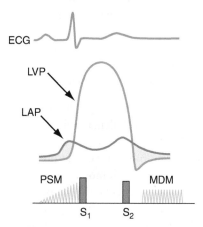

FIGURE 8-9 ■ Left ventricle pressure (LVP) and left atrium pressure (LAP) tracings shown with simultaneous electrocardiogram (ECG) and auscultatory characteristics in a patient with mitral stenosis. A murmur is heard during mid-diastole (mid-diastolic murmur [MDM]) during which time left atrial pressure exceeds left ventricular pressure due to inflow obstruction from mitral stenosis. A second murmur during late diastole (presystolic murmur [PSM]) can also be heard due to a pressure gradient between the left atrium and left ventricle during atrial contraction. (*Reproduced, with permission, from Fauci AS, Kasper DL, Braunwald E, et al.* Harrison's Principles of Internal Medicine. *17th ed. New York, NY: McGraw-Hill; 2008.*)

valve inflow can measure a pressure gradient between left atrium and left ventricle during diastole. A mean gradient of 5 to 10 mm Hg across the mitral valve in diastole suggests mild stenosis, a gradient of 11 to 15 mm Hg suggests moderate stenosis, and a gradient greater than 15 mm Hg indicates severe mitral obstruction.[7] Echocardiography is used to estimate the pulmonary artery pressure and assess right ventricular contractility. Cardiac catheterization can confirm echocardiographic pressure estimates and is sometimes used for this purpose in patients with MS. At catheterization, simultaneous left atrial and left ventricular pressures can be measured to determine if a gradient exists across the mitral valve. Pulmonary artery pressure can be measured directly, and pulmonary vascular resistance can be calculated.

Treatment. Diuretics to decrease pulmonary venous congestion are a mainstay of medical management, although care must be taken to avoid hypovolemia and further compromise of left ventricular output. Atrial arrhythmias secondary to left atrial hypertension and pulmonary infections must be managed appropriately. Indications for intervention include heart failure that is unresponsive to medical therapy (including poor weight gain in the infant) and/or significant pulmonary hypertension.[7] Patients with symmetrical chordal attachments and minimal mitral regurgitation are candidates for transcatheter balloon dilation of the mitral valve. This procedure is typically not curative but may reduce the mitral obstruction and left atrial hypertension such that symptoms of cardiac failure improve. Patients who have balloon dilation often undergo a surgical valve replacement later in life. Balloon valvuloplasty can lead to significant valve regurgitation. Failure of balloon dilatation or creation of severe mitral regurgitation is an indication for surgery.

Mitral valve replacement in infants and young children is fraught with challenges. Due to the small size of the mitral annulus in the pediatric age group, mechanical valve options are limited. The implanted mechanical valve also requires replacement as the child grows. Currently the standard of care is to use mechanical valves rather than tissue valves in the atrioventricular position because of their durability despite the requirement for anticoagulation with warfarin, which is necessary to prevent thromboembolic complications. Figure 8-10 shows a prosthetic St. Jude mechanical valve and a 3-dimensional echocardiographic image of a patient in whom such a valve was implanted. Depending on the valve pathology, repair may be possible, sparing the child valve replacement. In infants and small children, placement of an appropriate-sized valve in the supra-annular position may be required. Here, the prosthetic mitral valve is inserted within the left atrium above the mitral annulus where there is more room. Most of the above concerns apply to the older child as well, and mitral valve

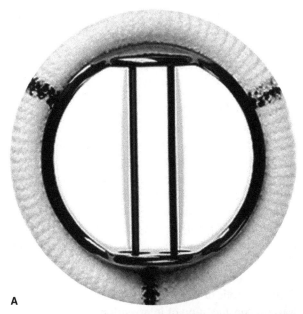

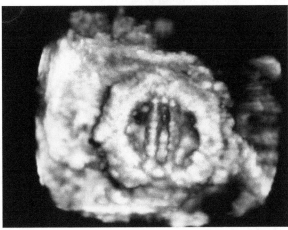

FIGURE 8-10 ■ **A.** Prosthetic St. Jude's Regent Mechanical Heart Valve is shown with the 2 metallic leaflets in the "open" position. (Acknowledgement: Regent is a trademark of St. Jude Medical, Inc. Reprinted with permission of St. Jude Medical, copyright 2011. All rights reserved.) **B.** Three-dimensional transesophageal echocardiogram images obtained in a 15-year-old female showing a 23-mm prosthetic St. Jude's valve that was placed in the mitral position. The image is frozen during diastole, when the metallic leaflets are in the "open" position.

replacement in a child should only be contemplated when repair is not a viable option. Mitral valve stenosis in the child seldom occurs in isolation, but usually is associated with other left-sided obstructive lesions, as in Shone complex (supravalvular mitral ring, parachute mitral valve, subaortic stenosis, and aortic coarctation). When surgical intervention is warranted for other associated left-sided lesions, a concomitant mitral valve repair or replacement should be considered.

Exercise guidelines for those with MS exist. Patients with mild stenosis and low pulmonary arterial pressures can participate in competitive sports. Those with higher degrees of obstruction or pulmonary arterial hypertension should be limited. It is important to recognize that valve function is likely to change over time, and therefore, exercise recommendations must be reassessed at each visit. Patients who are on systemic anticoagulation (eg, those with prosthetic mitral valve or recurrent atrial arrhythmias) should not engage in competitive sports that involve the risk of body contact and trauma.[4] Exercise guidelines for those with a prosthetic mitral valve are outlined in the mitral regurgitation section.

Mitral regurgitation

Definitions and epidemiology. Congenital mitral regurgitation (MR) is uncommon and occurs with primary valve abnormalities such as congenital mitral valve prolapse, a mitral arcade, or parachute mitral valve. In addition, MR is seen with cardiac inflammation, as in endocarditis, myocarditis, rheumatic fever, and collagen vascular diseases, or secondary to an infiltrative process such as metabolic diseases like Hurler disease. Ischemia from any cause can lead to mitral injury (ie, papillary muscle infarction) and resultant insufficiency. MR can result from annular dilatation, as in connective tissue diseases like Marfan and Ehlers-Danlos syndromes, or in the setting of a dilated cardiomyopathy, where there is incomplete leaflet coaptation.[8]

Pathogenesis. When the mitral valve works properly, coaptation of the leaflets effectively closes the valve inlet and prevents the "backflow" or regurgitation of blood from the left ventricle to the left atrium in systole. Primary or secondary abnormalities of the leaflets and/or annular dilation allow regurgitation of blood because the leaflets no longer coapt completely. MR decreases cardiac output because the blood that regurgitates from the ventricle to the atrium "steals" blood that should be flowing antegrade to the aorta. In acute, severe mitral insufficiency, left atrial pressure is increased, and the forward flow to the aorta is compromised with resultant pulmonary edema and low cardiac output. Conversely, in chronic or slowly progressive MR, the left atrium dilates to accommodate the additional blood, and left atrial and pulmonary hypertension can gradually develop. The left ventricle also accommodates to this increased volume by dilating. The compensatory mechanism of the left ventricle is initially to hypertrophy and increase systolic shortening to preserve cardiac output. Over time, however, the additional diastolic volume not only leads to left ventricular dilatation but eventually to left ventricular systolic failure.

Clinical presentation. Symptoms of MR result from left atrial hypertension and left ventricular diastolic and, eventually, systolic dysfunction. Quiet tachypnea (increased respiratory rate without other signs of respiratory compromise) is often an early sign. Infants and children may exhibit failure to thrive, diaphoresis with feeds, tachycardia, pallor, or decreased activity. As in MS, left atrial hypertension and pulmonary venous congestion can lead to wheezing and frequent pulmonary infections. Older children and adolescents may describe exercise intolerance.

On physical examination, patients with acute MR are usually tachypneic and tachycardic. If significant left ventricular dilatation is present, the apical impulse can be diffuse and displaced laterally. Typically, the first heart sound is blurred by a holosystolic, blowing murmur that is heard at the apex with radiation to the back (Figure 8-11). In severe MR, a diastolic murmur can be present due to the increased volume of blood flowing across the mitral valve during diastole.

Diagnostic tests. CXR can show left atrial enlargement, cardiomegaly, and pulmonary venous congestion in patients with long-standing regurgitation. ECG findings can be normal but also may include left atrial enlargement and left ventricular hypertrophy in the setting of chronic mitral insufficiency. Echocardiography is essential for visualizing the anatomy of the mitral valve and identifying the mechanism of the regurgitation. Color Doppler allows visualization of the regurgitant jets. Left atrial and ventricular sizes should be evaluated to help assess the burden of regurgitation. Precise determination of the regurgitant volume is difficult with echocardiography, but several factors are used to characterize the severity of leakage (ie, width and extent of the regurgitant jet, left atrial size). Cardiac MRI can quantify

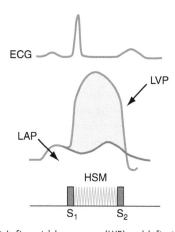

FIGURE 8-11 ■ Left ventricle pressure (LVP) and left atrium pressure (LAP) tracings shown with simultaneous electrocardiogram (ECG) and auscultatory characteristics in a patient with mitral regurgitation. The murmur is holosystolic (HSM) as it begins with the first heart sound (S_1) and terminates with the second heart sound. There is a pressure gradient between the left ventricle and left atrium throughout systole, and the regurgitant orifice allows blood to flow from ventricle to atrium. (*Reproduced, with permission, from Fauci AS, Kasper DL, Braunwald E, et al. Harrison's Principles of Internal Medicine. 17th ed. New York, NY: McGraw-Hill Companies; 2008.*)

the mitral valve regurgitant volume and left ventricular volume. Cardiac catheterization is uncommonly needed to assess MR but can be used when questions exist regarding left atrial and pulmonary arterial pressures, cardiac index, and pulmonary vascular resistance.

Treatment. Medical management of MR includes systemic afterload reduction to encourage forward rather than regurgitant flow. Diuretics are used to manage tachypnea and pulmonary edema. Infants and children with moderate to severe MR are treated with ACE inhibitors, although efficacy data in children are limited. Tachyarrhythmias can also occur due to left atrial and/ or left ventricular enlargement and must be aggressively treated. Indications for mitral valve intervention are not clearly established in children. Nonetheless, increasing left atrial or left ventricular size, decreasing left ventricular systolic function, and symptoms of heart failure warrant consideration of intervention.[8]

The only available intervention for MR in pediatric patients is surgery. Following the same surgical principles as for stenotic mitral valves, repair is favored over replacement. Repair techniques for regurgitant mitral valves are variable depending on the underlying mechanism of leakage. In all forms or repair for MR, care must be taken to not create valve stenosis. For durability purposes, if valve replacement is indicated, mechanical valves are preferred in the mitral position, and these patients require anticoagulation with warfarin.

Patients with mild to moderate MR that are in sinus rhythm with normal left ventricular size and systolic function and no evidence of elevated pulmonary artery pressures can engage in all competitive sports. Patients who have undergone mitral valve replacement with a bioprosthetic valve (not taking anticoagulation) who have normal valve function and normal left ventricular function can participate in moderate static and moderate dynamic sports. Those with a mechanical or bioprosthetic valve who are systemically anticoagulated should not participate in activities involving the risk of body contact or trauma.[4]

Mitral valve prolapse

Definitions and epidemiology. Mitral valve prolapse (MVP) is defined as the displacement of a portion of 1 or both of the mitral valve leaflets into the left atrium during systolic ventricular contraction. It occurs more often in women than in men, and the incidence increases with age; MVP is estimated to occur in 0.3% of people age 0 to 19 years and 2% of patients age 20 to 39 years. Patients with MVP have a histologically abnormal mitral valve that is often described as "floppy." The normal collagenous fibrosa is replaced by myomatous mucopolysaccharide. As a result, the leaflets are thickened and redundant, and the chordae are elongated and prone to rupture. MVP can occur in isolation or can occur in association with syndromes, especially connective tissue disorders such as Marfan syndrome, Ehlers Danlos syndrome, polycystic kidney disease, and pseudoxanthoma elasticum.[9]

Pathogenesis. Leaflet prolapse can cause regurgitation because the valve orifice is not completely sealed during systole. Sometimes, chordal rupture occurs, causing a flail leaflet and severe mitral leakage. The physiology of this regurgitation is discussed in the previous section on MR.

Clinical presentation. Most children and adolescents with MVP have minimal regurgitation. Many are asymptomatic and referred for evaluation of a murmur. Even in the absence of valvar regurgitation, some patients do have symptoms during childhood. Patients may complain of palpitations that may be due to premature atrial or ventricular contractions or supraventricular or ventricular tachycardia. Sudden death in the absence of significant MR is very rare.

The physical examination is characteristic in patients with MVP. The first and second heart sounds are normal. In cases of significant prolapse, a midsystolic click is heard that is often high pitched and corresponds to the prolapsing leaflet. If MR is present, the click will be accompanied by a systolic regurgitant murmur. Maneuvers that limit left ventricular volume, such as standing (decreased preload), will cause the click and murmur to occur earlier in systole (leaflets prolapse earlier). Conversely, maneuvers that increase ventricular volume such as squatting cause the click and murmur to occur later in systole.

Diagnostic tests. ECG and CXR are typically normal. Echocardiography is used to diagnose MVP and to characterize the degree of MR (Figure 8-12). Catheterization is uncommonly used. MRI is often not needed but can quantify the amount of MR if needed.

Treatment. Serial follow-up is recommended. The indications for surgery are based on the degree of MR and are described in the preceding section. Patients with MVP should be screened for underlying connective tissue disorders if clinically indicated.

Exercise guidelines for patients with MVP exist. Patients can participate in all competitive sports if they do not have any of the following: a history of prior syncope, a history of repetitive supraventricular or ventricular tachycardia, severe MR, left ventricular ejection fraction less than 50%, a prior embolic event, or a family history of MVP-related sudden death.[10]

Rheumatic heart disease

Rheumatic fever and its cardiac sequelae are a major cause of mitral and aortic valve disease worldwide.

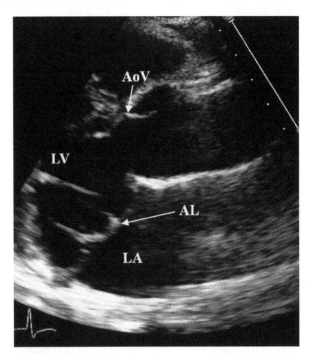

FIGURE 8-12 ■ Echocardiogram showing parasternal long axis view in an adolescent with Marfan syndrome and prolapse of the anterior mitral valve leaflet into the left atrium during ventricular systole. AL, anterior leaflet of the mitral valve; AoV, aortic valve; LA, left atrium; LV, left ventricle.

Carditis occurs in 30% to 70% of cases of acute rheumatic fever and is the most common cause of acquired heart disease in children and adolescents worldwide. Specifically, valvulitis leads to MR in nearly 95% and AR in 25% of patients with acute rheumatic carditis. If present, these hemodynamic lesions can progress with age. MS and AS are typically not associated with acute carditis but, instead, represent forms of chronic rheumatic heart disease, occurring 20 to 40 years after acute rheumatic fever.[11] Rheumatic heart disease is extensively discussed in Chapter 14.

Tricuspid Valve

Whereas the mitral valve has 2 leaflets, the tricuspid valve has 3 leaflets. The anterior leaflet acts to separate inflow from outflow portions of the right ventricle, the posterior leaflet lies against the inferior wall of the ventricle, and the septal leaflet lies against the ventricular septum. The tricuspid valve subapparatus consists of chordae tendineae and 3 papillary muscles. Like the mitral valve, the subvalvar apparatus prevents leaflet prolapse into the atria and aids in leaflet coaptation.

Tricuspid stenosis

Isolated congenital tricuspid stenosis is very rare and is more commonly associated with right ventricular hypoplasia (hypoplastic right heart variants) or right ventricular outflow tract obstruction. The pathophysiology and clinical manifestations of congenital tricuspid stenosis are the same as tricuspid atresia; tricuspid stenosis might even be a mild form of tricuspid atresia. Tricuspid atresia is discussed in Chapter 5.

Ebstein anomaly

Definitions and epidemiology. Ebstein anomaly is a rare congenital malformation of the tricuspid valve originally described in 1866 by Wilhelm Ebstein that accounts for less than 1% all congenital heart disease. The septal and posterior leaflets of the tricuspid valve are tethered and adherent to the right ventricle myocardium due to a failure of complete delamination during development. The anterior leaflet is not displaced but is often redundant or "sail-like." As a result, the *functional* valve annulus is displaced downward (toward the right ventricular apex). This creates a portion of right ventricle that is above the *functional* annulus but below the *true* annulus and is referred to as "atrialized right ventricle." The wall of the atrialized right ventricle is often thin and functionally integrated with the right atrium, thereby reducing the size of the *functional* right ventricle.[12]

The degree of valve deformity in Ebstein anomaly varies significantly. In some patients, there is mild tethering of the septal and posterior leaflets to the right ventricle and minimal apical displacement of the functional annulus. These patients may be asymptomatic and survive into adulthood without symptoms. However, in others, the septal and posterior leaflets are rudimentary and there is severe displacement of functional annulus, resulting in severe tricuspid insufficiency and a reduced size of the functional right ventricle.

The displacement of the septal leaflet predisposes patients to the formation of accessory connections between the atria and ventricles. Thus, ventricular preexcitation can occur, and many patients with Ebstein anomaly have Wolff-Parkinson-White syndrome. Atrial fibrillation, atrial flutter, and ventricular arrhythmias can also occur. Many patients with Ebstein anomaly have a patent foramen ovale.

Pathogenesis. The adherence of the septal and posterior valve leaflets causes abnormal tricuspid valve coaptation and, thus, tricuspid regurgitation during ventricular systole. The redundant anterior leaflet can prolapse into the atrium during systole and contribute to regurgitation. Valve regurgitation leads to right atrial enlargement including dilatation of the atrialized portion of the right ventricle. In addition, the atrialized right ventricle can impede ventricular filling. During atrial contraction, blood flows from the atrium into the atrialized ventricle. However, during ventricular systole, the atrialized ventricle contracts and propels blood back into the true right atrium.

Patients with mild forms of Ebstein anomaly may have very little tricuspid regurgitation. More severe forms are associated with significant tricuspid insufficiency and right atrial enlargement. The regurgitant volume may cause progressive dilatation of the true right ventricle. Right ventricular systolic failure with associated symptoms can occur. In some cases, left ventricular mechanics can be abnormally affected because the ventricular septum bulges leftward and impinges on the left ventricle and its outflow tract. Cyanosis can occur due to right-to-left shunting at atrial level. Abnormal right ventricular compliance, tricuspid regurgitation, and right ventricular inflow obstruction due to contraction of the atrialized right ventricle all contribute to elevation in right atrial pressure and right-to-left atrial shunting.

Clinical presentation. Newborns with severe Ebstein anomaly exhibit cyanosis due to right-to-left atrial shunting and limited antegrade pulmonary blood flow. In the setting of severe tricuspid insufficiency and increased pulmonary vascular resistance, the right ventricle may be unable to generate enough pressure to open the pulmonary valve. These patients have "functional" pulmonary atresia and may be ductal dependent for pulmonary blood flow. As the pulmonary vascular resistance decreases, antegrade flow from the right ventricle can occur, and right-to-left atrial shunting and cyanosis may decrease.

Other patients may present in childhood or adolescence with symptoms from tricuspid regurgitation and right ventricular failure including exercise intolerance, dyspnea on exertion, fatigue, and cyanosis. Patients with mild Ebstein anomaly may not present until adulthood, and the defect has even been diagnosed at autopsy. Arrhythmias may be the presenting symptom at any age, although it is a common presentation in adolescence.

The physical examination in patients with Ebstein anomaly depends on the lesion's severity. Neonates with severe disease and functional pulmonary atresia will exhibit cyanosis and a single second heart sound. In any patient with significant tricuspid regurgitation, a holosystolic murmur is heard at the left lower sternal border. Because the regurgitation increases right ventricular volume, a systolic ejection murmur (crescendo–decrescendo) can be present at the left upper sternal border representing increased flow across the pulmonary valve. The second heart sound typically is normal.[13]

Diagnosis. The ECG is typically abnormal in patients with Ebstein anomaly. Right atrial enlargement may be present and is suggested by tall, peaked P waves in lead II. Right ventricular hypertrophy may also be observed. One should look for a pre-excitation pattern

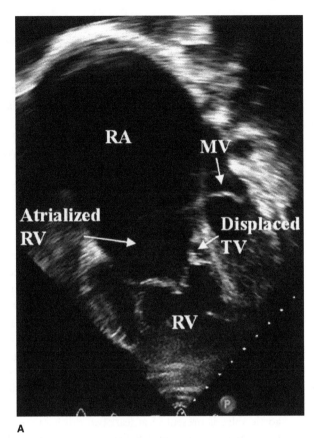

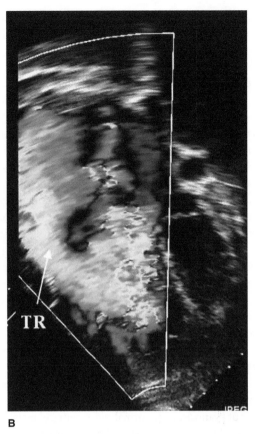

FIGURE 8-13 ■ **A.** Echocardiogram showing an apical 4-chamber view in a 15-year-old with severe Ebstein anomaly of the tricuspid valve. The functional annulus of the tricuspid valve is severely displaced toward the right ventricular apex creating a significant amount of atrialized right ventricle. The right atrium is severely enlarged. **B.** Echocardiogram in the same patient showing an apical 4-chamber view with color Doppler over the tricuspid valve and severe tricuspid regurgitation. MV, mitral valve; RA, right atrium; RV, right ventricle; TR, tricuspid regurgitation; TV, tricuspid valve.

(delta wave), which is present in a significant number of patients. Severe cardiomegaly is a pathognomonic finding in neonates with severe disease. Echocardiography is crucial in making the diagnosis of Ebstein anomaly (Figure 8-13). The structure of the tricuspid valve, right atrium, and right ventricle and the degree of tricuspid regurgitation can be characterized. In neonates with severely abnormal physiology, it is important to determine whether there is antegrade blood flow across the pulmonary valve. Catheterization is rarely indicated.

Treatment. Neonates with severe Ebstein anomaly, minimal or no antegrade blood flow across the pulmonary valve, and ductal-dependent pulmonary blood flow are stabilized with prostaglandins. As pulmonary vascular resistance drops, antegrade flow across the pulmonary valve increases such that pulmonary blood flow is no longer ductal dependent. Inhaled nitric oxide has been used in some neonates to assist in decreasing the pulmonary vascular resistance. If oxygen saturations improve, then intervention (ie, a modified Blalock-Taussig shunt or ductal stenting) can be deferred. Patients who survive infancy without an operation can do well

for several years and repair is deferred until symptoms arise or cyanosis occurs.[14]

Older patients with significant tricuspid regurgitation and signs of right ventricular failure can be managed with diuretics. ACE inhibitors have unproven benefit in patients with tricuspid regurgitation.[12] Observation and medical management are recommended for asymptomatic patients with no cyanosis and minimal cardiomegaly. Indications for surgery are significant exercise intolerance and/or cyanosis. Also, surgery should be considered in asymptomatic patients if right ventricular size is progressively increasing, systolic function is decreasing, or significant tachyarrhythmia occurs.[12]

Ebstein anomaly has long been a surgical challenge. Several surgical techniques and modifications have been used over the years. Most include some combination of a tricuspid valve repair or replacement, closure of the atrial septal defect, plication of the atrialized portion of the right ventricle, reduction atrioplasty of the right atrium, and an antiarrhythmia procedure.[12] A more recent procedure that has shown significant promise is the cone reconstruction; this procedure mobilizes the anterior and posterior tricuspid valve leaflets from their aberrant ventricular attachments. A cone is then created from the valve apparatus as the free edge of the mobilized leaflets are rotated in a clockwise fashion and sutured to the septal leaflet and septal border of the anterior leaflet.[14]

Other surgical approaches include a bidirectional superior cavopulmonary anastomosis that results in a decrease in the volume overload on the right ventricle in patients with poor right ventricular function. Alternatively, the Starnes procedure may be used as the first stage in a single-ventricle approach. This procedure consists of closing the tricuspid valve orifice with a fenestrated patch (limiting tricuspid regurgitation but enabling right ventricular decompression via controlled tricuspid regurgitation through the fenestration), excising the atrial septum, plicating the atrialized portion of the right ventricle, and creating a systemic-to-pulmonary artery shunt. The patient is then staged down a single ventricle pathway, with subsequent bidirectional superior cavopulmonary anastomosis and eventually Fontan palliation. Finally, heart transplantation remains an option for patients with severe biventricular dysfunction.

Exercise guidelines for patients with Ebstein anomaly do exist. Those with mild Ebstein anomaly without cyanosis, with normal right ventricular size, and with no history of tachyarrhythmias can participate in all sports.[2]

Tricuspid regurgitation

Congenital tricuspid insufficiency that is not caused by Ebstein anomaly of the tricuspid valve is very rare. It is caused by a dysplastic valve with thickened leaflets and short chordae. The papillary muscles may be hypoplastic. Unlike Ebstein anomaly, the valve leaflets and functional annulus are not displaced, and there is no atrialized right ventricle. The pathophysiology, clinical presentation, and diagnosis of isolated tricuspid insufficiency are similar to those described earlier for Ebstein anomaly and depend largely on the degree of regurgitation.

Surgical options for addressing tricuspid valve regurgitation are similar to those discussed previously for MR and generally include repair or replacement. As in the mitral position, repair is favored over replacement. If required, replacement is usually well tolerated due to the associated annular dilatation allowing a reasonable-sized valve to be placed in the annular position.

VASCULATURE

The normal thoracic aorta can be divided into the ascending aorta, transverse aortic arch, aortic isthmus, and proximal descending aorta. Typically, the transverse aortic arch courses over the left mainstem bronchus, defining it as a left aortic arch. The normal aorta first gives rise to the innominate artery, next the left common carotid artery, and finally the left subclavian artery. The innominate artery subsequently divides into the right subclavian and right common carotid arteries. In a normal aortic arch, the aortic isthmus is the region distal to the left subclavian but proximal to the entrance of the PDA in the proximal descending aorta. A right aortic arch is present if the aorta courses over the right mainstem bronchus.

Aortic Coarctation

Definitions and epidemiology

Most commonly, aortic coarctation is a discrete narrowing of the proximal thoracic aorta in the area of ductus arteriosus insertion (juxtaductal). Occasionally, instead of discrete narrowing, long segment hypoplasia of the proximal thoracic aorta may be present that may or may not be accompanied by hypoplasia of the transverse aortic arch. Coarctation represents 5% to 8% of congenital heart defects and is slightly more common in males. Coarctation frequently accompanies other left-sided obstructive lesions including MS and AS. A bicuspid aortic valve is present in at least two thirds of patients with aortic coarctation.[15] Patients who present within the first year of life are more likely to have associated intracardiac anomalies. Aortic coarctation is the most common cardiac lesion in Turner syndrome, in which roughly 35% of patients have the anomaly. In addition, up to 10% of patients with coarctation will have intracranial aneurysms that typically are located in the circle of Willis.[16]

Pathologically, discrete coarctation is caused by a prominent infolding in the aortic wall opposite to the entrance of the ductus arteriosus (posterior shelf). Histologically, this area has thickened media and intima. Some hypothesize that coarctation develops due to any disturbance that decreases blood flow from the left ventricle through the fetal aortic arch, with isthmus hypoplasia postulated to be secondary to decreased antegrade flow around the arch. Others hypothesize that coarctation develops because ductal tissue migrates into the juxtaductal aorta and constricts postnatally.[16]

Pathogenesis

Coarctation increases afterload on the left ventricle as the ventricle overcomes the obstruction in the proximal thoracic aorta. A pressure gradient will exist across the narrowed segment that, depending on cardiac output and collaterals, will increase with degree of obstruction. The blood pressure in the upper extremities will be elevated because these vessels originate from the arch proximal to the coarctation. However, hypertension can persist after repair, likely because patients have abnormal vascular reactivity, arterial compliance, and baroreceptor function.

In the immediate postnatal period, significant coarctation can be masked by a PDA. If coarctation is severe, lower extremity blood flow can occur via right-to-left shunting at the ductus arteriosus (critical or ductal-dependent coarctation). In others, the ductal ampulla (area of insertion of ductus into aorta) will decrease in size after the ductus closes, revealing the presence of a juxtaductal coarctation. In neonates with severe coarctation, the increased afterload can lead to left ventricular systolic dysfunction and cardiac failure. As left ventricular ejection diminishes, left atrial pressure increases, leading to pulmonary edema. In patients with less severe coarctation, left ventricular systolic dysfunction will not occur in the neonatal period. Instead, the patient will develop left ventricular hypertrophy over time to accommodate the increased afterload. After years, left ventricular systolic dysfunction may occur. In those with long-standing coarctation, intercostal collateral arteries dilate and carry blood to the aorta beyond the narrowing.

Clinical presentation

The presentation of aortic coarctation depends on age. In infants with critical coarctation and a wide open ductus arteriosus, blood pressures will be equal, although lower extremity pulse oximetry will be decreased compared to the upper extremity secondary to right-to-left flow at PDA. If not recognized while the ductus arteriosus is still patent, these infants will present with congestive heart failure and shock when the ductus arteriosus closes. On physical examination, the infant will appear ill with pallor, tachycardia, tachypnea, and hepatomegaly. Lower extremity pulses will be diminished and delayed compared to upper extremity pulses. When comparing upper and lower extremity pulses, it is best to compare the right arm pulse with either leg. The left subclavian artery originates immediately proximal to the coarctation, and its orifice may be stenotic, thus confusing blood pressure comparisons. Systolic blood pressure in the right arm can be compared to that in either leg to estimate the pressure gradient across the coarctation. Rarely, an aberrant right subclavian artery will arise distal to the coarctation, so all measurable blood pressures and pulses will be distal to the coarctation. Auscultation may reveal a harsh systolic ejection murmur due to turbulence across the coarctation. This murmur is typically appreciated at the left upper sternal border and between the scapulae in the patient's back.

Children and adolescents typically present with asymptomatic, upper extremity hypertension or with an isolated cardiac murmur. Physical examination can reveal elevated blood pressure in the right arm. As in infants, right arm systolic blood pressure should be compared to systolic blood pressure in either leg to estimate the pressure gradient across the lesion. (In normal patients, blood pressure in the leg is roughly 10 mmHg higher than the arm.) Lower extremity pulses will be diminished in amplitude. If there is significant collateral flow to the descending aorta via intercostals arteries; however, then a delay in the upstroke of the lower extremity pulses will not be present. Similar to infants, auscultation can reveal a systolic ejection murmur. If significant arterial collateral flow is present, a continuous murmur may be present throughout the chest anteriorly and posteriorly. If associated intracardiac anomalies are present such as a bicuspid aortic valve, then examination will reflect these defects. Females with Turner syndrome can have short stature, widely spaced nipples, and a webbed neck.

Diagnosis

ECG may be normal but often shows left ventricular hypertrophy in children and adolescents. CXR can show cardiomegaly and pulmonary edema in infants who present with heart failure. In children or adolescents, mild cardiomegaly may be present, and rib notching may be seen below the level of coarctation due to erosion of inferior surfaces of ribs by dilated intercostals arteries. Rib notching is uncommon in children less than 5 years of age. The aortic arch contour is abnormal and the "3 sign" can be present on frontal chest radiogram due to indentation at the coarctation site. Echocardiography is important for demonstrating the aortic abnormality, determining if transverse arch hypoplasia or long segment coarctation is present and evaluating for other associated heart defects. Doppler is used to estimate the pressure gradient across the coarctation. In neonates, the echocardiogram can image ductal patency and the direction of blood flow across the duct. Echocardiography is often sufficient to delineate aortic coarctation, but MRI can be used to illustrate the level of coarctation (Figure 8-14), especially in older patients with difficult echocardiographic windows. Cardiac catheterization can be diagnostic and therapeutic (see next section). The pressure gradient across the area of narrowing can be measured, and angiography definitively shows the vascular abnormality. In the setting of normal cardiac output, a peak-to-peak systolic pressure gradient of greater than 20 mm Hg at catheterization is considered hemodynamically significant.[16] Unless transcatheter intervention is being considered, cardiac catheterization is often not needed.

Treatment

Intervention is indicated for virtually all patients with coarctation, and the timing of repair or transcatheter therapy depends on the patient's presentation. Infants who present with shock or congestive heart failure

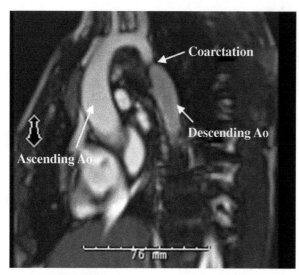

FIGURE 8-14 ■ Lateral view from cardiac magnetic resonance imaging in a 6-year-old male with upper extremity hypertension who was found to have coarctation of the aorta (Ao).

require aggressive treatment and near-immediate intervention. In addition, neonates may present with hepatic, renal, and/or intestinal compromise. A prostaglandin infusion should also be started immediately in neonates; if the duct opens, right-to-left flow can improve perfusion distal to the coarctation. Medical resuscitation also includes the use of diuretics and inotropes.

The preferred surgical technique for repair of discrete aortic coarctation in infants and young children remains resection with extended end-to-end anastomosis. In this technique, the aorta is mobilized from pleural and fascial attachments to enable aortic clamps to be placed proximal to the origin of the left common carotid artery and postductally on the descending aorta. The ductus is ligated and divided, with the coarctation segment resected. The incision is commonly extended on the inner curvature of the aortic arch and the outer curvature of the descending aorta to create the "extended end-to-end" anastomosis. The procedure is performed through a left posterolateral thoracotomy. However, aortic coarctation associated with severe arch hypoplasia requiring arch augmentation is done through a median sternotomy incision.

In children and adolescents who present with upper extremity hypertension or with a murmur, surgical repair is a commonly used treatment. In patients who are asymptomatic without severe upper extremity hypertension, the repair is elective.

Transcatheter strategies to treat aortic coarctation also exist. Balloon angioplasty is widely used to treat recurrent coarctation following surgical repair but is less often used to treat native coarctation due to concerns about recurrent narrowing and aneurysm formation. Balloon expandable stents can also be used to treat native or recurrent coarctation. Stent use is uncommon in

small children because it requires a large arterial sheath and the stent will not "grow," with the child necessitating repeat intervention over time. Typically, stent placement is reserved for adolescents and adults.[16]

Patients with treated coarctation may participate in aerobic sports several months after surgical or transcatheter intervention if a less than 20-mm Hg blood pressure gradient exists between the right arm and leg and if a normal peak systolic blood pressure exists at rest and with exercise.[2]

Interrupted Aortic Arch

Definitions and epidemiology

Interrupted aortic arch (IAA) is a complete interruption of the aorta that most commonly occurs between the left common carotid and left subclavian arteries (type B). Less often, the interruption will occur distal to the left subclavian artery (type A). Interruption between the 2 common carotid arteries (type C) is extremely rare (Figure 8-15). Many patients with IAA will have 22q11 microdeletion. Left-sided obstructive lesions are commonly associated with IAA, including bicuspid aortic valve, posterior malalignment VSD, and subaortic membrane.[17]

Pathogenesis

In patients with IAA, right-to-left shunting across the PDA supplies the aorta distal to the level of interruption. After birth, lower extremity perfusion persists as long as the ductus arteriosus is patent and the pulmonary vascular resistance is high. Once ductal closure occurs, the vascular supply distal to the interruption becomes ischemic.[17]

Clinical presentation

Infants without prenatal diagnosis will present in the first week of life with shock and congestive heart failure as the ductus arteriosus closes. In type B interruption, the lower body and left subclavian artery will be underperfused. Thus, pulses in the left arm and both legs will be markedly diminished compared to the right arm. In type A interruption, lower extremity perfusion will be compromised, similar to aortic coarctation. At presentation, infants will have significant metabolic acidosis and anuria. Prior to ductal closure, differential cyanosis will be present, as vascular territories distal to the interruption will be desaturated compared to the right arm. Much less commonly, the ductus arteriosus will remain patent during the neonatal period; as pulmonary vascular resistance falls, the ductus arteriosus will shunt less right to left, and such infants will present with heart failure and failure to thrive.[17]

Diagnosis

The ECG is commonly normal in neonates with IAA. The echocardiogram is the diagnostic test of choice. The

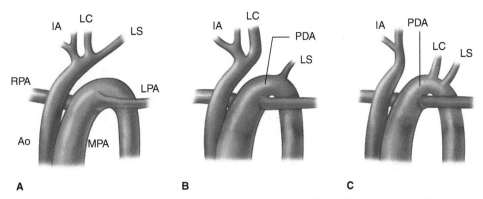

FIGURE 8-15 ■ Graphic images showing the anatomic types of interrupted aortic arch. **A.** The interruption is distal to the left subclavian artery. **B.** The interruption occurs between the left subclavian and left carotid arteries. **C.** The interruption occurs between the left carotid and innominate arteries. Ao, aorta; IA, innominate artery; LC, left carotid artery; LPA, left pulmonary artery; LS, left subclavian artery; MPA, main pulmonary artery; PDA, patent ductus arteriosus; RPA, right pulmonary artery. (*Reproduced, with permission, from Jonas RA. Interrupted aortic arch. In: Mavroudis C, Backer CL, eds.* Pediatric Cardiac Surgery. *2nd ed. St. Louis, MO: Mosby; 1994:184. Copyright Elsevier.*)

level of interruption and patency of the ductus arteriosus are determined, as well as associated intracardiac anomalies. Further aortic arch imaging may be necessary and computed tomography angiography or MRI can be used.

Treatment

Infants with IAA require a prostaglandin infusion to maintain ductal patency to maintain systemic blood flow distal to the interruption. All infants with IAA require surgical repair. Repair should follow after complete resuscitation has taken place. The preferred surgery is a single-stage neonatal repair. Arch repair can usually be accomplished with direct anastomosis, although patch aortoplasty can occasionally be required. Because many cases also have large VSDs, these are repaired simultaneously.

Vascular Rings

Definitions and epidemiology

A vascular ring is an anomaly of the aortic arch in which both the trachea and esophagus are surrounded by vascular structures. Importantly, all of the structures do not have to be patent; an atretic segment of a double aortic arch or the ligamentum arteriosum can complete a vascular ring. Multiple aortic arch anomalies are called vascular rings, but the 2 most common malformations that create a ring are discussed here—double aortic arch and right aortic arch with aberrant left subclavian artery.[18]

A double aortic arch consists of 2 arches, an anterior and leftward arch and a posterior and rightward arch (Figure 8-16). Both branch from the ascending aorta and then reconnect to constitute a single descending aorta. Typically, the right arch is dominant and gives rise to the right common carotid and right subclavian

arteries. The left arch is smaller and gives rise to the left common carotid and left subclavian arteries. Often the left arch is atretic distal to the left subclavian artery; only a fibrous cord attaches to the descending aorta. Double aortic arch is rarely associated with intracardiac abnormalities.[18]

A right aortic arch with aberrant left subclavian artery and left ligamentum arteriosum is the second most common form of a vascular ring. In this anomaly, a right arch is present and the arch branches emerge in the following order: left common carotid, right common carotid, right subclavian, and, finally, left subclavian. The left subclavian artery courses behind the esophagus and gives rise to the ligamentum arteriosum, which courses anteriorly to connect to the left pulmonary artery with completion of the ring. Even though the ligamentum is

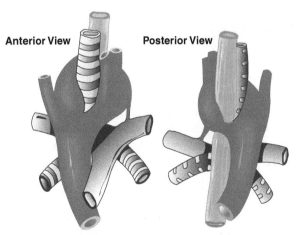

FIGURE 8-16 ■ Graphic representation of a double aortic arch forming a vascular ring around the trachea and esophagus. (*Adapted, with permission, from Doherty GM.* Current Diagnosis & Treatment: Surgery. *13th ed. New York, NY: McGraw-Hill; 2010.*)

not patent, a dimple or diverticulum (diverticulum of Kommerell) in the proximal left subclavian artery can be appreciated, indicating that the ligamentum arises from that vessel.

Pathogenesis

Because rings encircle the trachea and esophagus, both experience intermittent obstruction. However, the presence of a ring does not always mean that obstruction will occur. Some patients with a "loose ring" may never experience obstruction of the trachea and esophagus and remain asymptomatic throughout their lifetime.

Clinical presentation

Patients typically present in the first few years of life with stridor or "noisy breathing" that worsens with upper respiratory infections. These patients also may vomit solid foods. Toddlers or older children may present with dysphagia or choking with feeding, but these patients will often have a history of recurrent pulmonary infections. Rarely, adolescents and even adults who carry a diagnosis of asthma for years may ultimately be diagnosed with a ring. Importantly, some patients with a vascular ring never develop symptoms.

Diagnosis

Various tests can contribute to the diagnosis of a vascular ring. A CXR may suggest a right aortic arch and prompt consideration of a ring in a patient with respiratory symptoms. Barium swallow may show posterior indentation of the esophagus; a vascular ring should strongly be considered if this finding is present. Echocardiography can outline aortic arch anatomy but cannot visualize atretic vascular segments. However, the contours of the arch and its vessels can strongly suggest a double aortic arch or right aortic arch with aberrant left subclavian artery. MRI is particularly helpful in diagnosing vascular rings, as the aortic arch anatomy can be outlined and the trachea well visualized. The level and degree of tracheal obstruction can be described using MRI. Like echocardiography, MRI cannot visualize atretic vascular segments, but suspicion for an atretic arch or ligamentum arteriosum can be raised based on the contours of the arch and its branches as well as compression of the trachea. MRI often requires sedation in small children. Bronchoscopy is not routinely used but can show external tracheal compression from the ring.

Treatment

The presence of symptoms is an indication for surgical division of a vascular ring. In some patients with mild or vague symptoms, the decision to intervene can be challenging. For a double aortic arch, surgery involves division of the nondominant arch with the ends oversewn

or ligated. In the vast majority of cases, this will be the left aortic arch, and the approach will be through the left chest. Preoperative confirmation of arch dominance is therefore essential for proper surgical planning. For the vascular ring due to a right aortic arch with aberrant left subclavian artery and left ligamentum arteriosum, relief of the ring is simply by division of the ligamentum through the left chest.

Peripheral Pulmonary Stenosis

Definitions and epidemiology

Stenosis of the pulmonary arteries can affect the main pulmonary artery or either of its branches. Peripheral PS can occur in isolation or can be associated with other congenital cardiac defects such as tetralogy of Fallot. It is also often associated with congenital syndromes including congenital rubella, Williams syndrome, Noonan syndrome, and Alagille syndrome. In neonates, mild physiologic peripheral PS due to the small size of the branch pulmonary arteries after birth can create a systolic ejection murmur. This murmur does not represent significant pathology because it typically disappears by 6 to 12 months of age with arterial growth. If the murmur persists, then pathologic peripheral PS should be considered.[5]

Pathogenesis

Pathologic peripheral PS increases the afterload on the right ventricle. In cases of main pulmonary artery or bilateral branch pulmonary artery stenosis, right ventricular systolic pressure will be elevated to overcome the obstruction. Right ventricular hypertrophy will ensue, and right ventricular systolic failure can rarely result. If unilateral branch pulmonary artery stenosis is present, then right ventricular pressure will be normal because the unobstructed arterial tree can accommodate the increased flow without increasing pressure. However, over time, the increased flow to the unobstructed arterial tree may lead to pulmonary vascular disease.

Clinical presentation

Patients with unilateral stenosis or with mild to moderate bilateral pulmonary artery stenosis are typically asymptomatic. Severe obstruction can lead to symptoms of right ventricular failure including dyspnea on exertion and exercise intolerance. On physical examination, the first heart sound is normal and the second heart sound usually is normally split with increased intensity. A systolic ejection murmur (crescendo–decrescendo) may be present at the left upper sternal border that radiates to the axilla (both axilla if bilateral obstruction is present) and back.

Diagnosis

ECG is typically normal but may suggest right ventricular hypertrophy if severe obstruction is present. CXR commonly is normal. Echocardiography will delineate the anatomy of the main pulmonary artery and proximal left and right pulmonary arteries. Doppler can be used to localize and quantify the degree of obstruction. Likewise, echocardiography can estimate right ventricular pressure and can describe right ventricular size, function, and hypertrophy. Cardiac catheterization can be used to confirm concerning echocardiographic findings. The pressure gradient across the stenosis can be measured, right ventricular pressure can be measured, and angiography can determine the location and extent of stenosis. Likewise, catheterization can characterize distal stenoses that are poorly seen by echocardiogram. MRI can also be used to evaluate the pulmonary vascular tree.

Treatment

Patients with mild to moderate pulmonary arterial branch obstruction can typically be followed expectantly. Patients with significant obstruction, however, do require intervention. Transcatheter balloon angioplasty is a widely accepted therapy for peripheral PS. Complications include arterial rupture, aneurysm formation, and obstruction of small branch vessels. Balloon dilation is ineffective in many patients, and recurrent stenosis is common. As a result, balloon expandable stent placement has emerged as a therapy for some patients.[19] If transcatheter interventions fail, surgery may be needed. This involves proximal patch arterioplasty to augment the narrowed proximal branch pulmonary arteries in the hilum. For more distal vessel involvement, the application of intraoperative catheter-based techniques can be a useful adjunct.

Clinical Pearls

- Chest pain or syncope with exercise in a patient with AS should prompt immediate evaluation.
- Patients with AI and dilated aortic root should be evaluated for connective tissue disorder.
- An enlarged heart on CXR in a neonate with cyanosis likely represents Ebstein anomaly.
- Decreased lower extremity oxygen saturation can help identify a neonate with significant coarctation and right-to-left flow across the PDA.
- Neonates with Type B IAA (most common type) with a closing ductus arteriosus will have decreased left upper extremity and lower extremity pulses compared to the right upper extremity.

REFERENCES

1. Schneider DJ, Moore J. Aortic stenosis. In: Allen HD, Driscoll DJ, Shaddy RE, Feltes TF, eds. *Moss and Adams' Heart Disease in Infants, Children, and Adolescents: Including the Fetus and Young Adult.* 7th ed. Philadelphia, PA: Lippincott Williams & Wilkins; 2008:968-987.
2. Graham TP Jr, Driscoll DJ, Gersony WM, Newburger JW, Rocchini A, Towbin JA. Task Force 2: congenital heart disease. *J Am Coll Cardiol.* 2005;45:1326-1333.
3. Jonas R. Valve surgery. In: Jonas R, ed. *Comprehensive Surgical Management of Congenital Heart Disease.* London, United Kingdom: Hodder Arnold; 2004:301-319.
4. Bonow RO, Cheitlin MD, Crawford MH, Douglas PS. Task Force 3: valvular heart disease. *J Am Coll Cardiol.* 2005;45:1334-1340.
5. Prieto LR, Latson L. Pulmonary stenosis. In: Allen HD, Driscoll DJ, Shaddy RE, Feltes TF, eds. *Moss and Adams' Heart Disease in Infants, Children, and Adolescents: Including the Fetus and Young Adult.* 7th ed. Philadelphia, PA: Lippincott Williams & Wilkins; 2008:835-858.
6. Bruce CJ, Connolly HM. Right-sided valve disease deserves a little more respect. *Circulation.* 2009;119:2726-2734.
7. Baylen BG, Atkinson D. Mitral inflow obstruction. In: Allen HD, Driscoll DJ, Shaddy RE, Feltes TF, eds. *Moss and Adams' Heart Disease in Infants, Children, and Adolescents: Including the Fetus and Young Adult.* 7th ed. Philadelphia, PA: Lippincott Williams & Wilkins; 2008:922-936.
8. Baylen BG, Atkinson D. Congenital mitral insufficiency. In: Allen HD, Driscoll DJ, Shaddy RE, Feltes TF, eds. *Moss and Adams' Heart Disease in Infants, Children, and Adolescents: Including the Fetus and Young Adult.* 7th ed. Philadelphia, PA: Lippincott Williams & Wilkins; 2008:937-945.
9. Boudoulas H, Sparks E, Wooley, CF. The floppy mitral valve, mitral valve prolapse, and mitral valvular regurgitation. In: Allen HD, Driscoll DJ, Shaddy RE, Feltes TF, eds. *Moss and Adams' Heart Disease in Infants, Children, and Adolescents: Including the Fetus and Young Adult.* 7th ed. Philadelphia, PA: Lippincott Williams & Wilkins; 2008:946-967.
10. Maron BJ, Ackerman MJ, Nishimura RA, Pyeritz RE, Towbin JA, Udelson JE. Task Force 4: HCM and other cardiomyopathies, mitral valve prolapse, myocarditis, and Marfan syndrome. *J Am Coll Cardiol.* 2005;45:1340-1345.
11. Tani L. Rheumatic fever and rheumatic heart disease. In: Allen HD, Driscoll DJ, Shaddy RE, Feltes TF, eds. *Moss and Adams' Heart Disease in Infants, Children, and Adolescents: Including the Fetus and Young Adult.* 7th ed. Philadelphia, PA: Lippincott Williams & Wilkins; 2008:1256-1280.
12. Attenhofer Jost CH, Connolly HM, Dearani JA, Edwards WD, Danielson GK. Ebstein's anomaly. *Circulation.* 2007;115:277-285.
13. Epstein M. Tricuspid atresia, stenosis, and regurgitation. In: Allen HD, Driscoll DJ, Shaddy RE, Feltes TF, eds. *Moss and Adams' Heart Disease in Infants, Children, and Adolescents: Including the Fetus and Young Adult.* 7th ed. Philadelphia, PA: Lippincott Williams & Wilkins; 2008:817-834.
14. da Silva JP, Baumgratz JF, da Fonseca L, et al. The cone reconstruction of the tricuspid valve in Ebstein's anomaly. The operation: early and midterm results. *J Thorac Cardiovasc Surg.* 2007;133:215-223.

15. Rao PS. Coarctation of the aorta. *Curr Cardiol Rep.* 2005;7:425-434.

16. Beekman R. Coarctation of the aorta. In: Allen HD, Driscoll DJ, Shaddy RE, Feltes TF, eds. Moss and Adams' Heart Disease in Infants, Children, and Adolescents: *Including the Fetus and Young Adult.* 7th ed. Philadelphia, PA: Lippincott Williams & Wilkins; 2008:987-1004.

17. Jonas R. Interrupted aortic arch. In: Jonas R, ed. *Comprehensive Surgical Management of Congenital Heart Disease.* London, United Kingdom: Hodder Arnold; 2004: 470-482.

18. Jonas R. Vascular rings, slings, and tracheal anomalies. In: Jonas R, ed. *Comprehensive Surgical Management of Congenital Heart Disease.* London, United Kingdom: Hodder Arnold; 2004:497-509.

19. McMahon CJ, El Said HG, Vincent JA, et al. Refinements in the implantation of pulmonary arterial stents: impact on morbidity and mortality of the procedure over the last two decades. *Cardiol Young.* 2002;12:445-452.

CHAPTER 9

Conotruncal Abnormalities

Lindsay S. Rogers and
Chitra Ravishankar

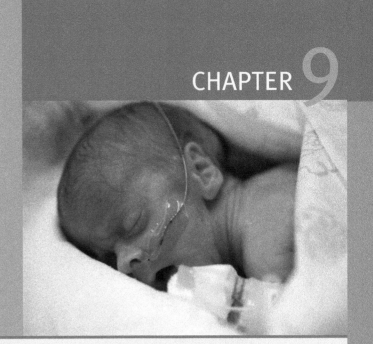

TRANSPOSITION OF THE GREAT ARTERIES

Background

Transposition of the great arteries (TGA) is a form of congenital heart defect (CHD) defined by ventricular–arterial discordance with the aorta arising from the right ventricle and the pulmonary artery (PA) arising from the left ventricle. Overall TGA accounts for 5% to 7% of all forms of CHD. The incidence ranges from 21.1 to 30.3 per 100,000 live births. Males are more commonly affected then females, accounting for 60% to 70% of cases. Untreated, 90% of infants will die within the first year of life, and 30% will die within the first week. In 1966, Rashkind and Miller performed the balloon atrial septostomy for the first time in a baby with TGA; this intervention dramatically influenced the survival of neonates with TGA.[1] Unlike other forms of CHD that have a high association with extracardiac anomalies, only 10% of patients with TGA have a coexisting extracardiac defect.[2]

TGA can take on many different anatomic forms with an assorted range of physiologic characteristics. Two of the most common forms of transposition are often referred to as dextro-TGA (d-TGA), or classic transposition, and levo-TGA (l-TGA). The letters d (dextro or rightward) and l (levo or leftward) stem from the Van Praagh segmental nomenclature system and refer to the anatomic position of the aortic valve in relation to the pulmonary valve.

The term d-TGA represents patients who have atria and ventricles in their correct anatomic position but have an aorta arising from the morphologic right ventricle (RV) and a PA originating from the morphologic left ventricle (LV). Patients with d-TGA most commonly have an aorta that is rightward and anterior to the PA (Figure 9-1).

In l-TGA, also known as congenitally corrected TGA (ccTGA), the right atrium drains into the anatomic LV (which is right-sided), and the left atrium drains to the anatomic RV (on the left side of the heart). The aorta arises from the left-sided morphologic RV, and the PA arises from the right-sided morphologic LV (Figure 9-2). Although these patients have the anatomic diagnosis of TGA, patients with l-TGA have "normal physiology," with an LV pumping deoxygenated blood to the lungs and an RV providing oxygenated blood to the body.

Dextro-Transposition of the Great Arteries

Definition and epidemiology

d-TGA is the most common form of transposition. Approximately one half of patients with TGA have another cardiac defect, not including patent foramen ovale (PFO) or patent ductus arteriosis (PDA). The most common associated cardiac defect is a ventricular septal defect (VSD), occurring in 40% to 45% of patients with TGA. However, only about one third of these VSDs are hemodynamically insignificant.[2] Other associated cardiac defects seen with TGA and their relative frequencies are listed in Table 9-1.

Pathophysiology

In d-TGA, the pulmonary and systemic circulations are in parallel, rather than series. Therefore, deoxygenated blood returning from the body to the right

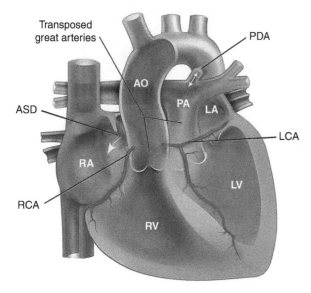

FIGURE 9-1 ■ Dextro-transposition of the great arteries (d-TGA). The aorta (AO) arises from the right ventricle (RV), and the pulmonary artery (PA) arises from the left ventricle (LV). An atrial septal defect (ASD) and patent ductus arteriosus (PDA) are commonly present. The left coronary artery (LCA) and right coronary artery (RCA) can be seen arising from the aorta. LA, left atrium; RA, right atrium. (© *2011 The Children's Hospital of Philadelphia, All Rights Reserved.*)

Cardiac Defects Associated with d-TGA

Associated Cardiac Defect	Frequency Seen with d-TGA
Patent ductus arteriosus	50%
Ventricular septal defect	40%-45%
Left ventricular outflow tract obstruction (PS)	25%
Tricuspid valve anomaly	31%
Mitral valve anomaly	20%
Aortic arch coarctation, hypoplasia, interruption	5%
Leftward juxtaposition of atrial appendages	2%-5%
Right aortic arch	4%

d-TGA, dextro-transposition of the great arteries; PS, pulmonary stenosis.

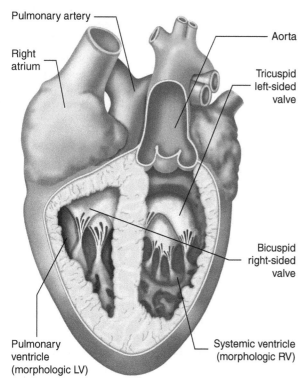

FIGURE 9-2 ■ Levo-transposition of the great arteries (l-TGA). The right atrium drains via the mitral valve to the morphologic left ventricle (LV), which gives rise to the pulmonary artery. The left atrium drains through the tricuspid valve to the morphologic right ventricle (RV), which gives rise to the aorta. (*Redrawn with permission from Icon Learning Systems division of MediMedia USA, Inc.*)

atrium (RA) crosses the tricuspid valve into the RV and exits the RV into the aorta, back out to the body and completely bypassing the lungs. Likewise, pulmonary venous return to the left atrium (LA) crosses the mitral valve into the LV and exits into the PA, headed back to the lungs. Without mixing of oxygenated and deoxygenated blood, it is easy to see how this physiology will quickly lead to profound cyanosis, acidosis, and death. In infants with a sizeable VSD, mixing at the ventricular level will provide more oxygenated blood to the body. In the absence of a VSD, newborns with TGA have 2 other potential areas for circulatory mixing, a PFO and PDA (Figure 9-1).

After fetal transition and a resultant drop in pulmonary vascular resistance, blood will shunt through the PDA mostly from aorta to PA. Although this shunt will not directly provide oxygenated blood to the body, increasing pulmonary blood flow will increase the overall amount of oxygenated blood and increase the amount of pulmonary venous return to the LA. This increase in blood volume will increase LA size and pressure, promoting mixing at the PFO.

The PFO itself can be very small to quite large in the newborn. In neonates with TGA and no VSD, mixing of oxygenated blood in the LA and deoxygenated right atrial blood via the PFO is the most important determinant of systemic saturation and overall stability. If the mixing is inadequate, as reflected by a low arterial saturation and partial pressure of oxygen in arterial blood (PaO$_2$), a procedure to enlarge the PFO must be undertaken. This procedure is known as a balloon atrial septostomy, or Rashkind procedure. For more information, see Chapter 5.

Clinical presentation and diagnosis

In some cases, d-TGA is diagnosed prenatally by fetal echocardiography. However, prenatal diagnosis can be challenging because the intracardiac anatomy can look essentially normal, with 4 chambers and 2 great vessels. In addition, TGA often occurs in isolation; therefore, it is uncommon for extracardiac anomalies to prompt more specialized evaluation and fetal echocardiography.

In the absence of prenatal diagnosis, patients with d-TGA almost always present in the newborn period with cyanosis. The degree of cyanosis is completely dependent on the amount of mixing between the systemic and pulmonary circulations as discussed earlier. Fifty-six percent of newborns with TGA (without VSD) are recognized within the first hour of life and 92% within the first day.[2] Table 9-2 describes physical examination, electrocardiogram, and chest x-ray findings seen in d-TGA. Echocardiography is the diagnostic modality of choice and should be sought for any infant in whom TGA is suspected.

Clinical Findings in Conotruncal Anomalies

	Tetralogy of Fallot	Truncus Arteriosus	d-TGA Without VSD	d-TGA with VSD	l-TGA
Physical Exam					
Overall	■ Variable degrees of cyanosis	■ Mild cyanosis	■ Cyanosis	■ Mild cyanosis	■ Normal
Respiratory	■ Normal	■ Tachypnea within the first week of life	■ Usually normal	■ Tachypnea at 2-6 weeks	■ Normal ■ If VSD, similar to d-TGA/VSD
Cardiac	■ Accentuated precordial RV impulse ■ S_2 single and often loud ■ Harsh SEM (crescendo-decrescendo) at LUSB	■ Bounding peripheral pulses ■ Bounding precordium ■ Ejection click and single S_2 ■ Apical S_3 ■ Loud pansystolic murmur at LLSB with diffuse radiation ■ Apical diastolic rumble ■ ± High-pitched diastolic murmur (TI)	■ First heart sound can be loud ■ Rarely murmur from: ■ LVOTO: SEM ■ PDA: continuous	■ Unremarkable at birth ■ 2-6 weeks (CHF): ■ Tachycardia ■ Pansystolic murmur ■ S_3 gallop ■ Mid-diastolic rumble	■ Loud S_2 ■ If VSD, similar to d-TGA/VSD
Ancillary Testing					
Chest x-ray	Boot-shaped heart ■ RVH with upturned apex ■ Decreased pulmonary vascular markings ■ RAA (25%)	■ Cardiomegaly ■ Increased pulmonary vascular markings ■ ± RAA	■ "Egg on a shoestring" ■ Narrow superior mediastinum ■ Mild cardiomegaly ■ Increased pulmonary vascular markings	■ Same as TGA/no VSD except with increase in pulmonary vascular markings as PVR falls	■ Dextrocardia and mesocardia 25% ■ Deformity of left mediastinal border
ECG	■ Isolated RVH ■ Fontal axis more rightward than usual	■ Normal axis ■ NSR ■ Normal intervals ■ Biventricular hypertrophy	■ Normal at birth ■ Can develop RAD and RVH ± LVH	■ Normal at birth ■ RAD and RVH ± LVH	■ Presence of Q waves in right precordial leads (absent on left) ■ Large Q waves in III and aVF ■ LAD

CHF, congestive heart failure; d-TGA, dextro-transposition of the great arteries; ECG, electrocardiogram; l-TGA, levo-transposition of the great arteries; LAD, left axis deviation; LLSB, left lower sternal border; LUSB, left upper sternal border; LVH, left ventricular hypertrophy; LVOTO, left ventricular outflow tract obstruction; NSR, normal sinus rhythm; PDA, patent ductus arteriosus; PVR, pulmonary vascular resistance; RAA, right aortic arch; RAD, right axis deviation; RV, right ventricle; RVH, right ventricular hypertrophy; SEM, systolic ejection murmur; TGA, transposition of the great arteries; TI, truncal insufficiency; VSD, ventricular septal defect.

Treatment

Medical. Once the diagnosis is made, infants are maintained on prostaglandin E_1 to ensure the patency of the PDA. However, they need to be closely monitored for side effects such as apnea, vasodilation, fever, rash, and edema. In addition, as mentioned earlier, balloon atrial septostomy (Rashkind procedure) may be necessary to enlarge the PFO, promoting mixing of the pulmonary venous and systemic venous blood, if persistently low arterial PaO_2 levels are present in the newborn period.

Surgical. Corrective surgery for d-TGA is usually undertaken in the first 1 to 2 weeks of life, after the pulmonary vascular resistance has fallen. In the current era, the most commonly performed operation for d-TGA is called the arterial switch operation (ASO) and involves translocation of the great vessels back to their appropriate positions. This surgery was first described in 1975 by Adib Jatene, a Brazilian surgeon, and became widely used in the 1980s. The ASO is now the procedure of choice for d-TGA.

The ASO is performed by first transecting the aorta and PA, just above the sinuses of each valve. The coronary arteries are then excised from the aortic sinus, taking a rim of tissue surrounding each coronary os (these are known as the coronary buttons). The distal main pulmonary (with attached branch PAs) is passed anterior to the aorta (LeCompte maneuver) and connected to the proximal aortic root, becoming the neopulmonary root. The coronary buttons are sewn to the proximal pulmonary root or the neoaortic root, and the distal ascending aorta (which is now behind the PA) is connected to the neoaortic root (Figure 9-3).

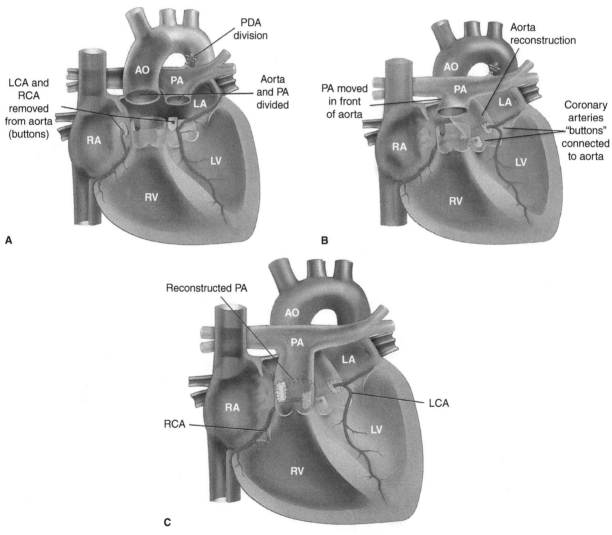

FIGURE 9-3 ■ **A.** Arterial switch operation (ASO), part 1. The patent ductus arteriosus (PDA) is ligated (if present). The aorta (AO) and pulmonary artery (PA) are divided. The left coronary artery (LCA) and right coronary artery (RCA) are removed from the aorta with surrounding tissue (buttons). **B.** ASO, part 2. The aorta (AO) is connected to the native pulmonary root, and the coronary buttons are connected to neoaorta. The pulmonary artery (PA) is moved in front of the aorta (LeCompte maneuver). **C.** Transposition of the great arteries after ASO, finished product. The pulmonary artery (PA) has been reconstructed and connected to the native aortic root. The right and left coronary arteries (RCA and LCA) can be seen, reimplanted onto the neoaorta. LA, left atrium; LV, left ventricle; RA, right atrium; RV, right ventricle. (© 2011 The Children's Hospital of Philadelphia, All Rights Reserved.)

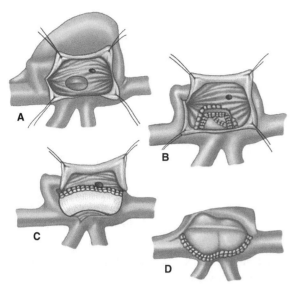

FIGURE 9-4 ■ The Senning operation. **A.** The atrial septum is cut near the tricuspid valve, creating a flap attached posteriorly between the caval veins. **B.** The flap of atrial septum is sutured to the anterior lip of the orifices of the left pulmonary veins, effectively separating the pulmonary and systemic venous channels. **C.** The posterior edge of the right atrial incision is sutured to the remnant of the atrial septum, diverting the systemic venous channel to the mitral valve. **D.** The anterior edge of the right atrial incision (lengthened by short incisions at each corner) is sutured around the cava above and below to the lateral edge of the left atrial incision, completing the pulmonary channel and diversion of pulmonary venous blood to the tricuspid valve area. (*Reproduced with permission from Mavroudis C, Backer CL, eds. D-Transposition of the great arteries. In:* Pediatric Cardiac Surgery. *2nd ed. St. Louis, MO: Mosby; 1994:345.*)

Prior to the introduction of the ASO, patients with d-TGA underwent an atrial-level switch operation that redirected systemic venous return to the LA and pulmonary venous return to the RA. This was accomplished by 1 of 2 methods, the Mustard or Senning operation (Figure 9-4). The Senning operation constructed an atrial baffle made from native atrial tissue, using the atrial septum. The Mustard procedure used baffle made from the pericardium and cut away most of the atrial septum. Both surgeries redirected blood to the appropriate outlet, while leaving the RV as the systemic pumping ventricle. Because of atrial size and the complexity of the surgery, patients often did not have surgery until a few weeks to several months after birth.

Most early and midterm follow-up studies comparing the ASO to the Mustard or Senning operation show the ASO to be superior when comparing ventricular performance, development of arrhythmias, and incidence of early sudden death.[3] Therefore, the atrial switch operation has been largely abandoned for the ASO in the current era.

In patients who have significant LV outflow tract obstruction (or pulmonary stenosis), an ASO may not be feasible because patients would be left with significant obstruction to systemic outflow (neoaorta). These patients often have large VSDs and can undergo a Rastelli procedure. In this operation, the VSD is closed to the native aorta with oversewing of the pulmonary valve. The RV is then connected to the PA via a homograft conduit.

Outpatient management

Postoperative management of patients after surgical repair of TGA should be focused on identification of potential short-, mid-, and long-term sequelae known to occur after ASO. A list of the more common morbidities associated with the ASO is provided in Table 9-3.[2-5]

Postoperative complications after ASO. Early mortality for patients after ASO is less than 10% and often associated with anatomic abnormalities, such as unusual coronary artery course, multiple VSDs, abnormal aortic arch, or atrioventricular valve malformations.[2]

Supravalvar pulmonary stenosis (PS) is the most common short-term complication following the ASO, with 5% to 30% of patients requiring reintervention by balloon angioplasty/stent placement via cardiac catheterization or rarely surgical repair with PA plasty. The etiology of supravalvar PS can be from compression of the PAs by the posterior aorta (with the LeCompte maneuver), circumferential narrowing at the suture line, or branch PA stenosis (stretching around the neoaorta).

Neoaortic root dilation is a known phenomenon after ASO and can be progressive. Progressive neoaortic root dilation can lead to aortic insufficiency. However, the number of patients needing surgical reintervention in childhood for root dilation or aortic insufficiency is small (<5%).[4]

Coronary artery patency is a major concern after ASO, given that the coronary arteries are moved from the aorta to the PA (neoaorta) at the time of the operation. Mechanical occlusion of the coronary arteries can occur in several forms, with a range of clinical manifestations (Table 9-3). In addition, the long-term effects that the ASO may have on development of coronary artery disease, long-term ventricular function, and development of arrhythmia are not yet known. The oldest survivors are currently in their third decade, and it is unknown whether coronary artery disease will occur prematurely in this patient population.[3] However, it is important to keep in mind that the presentation of myocardial ischemia in this patient population may not be classic chest pain, because their hearts have been effectively deinnervated as a result of surgical suture lines. Therefore, a high suspicion of coronary artery pathology is always warranted when caring for these patients at any stage in their life.

Postoperative complications of the atrial switch operation. The atrial switch procedures, the Mustard and Senning operations, were routinely performed through the early 1990s. Therefore, there are a large

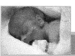

Complications of ASO

Complication	Incidence	Time Course	Clinical Presentation	Treatment
Supravalvar pulmonary stenosis	5%-30%	Immediate to midterm	Asymptomatic RV failure	BDA Stent placement Surgery
Neoaortic root dilation	3% at 1 year 49% at 10 years[4]	Intermediate to long term	Asymptomatic	Surgical repair: timing unknown as dissection is rare
Neoaortic valve regurgitation	0%-50%	Immediate to long term	Typically asymptomatic	Surgery if hemodynamically significant (rarely necessary)
Coronary Artery Occlusion				
Intraoperative occlusion		Immediate	Ventricular dysfunction and inability to separate from bypass	Surgical revision if possible
Subacute kinking	Late myocardial infarction in 1%-2%	Weeks to months after surgery	Chronic low output presenting with poor feeding and sweating Risk for circulatory collapse and late myocardial infarction	Surgical revision if significant dysfunction
Asymptomatic occlusion	1%-2% of hospital survivors	Likely gradual progression	None	None; adequate collateralization present

Complications after arterial switch operation (ASO).[2-5] The complication, incidence, expected timing of presentation, presenting symptoms and the currently accepted treatments are outlined above. RV, right ventricle; BDA, balloon dilating angioplasty; MI, myocardial infarction; ASO, arterial switch operation.

number of patients in their late teens and adulthood who are living with this type of anatomic correction. Long-term sequelae after the atrial switch operation are listed in Table 9-4. One of the most well-described effects of the atrial switch operation is RV dysfunction. The RV was not designed to perform as the systemic ventricle.

Complications of the Atrial Switch Operation

Complication	Clinical Manifestation
Right ventricular dysfunction	Exercise intolerance, orthopnea, cough, respiratory distress
Arrhythmias	
Tachyarrhythmia	Palpitations, episodic dizziness, syncope
Bradyarrhythmia	Fatigue, exercise intolerance, syncope
Baffle leaks	Cyanosis
Systemic venous pathway obstruction	Peripheral edema, ascites, portal-venous congestion
Pulmonary venous pathway obstruction	Respiratory distress, exercise intolerance

Complications following the atrial level switch operation. Short and long-term complications following Mustard or Senning operations are outlined along with their clinical presentation. RV, right ventricle.[2,4,6]

Tricuspid regurgitation often accompanies RV dysfunction and tends to progressively worsen as RV function deteriorates. Treatment of RV dysfunction is challenging, and clinicians are often tempted to use β-blockers and angiotensin-converting enzyme inhibition given their known benefits in acquired heart disease. However, to date, there have been no convincing data that these, or other medications, provide any survival benefit for patients with RV dysfunction after atrial switch.[5]

Arrhythmia is another well-known complication after atrial switch operation and is predominated by atrial arrhythmia, given the degree of atrial manipulation that occurs with this surgery. These rhythm disturbances include bradycardia due to sinus node dysfunction, which can occur with a slow junctional rhythm. Tachyarrhythmias commonly include ectopic atrial tachycardia or atrial flutter, which occurs in 5% to 15% of patients.[2] Surgical complete heart block and ventricular arrhythmias can also occur. Pacemaker implantation for atrial or atrioventricular (AV) nodal disease was not uncommon and was required in 11% of patients in 1 large series.[4] Late sudden death is seen in 2% to 10% of patients, and sinus node dysfunction and rapid atrial arrhythmias are thought to play a role.

Leaks between the systemic and pulmonary venous baffles can occur, and resultant shunting can lead to systemic desaturation. In addition, obstruction to either the pulmonary venous or systemic venous pathway can also occur and may require intervention in the cardiac catheterization laboratory or surgical correction.

Overall long-term management

All patients with TGA require routine evaluation by a pediatric or adult congenital cardiologist throughout their entire life. Once out of the immediate postoperative period, annual follow-up is usually recommended. However, routine primary care evaluations play an important role in identification of new symptoms that may prompt more immediate cardiology evaluation. As described earlier, surgical repair of TGA is associated with morbidities that may require further catheter-based or surgical intervention.

Overall, patients with TGA tend to live healthy and productive lives. Neurodevelopmental outcome of patients with d-TGA undergoing the ASO has also been very well described thanks to the Boston Circulatory Arrest trial (for more information, see Chapter 11). Our hope is that patients with the ASO will not face as many long-term sequelae as those who underwent the atrial switch operation. So far, this has proven true; however, longer term follow-up is needed as patients with ASO progress into older adulthood.

Levo-Transposition of the Great Arteries

Definition and epidemiology

l-TGA is a rare form of CHD, with a prevalence of about 0.03 per 1000 live births, and accounts for only 0.05% of congenital heart lesions. It is thought that l-TGA occurs secondary to inverse looping of the primitive cardiac tube during early fetal development.[6] This results in ventricular inversion, with the RV on the patient's left and the LV on the patient's right. The atria are usually normally positioned, and there is transposition of the great arteries, with the PA arising from the morphologic LV and the aorta arising from the morphologic RV. Therefore, normal physiology ensues as blue blood is transported to the lungs and oxygenated blood is pumped to the body, albeit by the RV. Given the resultant normal physiology, despite the abnormal morphology, this form of CHD has been referred to as "congenitally corrected transposition of the great arteries."

As with d-TGA, patients with l-TGA can have several commonly associated cardiac defects. In fact, well over 90% of patients will have some other cardiac anomaly (Table 9-5). The 3 most common associated abnormalities are VSD, abnormalities of the AV valve such as Ebstein anomaly of the tricuspid valve, and PS. A dysplastic tricuspid valve is often regurgitant, and tricuspid regurgitation is a well-known risk factor for RV dysfunction and overall poor outcome in patients with l-TGA.[5]

Another clinically important associated defect is complete heart block. Patients with l-TGA have an abnormally placed AV node and conduction system (ie,

Defects Associated with l-TGA

Associated Cardiac Defect	Frequency Seen with l-TGA
Tricuspid valve abnormality	Up to 90%
VSD	80%-90%
Pulmonary outflow obstruction	30%-50%
Isolated dextrocardia or mesocardia	25%
Situs inversus	5%
Mitral valve abnormality	10%
Complete heart block	10% (at initial presentation)

l-TGA, levo-transposition of the great arteries; VSD, ventricular septal defect.

His bundle). The abnormal location of the His bundle seems to make it more vulnerable to fibrosis, often resulting in varying degrees of AV block. Consequently, complete heart block is common in l-TGA with a progressive incidence of about 2% per year.[5] Surgical or catheter intervention can also precipitate compete heart block in these patients. In addition, Wolff-Parkinson-White syndrome or pre-excitation also occurs commonly with l-TGA and can lead to the occurrence of supraventricular tachycardia.[7]

Clinical presentation and diagnosis

Clinical, radiographic, and electrocardiogram abnormalities seen in patients with l-TGA are listed in Table 9-2. Definitive diagnosis can be made with echocardiogram if clinical suspicion exists. However, children with isolated l-TGA are usually asymptomatic in childhood. Therefore, patients with l-TGA and no other cardiac anomalies can go undiagnosed until they become symptomatic in adult life; one third of these patients manifest congestive heart failure by the fifth decade secondary to RV failure. It has been reported that a minority of patients with isolated l-TGA will be functionally normal into their seventh and eighth decades. In contrast, prior to surgical intervention, two thirds of patients with associated cardiac defects manifested congestive heart failure by the age of 45 years.[5]

Infants with associated cardiac defects will have clinical manifestations of those lesions. For example, infants with l-TGA and VSD may begin to show heart failure symptoms at a few weeks of life, when pulmonary vascular resistance falls.

Treatment

Medical. As mentioned earlier, early management of patients with l-TGA is usually focused on their associated anomalies. Infants with significant pulmonary outflow obstruction, coarctation, or interrupted aortic arch are ductal dependant, requiring prostaglandin at birth until surgical intervention can be performed. Later, medical management is focused on treatment of systemic AV valve regurgitation and RV failure.

Surgical. Appropriate surgical management of l-TGA is an area of continued debate, and details are beyond the scope of this chapter. There are 3 broad approaches: (1) "anatomic" repair leaving the RV as the systemic ventricle; (2) making the LV the systemic ventricle using the "double-switch" operation (a combination of atrial-level and arterial-level switch); and (3) single-ventricle palliation to Fontan completion if 1 of the ventricles is considered to be hypoplastic.

In adolescence and adulthood, surgical management of l-TGA is often focused on tricuspid valve repair or replacement. As the RV begins to fail, there is progressive tricuspid regurgitation with RV volume loading and annular dilation, further worsening RV function in a progressive manner. In the adult population, surgical tricuspid valve replacement can be accomplished with a relatively low mortality rate at experienced centers with improvement in functional status for most survivors.[5]

Outpatient management

The short- and long-term complications for patients who undergo a double-switch operation are outlined earlier in the section on atrial switch and ASO. Because the double-switch operation has been a recently adopted management strategy for this disease, only short- and midterm outcomes are available, with early mortality of 5.6% and 7-year survival rates of 85% for ASO and 95.5% for the Rastelli procedure in 1 study.[6]

Regardless of operative management, patients with l-TGA should have routine follow-up with a pediatric or adult congenital heart disease specialist. Evaluation will often include imaging via echocardiography or magnetic resonance imaging, exercise testing, and arrhythmia monitoring. Any change in functional capacity, new-onset palpitations, chest pain, shortness of breath, or peripheral edema should prompt more immediate referral for cardiology follow-up.

Overall outcome

l-TGA is an uncommon form of CHD with a wide range of clinical manifestations that are dependent on the coexisting cardiac defects. Optimal surgical management for these patients is unclear. However, we do know that in the majority of patients, the systemic RV will eventually manifest RV failure with significant tricuspid regurgitation. It remains unclear whether the double-switch operation will offer less long-term morbidity than having a systemic RV. More information is needed to guide treatment for this unusual form of CHD.

TETRALOGY OF FALLOT

Definitions and Epidemiology

Tetralogy of Fallot (TOF) is one of the most common cyanotic CHDs. A French physician by the name of Etienne-Louis Fallot made the pathologic and clinical connection in 1888 by performing autopsies on 2 patients who had long-standing cyanosis, terming the disease "la maladie bleue" or "the blue disease." In addition, TOF has significant importance in the history of surgical palliation in congenital heart disease. The first surgical aortopulmonary shunt (classic Blalock-Taussig shunt) was placed in a young girl with TOF for palliation of cyanosis in 1945. This surgical procedure was life-saving in children with TOF and heralded the beginning of pediatric cardiac surgery.[8]

The 4 major anatomic features of TOF are large "malalignment-type" VSD, overriding of the aorta over the ventricular septum, RV outflow tract (RVOT) obstruction and RV hypertrophy (Figure 9-5). Although every patient diagnosed with TOF has these 4 anatomic characteristics, there is a diverse spectrum of disease. Patients can have severe RV outflow obstruction to the degree of pulmonary valve atresia, or as in TOF with "absent pulmonary valve" syndrome, they can have minimal RV outflow obstruction but free regurgitation. The degree of RVOT obstruction varies from minimal PS as in "pink TOF" to complete atresia of the pulmonary valve.

The prevalence of TOF ranges from 0.26 to 0.48 per 1000 live births. It accounts for 6.8% of all forms of

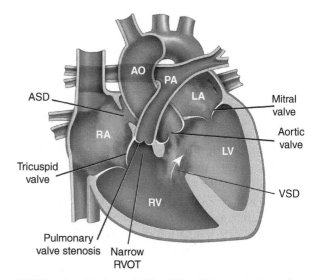

FIGURE 9-5 ■ Tetralogy of Fallot (TOF). Right ventricular outflow tract (RVOT) narrowing with valvar pulmonary stenosis, ventricular septal defect (VSD), overriding aorta (AO), and right ventricular (RV) hypertrophy are the 4 classic findings associated with TOF. Note that the pulmonary artery (PA) is much smaller than the aorta, which is typical in TOF. ASD, atrial septal defect; LA, left atrium; LV, left ventricle; RA, right atrium. (© *2011 The Children's Hospital of Philadelphia, All Rights Reserved.*)

CHD and is one of the most common forms of cyanotic CHD. Approximately 80% of patients with TOF have PS, whereas about 20% have TOF with pulmonary atresia.[8] In TOF with pulmonary atresia, the branch pulmonary arteries are supplied either by a PDA or collateral arteries from the descending aorta, known as TOF with multiple aortopulmonary collateral arteries. TOF/pulmonary atresia with multiple aortopulmonary collateral arteries is a rare form of TOF and will not be further discussed in this chapter.

Pathophysiology

The exact mechanism of malformation that leads to TOF is uncertain. There are several theories about how this abnormal conotruncal arrangement forms. In embryonic life, the great arteries form from a common truncus arteriosus, whereas the ventricular outflow tracts form from the distal bulbus cordis. Together, these regions become the conotruncus. It is thought that malrotation and faulty partitioning of the conotruncus results in the misplacement of the aorta over the VSD and a narrow pulmonary outflow. Alternatively, others have theorized that underdevelopment of the pulmonary infundibulum (subpulmonary outflow) causes this RVOT narrowing and malalignment of the conal (or outlet) septum.[8] However, despite these theories, the exact pathogenesis of this disease is unknown.

Although the molecular basis of TOF is not well understood, there are proven associations of TOF with certain genetic syndromes. In fact, one study found that 12% of patients with TOF have some type of identified chromosomal abnormality. Trisomy 21 is one of the more commonly described genetic syndromes associated with TOF. In addition, DiGeorge syndrome, or 22q11 deletion, is becoming more widely recognized in its association with TOF. In some studies, up to 25% of patients with TOF have a microdeletion on 22q11.[9] Patients with TOF and an associated aortic arch anomaly (such as right aortic arch or an aberrant subclavian artery) or vascular anomaly more commonly have 22q11 deletion than those without these arterial anomalies. Alagille syndrome is also known to be associated with TOF. For more in-depth information about known genetic associations of CHD, see Chapter 4.

Clinical Presentation and Diagnosis

An overview of clinical presentation and diagnostic characteristics of patients with TOF is provided in Table 9-2. Currently, most patients with TOF are diagnosed by fetal echocardiogram. When prenatal diagnosis is made, preparations can be made for immediate postnatal assessment and stabilization if it is deemed necessary.

In the absence of prenatal diagnosis, patients with TOF usually come to clinical attention in the newborn period secondary to a harsh systolic ejection murmur with or without cyanosis. Overall, the clinical presentation of patients with TOF is strongly dependent on the degree of RVOT obstruction. The greater the degree of RVOT obstruction, secondary to subpulmonary and pulmonary stenosis, the smaller the amount of pulmonary blood flow and the greater the degree of right-to-left shunting at the level of the VSD, leading to increased cyanosis. Chest radiography and electrocardiogram can help with the diagnosis (Table 9-2), but an echocardiogram is required to make the definitive diagnosis.

Most newborns with TOF do not require any immediate intervention and can be discharged from the normal nursery with close cardiology follow-up. However, there is a subset of patients with TOF who have significant cyanosis at birth secondary to severe PS or pulmonary atresia. These patients require prostaglandin infusion to maintain patency of the ductus arteriosis in order to supplement pulmonary blood flow. This group of patients requires surgical or catheter-related intervention in the newborn period. In addition, patients with TOF/absent pulmonary valve syndrome can have significant respiratory distress in the newborn period secondary to severe branch PA dilation and resultant bronchial airway compression.

The majority of infants with TOF have a mild to moderate degree of RVOT obstruction and can be scheduled for an elective repair at 3 to 6 months of life. These infants require close follow-up by a pediatric cardiologist for signs of intermittent cyanosis (hypercyanotic spells) or progressive baseline cyanosis. Either of these findings is an indication for earlier surgical intervention. Patients with minimal RVOT obstruction may have normal saturations at birth secondary to minimal right-to-left shunting across the VSD. Uncommonly, patients will have so little RVOT obstruction that they will begin to develop heart failure symptoms as their pulmonary vascular resistance falls at a few weeks of life (for more information, see Chapter 7).

Hypercyanotic spells

Hypercyanotic episodes, commonly referred to as "Tet spells," are a well-described phenomenon in infants with unrepaired TOF. These episodes are characterized by severe and progressive cyanosis. The cause is thought to be secondary to an acute increase in the degree of subpulmonic obstruction, resulting in a decreased amount of pulmonary blood flow and an increase in right-to-left flow across the VSD. However, given that these spells can occur in patients with pulmonary atresia, it has been hypothesized that a decrease in systemic vascular resistance or increase in pulmonary vascular resistance can also lead to this clinical phenomenon. These spells can be precipitated by high fever, dehydration, noxious stimuli, and sedation (decrease in systemic vascular resistance). In addition to severe cyanosis, a typical spell is also characterized by a decrease in the intensity or complete disappearance of the systolic murmur.

Interventions should be directed at increasing pulmonary blood flow by decreasing pulmonary vascular resistance and infundibular narrowing and increasing systemic vascular resistance. Systemic vascular resistance and venous return, or preload, is increased by assuming the "knee-chest" position. Therefore, the majority of spells can be terminated by placing the child in the most comfortable position, usually in a parent's arms, bending the knees to the chest, and using supplemental oxygen with a mask. If these noninvasive interventions fail, pharmacologic therapy should be used. Sedatives like morphine or ketamine (ketamine has the advantage of increasing systemic vascular resistance), α-agonists such as phenylephrine, and β-blockers such as propranolol can all be effective treatment. Overall attention should also be paid to adequate hydration and correction of acidosis.

Associated defects

In addition to the 4 coexisting lesions that define TOF, other cardiac defects can also be present in these patients.[8,10] These defects are outlined in Table 9-6. Atrial septal defects (ASDs) are by far the most commonly associated lesion, occurring in over 80% of patients with TOF. Furthermore, the presence of additional VSDs or an aortic arch anomaly occurs in over 10% of patients. Common AV canal defects with TOF

are most commonly seen in association with trisomy 21. Coronary artery anomalies common to TOF are important to the surgeon, because a large conal branch from the right coronary artery or a left anterior descending artery arising from the right coronary artery both cross the RVOT and preclude a transannular repair (see later surgical section).

Treatment

Complete repair

The definitive treatment for TOF is full surgical repair, which consists of relief of RVOT obstruction and closure of the VSD. The VSD is closed with a Dacron or Gore-Tex patch, the RVOT obstruction is relieved by resection of RV muscle bundle underneath the pulmonary valve followed by augmentation of the RVOT with a patch. If the pulmonary valve annulus itself is deemed to be too small, the incision is carried across the valve annulus into the main PA; this is called a "transannular patch repair" (Figure 9-6). If present, the ASD is frequently partially closed, leaving a small ASD/PFO for right-to-left shunting in the immediate postoperative period as the RV compliance improves.

In cases of TOF with pulmonary atresia, patients require a tube graft from the RV to the PA (RV-PA conduit) (Figure 9-7). In addition, patients with certain coronary artery abnormalities (see associated lesions) that preclude an incision across the RVOT may also require RV-PA conduit placement. In the long term, an RV-PA conduit is less desirable than an outflow patch because the conduit will not grow with the child. Therefore, the conduit will need to be replaced at least 2 to 3 times as the child grows to adult size.

Cardiac Defects Associated with Tetralogy of Fallot	
Associated Cardiac Defect	Incidence
PFO or ASD	83%
Additional VSDs	5%
Common AV canal defect	3.4%
Right aortic arch	25%
LSVC	11%
Anomalous muscle bundles	3% (s/p repair)
Anomalous pulmonary venous drainage, Ebstein anomaly of TV, left heart abnormalities	Rare
Coronary Abnormalities	
Large conal branch/accessory LAD	15%
LAD from RCA	5%
Single origin of coronaries	4%

ASD, atrial septal defect; AV, atrioventricular; LAD, left anterior descending artery; LSVC, left superior vena cava; PFO, patent foramen ovale; RCA, right coronary artery; TV, tricuspid valve; VSD, ventricular septal defect.

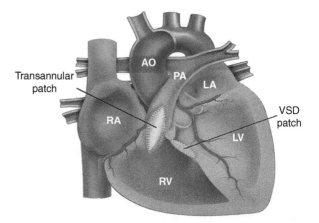

FIGURE 9-6 ■ Repair of tetralogy of Fallot (TOF) with a transannular outflow tract patch. In this type of TOF repair, the right ventricular outflow tract patch extends from the right ventricle (RV), across the pulmonary valve, to the main pulmonary artery (PA; ie, transannular patch). In addition, the ventricular septal defect (VSD) is closed with a patch. AO, aorta; LA, left atrium; LV, left ventricle; RA, right atrium. (© 2011 The Children's Hospital of Philadelphia, All Rights Reserved.)

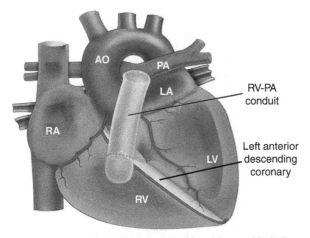

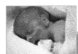

FIGURE 9-7 ■ Tetralogy of Fallot repair with a right ventricle (RV) to pulmonary artery (PA) conduit. In this case, the left anterior descending coronary originates from the right coronary artery and crosses the right ventricular outflow tract, precluding a transannular patch repair. AO, aorta; LA, left atrium; LV, left ventricle; RA, right atrium. (© 2011 The Children's Hospital of Philadelphia, All Rights Reserved.)

Palliative surgery

When persistent cyanosis is present in the newborn period, an intervention may be necessary to augment pulmonary blood flow. Palliative procedures can be either surgical or catheter-based interventions. Surgical palliation usually consists of placement of an aortopulmonary shunt such as a modified Blalock-Taussig shunt, a Gore-Tex tube that connects the innominate artery to the PA. In the current era, catheter-based interventions such as balloon dilation of the pulmonary valve and stenting of the RVOT or ductus arteriosis can be performed to increase pulmonary blood flow. Patients with initial palliative procedures as neonates will typically return at 3 to 6 months for full repair.

In some centers, complete TOF repair (as described earlier) is performed with good success in the neonate; however, smaller infants remain at increased risk for postoperative morbidity.

Surgical outcomes

Overall outcomes for patients with TOF are excellent. Postoperative survival to hospital discharge is greater than 95%. Twenty-year survival for patients discharged after surgery was 98% in one study.[9] However, there are long-term morbidities associated with TOF after complete repair, and lifelong cardiology follow-up is essential. Our current understanding of long-term outcomes in this disease is based on operative techniques from the 1980s and earlier. Since that time, surgical techniques have evolved to minimize the extent of the incision on the RV (minimizing RV scar) and maintain pulmonary valve competency when possible. We hope that these changes in surgical approach will have a positive impact on the long-term morbidities discussed in the next section.

Outpatient Management

There are several well-described morbidities associated with TOF repair (Table 9-7). The most pervasive postoperative issue after TOF repair is pulmonary insufficiency or regurgitation. Pulmonary regurgitation increases the RV volume load, leading to RV dilation and eventually RV dysfunction. RV dilation can in turn lead to arrhythmias, LV dysfunction, and progressive right and left heart failure. Symptoms are unusual in childhood and may not manifest until the third decade or later. This can have a significant impact on quality of life and may even contribute to a small but present incidence of sudden death in these patients. In the current era, in addition to echocardiography, exercise stress test, Holter evaluation, and magnetic resonance imaging (MRI) are routinely used to assess RV volume and function.

Patients with significant RV dilation, new-onset ventricular tachycardia, and/or overt exercise intolerance are candidates for pulmonary valve replacement. Traditionally, pulmonary valve replacement has required surgical intervention. However, recent development of percutaneous pulmonary valve replacement in the cardiac catheterization lab has revolutionized the management of these patients. Currently, this technology is approved by the Food and Drug Administration for placement in an existing RV-PA conduit, but not for the native RVOT (ie, patients who had a patch repair).

Long-Term Morbidity After Tetralogy of Fallot Repair	
Morbidity	Potential Treatment
Pulmonary valve insufficiency with secondary RV dilation	PV replacement Common indications: ■ Severe RV dilation ■ New, symptomatic ventricular tachycardia ■ Overt exercise intolerance
Pulmonary artery stenosis and/or RV-PA conduit stenosis	■ Balloon dilation angioplasty/ stenting ■ Surgical correction
Ventricular arrhythmias	■ Catheter or surgical ablation ■ AICD placement
Atrial arrhythmias	■ Catheter ablation ■ Medical management
Aortic root dilation	Surgical aortic root replacement Common indications: ■ Significant aortic insufficiency ■ Aortic root >5.5 cm (relative indication)

AICD, automatic implantable cardioverter-defibrillator; PA, pulmonary artery; PV, pulmonary valve; RV, right ventricle.

This will likely change in the next several years as new technology emerges.

Another known entity in adult patients after TOF repair is ventricular arrhythmias, which are a risk factor for sudden death. One of the identified risk factors for symptomatic ventricular tachycardia and sudden death is a QRS duration of greater than 180 ms.[9] Pulmonary valve replacement before the onset of RV dysfunction may have a role in decreasing RV size and therefore decrease the incidence of ventricular tachycardia. However, some patients will require catheter ablation and/or placement of implantable cardioverter-defibrillators given the association of symptomatic ventricular tachycardia, wide QRS duration, and sudden death.

Aortic root dilation is a late postoperative complication in adults with TOF. Dissections have been rarely reported. The underlying mechanism is unclear but differs from other forms of aortic aneurysms. Although there are no true guidelines for intervention, progressive aortic insufficiency and aortic root dilation greater than 5.5 cm are typically agreed upon as indications for aortic root replacement.[9]

Quality of life in patients with TOF is typically very good. However, although no overt symptoms of exercise intolerance may exist, most patients with TOF have an exercise capacity (maximal oxygen consumption and working capacity) that is 80% to 85% normal. Therefore, routine evaluations to detect subtle changes in exercise tolerance may help prompt interventions such as pulmonary valve replacement before symptoms impact quality of life.

TOF is one of the most common forms of cyanotic congenital heart disease. Fortunately, advances in surgical technique and postoperative care have allowed for excellent long-term survival in this patient population. Given the associated morbidities seen in the adult patient population, lifelong routine cardiology follow-up is imperative to maintain maximal functional capacity. With advances in surgical technique, catheter-based interventions, and a more broad understanding of long-term outcomes, we hope overall survival and quality of life in patients with TOF will continue to improve.

TRUNCUS ARTERIOSUS

Definitions and Epidemiology

Truncus arteriosus (TA) is relatively uncommon, representing approximately 2% to 4% of all forms of CHD. TA is defined by having a single arterial trunk that gives rise to the coronary, pulmonary, and systemic circulations. This trunk occurs in conjunction with a VSD, giving both ventricles an outlet to this single arterial trunk (Figure 9-8).

TA has 4 major types, distinguished by the origin of the pulmonary arteries and the distal arch anatomy. The

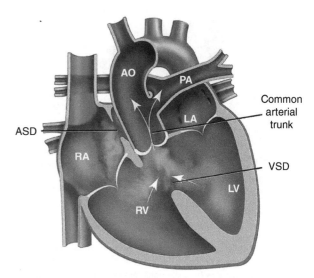

FIGURE 9-8 ■ Truncus arteriosus (TA). There is a common arterial trunk arising from both ventricles. The pulmonary arteries (PA) and ascending aorta (AO) both arise from this common arterial trunk. A ventricular septal defect (VSD) is present below the common truncus. An atrial septal defect (ASD) is also shown and is common in TA. LA, left atrium; LV, left ventricle; RA, right atrium; RV, right ventricle. (© *2011 The Children's Hospital of Philadelphia, All Rights Reserved.*)

4 major types of TA, classified by Collett and Edwards and modified by Van Praagh, are shown in Figure 9-9. The most common types of TA are Van Praagh A1 and A2, where both pulmonary arteries arise from the common arterial trunk. Type IV TA, as defined by Collett and Edwards, is now commonly accepted as a form of TOF with pulmonary valve atresia. Aside from their anatomic distinctions, classification of TA has clinical importance; types A3 and A4 (Van Praagh) are dependent on the patency of the ductus arteriosis after birth, and initiation of prostaglandin is essential in management of these patients.

Pathophysiology

In fetal life, the TA is a normally occurring structure that sits between the primitive outflow tracts (bulbus cordis) and the aortic sac and aortic arch system. Division of the TA during fetal development leads to the formation of the proximal ascending aorta and pulmonary trunk. The endocardial cushions, responsible for this partitioning, fuse with the developing conal septum (the portion of the septum that sits between the aortic and pulmonary valves) forming both ventricular outflow tracts. When this truncal septation does not occur in a normal fashion, persistence of the TA can occur. In addition, this failure of septation includes underdevelopment or malposition of the conal septum, resulting in a VSD.[11]

Clinical Presentation and Diagnosis

Most patients with TA are diagnosed in fetal life or the early neonatal period. Fetuses with TA and severe truncal

Collett & Edwards

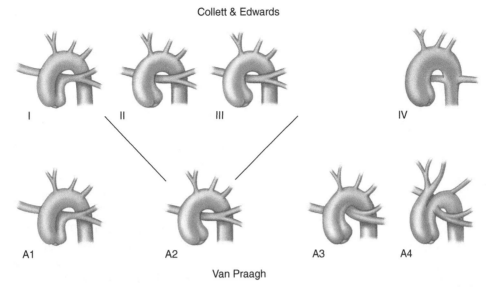

Van Praagh

FIGURE 9-9 ■ Anatomic classification of truncus arteriosus. Collett and Edwards' class I is similar to Van Praagh's A1 with the appearance of a partial main pulmonary artery (MPA) segment arising from the common trunk. Collett and Edwards' classes II and III are almost indistinguishable from each other and similar to the Van Praagh A2, with the pulmonary arteries coming directly off the ascending aorta, without an MPA segment. Van Praagh A3 is defined by absence of 1 pulmonary artery, usually arising from a patent ductus arteriosus (PDA). A4 has a hypoplastic or interrupted aortic arch with the PDA supplying the descending aorta. (*Reproduced with permission from Fyler DC. Truncus arteriosis. In: Fyler DC, ed. Nadas' Pediatric Cardiology. Philadelphia, PA: Hanley and Belfus; 1992:676. Copyright Elsevier. As adapted with permission from Hernanz-Schulman M, Fellows KE. Persistent truncus arteriosis: Pathologic, diagnostic and therapeutic considerations. Semin Roentgenol. 1985;20:121. Copyright Elsevier.*)

valve stenosis or insufficiency have been described to develop hydrops fetalis.

The clinical, radiographic, and electrocardiographic features commonly seen in infants with TA are outlined in Table 9-2. In general, these neonates present with severe congestive heart failure within the first few days of life, because the PA is directly connected to the aorta. Echocardiography is usually sufficient to diagnose TA and define all associated cardiac malformations.

The semilunar valve (truncal valve) in patients with TA is commonly abnormal. In a review of several studies, truncal valve anatomy was tricuspid in 69%, quadricuspid in 22%, bicuspid in 9%, and pentacuspid or unicommissural in 0.3% of patients.[11] In addition, the truncal valve can be thickened and dysplastic, leading to variable degrees of stenosis and insufficiency. Truncal valve stenosis is often associated with truncal root dilation.

Additional cardiac malformations seen in association with TA are listed in Table 9-8. The incidence of 22q11 deletion, DiGeorge syndrome, is 20% to 41% in infants with TA, occurring more commonly in those with a discontinuous PA or aortic arch anomaly (such as right aortic arch with abnormal branching pattern).[12] Extracardiac anomalies are present in 21% to 30% of patients with TA and include skeletal malformations, hydroureter, bowel malrotation, and other multiple complex anomalies.

Cardiac Defects Associated with Truncus Arteriosus

Associated Cardiac Defect	Incidence
Absent PDA	~50%
Anomalies in coronary artery origin	37%-49%
Unilateral absence of pulmonary artery	16%
Right aortic arch (mirror image branching)	21%-36%
Interrupted aortic arch	11%-19%
Aberrant subclavian artery	4%-10%
Arch hypoplasia ± coarctation	3%
Secundum ASD	9%-20%
Mild tricuspid stenosis	6%
Left superior vena cava to coronary sinus	4%-9%
Anomalous pulmonary venous return, tricuspid and mitral atresia, ventricular inversion, complete atrioventricular canal	Rare

Cardiac defects seen in association with TA and their relative incidence are listed above [12]. PDA, patent ductus arteriosus; ASD, atrial septal defect.

Treatment

Surgical repair of TA in early infancy is imperative to prevent the development of pulmonary vascular disease that results from excessive, unrestrictive pulmonary blood flow. Without surgical correction, one series reported a mean age of death at 5 weeks of age, and

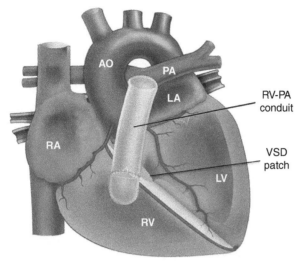

FIGURE 9-10 ■ Truncus arteriosus after repair. The ventricular septal defect (VSD) has been closed to the ascending aorta (AO). The branch pulmonary arteries (PA) have been disconnected from the common trunk and sewn to the right ventricular–pulmonary artery (RV-PA) conduit. The common trunk is patched where the pulmonary arteries have been removed and is now an exclusive aorta. LA, left atrium; LV, left ventricle; RA, right atrium; RV, right ventricle. (© *2011 The Children's Hospital of Philadelphia, All Rights Reserved*.)

another reported 15% survival beyond 1 year of age. Death occurred from heart failure, complications of pulmonary hypertension, or infective endocarditis.[11]

Surgical repair begins with detaching the pulmonary arteries from the truncal root, followed by patching the truncal root in the area of the detached pulmonary arteries to make that vessel an exclusive ascending aorta. The VSD is closed with a patch, creating an LV outflow tract to the common trunk, or ascending aorta. A conduit or tube graft is usually required to establish continuity between the RV and the PA (RV-PA conduit) (Figure 9-10). If there is significant truncal valve stenosis or insufficiency present, a truncal valve repair or, rarely, replacement may be undertaken at the time of the initial surgery.

Over the past 3 decades, there have been significant advances in cardiac surgery in infants including the management of TA, with decreasing mortality. One recent report showed an early postoperative mortality rate of 5%.[13] In some cases, extracardiac malformations can complicate the postoperative course, but overall, patients with TA do relatively well after neonatal repair.

Outpatient Management

Reoperation

All patients who have a TA repair in infancy will require conduit replacement in childhood, because the RV-PA homograft conduit size remains fixed as the child grows. Patients will experience increasing RV pressures secondary to conduit stenosis, and conduit replacement must be undertaken to prevent excessive RV work and

potential dysfunction. Often patients require 2 to 3 conduit replacements by the time they reach adult size.

It has been well described that long-term morbidity and mortality are increased in patients with moderate to severe truncal valve insufficiency.[14] Patients with significant truncal valve regurgitation may need to undergo truncal valve repair or replacement in childhood or adult life. In addition, reoperation or catheter-based intervention may be required in some patients for closure of residual VSD or ASD or PA angioplasty (secondary to narrowing of 1 or both pulmonary arteries).[15]

Finally, all repaired patients with TA are left with free pulmonary insufficiency. Although the homograft conduits used to connect the RV to the branch pulmonary arteries contain a semilunar valve, these valves often become incompetent within a year after surgery. Therefore, like patients with TOF (discussed earlier), they are at risk for RV dilation and dysfunction. Pulmonary valve replacement, percutaneous or surgical, should be considered in older patients who have exercise intolerance, severe RV dilation, or a significant ventricular tachyarrhythmia.

Overall Long-Term Management

Overall 15-year survival after hospital discharge was 83% in one series, which included patients operated on in the mid-1970s to the late 1990s.[14] Therefore, it is likely that patients who have TA repair in the current era will have improved long-term survival given advances in surgical technique and postoperative care. Functional status has been reported as good, with the majority of patients in New York Heart Association functional class I.

Long-term follow-up with a pediatric and/or an adult congenital heart disease specialist is imperative to optimizing outcome. Cardiac follow-up will focus on identification of conduit dysfunction, PA stenosis, ventricular dysfunction, progression of truncal valve stenosis/insufficiency, and changes in exercise capacity. Echocardiography and MRI are useful tools used for detection and progression of the above factors.

Clinical Pearls

■ Most forms of conotruncal heart disease present with cyanosis in infancy.
■ "Big, blue, baby boy" is typical of dextro-transposition of the great arteries (d-TGA); TGA affects males more commonly than females.
■ d-TGA is usually an isolated anomaly.
■ Congenitally corrected transposition of the great arteries can present in infancy if associated with other cardiac anomalies such as ventricular septal defects, pulmonary stenosis, or tricuspid regurgitation but can otherwise go undetected into adulthood. Adults can present with symptoms of congestive heart failure as their systemic right ventricle begins to fail.

- In tetralogy of Fallot, the degree of cyanosis is dependent on the amount of right ventricular outflow tract obstruction.
- "Tet spells" or hypercyanotic spells can be terminated in most instances by placing the infant in the most comfortable position such as a parent's arms, gently putting their knees to chest, and giving supplemental oxygen with a mask.
- Tetralogy of Fallot and truncus arteriosis are both associated with 22q11 microdeletion.
- Truncus arteriosus is the most likely form of conotruncal heart disease to be associated with extracardiac congenital anomalies.
- Most patients with conotruncal heart disease undergo infant repair, with good outcomes in the current era. Therefore, long-term sequelae of congenital heart defects are becoming more common in adult patients, making follow-up with cardiologists who have expertise in congenital heart disease imperative.

REFERENCES

1. Jonas RA. Transposition of the great arteries. In: Jonas RA, ed. *Comprehensive Surgical Management of Congenital Heart Disease*. London, United Kingdom: Hodder and Arnold; 2004:256-300.
2. Wernovsky G. Transposition of the great arteries. In: Allen HD, Driscoll DJ, Shaddy RE, Feltes TF, eds. *Moss and Adams' Heart Disease in Infants, Children, and Adolescents: Including the Fetus and Young Adult*. 7th ed. Philadelphia, PA: Lippincott Williams & Wilkins; 2008:1039-1087.
3. Cohen MS, Wernovsky G. Is the arterial switch operation as good over the long term as we thought it would be? *Cardiol Young*. 2006;16(Suppl 3):117-124.
4. Skinner J, Hornung T, Rumball E. Transposition of the great arteries: from fetus to adult. *Heart*. 2008;94: 1227-1235.
5. Warnes CA. Transposition of the great arteries. *Circulation*. 2006;114:2699-2709.
6. Dyck J, Atallah J. Congenitally corrected transposition of the great arteries. In: Allen HD, Driscoll DJ, Shaddy RE, Feltes TF, eds. *Moss and Adams' Heart Disease in Infants, Children, and Adolescents: Including the Fetus and Young Adult*. 7th ed. Philadelphia, PA: Lippincott Williams & Wilkins; 2008.
7. Blaufox AD, Saul JP. *Accessory Pathway-Mediated Tachycardias*. Philadelphia, PA: Lippincott Williams & Wilkins; 2001.
8. Siwik E, Erenberg F, Zahka K, Goldmuntz E. Tetralogy of fallot. In: Allen HD, Driscoll DJ, Shaddy RE, Feltes TF, eds. *Moss and Adams' Heart Disease in Infants, Children, and Adolescents: Including the Fetus and Young Adult*. 7th ed. Philadelphia, PA: Lippincott Williams & Wilkins; 2008.
9. Apitz C, Webb GD, Redington AN. Tetralogy of Fallot. *Lancet*. 2009;374:1462-1471.
10. Breitbart R, Fyler D. *Tetralogy of Fallot*. 2nd ed. Philadelphia, PA: Saunders Elsevier; 2006.
11. Cabalka AK, Edwards WD, Dearani JA. *Truncus Arteriosus*. 7th ed. Philadelphia, PA: Lippincott Williams & Wilkins; 2008.
12. Momma K. Cardiovascular anomalies associated with chromosome 22q11.2 deletion syndrome. *Am J Cardiol*. 2010;105:1617-1624.
13. Thompson LD, McElhinney DB, Reddy M, Petrossian E, Silverman NH, Hanley FL. Neonatal repair of truncus arteriosus: continuing improvement in outcomes. *Ann Thorac Surg*. 2001;72:391-395.
14. Rajasinghe HA, McElhinney DB, Reddy VM, Mora BN, Hanley FL. Long-term follow-up of truncus arteriosus repaired in infancy: a twenty-year experience. *J Thorac Cardiovasc Surg*. 1997;113:869-878.
15. Brown JW, Ruzmetov M, Okada Y, Vijay P, Turrentine MW. Truncus arteriosus repair: outcomes, risk factors, reoperation and management. *Eur J Cardiothorac Surg*. 2001;20:221-227.

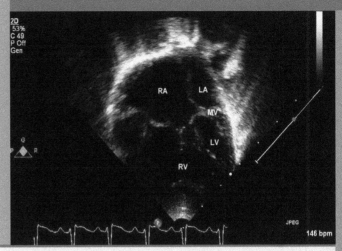

CHAPTER 10

Single-Ventricle Congenital Heart Disease

Matthew J. O'Connor,
David J. Goldberg and Jack Rychik

INTRODUCTION

In general, the most complex forms of congenital heart disease (CHD) fall into the category of single-ventricle defects. Only in recent decades has survival beyond the neonatal period become the norm in the developed world, owing to a number of factors, namely the introduction of prostaglandin infusion, innovative surgical strategies such as the Norwood procedure, accurate post-natal noninvasive assessment through echocardiography, and improvements in prenatal diagnosis. Today, surgical palliation of single-ventricle CHD is expected to result in favorable short- and long-term outcomes into early adulthood for most patients. With the improvement in survival in recent decades, attention is now being turned toward optimizing long-term outcomes and addressing the many functional limitations still experienced by sur-vivors of single-ventricle CHD.

DEFINITIONS AND EPIDEMIOLOGY

Anatomic Definition

Broadly speaking, single-ventricle CHD can be defined as any congenital heart defect in which there is admix-ture of systemic and pulmonary venous return in association with atresia (absence of a normally patent structure) or significant hypoplasia (smaller size than normal) of a cardiac valve or chamber.[1] Depending on the defect, admixture can occur at 1 or multiple ana-tomic locations within the heart. Single-ventricle CHD results from atresia or hypoplasia of either an atrioven-tricular valve or semilunar valve; atresia or hypoplasia of the ventricle associated with the affected atrioventricular

or semilunar valve typically exists in conjunction with the valve abnormality. For example, a common form of single-ventricle CHD affecting the right side of the heart is tricuspid atresia, wherein a hypoplastic or imperforate tricuspid valve is associated with underdevelopment of the right ventricle and right ventricular outflow tract. Pulmonary blood flow is provided by antegrade flow from the left ventricle (via a ventricular septal defect) or, in the absence of a ventricular septal defect, via the ductus arteriosus. In either situation, admixture of sys-temic and pulmonary venous return occurs via obliga-tory right-to-left shunting at the atrial level. The pro-totypic form of single ventricle affecting the left side of the heart is hypoplastic left heart syndrome (HLHS).[2] In HLHS, atresia or hypoplasia of the mitral valve and/ or aortic valves is associated with atresia or hypoplasia of the entire ensemble of left heart structures. Systemic output is provided by the right ventricle and ductus arteriosus, with admixture of systemic and pulmonary venous return occurring via left-to-right shunting at the atrial level. From an anatomic standpoint, it is impor-tant to recognize that abnormalities of the systemic and pulmonary veins with respect to their number, size, and site of drainage are frequently associated with single-ventricle CHD and that these additional defects can increase the complexity of surgical approaches and affect outcomes.[3,4]

It should be noted that "true" single ventricle (ie, the situation in which there is only 1 ventricle) is quite rare.[5] In most cases of single-ventricle CHD, there is a dominant ventricle of either left or right ventricular morphology, and the secondary ventricle is typically hypoplastic or rudimentary. Due to the relative rar-ity of anatomic single ventricle, many authors prefer the terms "functional single ventricle" or "functionally univentricular heart" when describing the physiology of single-ventricle CHD. For consistency throughout this chapter, however, the term single-ventricle CHD will be used. In addition, it should be recognized that single-ventricle CHD can result from a large number of individual defects. For the purposes of simplicity, only the most commonly encountered lesions causing single-ventricle CHD will be discussed in this chapter.

A discussion of the anatomy of single-ventricle CHD would not be complete without brief mention of the heterotaxy syndrome. Heterotaxy syndrome is a disorder of visceroatrial situs, that is, the position and orientation of the thoracic and abdominal organs. Heterotaxy syndrome has been described as the coexistence of situs solitus (normal position and orientation of the thoracic and abdominal organs) and situs ambiguus (abnormal position and orientation of the thoracic and abdominal organs) within an individual.[6] Single-ventricle CHD is common in patients with heterotaxy, typically in the form of unbalanced atrioventricular canal defects or double-outlet right ventricle with pulmonary outflow tract obstruction, although up to 25% of affected patients may be candidates for biventricular repair.[7] In addition to the complex underlying cardiac anatomy, abnormalities of cardiac position, systemic venous drainage, and pulmonary venous drainage occur in a sizeable proportion of patients.[8] Profound rhythm disturbances such as complete heart block are seen in nearly 20% of patients with heterotaxy[8] and confer a poor prognosis.[9,10] A number of extracardiac abnormalities are also associated with heterotaxy, including ciliary dyskinesia, abnormal splenic function, and intestinal malrotation, all of which impact morbidity and mortality following treatment of complex single-ventricle CHD.

Physiologic Definition

As discussed earlier in the previous examples, single-ventricle CHD can be conceptually grouped according to the underlying physiology. It is important to understand that the usual categorization of CHD into "cyanotic" and "acyanotic" forms does not allow for a full understanding of single-ventricle physiology. Rather, single-ventricle CHD is best characterized from a physiologic perspective by grouping the anatomic subtypes according to the presence of obstruction to either systemic or pulmonary blood flow. Within this conceptual framework, the presence or absence of cyanosis is a secondary determination that is in turn dependent on the balance of pulmonary and systemic blood flow within an individual patient. In the setting of single-ventricle physiology, the factors determining the balance of pulmonary and systemic blood flow depend on 3 factors:

(1) the magnitude of pulmonary or systemic obstruction; (2) patency of the ductus arteriosus; and (3) the relative resistances between the systemic and pulmonary vascular beds. The latter 2 factors may be manipulated through pharmacologic means and therefore serve as therapeutic targets in the preoperative phase for neonates with single-ventricle physiology.

In single-ventricle physiology, the oxygen saturation in the pulmonary artery is equal to the oxygen saturation in the aorta, due to the admixture of systemic and pulmonary venous return. This is in contrast to both normal physiology, in which the pulmonary artery oxygen saturation is less than that of the aorta, and to transposition physiology, in which the pulmonary artery oxygen saturation is higher than that in the aorta. Each form of obstructed blood flow (systemic or pulmonary) in single-ventricle CHD has distinct physiology, anatomic substrates, and clinical presentation. Simultaneous obstruction to both systemic and pulmonary blood flow is quite rare and is typically incompatible with survival apart from orthotopic heart transplantation.

Lesions with Obstruction to Pulmonary Blood Flow

In lesions with obstruction to pulmonary blood flow, atresia or hypoplasia of the tricuspid valve, the right ventricle, the right ventricular outflow tract, and the pulmonary valve (alone or in combination) leads to inadequate pulmonary blood flow. This results in cyanosis in the absence of a patent ductus arteriosus or aortopulmonary collateral vessels, both of which can provide pulmonary blood flow from the aorta. Low cardiac output may occur if there is any element of obstruction to systemic venous return (described in detail later in the Clinical Presentation section). The major forms of such defects are outlined in Table 10-1. Commonly encountered lesions with this physiology include tricuspid atresia, pulmonary atresia with intact ventricular septum, double-inlet left ventricle, pulmonary atresia with right ventricular aorta, and complete common atrioventricular canal defects unbalanced favoring the left ventricle.

Lesions with Obstruction to Systemic Blood Flow

Similarly, in lesions with obstruction to systemic blood flow, atresia or hypoplasia of the mitral valve, the left ventricle, the left ventricular outflow tract, and the aortic valve (alone or in combination) leads to inadequate systemic blood flow. In the absence of a patent ductus arteriosus, low cardiac output and circulatory collapse will ensue. However, cyanosis may also be a presenting

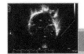

Single-Ventricle Defects Causing Obstruction to Pulmonary Blood Flow

- Pulmonary atresia with intact ventricular septum*
- Tricuspid atresia with normally related great vessels*
- Right ventricular aorta with pulmonary atresia
- Tetralogy of Fallot with pulmonary atresia and major aortopul-monary collateral vessels†
- Double-outlet right ventricle†
- Severe Ebstein malformation of the tricuspid valve
- Unbalanced atrioventricular canal defect favoring the left ventricle
- Double-inlet left ventricle with normally related great vessels (Holmes heart)
- Unspecified single ventricle with severe pulmonary stenosis or atresia

*Most common.
†Some forms.

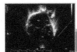

Single-Ventricle Defects Causing Obstruction to Systemic Blood Flow

- Hypoplastic left heart syndrome and variants
  Mitral stenosis and aortic stenosis
  Mitral atresia and aortic atresia
  Mitral stenosis and aortic atresia
  Mitral atresia and aortic stenosis
  Double-outlet right ventricle with mitral and aortic atresia
  Unbalanced atrioventricular canal defect favoring the right ventricle
- Mitral valve dysplasia with severe aortic stenosis
- Tricuspid atresia with dextro-transposition of the great vessels
- Double-inlet left ventricle with levo-transposition of the great vessels

feature if there is any obstruction to pulmonary venous return (described in detail later in the Clinical Presentation section). Obstruction to pulmonary venous return occurs when either the pulmonary veins drain anomalously in an obstructed fashion or, more commonly, when there is restriction to egress of pulmonary venous return at the atrial septum. In either case, infants with single-ventricle CHD, obstructed systemic blood flow, and obstructed pulmonary venous return present with early-onset, profound cyanosis and have significant morbidity and mortality.[4,11] The major forms of single-ventricle defects causing obstruction to systemic blood flow are listed in Table 10-2. Because HLHS is the most commonly encountered single-ventricle defect, much of the content in this chapter focuses on HLHS, reflecting the exhaustive efforts undertaken in recent decades to improve survival for this once uniformly fatal lesion.

Incidence and Prevalence of Single-Ventricle CHD

The overall incidence of CHD reported in the literature is quite variable, due to academic variations in the categorization of the various forms of CHD and changing patterns of diagnosis in recent decades.[12] It is generally recognized, however, that CHD affects approximately 0.8% of all births when bicuspid aortic valve and patent foramen ovale are excluded from consideration. The incidence of single-ventricle CHD is significantly less, although its exact incidence is once again difficult to pinpoint given the lack of a standardized definition of single-ventricle CHD in the literature and

the significant anatomic variability within the subgroup of single-ventricle lesions. In the landmark "Report of the New England Regional Infant Cardiac Program,"[13] published in 1980, the incidence of single-ventricle CHD, which for the purposes of this study included tricuspid atresia, HLHS, pulmonary atresia with intact ventricular septum, and undifferentiated single-ventricle lesions, was approximately 0.05% of live births (0.5 cases per 1000 live births). A narrower definition of single-ventricle CHD was used for the Baltimore-Washington Infant Study (1981-1989), wherein HLHS, tricuspid atresia, and pulmonary atresia with intact ventricular septum were excluded. In this study, the *prevalence* of single ventricle was far lower at 0.006% of live births, or 1.25% of all cases of CHD.[14] Regardless of these varying definitions, it is unlikely that the *incidence* of single-ventricle CHD in live births has changed significantly over time, as asymptomatic single-ventricle CHD evading detection in the newborn period is quite rare. However, the *prevalence* of single-ventricle CHD continues to increase commensurate with improved survival.[15] The most common form of single-ventricle CHD is HLHS, with an incidence of approximately 266 per 1,000,000 live births (approximately 1000 births/year in the United States).[16]

PATHOGENESIS AND GENETICS

The genetic causes of single-ventricle CHD are not yet entirely understood. Although approximately 40 genes have been implicated in nonsyndromic CHD (ie, the presence of CHD in the absence of a known identified genetic syndrome), most cases of CHD appear to be sporadic with multiple risk factors.[17] For single-ventricle CHD, mutations in *HAND1*,[18] *GJA1*,[19] and *NKX2.5*[20] have been reported in patients with HLHS, with an even larger number of individual gene mutations reported in patients with heterotaxy syndrome.[17,21] Several genetic syndromes are well known to be associated with single-ventricle forms of CHD, particularly HLHS: The Turner,[22] Rubenstein-Taybi,[23] Holt-Oram,[24] and Jacobsen syndromes[25] are all observed with an increased incidence of HLHS compared to the general population. In a recent report of 240 fetuses with HLHS evaluated at our center over a 5-year period, 9.2% had a major extracardiac genetic or chromosomal abnormality with the most commonly encountered syndromes being Turner syndrome, trisomy 18, and trisomy 13.[26] This incidence of major chromosomal abnormalities in HLHS is consistent with the incidence of chromosomal abnormalities (12.9%) in the large, albeit older, Baltimore-Washington Infant Study from the 1980s.[27] No specific environmental, infectious, or pharmacologic agent exposure has been implicated as a cause of single-ventricle CHD.

Although most occurrences of CHD are felt to be sporadic, an emerging body of evidence is beginning to decipher the heritable nature of some forms of single-ventricle CHD, particularly HLHS. Relationships between complex single-ventricle defects and less severe manifestations of CHD are coming to attention through careful family studies of patients with HLHS. As an example, less severe yet clinically significant left-sided heart abnormalities appear to exist with increased frequency in first-degree relatives of patients with HLHS. In 2004, Lewin et al.[28] reported the results of a study where the first-degree relatives of nonsyndromic patients with congenital aortic valve stenosis, coarctation of the aorta, bicuspid aortic valve, or HLHS underwent screening echocardiography for abnormalities of left ventricular outflow. In the 30 patients with HLHS in this study, 8 first-degree relatives had abnormalities of the mitral valve and left ventricular outflow tract. Recently, a study using genome-wide linkage analysis demonstrated that HLHS maps to multiple chromosomal loci, with a clear relationship of these loci to bicuspid aortic valve.[29] These studies suggest that there is a certain degree of heritability to left ventricular outflow tract obstruction. It is therefore reasonable to perform echocardiographic screening of first-degree relatives with HLHS in order to evaluate for bicuspid aortic valve and other left ventricular outflow tract abnormalities.

Due to the well-known incidence of familial clustering of CHD, the recurrence risk of CHD for first-degree relatives has been studied extensively.[30] Such information is obviously of great interest to parents of children with single-ventricle CHD as they assess their individual risk of CHD recurrence in future pregnancies.

A recent study of a large population from Denmark sheds light on this important question. For any pregnancy affected by CHD, the relative risk of recurrence of the same form of CHD in first-degree relatives was approximately 3, with significantly higher relative risks for specific defects such as heterotaxy syndrome, atrioventricular canal defects, and left ventricular outflow tract obstruction.[31] In a follow-up study from the same group, the relative risk of recurrence of another form of CHD in first-degree relatives was approximately 2 to 4 times above the background risk of CHD, depending on the specific defect found in the proband.[32] Nonetheless, in both studies, the proportion of CHD accounted for by familial recurrence was less than 5%, again suggesting that most cases of CHD are sporadic. In a large fetal series of approximately 6000 pregnancies, recurrence of CHD in fetuses of first-degree relatives with CHD was 2.7%.[33] Therefore, the occurrence of single-ventricle CHD in a family should prompt the performance of a fetal echocardiogram in any future pregnancies, with consideration given to early second-trimester fetal echocardiographic imaging.[34]

CLINICAL PRESENTATION

The clinical presentation of single-ventricle CHD is dependent on the specific defect and age at presentation. In the following text, common clinical presentations of single-ventricle CHD will be presented according to the following age groups: fetus, neonate, infant, and child. The clinical presentation of single-ventricle CHD is presented in additional detail in Chapter 5 (Evaluation and Therapy: Neonatal Critical Heart Disease). Signs and symptoms associated with single-ventricle CHD are listed in Table 10-3.

Fetal Diagnosis of Single-Ventricle CHD

Routine ultrasonographic screening of pregnant women in the United States during the second trimester (approximately 20 weeks of gestation) allows for identification of most forms of CHD. However, the rate of prenatal detection of CHD remains surprisingly low (<50%), although the rate of prenatal diagnosis appears to be increasing in recent decades.[35-37] Interestingly, single-ventricle forms of CHD, despite their relative rarity, may be more easily diagnosed than other forms of CHD (eg, transposition of the great vessels and other conotruncal defects) because single-ventricle CHD usually results in an obviously abnormal standard 4-chamber view of the heart.[35,38] Figure 10-1 demonstrates a normal fetal heart on echocardiography, and Figure 10-2 demonstrates an abnormal fetal heart with HLHS. The effect, if any, of

Presenting Signs and Symptoms of Single-Ventricle Congenital Heart Disease

- Single-ventricle defects with obstruction to systemic blood flow

  Poorly palpable femoral pulses

  Cool extremities

  Poor feeding

  Lethargy

  Hypothermia

  Acidosis

  Hypoglycemia

  Single second heart sound

- Single-ventricle defects with obstruction to pulmonary blood flow

  Cyanosis

  Single second heart sound

prenatal diagnosis of CHD on postnatal mortality from CHD is not yet clear. Although some studies have shown less short-term morbidity in infants prenatally diagnosed with CHD, there does not appear to be a measurable effect on survival.[39] Similar findings have been borne out by other studies from the past decade.[40-42]

In the fetus, single-ventricle CHD is typically well tolerated from a hemodynamic standpoint unless there are coexisting anatomic abnormalities such as significant atrioventricular valve regurgitation, ventricular dysfunction, or dysrhythmias. However, blood flow patterns through the fetus are altered in the presence

of single-ventricle CHD, as has been documented by a number of studies evaluating Doppler flow patterns in sites such as the fetal middle cerebral artery.[43,44] In the case of HLHS, the most highly saturated blood from the placenta (umbilical venous return passing through the ductus venosus) is directed from the right ventricle to ductus arteriosus and descending aorta, in comparison to the normal fetus, where umbilical venous return is directed across the foramen ovale to the mitral valve, left ventricle, and ascending aorta. This may have implications for neurologic development; several recent studies have shown that fetuses[45] and infants with HLHS[46] have smaller brain volumes and maturation than gestational age-matched controls. Infants with single-ventricle CHD also have been shown to have a high incidence of frank microcephaly as well as head circumferences disproportionately small when compared to weight.[47]

Although the effects on overall mortality from CHD are debatable, a prenatal diagnosis of single-ventricle CHD clearly offers significant benefits to the fetus and parents. First, prenatal recognition of the defect allows for the timely delivery of appropriate medical care to the infant upon delivery. Most infants with single-ventricle CHD will require prostaglandin infusion to maintain patency of the ductus arteriosus. It is clearly preferable for an intravenous prostaglandin infusion to be initiated in a controlled setting, in an infant not yet compromised by profound cyanosis or low cardiac output. In addition, the fetus with single-ventricle CHD may occasionally have additional anatomic features that, if unrecognized, quickly lead to hemodynamic instability. Given the relative rarity of these complicating features layered on top of an already

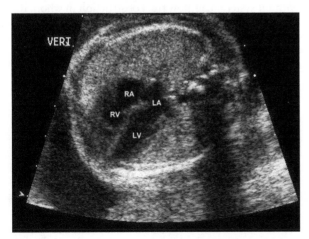

FIGURE 10-1 ■ Fetal echocardiogram at 22 weeks of gestation demonstrating normal heart position and structure from 4-chamber view. LA, left atrium; LV, left ventricle; RA, right atrium; RV, right ventricle.

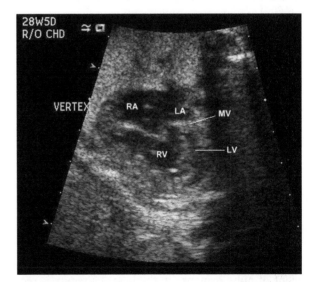

FIGURE 10-2 ■ Fetal echocardiogram at 25 weeks of gestation demonstrating size discrepancy of the left and right ventricles in a fetus with hypoplastic left heart syndrome HLHS. The mitral valve is atretic (imperforate), and the left ventricle is severely hypoplastic. LA, left atrium; LV, left ventricle; MV, mitral valve; RA, right atrium; RV, right ventricle.

uncommon disease, delivery of a fetus with single-ventricle CHD at a facility unfamiliar with or unprepared for a hemodynamically compromised infant may prove fatal. Examples of these additional anatomic features include restrictive or intact atrial septum in HLHS,[48] obstructed pulmonary venous return in forms of single-ventricle CHD associated with the heterotaxy syndrome,[49] and complete heart block associated with heterotaxy syndrome.[9] Ideally, all fetuses identified with single-ventricle CHD will be delivered at a tertiary center familiar with neonatal CHD. Early evaluation and treatment of infants with single-ventricle CHD may prevent or mitigate the potentially adverse consequences of postnatally diagnosed CHD that may manifest upon ductal closure, including profound cyanosis, circulatory collapse, shock, end-organ dysfunction, and even death. Additionally, identification of single-ventricle CHD allows the family time to prepare for the delivery of an infant with complex disease, to learn about the anatomy and anticipated postnatal treatment strategy, and importantly, to discuss options regarding continuation of the pregnancy.

Neonatal Presentation

Despite the increasing likelihood of prenatal diagnosis of single-ventricle CHD, a significant proportion are still identified postnatally, even following discharge from the newborn nursery.[50] Late neonatal presentation (ie, following discharge from the nursery) of single-ventricle CHD can occur for several reasons. First, ductal patency is frequently prolonged in infants with single-ventricle CHD; thus, the adverse hemodynamics conferred by ductal closure may not be immediately apparent. On physical examination, many infants with single-ventricle CHD have no cardiac murmurs. Although a single second heart sound may indicate hypoplasia or atresia of a semilunar valve, the presence or absence of splitting of the second heart sound can be difficult to appreciate at the higher heart rates present in the newborn. Finally, cyanosis is generally not apparent unless the oxygen saturation is less than 85%, and this threshold will be lower if the baby is anemic. Screening of all newborns with pulse oximetry in the lower extremity prior to discharge from the newborn nursery will detect cyanosis from both left and right heart obstructive lesions; however, this relatively inexpensive modality is not yet universally practiced in the United States.[36] It is important to note that the location of pulse oximetry measurement is vital in obtaining clinically relevant information. Measurement of pulse oximetry in the lower extremity is recommended because hypoxemia from lesions causing obstruction to both pulmonary and systemic blood flow will be detected. If pulse oximetry were measured from the upper extremity in a patient with duct-dependent systemic blood flow, relatively well-saturated blood

from the ascending aorta may lead to a falsely reassuring clinical picture.

The neonate with duct-dependent systemic blood flow from a left heart obstructive lesion (eg, HLHS) will typically present with signs and symptoms of low cardiac output. Clinically, this often manifests as lethargy, poor feeding with vomiting, and decreased urine output. On examination, the infant may be mottled, with cool extremities, hepatomegaly, and poorly palpable femoral and pedal pulses. Cyanosis may not be a cardinal presenting symptom unless there is obstruction to egress of pulmonary venous return (ie, restrictive or intact atrial septum in HLHS and other left heart obstructive lesions). These signs and symptoms of low cardiac output can easily be missed[51] and may be incorrectly attributed to sepsis; therefore, consideration of critical CHD and initiation of prostaglandin infusion must be given to any ill-appearing neonate.

In contrast, the neonate with duct-dependent pulmonary blood flow from a right heart obstructive lesion (eg, pulmonary atresia with intact ventricular septum) will present predominantly with cyanosis, which may be profound upon ductal closure. In the absence of ventricular dysfunction or atrioventricular valve regurgitation, cardiac output will typically be preserved, and acidosis is not frequently encountered.

Clinical Presentation in the Older Infant or Young Child

It is rare for single-ventricle CHD to present outside the neonatal period. However, there have been case reports of older children and adults presenting with HLHS in whom ductal patency persisted.[52,53] Late presentation of single-ventricle CHD may occur in instances of double-inlet left ventricle or other complex forms of CHD without systemic outflow tract obstruction in whom the balance of systemic and pulmonary artery blood flow is such that cyanosis is minimized, yet symptoms of pulmonary overcirculation are avoided as well. This group of patients can be difficult to manage surgically because they frequently have developed pulmonary vascular disease, making surgical palliative strategies along the single-ventricle pathway problematic.

DIFFERENTIAL DIAGNOSIS

The major differential diagnoses of single-ventricle CHD include sepsis (bacterial, viral, or fungal), pulmonary hypertension, cardiomyopathy, lung disease, shock, ingestion of toxic substances, and other forms of CHD. The most useful tool available to all clinicians to effectively screen for single-ventricle CHD among

Differential Diagnosis of Single Ventricle Congenital Heart Disease, Listed in Order of Severity

- Common conditions
  Other forms of congenital heart disease
  Pulmonary hypertension
  Cardiomyopathy
  Sepsis (bacterial, viral, fungal)
  Parenchymal lung disease
  Hypoglycemia
- Rare conditions
  Poisonings/intoxications (methemoglobinemia)

these conditions is the hyperoxia test. The hyperoxia test will distinguish cyanosis caused by lung disease from cyanosis caused by intracardiac mixing. The hyperoxia test is based on the principle that provision of supplemental oxygenation will improve or normalize systemic oxygenation in the setting of hypoxemia from lung disease, but will not improve or normalize in the setting of single-ventricle CHD. Specialized tools such as echocardiography, cardiac catheterization, and cardiac magnetic resonance imaging (MRI) are required to establish the specific diagnosis (see below). The major differential diagnoses of single-ventricle CHD are presented in Table 10-4. Until the diagnosis of single-ventricle CHD is excluded with certainty, it is recommended that prostaglandin infusion be initiated along with stabilization efforts in any infant in whom CHD is suspected.

DIAGNOSIS

Absent the history of a prenatal diagnosis, a history and physical examination can frequently lend important insights into the cardiac diagnosis after noncardiac disease processes are excluded. Even in the era of prenatal diagnosis, confirmation of the prenatal findings is important because the accuracy of fetal echocardiography is not 100%[54] and may vary from center to center depending on the skill and expertise of those making the diagnosis.[55] In cases of left heart obstruction, as outlined earlier, the history often elicits symptoms of poor feeding, lethargy, a weak cry, mottling, and cool extremities. Right heart obstructive lesions are notable for cyanosis of a varying degree. The physical examination should involve a complete set of vital signs, including 4-extremity blood pressures and an oxygen saturation measurement in the lower extremity. The cardiac physical examination may demonstrate several significant findings. The precordium is typically hyperdynamic on palpation, due to 1 ventricle

pumping both the systemic and pulmonary output. The first heart sound is typically normal, but in cases of single-ventricle CHD in which there is atresia or hypoplasia of a semilunar valve, the second heart sound is typically single. Normal splitting of the second heart sound virtually rules out single-ventricle CHD. As stated previously, murmurs are unusual; holosystolic murmurs may indicate clinically significant atrioventricular valve regurgitation.

The chest radiograph may be beneficial, although no specific shape or contour to the cardiothoracic silhouette is specific for single-ventricle CHD. The lung fields frequently appear oligemic in patients with right heart obstructive lesions, whereas congestion predominates in those with left heart obstructive lesions, particularly in the setting of a closing ductus. The electrocardiogram is rarely if ever diagnostic, but can confirm sinus rhythm and eliminate dysrhythmias that may complicate the clinical picture. In the current era, most if not all forms of single-ventricle CHD can be accurately diagnosed with 2-dimensional echocardiography with color flow and spectral Doppler analysis. Echocardiography has the advantage of being noninvasive and portable and can delineate anatomic information with high fidelity. Additionally, echocardiography can noninvasively assess ventricular function, and Doppler color flow analysis lends important information regarding valve function. In previous decades, most forms of CHD required cardiac catheterization with angiography for confirmation of diagnosis. Cardiac catheterization remains an important tool for obtaining hemodynamic data and performing interventions and is necessary for diagnostic purposes in rare instances in which there are multiple sources of pulmonary blood flow (eg, major aortopulmonary collaterals in the setting of tetralogy of Fallot with pulmonary atresia), uncertainties with respect to the systemic or pulmonary venous anatomy, or unexpected physiology. The role of cardiac MRI in the diagnosis of CHD remains an evolving process. Cardiac MRI has several advantages over echocardiography as a noninvasive diagnostic tool, particularly with respect to obtaining hemodynamic data and imaging of regions not well imaged by echocardiography (eg, distal branch pulmonary arteries). However, it requires specialized, nonportable equipment; in young children, it requires deep sedation and/or general anesthesia. A generalized algorithm for the diagnosis of single-ventricle CHD is presented in Figure 10-3.

TREATMENT

The general principles of treatment of single-ventricle CHD will be discussed below, whereas specific treatment pathways for each lesion will be discussed in the lesion-specific sections. A treatment algorithm for

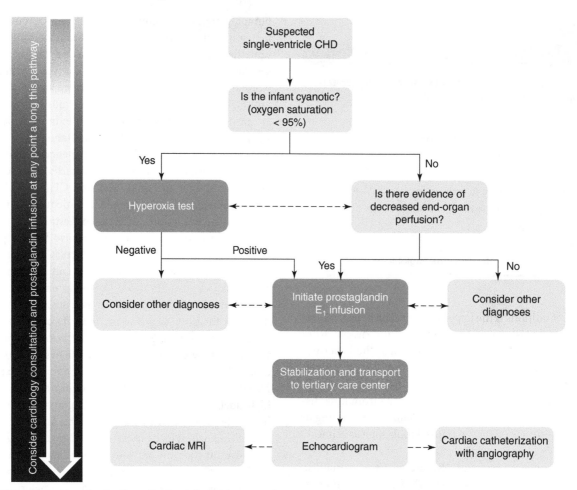

FIGURE 10-3 ■ Algorithm for diagnosis of an infant with suspected single-ventricle congenital heart disease (CHD). MRI, magnetic resonance imaging.

patients diagnosed with single-ventricle CHD is shown in Figure 10-4.

In single-ventricle CHD, a biventricular circulation frequently cannot be achieved on account of atresia or hypoplasia of atrioventricular valves, ventricles, and/or semilunar valves. In general, single-ventricle CHD is readily apparent on diagnostic investigation, and the decision to pursue a treatment strategy appropriate for the diagnosis is obvious. In some cases, however, the determination of suitability for a biventricular circulation is not apparent; these cases can be quite challenging for both the cardiologist and surgeon.[56-59] Treatment strategies for the so-called "borderline" left or right ventricle are beyond the scope of this chapter.

The major principle in treating single-ventricle CHD is to provide unobstructed systemic blood flow along with a stable source of pulmonary blood flow.[60] At the time of diagnosis, these goals can be accomplished with the use of prostaglandin to maintain patency of the ductus arteriosus. However, prolonged therapy with prostaglandin infusion is not a viable strategy. First, prostaglandin must be administered by continuous infusion,

making long-term treatment impractical. Prostaglandin infusion is also associated with important adverse side effects, including fever, rash, irritability, hypotension, and apnea.[61] Prolonged medical management of single-ventricle CHD is not desirable, and more durable surgical strategies are required.

In general, patients with single-ventricle CHD are subjected to a 3-stage surgical strategy culminating in the Fontan procedure; this strategy is frequently referred to as single-ventricle palliation or, more colloquially, as the "single-ventricle pathway." The details of single-ventricle palliation will be outlined below. It is important to recognize that the conduct, timing, and order of single-ventricle palliation are frequently individualized between individual centers and for individual patients. The first stage typically occurs in the neonatal period and involves a Norwood operation (for lesions with critically obstructed or ductal-dependent systemic blood flow), Blalock-Taussig shunt (for lesions with critically obstructed pulmonary blood flow), or pulmonary artery band (for lesions with unobstructed systemic and pulmonary blood flow). In some patients, pulmonary

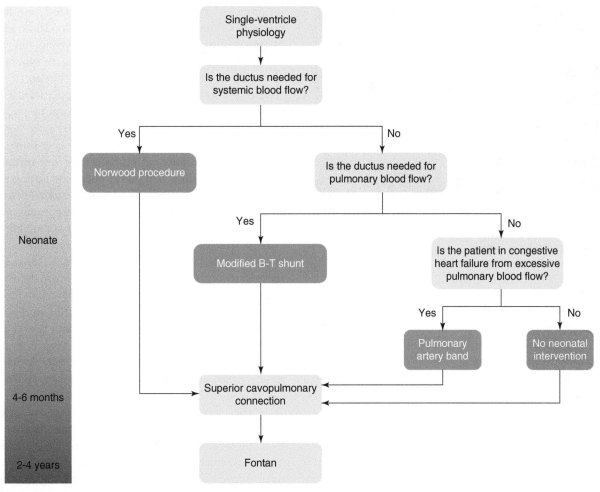

FIGURE 10-4 ■ Algorithm for treatment of an infant with confirmed single-ventricle congenital heart disease. B-T, Blalock-Taussig.

and systemic blood flows are well balanced, and no neonatal intervention may be required. Regardless of the neonatal approach, later in infancy (between 4 and 6 months of age), a superior cavopulmonary anastomosis is performed with removal of the Blalock-Taussig shunt. In this procedure, the superior vena cava is disconnected from the right atrium and is anastomosed in an end-to-side fashion with the right pulmonary artery. Following a superior cavopulmonary anastomosis, pulmonary blood flow is derived from passive flow from the superior vena cava into the pulmonary artery. The third and final stage of single-ventricle palliation involves an inferior cavopulmonary anastomosis, which is termed the Fontan procedure. In a Fontan procedure, the inferior vena cava is directly anastomosed to the right pulmonary artery such that systemic venous return from the lower half of the body is directed to the pulmonary arteries without an interposed pumping chamber. Regardless of the underlying defect, patients who have completed all 3 stages of single-ventricle palliation share the following characteristics: (1) passive return of systemic venous blood to the pulmonary arteries without an interposed

ventricle and (2) systemic cardiac output provided by the single ventricle.

LESION-SPECIFIC PATHWAYS

Lesions with Obstructed Systemic Blood Flow (Hypoplastic Left Heart Syndrome)

As discussed previously, the most common form of single-ventricle CHD leading to obstructed systemic blood flow is HLHS. Prior to the early 1980s, HLHS was a uniformly fatal diagnosis, with comfort care routinely provided to infants postnatally. The advent of the Norwood procedure, promulgated by Dr. William I. Norwood in 1983,[62] as well as infant heart transplantation, advocated by Dr. Leonard Bailey,[63] have radically changed the outlook for this group of patients from nearly certain neonatal mortality to approximately 90% survival beyond the neonatal period. In HLHS, atresia

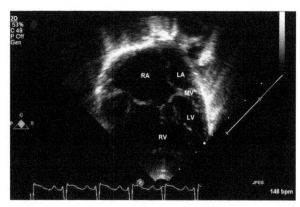

FIGURE 10-5 ■ Apical 4-chamber echocardiographic view of infant with hypoplastic left heart syndrome. Note the marked size discrepancy between the right ventricle (RV) and left ventricle (LV). LA, left atrium; MV, mitral valve; RA, right atrium.

or hypoplasia of the mitral and/or aortic valves is associated with severe underdevelopment of the left ventricle, such that it is unable to maintain adequate systemic cardiac output without assistance from the right ventricle via the ductus arteriosus.[2]

In the "classic" form of HLHS, the mitral and aortic valves are present but imperforate. The left ventricle is tiny or nearly entirely absent (Figure 10-5). It is important to recognize that a variable spectrum of hypoplasia of the left heart structures is encountered in HLHS. The left atrium is usually small, and the entire aortic arch is hypoplastic with coarctation. Important variations of HLHS include severely unbalanced atrioventricular canal defects, double-outlet right ventricle with mitral atresia, critical aortic valve stenosis, and dysplasia of the mitral valve with left ventricular dysfunction. The right heart structures are typically normal; however, the tricuspid valve may demonstrate abnormalities in 25% of patients,[64] occasionally leading to clinically important tricuspid regurgitation. In the fetus, HLHS is typically well tolerated as the right ventricle maintains cardiac output, albeit at a value lower than normal.[65] Following birth and closure of the ductus, however, low cardiac output and death will ensue unless prostaglandin infusion and proper resuscitative measures are taken. Typically, a patent foramen ovale allows pulmonary venous return to the left atrium to pass in an unobstructed fashion to the right atrium in HLHS. However, in approximately 5% of cases of HLHS, the atrial septum is intact or severely restrictive, leading to refractory cyanosis and hypoxemia if not treated promptly via balloon atrial septostomy.[48] These infants have a particularly high mortality, and survivors frequently are afflicted with pulmonary vascular disease.

Following stabilization of the infant, the Norwood procedure is typically performed at several days of age as a means of surgical palliation. There are 3 main objectives to the Norwood procedure when applied to HLHS:

(1) provision of unobstructed systemic blood flow; (2) provision of a stable source of pulmonary blood flow; and (3) provision of unobstructed pulmonary venous return. In HLHS, the right ventricle is recruited as the systemic ventricle. In the Norwood procedure, a "neoaorta" is created by disconnecting the branch pulmonary arteries from the main pulmonary artery and performing a side-to-side anastomosis of the main pulmonary artery with the hypoplastic ascending aorta.[66] Figure 10-6 shows a depiction of the Norwood procedure. At our institution, this anastomosis is typically augmented using an allograft (cadaveric human blood vessel material) patch. Pulmonary blood flow is then established by means of a systemic-to-pulmonary artery shunt, such as a modified Blalock-Taussig shunt or right ventricular-to-pulmonary artery conduit (Sano modification).[67] Finally, an atrial septectomy is performed to ensure unobstructed egress of pulmonary venous return from the left atrium. Following the Norwood procedure, the right ventricle pumps cardiac output to both the lungs and body, and the oxygen saturation typically ranges from 80% to 90%. By limiting pulmonary blood flow, the systemic-to-pulmonary artery shunt prevents symptoms of heart failure from excessive pulmonary blood flow.

The Norwood operation was initially associated with very high mortality. In the recent era, however, short-term outcomes have improved dramatically, with survival to hospital discharge now approximately 90% in experienced centers.[68-70] Between 4 and 6 months of age, the second stage of single-ventricle palliation is performed. The period between the Norwood procedure and second-stage palliation ("interstage period") is a high-risk time for the infant. Infants palliated with a Norwood procedure have an inherently unstable circulation in that pulmonary blood flow is provided solely from a shunt; distortion or thrombosis of the shunt occurs in approximately 10% of patients and may lead to unacceptable cyanosis and even sudden death.[71] Infants between the first and second stage of single-ventricle palliation tolerate normal physiologic stressors (eg, fever, dehydration, intercurrent respiratory infections) poorly; there remains an approximately 15% risk of death in this population during the interstage period.[72] In response to this high interstage attrition, many centers have instituted intensive home monitoring programs for these fragile infants between the first and second stages of single-ventricle palliation.[73]

The second stage of single-ventricle palliation is the superior cavopulmonary anastomosis (Figure 10-7). The term "second stage" is somewhat of a misnomer, because patients with well-balanced systemic and pulmonary blood flow may have a superior cavopulmonary connection performed as their first surgical intervention. A cardiac catheterization is typically performed prior to second-stage palliation for a full hemodynamic evaluation. Cardiac MRI is playing an emerging role in

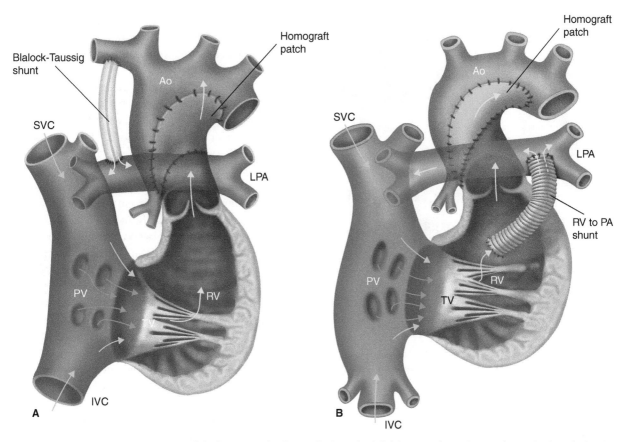

FIGURE 10-6 ■ Pictorial representation of the first stage of palliation for hypoplastic left heart syndrome (Norwood procedure). Both the classic Norwood procedure using a right modified Blalock-Taussig shunt **(A)** and the Sano modification using a right ventricle-to-pulmonary artery conduit **(B)** are shown. Note how homograft patch material is used to create a "neoaorta" comprising elements of the main pulmonary artery and hypoplastic ascending aorta. Ao, aorta; IVC, inferior vena cava; LPA, left pulmonary artery; PA, pulmonary artery; PV, pulmonary veins; RV, right ventricle; SVC, superior vena cava; TV, tricuspid valve. (*Adapted with permission, from Barron DJ, Kilby MD, Davies B, et al. Hypoplastic left heart syndrome.* Lancet. *2009;374:551-564. Copyright Elsevier.*)

the evaluation of anatomy and hemodynamics in this patient population and may obviate the need for invasive cardiac catheterization in the future.[74] At the time of the superior cavopulmonary anastomosis, the superior vena cava is connected to the right pulmonary artery in an end-to-side fashion. Variations in surgical technique have led to various eponymously named procedures common in clinical practice; the most frequently encountered terms for the second stage include the Glenn and hemi-Fontan procedures.[75,76] Regardless of surgical technique, following the superior cavopulmonary anastomosis, systemic venous return from the upper half of the body returns directly to the lungs without passing through the right ventricle. This has the effect of reducing the volume load imposed upon the right ventricle following the Norwood procedure,[77] although systemic oxygen saturation typically remains similar to that following the Norwood procedure. Low pulmonary artery pressures are necessary for a successful superior cavopulmonary anastomosis; therefore, the procedure is typically not performed until 3 to 6 months of age, when pulmonary vascular resistance has fallen to normal adult levels.

Survival following the superior cavopulmonary anastomosis is expected, with postoperative mortality being uncommon.[78,79] However, with growth, cyanosis becomes more prominent as the lower half of the body contributes a higher proportion of systemic venous return. As such, the third stage of single-ventricle palliation is typically performed between 2 and 4 years of age. This third stage is commonly referred to as the Fontan procedure. In the Fontan procedure, blood flow from the inferior vena cava is directed into the pulmonary arteries (Figure 10-8). Various techniques for the Fontan procedure have been described since its introduction in the early 1970s.[80] Currently, the Fontan procedure is performed by means of either an extracardiac conduit or an intra-atrial tunnel. Following the Fontan procedure, all systemic venous return enters the lungs passively, without an interposed pumping chamber. The right ventricle receives only oxygenated pulmonary venous return and serves as the systemic ventricle. This hemodynamic arrangement is accomplished at the expense of slightly higher central venous pressure and nonpulsatile pulmonary blood flow. In some patients, central venous pressure may be pathologically elevated postoperatively,

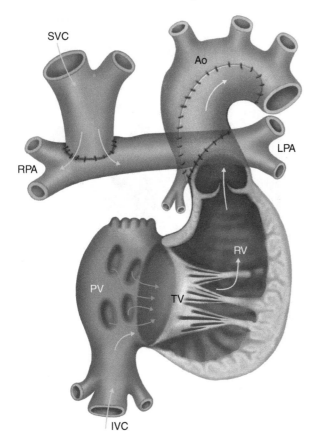

FIGURE 10-7 ■ Pictorial representation of the second stage of single-ventricle palliation. In this image, the anatomy is that of hypoplastic left heart syndrome following the Norwood procedure. Note the superior cavopulmonary connection, or end-to-side anastomosis of the superior vena cava to the right pulmonary artery. Ao, aorta; IVC, inferior vena cava; LPA, left pulmonary artery; PV, pulmonary veins; RV, right ventricle; RPA, right pulmonary artery; SVC, superior vena cava; TV, tricuspid valve. (*Adapted with permission, from Barron DJ, Kilby MD, Davies B, et al. Hypoplastic left heart syndrome.* Lancet. *2009;374:551-564. Copyright Elsevier.*)

leading to ascites and pleural effusions. To mitigate against the adverse effects of an acutely elevated central venous pressure, a fenestration is often placed within the Fontan pathway at the time of surgery,[81] although the decision to place a fenestration remains surgeon- and center-specific. Fenestration allows for decompression of the Fontan pathway into the right atrium if central venous pressures become elevated, thereby maintaining cardiac output in the event of increased impedance to flow through the pulmonary arterial bed. Fenestration maintains adequate cardiac output at the expense of cyanosis, however. In patients with a fenestration, oxygen saturations are approximately 85%; absent a fenestration, oxygen saturations in a patient with Fontan physiology are at the lower limit of normal (low 90% range). The oxygen saturation in patients with Fontan physiology is never completely normal, due to highly desaturated blood from the coronary sinus draining

into the right atrium (which has been excluded from the systemic venous return by the Fontan pathway),[81] as well as to microscopic pulmonary arteriovenous malformations.

Although staged surgical palliation culminating in the Fontan procedure is now the accepted standard of care for treatment of HLHS at most centers, alternative treatment pathways proposed during the early years of the Norwood procedure are still practiced, with newer approaches also being promulgated. Although comfort care remains advocated by some,[82] the continually improving outcomes in recent years has made this strategy more difficult to justify. In the first years following introduction of the Norwood procedure, very high mortality led to the concept of infant heart transplantation for HLHS.[63] Rather than undergoing the Norwood procedure, infants were listed for heart transplantation while maintained on prostaglandin infusion. Although the short-term outcomes of this approach are quite favorable, the limited pool of donor organs, limited life span of a transplanted heart due to chronic graft rejection, and steadily improving outcomes of the Norwood operation have led to diminished enthusiasm for this strategy as primary treatment for HLHS.[83] Nonetheless, heart transplantation retains a very important therapeutic role in treating life-threatening myocardial dysfunction at any point along the single-ventricle palliation pathway.

Due in part to increased recognition of the adverse effects of cardiopulmonary bypass on the neurodevelopmental outcomes of children with HLHS, a new strategy for the treatment of HLHS and similar lesions has been termed the "hybrid procedure."[84,85] In this approach, named as such due to the collaborative efforts of cardiac surgeons and pediatric interventional cardiologists, the neonate with HLHS undergoes pulmonary artery banding—a procedure not requiring cardiopulmonary bypass or deep hypothermic circulatory arrest—in conjunction with transcatheter stenting of the ductus arteriosus. Subsequently, a modified form of the superior cavopulmonary anastomosis is performed between 4 and 6 months of age. Whether this strategy represents an advantage over the traditional surgical approach for HLHS remains unanswered.

Lesions with Obstruction to Pulmonary Blood Flow

Single-ventricle lesions with obstruction to pulmonary blood flow represent a more diverse group than left heart obstructive lesions. The major variants of this lesion include pulmonary atresia with intact ventricular septum, tricuspid atresia, and double-inlet left ventricle. In addition, there are several rare lesions that defy easy attempts at categorization, including superoinferior

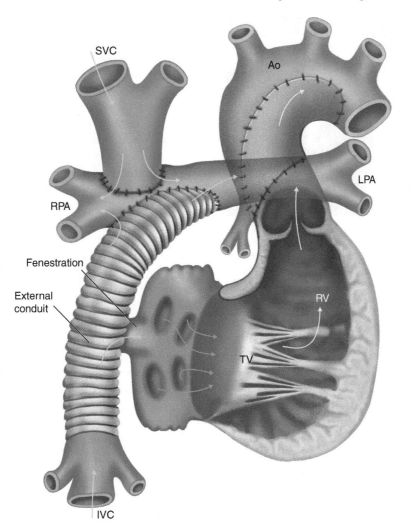

FIGURE 10-8 ■ Pictorial representation of the third stage of single-ventricle palliation (Fontan procedure). In this image, the anatomy is that of HLHS following the first 2 stages of single-ventricle palliation. Note how the inferior vena cava (IVC) is anastomosed to the right pulmonary artery via an extracardiac conduit. The lateral tunnel variation of the Fontan procedure is not shown. Ao, aorta; LPA, left pulmonary artery; RPA, right pulmonary artery; RV, right ventricle; SVC, superior vena cava; TV, tricuspid valve. (*Adapted with permission, from Barron DJ, Kilby MD, Davies B, et al. Hypoplastic left heart syndrome. Lancet. 2009;374:551-564. Copyright Elsevier.*)

ventricles, crisscross atrioventricular relationships, and "true" single ventricle; discussion of these lesions is beyond the scope of this chapter. In the paragraphs that follow, the relevant anatomic characteristics of pulmonary atresia with intact ventricular septum, tricuspid atresia, and double-inlet left ventricle will be briefly described, followed by a discussion regarding their surgical management.

Tricuspid Atresia

Tricuspid atresia was one of the earliest single-ventricle lesions treated with successful surgical palliation. The first report of the Fontan procedure in 1972 concerned a patient with tricuspid atresia.[86] In tricuspid atresia, an atretic tricuspid valve leads to underdevelopment of the right ventricle (Figure 10-9). There are several different anatomic subtypes of tricuspid atresia, which are grouped according to the presence or absence of a ventricular septal defect as well as the relationship of the great arteries. The most common anatomic subtype of tricuspid atresia (70%-80%) is with a ventricular septal defect and normally related great vessels. Tricuspid atresia can occur with transposition of the great arteries, the physiology of which mimics that of HLHS (discussed earlier).

In tricuspid atresia with normally related great vessels and a ventricular septal defect, systemic venous return is shunted right to left across an obligatory atrial communication, which then completely mixes with pulmonary venous return in the left atrium. The size of the

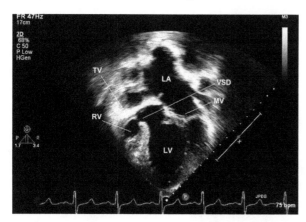

FIGURE 10-9 ■ Apical 4-chamber echocardiographic view of infant with tricuspid atresia. Note the muscular plate located in place of the normal tricuspid valve position and the hypoplastic right ventricle, which communicates to the normal size left ventricle by way of a ventricular septal defect. LA, left atrium; LV, left ventricle; MV, mitral valve; RV, right ventricle; TV, tricuspid valve; VSD, ventricular septal defect.

ventricular septal defect determines the physiology and clinical presentation. In patients with no ventricular septal defect, pulmonary atresia results, and the patient is entirely ductal-dependent for pulmonary blood flow. In patients with a large ventricular septal defect, pulmonary blood flow may be unrestricted and symptoms of congestive heart failure from excessive left-to-right shunting can occur as pulmonary vascular resistance falls during the newborn period. Many patients with tricuspid atresia and a ventricular septal defect have a moderate-sized ventricular septal defect, which confers some restriction to pulmonary blood flow and allows for balancing of systemic and pulmonary blood flow.

The treatment of tricuspid atresia and normally related great vessels is determined based on the anatomic subtype and the underlying physiology. In patients with a large ventricular septal defect and symptoms of congestive heart failure, pulmonary artery banding may be necessary in the neonatal period to control pulmonary blood flow and symptoms of congestive heart failure. In contrast, patients with a very small ventricular septal defect or pulmonary atresia will require an additional source of pulmonary blood flow (eg, modified Blalock-Taussig shunt) to prevent excessive cyanosis. Regardless of the neonatal treatment strategy (pulmonary artery band versus Blalock-Taussig shunt), these patients undergo superior cavopulmonary connection between 4 and 6 months of age, followed by Fontan completion between 2 and 4 years of age. The conduct of the superior cavopulmonary connection and Fontan completion in patients with right heart obstructive lesions is generally identical to that of patients with HLHS. Although reports from earlier series demonstrated worse outcomes in patients with a systemic right ventricle and a Fontan circulation (eg, patients with HLHS) than those

with a systemic left ventricle (eg, patients with tricuspid atresia), recent reports of long-term follow-up in patients with Fontan physiology have not demonstrated this association.[87,88]

It is important to reiterate the concept of "balancing" pulmonary and systemic blood flow in understanding the treatment strategies in patients with tricuspid atresia. While inadequate pulmonary blood flow leads to cyanosis and excessive pulmonary blood flow leads to congestive heart failure, some patients attain a physiologic balance between systemic and pulmonary blood flow such that neither extreme is reached. Patients with moderate-sized ventricular septal defects in the setting of tricuspid atresia may have well-balanced systemic and pulmonary blood flow, with no neonatal intervention required. These patients typically have moderately restrictive ventricular septal defects that limit pulmonary blood flow. This group of patients can undergo superior cavopulmonary connection as an initial procedure between 4 and 6 months of age, followed by Fontan completion at 2 to 4 years of age. It is also important to recognize that patients with moderate-sized ventricular septal defects and apparently well-balanced systemic and pulmonary blood flow must be followed carefully, because restriction to ventricular septal defect flow can occur insidiously or precipitously.

Pulmonary Atresia with Intact Ventricular Septum

In pulmonary atresia with intact ventricular septum (PA/IVS), sometimes referred to as "hypoplastic right heart syndrome," there is an atretic pulmonary valve in association with hypoplasia (of a variable degree) of the tricuspid valve and right ventricle.[89] PA/IVS is a rare condition, occurring in 0.07 per 1000 live births (approximately half the incidence of HLHS).[13] Extracardiac abnormalities in PA/IVS appear to be uncommon.

In PA/IVS, pulmonary blood flow is supplied solely by the ductus arteriosus. A hallmark of this lesion is a hypoplastic or dysplastic tricuspid valve, which is associated with a severely hypertrophied, hypertensive right ventricle (Figure 10-10). The degree of right ventricular hypertension is impressive, with right ventricular systolic pressure often significantly higher than the systemic blood pressure. Not infrequently, there is coronary artery involvement in this disease, which has important implications for management. In approximately 30% to 45% of patients, "sinusoids" or primitive vascular connections between the right ventricle and distal coronary arterial bed maintain distal coronary perfusion.[90,91] In a smaller proportion of patients, proximal interruptions of the coronary artery system are present in patients with PA/IVS. Coronary blood flow distal to these interruptions is of necessity provided from the hypertensive

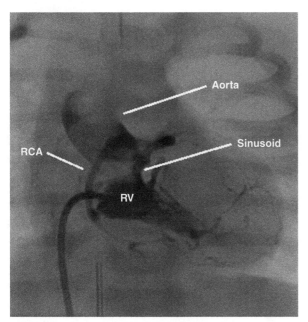

FIGURE 10-10 ■ Right ventricular angiogram in a patient with pulmonary atresia with intact ventricular septum. The catheter courses from inferior vena cava to the right atrium, through the hypoplastic tricuspid valve, and into the hypoplastic right ventricle (RV). There are several connections between the right ventricular cavity and coronary arteries; the largest (labeled sinusoid) leads to the right coronary artery (RCA).

right ventricle via sinusoids. The combination of proximal coronary artery interruptions, sinusoids, and a hypertensive right ventricle leads to the entity of "right ventricular-dependent coronary circulation," a unique physiologic situation in which distal coronary perfusion is maintained by a hypertensive right ventricle.

PA/IVS is typically identified prenatally by marked size discrepancy between the right and left ventricles.[92] Postnatally, profound cyanosis will occur in the absence of ductal patency. The diagnosis is confirmed by echocardiography; however, diagnostic cardiac catheterization is often required to document the status of the coronary arteries and to rule out right ventricular dependence of the distal coronary circulation. At our institution, PA/IVS represents one of the few remaining forms of CHD in which diagnostic cardiac catheterization remains mandatory prior to any interventions, as no other imaging modality is able to reliably determine the presence of right ventricular–dependent coronary circulation.

The treatment strategy for PA/IVS hinges on 2 factors: the size of the tricuspid valve annulus and the presence of right ventricular–dependent coronary circulation. If the tricuspid valve annulus diameter is less than 2 standard deviations below the mean normalized for age and body surface area, a successful biventricular circulation is unlikely and the patient should be palliated along the single-ventricle pathway.[91] This would include placement of a modified Blalock-Taussig shunt

in the neonatal period, followed by superior cavopulmonary connection at 3 to 6 months of age and Fontan completion at 2 to 4 years of age as described earlier for HLHS. If the tricuspid valve annulus diameter is larger than this threshold value, consideration can be given to surgical or transcatheter procedures aimed at re-establishing continuity between the right ventricle and main pulmonary artery, with the ultimate goal of attaining a biventricular circulation. Recent data demonstrate that approximately 30% of patients are candidates for a biventricular approach to repair, with approximately 80% to 90% 5-year survival.[93,94] Such an approach is contraindicated, however, in the presence of right ventricular–dependent coronary circulation. Re-establishing continuity between the right ventricle and pulmonary artery will decompress the hypertensive right ventricle and lead to a coronary steal phenomenon, coronary ischemia, and myocardial infarction.

Historically, survival in patients with PA/IVS was thought to be less favorable than other forms of single-ventricle CHD, possibly on account of the unique coronary artery abnormalities encountered in this population. In the current era, outcomes of patients with PA/IVS palliated along the single-ventricle pathway appear to be comparable to single-ventricle palliation for other lesions, excepting patients with coronary artery atresia, who continue to have very poor outcomes.[95]

Double-Inlet Left Ventricle

In double-inlet left ventricle (DILV), both the mitral and tricuspid valves enter the left ventricle. In DILV, the left ventricle is the dominant ventricle. A ventricular septal defect is typically present, leading to a right ventricular outflow tract. In most cases of DILV, both ventricular inversion and transposition of the great vessels are present. The dominant left ventricle is rightward and posterior to the diminutive anterior and leftward right ventricle (Figure 10-11). Additionally, the aorta is leftward and anterior to the pulmonary artery and arises from the right ventricle. Rarely, DILV with normally related great vessels occurs and is eponymously referred to as Holmes heart. The anatomic subtypes of DILV are described in detail in several excellent references.[96,97]

DILV is rare, with an incidence similar to that of PA/IVS at 0.1 cases per 100,000 live births.[13] The clinical presentation and surgical strategy depend primarily on the degree of obstruction to flow through the ventricular septal defect and whether the great artery arising from the diminutive right ventricle exhibits obstruction. Ultimately, patients with DILV require single-ventricle palliation to a Fontan procedure as described earlier in this chapter, with long-term outcomes and complications similar to other patients undergoing single-ventricle palliation.

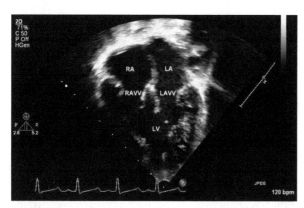

FIGURE 10-11 ■ Apical 4-chamber echocardiographic view of infant with double inlet left ventricle. Note the 2 atrioventricular valves emptying into the single left ventricle. The small right ventricle is not seen in this imaging plane. LA, left atrium; LAVV, left atrioventricular valve; RA, right atrium; RAVV, right atrioventricular valve.

Neurodevelopmental Outcomes, Quality of Life, and Exercise Capacity in Patients with Single Ventricle

The improvements in long-term survival following the Fontan procedure for all forms of single ventricle now mean that most patients born with single-ventricle physiology in the developed world can expect to live into adulthood. With these remarkable improvements, attention is increasingly being turned to maximizing the quality of life for these patients.

Neurodevelopmental abnormalities appear to be particularly common in patients with single-ventricle CHD. The substrate for abnormal brain development appears to begin in utero, as evidenced by the abnormal fetal and preoperative neuroimaging findings in patients with complex CHD described earlier in this chapter. Layered on top of this abnormal substrate are the neurologic insults conferred by cardiopulmonary bypass and deep hypothermic circulatory arrest. Patients with HLHS have been the most closely studied with respect to neurodevelopmental status among single-ventricle patients. Several studies from the past decade reveal that survivors of the Norwood procedure display abnormalities in motor and cognitive domains of child development.[98,99] Intelligence appears to be decreased slightly from population norms. In addition, more subtle deficiencies in attention and behavior have been observed in the HLHS population at a rate significantly higher than that expected in the general population.[100] Recognition of these abnormalities has led to attempts to mitigate their severity along all aspects of the care spectrum, including cardiopulmonary bypass strategies, postoperative monitoring in the intensive care unit, and targeted neurodevelopmental surveillance in the community.

Quality of life is also being closely studied in pediatric and adult survivors of single-ventricle palliation.

New cardiac-specific quality-of-life measurement tools have been validated and are currently being applied to the CHD population.[101] Many studies have evaluated quality-of-life characteristics in single-ventricle patients following Fontan, although the results are conflicting with respect to the existence and magnitude of patient- and parent-perceived deficiencies in quality-of-life measures.[102-109] One of the common themes in many of these studies, however, is decreased physical activity level that appears to be multifactorial in etiology. Although formal measures of exercise capacity in patients with a Fontan circulation are decreased compared to healthy controls,[110] a positive relationship between abnormalities in exercise testing and diminished quality of life are not apparent.[111]

CONCLUSION

Application of the single-ventricle palliation strategy has led to impressive increases in survival for what was recently considered a fatal disease. Long-term (>5 year) survival of patients with single-ventricle CHD following the Fontan procedure is approximately 85%,[87,88] and patients born with HLHS today can expect to live well into their 20s. However, when factors other than survival are considered, the long-term outcomes of single-ventricle palliation are far from certain. The physiology of the Fontan circulation is not normal, and patients and their providers are becoming increasingly aware of long-term morbidities such as atrial arrhythmias,[112] failure of the systemic right ventricle,[113] protein-losing enteropathy, and plastic bronchitis.[112,114,115] Once complications such as these have developed, heart transplantation may be the only viable strategy for long-term survival.[116,117] However, newer medical therapies[118,119] and mechanical assist devices[120] for the Fontan circulation are being developed, which may offer hope for maximizing the longevity of the Fontan circulation while maintaining acceptable quality of life. The serious problems encountered by long-term survivors of the Fontan procedure serve as a reminder that treatment of single ventricle is palliative rather than curative.

Clinical Pearls

- Infants with single-ventricle type of congenital heart disease in which there is increased pulmonary blood flow (ie, HLHS) may present with very little cyanosis at birth.
- Although supplemental oxygen may be detrimental to infants with single ventricle and obstruction to systemic flow, supplemental oxygen may be administered to infants with suspicion of single ventricle who are markedly hypoxic with arterial partial pressure of oxygen of less than 30 torr.

- The period of time between first-stage palliation of single ventricle with an aortopulmonary shunt and the second stage of superior cavopulmonary connection is a fragile one. Challenges in some infants may include difficulty feeding, poor weight gain, and decreased oxygenation.
- The surgical strategy for single ventricle allows for survival by mimicking the normal circulation. Desaturated venous blood is passively channeled to the lungs through the Fontan connections, and oxygenated blood is pumped to the body by the single ventricle. The absence of a pulmonary ventricle results in abnormal physiology and important negative long-term consequences.
- Factors that increase pulmonary vascular resistance such as lung disease or high altitude may hinder passive forward flow, diminish filling of the single ventricle, and limit cardiac output after Fontan operation.
- Sudden changes in weight, tight-fitting clothes, or swelling may be a sign of protein-losing enteropathy after Fontan operation.
- Recurrent, inexplicable cough with expectoration of thick mucus or bronchial casts may be a sign of plastic bronchitis after Fontan operation.
- Children and adolescents with single ventricle and Fontan circulation may be permitted to exercise; however, their capacity and endurance typically decline in the adolescent and early adult years.
- Creating a good quality and lengthy duration of life remains a challenging goal and is the next frontier for children with single-ventricle congenital heart disease.

REFERENCES

1. Nelson DP, Schwartz SM, Chang AC. Neonatal physiology of the functionally univentricular heart. *Cardiol Young.* 2004;14(Suppl 1):52-60.
2. Barron DJ, Kilby MD, Davies B, et al. Hypoplastic left heart syndrome. *Lancet.* 2009;374(9689):551-564.
3. Iyer GK, Van Arsdell GS, Dicke FP, et al. Are bilateral superior vena cavae a risk factor for single ventricle palliation? *Ann Thorac Surg.* 2000;70:711-716.
4. Lodge AJ, Rychik J, Nicolson SC, et al. Improving outcomes in functional single ventricle and total anomalous pulmonary venous connection. *Ann Thorac Surg.* 2004;78:1688-1695.
5. Khairy P, Poirier N, Mercier L. Univentricular heart. *Circulation.* 2007;115:800-812.
6. Cohen MS, Anderson RH, Cohen MI, et al. Controversies, genetics, diagnostic assessment, and outcomes relating to the heterotaxy syndrome. *Cardiol Young.* 2007;17:29-43.
7. Lim HG, Bacha EA, Marx GR, et al. Biventricular repair in patients with heterotaxy syndrome. *J Thorac Cardiovasc Surg.* 2009;137:371-379.
8. Cohen MS, Schultz AH, Tian Z, et al. Heterotaxy syndrome with functional single ventricle: does prenatal diagnosis improve survival? *Ann Thorac Surg.* 2006;82:1629-1636.
9. Glatz AC, Gaynor JW, Rhodes LA, et al. Outcome of high-risk neonates with congenital complete heart block paced in the first 24 hours after birth. *J Thorac Cardiovasc Surg.* 2008;136:767-773.
10. Kelle AM, Backer CL, Tsao S, et al. Dual-chamber epicardial pacing in neonates with congenital heart block. *J Thorac Cardiovasc Surg.* 2007;134:1188-1192.
11. Glatz JA, Tabbutt S, Gaynor JW, et al. Hypoplastic left heart syndrome with atrial level restriction in the era of prenatal diagnosis. *Ann Thorac Surg.* 2007;84:1633-168.
12. van der Bom T, Zomer AC, Zwinderman AH, et al. The changing epidemiology of congenital heart disease. *Nat Rev Cardiol.* 2011;8:50-60.
13. Report of the New England Regional Infant Cardiac Program. *Pediatrics.* 1980;65:377-461.
14. Steinberger EK, Ferencz C, Loffredo CA. Infants with single ventricle: a population-based epidemiological study. *Teratology.* 2002;65:106-115.
15. Warnes CA, Liberthson R, Danielson GK Jr, et al. Task Force 1: the changing profile of congenital heart disease in adult life. *J Am Coll Cardiol.* 2001;37:1170-1175.
16. Hoffman JIE, Kaplan S. The incidence of congenital heart disease. *J Am Coll Cardiol.* 2002;39:1890-1900.
17. Wessels M, Willems P. Genetic factors in non-syndromic congenital heart malformations. *Clin Genet.* 2010;78: 103-123.
18. Reamon-Buettner SM, Ciribilli Y, Inga A, Borlak J. A loss-of-function mutation in the binding domain of HAND1 predicts hypoplasia of the human hearts. *Hum Mol Genet.* 2008;17:1397-1405.
19. Dasgupta C, Martinez AM, Zuppan CW, et al. Identification of connexin43 (alpha$_1$) gap junction gene mutations in patients with hypoplastic left heart syndrome by denaturing gradient gel electrophoresis (DGGE). *Mutat Res.* 2001;479:173-186.
20. McElhinney DB, Geiger E, Blinder J, Woodrow Benson D, Goldmuntz E. NKX2.5 mutations in patients with congenital heart disease. *J Am Coll Cardiol.* 2003;42:1650-1655.
21. Belmont JW, Mohapatra B, Towbin JA, Ware SM. Molecular genetics of heterotaxy syndromes. *Curr Opin Cardiol.* 2004;19:216-220.
22. Reis PM, Punch MR, Bove EL, van de Ven CJ. Outcome of infants with hypoplastic left heart and Turner syndromes. *Obstet Gynecol.* 1999;93:532-535.
23. Stevens CA, Bhakta MG. Cardiac abnormalities in the Rubinstein-Taybi syndrome. *Am J Med Genet.* 1995;59:346-348.
24. Bruneau BG, Logan M, Davis N, et al. Chamber-specific cardiac expression of Tbx5 and heart defects in Holt–Oram syndrome. *Dev Biol.* 1999;211:100-108.
25. Grossfeld PD, Mattina T, Lai Z, et al. The 11q terminal deletion disorder: a prospective study of 110 cases. *Am J Med Genet A.* 2004;129A:51-61.
26. Rychik J, Szwast A, Natarajan S, et al. Perinatal and early surgical outcome for the fetus with hypoplastic left heart syndrome: a 5-year single institutional experience. *Ultrasound Obstet Gynecol.* 2010;36:465-470.
27. Ferencz C, Neill CA, Boughman JA, et al. Congenital cardiovascular malformations associated with chromosome abnormalities: an epidemiologic study. *J Pediatr.* 1989;114:79-86.
28. Lewin MB, McBride KL, Pignatelli R, et al. Echocardiographic evaluation of asymptomatic parental and sibling cardiovascular anomalies associated with congenital left

ventricular outflow tract lesions. *Pediatrics*. 2004;114: 691-696.

29. Hinton RB, Martin LJ, Rame-Gowda S, et al. Hypoplastic left heart syndrome links to chromosomes 10q and 6q and is genetically related to bicuspid aortic valve. *J Am Coll Cardiol*. 2009;53:1065-1071.

30. Calcagni G, Digilio MC, Sarkozy A, Dallapiccola B, Marino B. Familial recurrence of congenital heart disease: an overview and review of the literature. *Eur J Pediatr*. 2007;166:111-116.

31. Oyen N, Poulsen G, Boyd HA, et al. Recurrence of congenital heart defects in families. *Circulation*. 2009;120:295-301.

32. Øyen N, Poulsen G, Wohlfahrt J, et al. Recurrence of discordant congenital heart defects in families. *Circ Cardiovasc Genet*. 2010;3:122-128.

33. Gill HK, Splitt M, Sharland GK, Simpson JM. Patterns of recurrence of congenital heart disease: an analysis of 6,640 consecutive pregnancies evaluated by detailed fetal echocardiography. *J Am Coll Cardiol*. 2003;42:923-929.

34. Johnson B, Simpson LL. Screening for congenital heart disease: a move toward earlier echocardiography. *Am J Perinatol*. 2007;24:449-456.

35. Friedberg MK, Silverman NH, Moon-Grady AJ, et al. Prenatal detection of congenital heart disease. *J Pediatr*. 2009;155:26-31.

36. Mahle WT, Newburger JW, Matherne GP, et al. Role of pulse oximetry in examining newborns for congenital heart disease: a scientific statement from the AHA and AAP. *Pediatrics*. 2009;124:823-836.

37. Khoshnood B, De Vigan C, Vodovar V, et al. Trends in prenatal diagnosis, pregnancy termination, and perinatal mortality of newborns with congenital heart disease in France, 1983-2000: a population-based evaluation. *Pediatrics*. 2005;115:95-101.

38. Chew C, Halliday JL, Riley MM, Penny DJ. Population-based study of antenatal detection of congenital heart disease by ultrasound examination. *Ultrasound Obstet Gynecol*. 2007;29:619-624.

39. Levey A, Glickstein JS, Kleinman CS, et al. The impact of prenatal diagnosis of complex congenital heart disease on neonatal outcomes. *Pediatr Cardiol*. 2010;31:587-597.

40. Sivarajan V, Penny DJ, Filan P, Brizard C, Shekerdemian LS. Impact of antenatal diagnosis of hypoplastic left heart syndrome on the clinical presentation and surgical outcomes: the Australian experience. *J Paediatr Child Health*. 2009;45:112-117.

41. Tzifa A, Barker C, Tibby SM, Simpson JM. Prenatal diagnosis of pulmonary atresia: impact on clinical presentation and early outcome. *Arch Dis Child Fetal Neonatal Ed*. 2007;92:F199-F203.

42. Mahle WT, Clancy RR, McGaurn SP, Goin JE, Clark BJ. Impact of prenatal diagnosis on survival and early neurologic morbidity in neonates with the hypoplastic left heart syndrome. *Pediatrics*. 2001;107:1277-1282.

43. Szwast A, Tian Z, McCann M, Donaghue D, Rychik J. Vasoreactive response to maternal hyperoxygenation in the fetus with hypoplastic left heart syndrome. *Circ Cardiovasc Imaging*. 2010;3:172-178.

44. Kaltman JR, Di H, Tian Z, Rychik J. Impact of congenital heart disease on cerebrovascular blood flow dynamics in the fetus. *Ultrasound Obstet Gynecol*. 2005;25:32-36.

45. Limperopoulos C, Tworetzky W, McElhinney DB, et al. Brain volume and metabolism in fetuses with congenital heart disease: evaluation with quantitative magnetic resonance imaging and spectroscopy. *Circulation*. 2010;121:26-33.

46. Licht DJ, Shera DM, Clancy RR, et al. Brain maturation is delayed in infants with complex congenital heart defects. *J Thorac Cardiovasc Surg*. 2009;137:529-536.

47. Shillingford AJ, Ittenbach RF, Marino BS, et al. Aortic morphometry and microcephaly in hypoplastic left heart syndrome. *Cardiol Young*. 2007;17:189-195.

48. Rychik J, Rome JJ, Collins MH, DeCampli WM, Spray TL. The hypoplastic left heart syndrome with intact atrial septum: atrial morphology, pulmonary vascular histopathology and outcome. *J Am Coll Cardiol*. 1999;34: 554-560.

49. Heinemann MK, Hanley FL, Van Praagh S, et al. Total anomalous pulmonary venous drainage in newborns with visceral heterotaxy. *Ann Thorac Surg*. 1994;57:88-91.

50. Dorfman AT, Marino BS, Wernovsky G, et al. Critical heart disease in the neonate: presentation and outcome at a tertiary care center. *Pediatr Crit Care Med*. 2008;9:193-202.

51. Chang RK, Gurvitz M, Rodriguez S. Missed diagnosis of critical congenital heart disease. *Arch Pediatr Adolesc Med*. 2008;162:969-974.

52. Vargas-Barron J, Rijlaarsdam M, Romero-Cardenas A, et al. Hypoplastic left heart syndrome: report of a case of spontaneous survival to adulthood. *Am Heart J*. 1992;123:1713-1719.

53. Ehrlich M, Bierman FZ, Ellis K, Gersony WM. Hypoplastic left heart syndrome: report of a unique survivor. *J Am Coll Cardiol*. 1986;7:361-365.

54. Gottliebson WM, Border WL, Franklin CM, Meyer RA, Michelfelder EC. Accuracy of fetal echocardiography: a cardiac segment-specific analysis. *Ultrasound Obstet Gynecol*. 2006;28:15-21.

55. Meyer-Wittkopf M, Cooper S, Sholler G. Correlation between fetal cardiac diagnosis by obstetric and pediatric cardiologist sonographers and comparison with postnatal findings. *Ultrasound Obstet Gynecol*. 2001;17:392-397.

56. Jonas RA. Fontan or septation: when I abandon septation in complex lesions with two ventricles. *Semin Thorac Cardiovasc Surg Pediatr Card Surg Annu*. 2009:94-98.

57. Szwast AL, Marino BS, Rychik J, et al. Usefulness of left ventricular inflow index to predict successful biventricular repair in right-dominant unbalanced atrioventricular canal. *Am J Cardiol*. 2011;107:103-109.

58. Grosse-Wortmann L, Yun TJ, Al-Radi O, et al. Borderline hypoplasia of the left ventricle in neonates: insights for decision-making from functional assessment with magnetic resonance imaging. *J Thorac Cardiovasc Surg*. 2008;136:1429-1436.

59. Jegatheeswaran A, Pizarro C, Caldarone CA, et al. Echocardiographic definition and surgical decision-making in unbalanced atrioventricular septal defect: a Congenital Heart Surgeons' Society multiinstitutional study. *Circulation*. 2010;122(11 Suppl):S209-S215.

60. Jaquiss RD, Imamura M. Single ventricle physiology: surgical options, indications and outcomes. *Curr Opin Cardiol*. 2009;24:113-118.

61. Meckler GD, Lowe C. To intubate or not to intubate? Transporting infants on prostaglandin E1. *Pediatrics.* 2009;123(1):e25-e30.

62. Norwood WI, Lang P, Hansen DD. Physiologic repair of aortic atresia-hypoplastic left heart syndrome. *N Engl J Med.* 1983;308:23-26.

63. Razzouk AJ, Chinnock RE, Gundry SR, et al. Transplantation as a primary treatment for hypoplastic left heart syndrome: intermediate-term results. *Ann Thorac Surg.* 1996;62:1-8.

64. Martinez R. Assessment of the tricuspid valve in hypoplastic left heart syndrome. *Cardiol Young.* 2004;14:27-33.

65. Szwast A, Tian Z, McCann M, Donaghue D, Rychik J. Right ventricular performance in the fetus with hypoplastic left heart syndrome. *Ann Thorac Surg.* 2009;87:1214-1219.

66. Reemtsen BL, Pike NA, Starnes VA. Stage I palliation for hypoplastic left heart syndrome: Norwood versus Sano modification. *Curr Opin Cardiol.* 2007;22:60-65.

67. Ohye RG, Sleeper LA, Mahony L, et al. Comparison of shunt types in the Norwood procedure for single-ventricle lesions. *N Engl J Med.* 2010;362:1980-1992.

68. Mair R, Tulzer G, Sames E, et al. Right ventricular to pulmonary artery conduit instead of modified Blalock-Taussig shunt improves postoperative hemodynamics in newborns after the Norwood operation. *J Thorac Cardiovasc Surg.* 2003;126:1378-1384.

69. Tabbutt S, Dominguez TE, Ravishankar C, et al. Outcomes after the stage I reconstruction comparing the right ventricular to pulmonary artery conduit with the modified Blalock Taussig shunt. *Ann Thorac Surg.* 2005;80:1582-1591.

70. Azakie A, Martinez D, Sapru A, et al. Impact of right ventricle to pulmonary artery conduit on outcome of the modified Norwood procedure. *Ann Thorac Surg.* 2004;77:1727-1733.

71. O'Connor MJ, Ravishankar C, Ballweg JA, et al. Early systemic-to-pulmonary artery shunt intervention in neonates with congenital heart disease. *J Thorac Cardiovasc Surg.* 2011;142:106-112.

72. Hehir DA, Dominguez TE, Ballweg JA, et al. Risk factors for interstage death after stage 1 reconstruction of hypoplastic left heart syndrome and variants. *J Thorac Cardiovasc Surg.* 2008;136:94-99.

73. Ghanayem NS, Cava JR, Jaquiss RD, Tweddell JS. Home monitoring of infants after stage one palliation for hypoplastic left heart syndrome. *Semin Thorac Cardiovasc Surg Pediatr Card Surg Annu.* 2004;7:32-38.

74. Brown DW, Gauvreau K, Powell AJ, et al. Cardiac magnetic resonance versus routine cardiac catheterization before bidirectional Glenn anastomosis in infants with functional single ventricle: a prospective randomized trial. *Circulation.* 2007;116:2718-2725.

75. Jacobs ML, Pourmoghadam KK. The hemi-Fontan operation. *Semin Thorac Cardiovasc Surg Pediatr Card Surg Annu.* 2003;6:90-97.

76. Freedom RM, Nykanen D, Benson LN. The physiology of the bidirectional cavopulmonary connection. *Ann Thorac Surg.* 1998;66:664-667.

77. Donofrio MT, Jacobs ML, Spray TL, Rychik J. Acute changes in preload, afterload, and systolic function after superior cavopulmonary connection. *Ann Thorac Surg.* 1998;65:503-508.

78. Kogon BE, Plattner C, Leong T, et al. The bidirectional Glenn operation: a risk factor analysis for morbidity and mortality. *J Thorac Cardiovasc Surg.* 2008;136:1237-1242.

79. Scheurer MA, Hill EG, Vasuki N, et al. Survival after bidirectional cavopulmonary anastomosis: analysis of preoperative risk factors. *J Thorac Cardiovasc Surg.* 2007;134:82-89.

80. de Leval MR. Evolution of the Fontan-Kreutzer procedure. *Semin Thorac Cardiovasc Surg Pediatr Card Surg Annu.* 2010;13:91-95.

81. Gentles TL, Mayer JE Jr, Gauvreau K, et al. Fontan operation in five hundred consecutive patients: factors influencing early and late outcome. *J Thorac Cardiovasc Surg.* 1997;114:376-391.

82. Kon AA. Healthcare providers must offer palliative treatment to parents of neonates with hypoplastic left heart syndrome. *Arch Pediatr Adolesc Med.* 2008;162:844-848.

83. Chrisant MR, Naftel DC, Drummond-Webb J, et al. Fate of infants with hypoplastic left heart syndrome listed for cardiac transplantation: a multicenter study. *J Heart Lung Transplant.* 2005;24:576-582.

84. Chen Q, Parry AJ. The current role of hybrid procedures in the stage 1 palliation of patients with hypoplastic left heart syndrome. *Eur J Cardiothorac Surg.* 2009;36:77-83.

85. Galantowicz M, Cheatham JP, Phillips A, et al. Hybrid approach for hypoplastic left heart syndrome: intermediate results after the learning curve. *Ann Thorac Surg.* 2008;85:2063-2071.

86. Kreutzer GO, Schlichter AJ, Kreutzer C. The Fontan/Kreutzer procedure at 40: an operation for the correction of tricuspid atresia. *Semin Thorac Cardiovasc Surg Pediatr Card Surg Annu.* 2010;13:84-90.

87. Hirsch JC, Goldberg C, Bove EL, et al. Fontan operation in the current era: a 15-year single institution experience. *Ann Surg.* 2008;248:402-410.

88. Mitchell ME, Ittenbach RF, Gaynor JW, et al. Intermediate outcomes after the Fontan procedure in the current era. *J Thorac Cardiovasc Surg.* 2006;131:172-180.

89. Shinebourne EA, Rigby ML, Carvalho JS. Pulmonary atresia with intact ventricular septum: from fetus to adult: congenital heart disease. *Heart.* 2008;94:1350-1357.

90. Giglia TM, Mandell VS, Connor AR, Mayer JE Jr, Lock JE. Diagnosis and management of right ventricle-dependent coronary circulation in pulmonary atresia with intact ventricular septum. *Circulation.* 1992;86:1516-1528.

91. Hanley FL, Sade RM, Blackstone EH, et al. Outcomes in neonatal pulmonary atresia with intact ventricular septum. A multiinstitutional study. *J Thorac Cardiovasc Surg.* 1993;105:406-424.

92. Salvin JW, McElhinney DB, Colan SD, et al. Fetal tricuspid valve size and growth as predictors of outcome in pulmonary atresia with intact ventricular septum. *Pediatrics.* 2006;118:e415-e420.

93. Daubeney PE, Wang D, Delany DJ, et al. Pulmonary atresia with intact ventricular septum: predictors of early and medium-term outcome in a population-based study. *J Thorac Cardiovasc Surg.* 2005;130:1071e1-1071e9.

94. Odim J, Laks H, Tung T. Risk factors for early death and reoperation following biventricular repair of pulmonary

atresia with intact ventricular septum. *Eur J Cardiothorac Surg.* 2006;29:659-665.

95. Guleserian KJ, Armsby LB, Thiagarajan RR, del Nido PJ, Mayer JE Jr. Natural history of pulmonary atresia with intact ventricular septum and right-ventricle-dependent coronary circulation managed by the single-ventricle approach. *Ann Thorac Surg.* 2006;81:2250-2258.

96. Keane JF, Keane DC. Single ventricle. In: Keane JF, Lock JE, Fyler DC, eds. *Nadas' Pediatric Cardiology.* 2nd ed. Philadelphia, PA: Elsevier, 2006:743-750.

97. Cook AC, Anderson RH. The anatomy of hearts with double inlet ventricle. *Cardiol Young.* 2006;16(Suppl 1): 22-26.

98. Mahle WT, Visconti KJ, Freier MC, et al. Relationship of surgical approach to neurodevelopmental outcomes in hypoplastic left heart syndrome. *Pediatrics.* 2006;117: e90-e97.

99. Tabbutt S, Nord AS, Jarvik GP, et al. Neurodevelopmental outcomes after staged palliation for hypoplastic left heart syndrome. *Pediatrics.* 2008;121:476-483.

100. Shillingford AJ, Glanzman MM, Ittenbach RF, et al. Inattention, hyperactivity, and school performance in a population of school-age children with complex congenital heart disease. *Pediatrics.* 2008;121:e759-e767.

101. Marino BS, Tomlinson RS, Wernovsky G, et al. Validation of the pediatric cardiac quality of life inventory. *Pediatrics.* 2010;126:498-508.

102. McCrindle BW, Williams RV, Mitchell PD, et al. Relationship of patient and medical characteristics to health status in children and adolescents after the Fontan procedure. *Circulation.* 2006;113:1123-1129.

103. Lambert LM, Minich LL, Newburger JW, et al. Parent-versus child-reported functional health status after the Fontan procedure. *Pediatrics.* 2009;124:e942-e949.

104. McCrindle BW, Williams RV, Mital S, et al. Physical activity levels in children and adolescents are reduced after the Fontan procedure, independent of exercise capacity, and are associated with lower perceived general health. *Arch Dis Child.* 2007;92:509-514.

105. Manlhiot C, Knezevich S, Radojewski E, et al. Functional health status of adolescents after the Fontan procedure: comparison with their siblings. *Can J Cardiol.* 2009;25:e294-e300.

106. Uzark K, Jones K, Slusher J, et al. Quality of life in children with heart disease as perceived by children and parents. *Pediatrics.* 2008;121:e1060-e1067.

107. Muller J, Christov F, Schreiber C, Hess J, Hager A. Exercise capacity, quality of life, and daily activity in the long-term follow-up of patients with univentricular

heart and total cavopulmonary connection. *Eur Heart J.* 2009;30:2915-2920.

108. van den Bosch AE, Roos-Hesselink JW, Van Domburg R, et al. Long-term outcome and quality of life in adult patients after the Fontan operation. *Am J Cardiol.* 2004;93:1141-1145.

109. d'Udekem Y, Cheung MM, Setyapranata S, et al. How good is a good Fontan? Quality of life and exercise capacity of Fontans without arrhythmias. *Ann Thorac Surg.* 2009;88:1961-1969.

110. Paridon SM, Mitchell PD, Colan SD, et al. A cross-sectional study of exercise performance during the first 2 decades of life after the Fontan operation. *J Am Coll Cardiol.* 2008;52:99-107.

111. McCrindle BW, Zak V, Sleeper LA, et al. Laboratory measures of exercise capacity and ventricular characteristics and function are weakly associated with functional health status after Fontan procedure. *Circulation.* 2010;121:34-42.

112. Stephenson EA, Lu M, Berul CI, et al. Arrhythmias in a contemporary fontan cohort: prevalence and clinical associations in a multicenter cross-sectional study. *J Am Coll Cardiol.* 2010;56:890-896.

113. Lopez L, Cohen MS, Anderson RH, et al. Unnatural history of the right ventricle in patients with congenitally malformed hearts. *Cardiol Young.* 2010;20(Suppl 3):107-112.

114. Rychik J. Forty years of the Fontan operation: a failed strategy. *Semin Thorac Cardiovasc Surg Pediatr Card Surg Annu.* 2010;13:96-100.

115. Goldberg DJ, Dodds K, Rychik J. Rare problems associated with the Fontan circulation. *Cardiol Young.* 2010;20(Suppl 3):113-119.

116. Lamour JM, Kanter KR, Naftel DC, et al. The effect of age, diagnosis, and previous surgery in children and adults undergoing heart transplantation for congenital heart disease. *J Am Coll Cardiol.* 2009;54:160-165.

117. Jayakumar KA, Addonizio LJ, Kichuk-Chrisant MR, et al. Cardiac transplantation after the Fontan or Glenn procedure. *J Am Coll Cardiol.* 2004;44:2065-2072.

118. Reinhardt Z, Uzun O, Bhole V, et al. Sildenafil in the management of the failing Fontan circulation. *Cardiol Young.* 2010;20:522-525.

119. Thacker D, Patel A, Dodds K, et al. Use of oral budesonide in the management of protein-losing enteropathy after the Fontan operation. *Ann Thorac Surg.* 2010;89:837-842.

120. Rodefeld MD, Coats B, Fisher T, et al. Cavopulmonary assist for the univentricular Fontan circulation: von Karman viscous impeller pump. *J Thorac Cardiovasc Surg.* 2010;140:529-536.

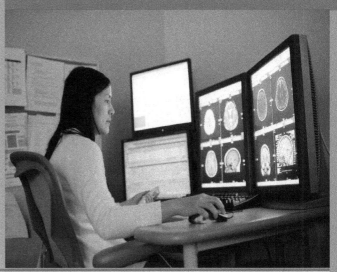

CHAPTER 11

Neurodevelopment in Children with Complex Congenital Heart Disease

*Marianne Glanzman,
Daniel Licht and Gil Wernovsky*

EPIDEMIOLOGY

Approximately 40,000 children are born in North America each year with congenital heart disease (CHD). Approximately half of these children require no therapy, because the defect is relatively minor (eg, a bicuspid aortic valve) or spontaneously heals (eg, a small ventricular septal defect). However, in the other half of these children, surgical or catheter intervention is necessary. For some of the children in this group, the CHD does not cause hypoxemia, circulatory insufficiency, or symptoms; these children typically undergo repair on an elective basis in childhood (eg, atrial septal defects or progressive valvar disease). In this group of school-age children, it has been shown that there is little to no impact on the central nervous system from either the unrepaired defect or from the effects of anesthesia, surgery, or postoperative care following the repair.[1]

In contrast, it is now increasingly recognized that the group of children with CHD severe enough to require surgery shortly after birth (eg, transposition of the great arteries [TGA], hypoplastic left heart syndrome [HLHS], total anomalous pulmonary venous return) or in early infancy (eg, tetralogy of Fallot, atrioventricular canal, large ventricular septal defects) are at increased risk for neurologic, behavioral, and psychological abnormalities as they mature. For the purposes of this chapter, we will discuss the findings on the group of children who require surgery in early infancy—those considered to have "complex congenital heart disease" (cCHD).

With improvements in diagnosis, surgery, and perioperative care, it is estimated that 95% of children born in 2010 with cCHD will survive into childhood and beyond. Current research discussed below suggests that approximately half will have neurologic, behavioral,

psychosocial, or cognitive abnormalities. Unless there is a decrease in the prevalence of these problems, over the next 2 decades it is estimated that an additional 130,000 children will enter the U.S. school system at significant risk for educational, interpersonal, and, ultimately, occupational impairment (Figure 11-1).

PATHOGENESIS

Initially, it was presumed that hypoxemia, intraoperative factors, or both were the likely causes of adverse developmental outcome, but current data suggest that the factors are multiple and probably interactive. Children with cCHD have an increased risk for congenital structural central nervous system (CNS) abnormalities and presurgical white matter injury, stroke, hemorrhage, and microcephaly. About 50% have neurologic or neurobehavioral abnormalities before their first surgery, including hyper- or hypotonia, motor asymmetry, micro- or macrocephaly, jitteriness, poor state regulation, and/or a weak suck reflex. The specific cardiac defect also plays a role in subsequent developmental risk. It appears that differences in fetal blood flow and substrate delivery that occur in the presence of cCHD lead to immaturity of brain development and render term infants with cCHD vulnerable to the types of brain injury seen in premature infants.[2,3]

Multiple factors can contribute to brain injury during and after surgical repair (Table 11-1). The type of support during surgery (deep hypothermic circulatory arrest versus continuous cardiopulmonary bypass) has been studied extensively, and although prolonged use of either is clearly disadvantageous, the nature of the defect that leads to the prolonged surgical time may be critical rather than the technique itself. Other factors

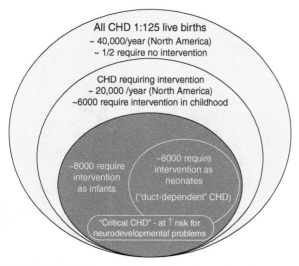

FIGURE 11-1 ■ Scope of the problem. Approximately 14,000 infants born each year are at risk for neurodevelopmental impairment secondary to complex congenital heart disease (CHD) requiring intervention early in life.

necessary because the nutritional and oxygen demands of the growing fetus can no longer be satisfied by diffusion alone. The development of the brain begins concurrent with cardiovascular development but continues throughout the pregnancy with a dramatic increase in brain size in the third trimester of gestation (Figure 11-2A) due to elaboration of neuronal microstructure (eg, dendrites, axons, synapses) and the onset of myelination, which continues for many years postnatally. The formation and refinement of connections in the brain require neuronal activity and glial maturation. These both lead to an increase in brain metabolism with dependence on heart function for oxygen and substrate delivery.

Down (trisomy 21), Williams (chromosome 7q11 deletion), Noonan (several genes), and DiGeorge (chromosome 22q microdeletion) syndromes are examples of known genetic causes of both cardiac malformations and neurodevelopmental deficits. There are likely additional, as yet unidentified, genetic effects on both heart and brain because similar morphogenetic events in brain and heart development engage many of the same genes such as sonic hedgehog[4] (progenitor proliferation and outflow tract development) and notch/jagged[7] (cardiac and neural progenitor cell fate, cardiac ventricle formation, and angiogenesis).

It has long been observed that the head circumferences in infants with cCHD are smaller than those of infants of similar gestational ages without cCHD[3,8] (Figure 11-2B). Not only are the head circumferences smaller, but infants with CHD are prone to a hypoxic-ischemic white matter injury that is not distinguishable from periventricular leukomalacia, an injury seen primarily in premature infants (Figure 11-3). Importantly, in mixed populations of infants with cCHD, this injury is seen in about 20% of patients before surgery and in over 50% after surgery.[2]

include the degree of cooling, use of hemodilution, and type of blood gas and pH management. Postoperative factors have been studied less frequently but appear to include hemodynamic lability leading to reduced cerebral blood flow and oxygen delivery, hyperthermia, and the length of the intensive care unit stay itself.[2,3]

Early brain and heart organogenesis occurs simultaneously in the human fetus. Similar developmental programs are invoked for both systems including stem and progenitor cell proliferation, cell fate commitment, migration, and left/right and dorsal/ventral patterning.[4-6] The cardiovascular system is the first organ system to function in the embryo and is complete at about 8 to 10 weeks of gestational age. This precocious development is

Potential Etiologies of Central Nervous System Abnormalities in Children with Complex Congenital Heart Disease

Fetal	Preoperative	Intraoperative	Postoperative	Other
Abnormal cerebral resistance	Decreased cerebral blood flow	Hypothermia	Hypoxemia	Parental stress
Decreased cerebral blood flow	Decreased oxygen delivery	Anesthetic agents	Hypotension	Socioeconomic status
Decreased oxygen delivery	Cardiac arrest	Cardiopulmonary bypass	Cardiac arrest	Genetic syndromes
Low birth weight	Paradoxical embolus	Circulatory arrest	Decreased cerebral blood flow	Genetic polymorphisms
Prematurity		Regional cerebral perfusion	Embolism	
		Glucose management	Hypothermia	

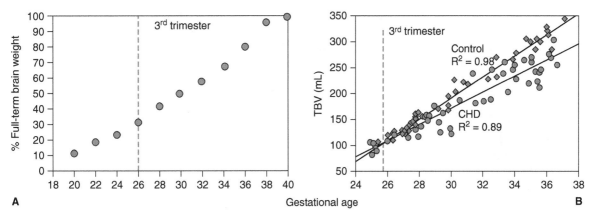

FIGURE 11-2 ■ **A.** Expected in utero brain growth as a percentage of full-term brain weight. There is a rapid rise in brain growth during the third trimester. **B.** A comparison of measured total brain volumes (TBV) from fetal brain magnetic resonance imaging in fetuses with congenital heart disease (CHD) (*open circles*) and fetuses without CHD (*filled squares*). (*Adapted with permission from Limperopoulos C, Tworetzky W, McElhinney DB, et al. Brain volume and metabolism in fetuses with congenital heart disease: evaluation with quantitative magnetic resonance imaging and spectroscopy.* Circulation. *2010;121:26-33.*).

Relative to the normal control newborns, newborns with cCHD had 10% lower N-acetylaspartate/choline ratios and 4.5% higher diffusivity on nuclear magnetic resonance spectroscopy.[9] Comparing these data to values obtained from normal fetuses suggests that term newborns with cCHD have a delay in brain development

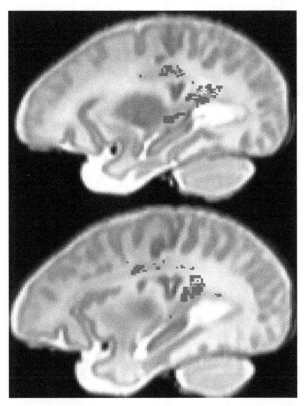

FIGURE 11-3 ■ Typical distribution of periventricular leukomalacia (PVL) lesions from 9 presurgical patients with either hypoplastic left heart syndrome (HLHS) or transposition of the great arteries (TGA). The tracings are overlaid on a brain atlas composed of a composite of 42 T2 volumetric brain magnetic resonance images (33 with HLHS and 19 with TGA).

of approximately 1 month, equivalent to an infant born prematurely at 34 to 36 weeks. Licht et al.[8] evaluated brain maturation in 42 full-term (average gestational age, 38.9 ± 1.1 weeks) infants born with CHD prior to surgery. Based on (1) degree of myelination, (2) degree of cortical folding, (3) the radiographic presence or absence of germinal matrix in the anterior and posterior horns of the lateral ventricles, and (4) the presence and number of migrating bands of glial cells, these infants had symmetric delays in brain development across all 4 areas assessed, appropriate for infants born at 35 weeks of gestation. Similarly, using fetal magnetic resonance images, Limperopoulos et al.[3] performed a cross-sectional study comparing brain volumes in fetuses with and without CHD. They concluded that there was divergence of brain growth starting at the beginning of the third trimester[3] (Figure 11-2B). Thus, the finding of a delay of 4 to 5 weeks is consistent across institutions and studies.

The areas of the affected white matter (Figure 11-3) are homologous to the periventricular areas rich in premyelinating oligodendrocytes in animal models. Failure of nutrient and oxygen delivery during late gestation, transition from fetal to neonatal blood flow, or postnatal/presurgical care results in white matter ischemia in the areas of brain (periventricular white matter) where premyelinating oligodendrocytes reside. Delayed brain development, at the biochemical, cellular, and structural levels, may underlie the preponderance of injury to periventricular white matter in term newborns with cCHD as well as the increased risk for an open operculum.[2,3,8,9]

More recently, it has been shown that the abnormal circulation in cCHD will cause significant abnormalities of cerebral blood flow in the fetus. In the fetus without CHD, gas exchange occurs in the placenta. Oxygenated blood returns through the umbilical vein and ductus venosus to the portal vein, inferior vena cava,

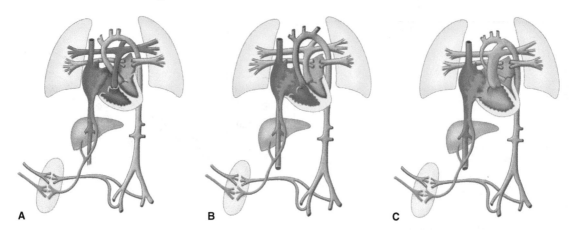

FIGURE 11-4 ■ **A.** Normal fetal circulation: Red (oxygenated) blood from the placenta is preferentially streamed from the ductus venosus through the right atrium to the left side of the heart and then pumped via the ascending aorta to the brain and body. **B.** Fetal circulation with transposition of the great arteries: Red blood circulates normally to the left heart structures but is then pumped via the common pulmonary artery to the ductus arteriosus and the descending aorta. Blue (low oxygen–containing) blood returns to the right atrium from the body and the brain and is pumped via the ascending aorta to the brain. **C.** Fetal circulation with hypoplastic left heart syndrome: Complete mixing of red and blue blood occurs at the level of the right atrium. Blood is pumped to the common pulmonary artery and the ductus arteriosus. Antegrade flow delivers blood to the lower body, and retrograde flow in the transverse arch delivers blood to the head and brain. (*Adapted with permission from Johnson, BA and Ades, A. Delivery room and early postnatal management of neonates who have prenatally diagnosed congenital heart disease.* Clinics in Perinatology. *2005;32:921-946.*).

and right atrium and deoxygenated blood returns to the placenta via the umbilical artery (Figure 11-4A). Prior to birth, blood flow to the lungs is very low due to elevated pulmonary vascular resistance and relatively low lung volumes. Two connections exist between the systemic and pulmonary circulations: the foramen ovale connecting the right and left atria, and the ductus arteriosus between the pulmonary trunk and descending aorta. Oxygenated umbilical venous blood is preferentially directed through the ductus venosus into the left lobe of the liver. As a result, the oxygen saturation is higher in the left hepatic veins as they join the inferior vena cava, resulting in streams of blood with different saturations. The higher saturated stream containing blood from the ductus venosus is preferentially directed across the foramen ovale to the left atrium. This blood mixes with the limited amount of pulmonary venous blood returning from the lungs. The resulting oxygen saturation in the fetal left ventricle, and thus to the brain, is approximately 65%. Blood ejected by the right ventricle consists of venous blood from the superior vena cava, as well as the relatively desaturated streams from the inferior vena cava and coronary sinus. The resulting oxygen saturation in the fetal right ventricle is approximately 55%.

In most forms of cCHD, the abnormal anatomy will lead to abnormalities of fetal oxygen content, differences in intravascular streaming, and/or changes in cerebral vascular resistance, all of which may lead to abnormalities of cerebral oxygen delivery. For example, in TGA and HLHS, specific alterations in fetal blood flow may lead to decreased brain oxygen delivery. In TGA, the aorta arises from the right ventricle and thus receives the relatively desaturated blood from the superior vena cava and lower saturation stream of blood in the inferior vena

cava (Figure 11-4B). The higher saturated stream from the left hepatic veins is directed normally across the foramen ovale to the morphologic left ventricle. The left ventricle, however, is connected to the pulmonary trunk, and this higher saturated blood (approximately 65%) is delivered to the lungs and lower body. In HLHS, the fetal circulation is characterized by obstructed antegrade flow at the level of the left atrium. This results in reversal of flow across the foramen ovale and reduced or absent flow through the left ventricle and into the ascending aorta. All systemic and placental venous return mixes in the right ventricle and is ejected into the pulmonary trunk and ductus arteriosus, the beneficial effects of streaming seen in the fetus without cCHD are absent. In addition, flow to the head and neck vessels primarily occurs by retrograde flow into the transverse aorta (Figure 11-4C). Fetuses with HLHS have been shown to have lower cerebral vascular resistance than normal fetuses, and in particular, neonates with HLHS and aortic atresia (with obligate retrograde flow to the brain) are the most likely to have microcephaly at birth.[10] In both TGA and HLHS, as well as most other forms of cCHD, disordered fetal circulation places the brain at risk for disrupted growth and development, particularly during the third trimester.[2,3,8-10]

CLINICAL PRESENTATION

Birth to Three Years of Age

Developmental scores discussed throughout this chapter refer to standard scores with a population mean of 100 and standard deviations (SD) of 15. Thus, a score of 85 is

1 SD below the mean, and approximately 16% of a normally distributed population would be expected to score below this. A score of 70 is 2 SD below the mean, and only about 2.5% of the population would be expected to score below this. Depending on the test, 1, 1.5, or 2 SD below the mean is considered delayed, or there may be a distinction between mild-moderate (1-1.5 SD) and severe delay (>2 SD below the mean). (See Appendix 11-1 for additional information about some commonly used developmental assessment tools.)

Cognitive abilities in infants and toddlers with cCHD are typically within the average or "normal" range but lower than the corresponding population mean. On the Mental Development Index (MDI) of the Bayley Scales of Infant Development, infants and toddlers with cCHD have an average MDI of 89 to 95 ± 9 to 17.[2,11-15] Approximately 5% to 11% of infants and toddlers have an MDI of less than 70.[14,16,17]

Motor delay is the most common and prominent finding in this age group. The same cohorts described earlier have Psychomotor Development Indices (PDI) from the Bayley Scales of 73 to 91 ± 13 to 23.[2,11-16] Approximately 14% to 48% have PDI scores less than 70. On a specific test of motor function, the Peabody Developmental Motor Scales, a similar percentage (42%) of children with cCHD showed delays (>1.5 SD below the mean) in gross and fine motor skills 12 to 18 months after surgery in the first 2 years of life.[17]

The single most important factor in predicting a lower MDI or PDI is the presence of a known genetic condition, such as trisomy 21 or chromosome 22q11 microdeletion.[12] When scores are separated based on the presence of a known genetic condition, these infants and toddlers have a mean MDI of 74 ± 14 and PDI of 60 ± 12, whereas subjects without a known genetic condition have a mean MDI of 93 ± 13 and PDI of 82 ± 16.[11]

Specific measures of speech and language demonstrate high rates of receptive and expressive language as well as phonologic (articulation) delays. Thirty-four percent of children with cCHD show language delays (primarily expressive) that are greater than 1.5 SD below the mean for age.[17] As early as 1 year of age, it can be observed that children are excessively quiet with rare use of recognizable words. At 2.5 years of age, delays in the development of vocabulary, word usage, word endings, and combining words are evident.[18] Approximately 25% of children are diagnosed with apraxia of speech,[19] a condition in which speech is limited by oral–motor planning and integration deficits.

Behavior and temperament are atypical prior to surgery in over one third of infants. They are described as being more irritable or lethargic.[20] On the Early Infancy Temperament Questionnaire, infants with a single-ventricle form of cCHD have more negative mood and are more difficult to soothe compared with controls.[21]

The Functional Independence Measure for Children (WeeFIM), the Vineland Adaptive Behavior Scale, and the Adaptive Behavioral Assessment System-II are commonly used, parent-report measures of children's function in a variety of domains of daily life. Children at 18 to 24 months of age who had a Norwood or arterial switch procedure at less than 6 weeks of age are 4 times as likely to have a delay on the General Adaptive Composite of the Adaptive Behavioral Assessment System-II compared with the norm group.[22] In a cohort specifically excluding children with HLHS, assessment at 12 to 18 months after the first open-heart surgery shows lower than average developmental quotients (77-92 ± 24-30) for self-care, mobility, and cognition on the WeeFIM, with only 21% functioning at age level. Standard scores for daily living skills and socialization are also in this range on the Vineland Adaptive Behavior Scale, with greater than half of the children exhibiting poor socialization skills.[20] These results suggest that social impairment may become apparent in toddlers and young children when a greater variety and complexity of social interaction is expected.

The presence of a life-threatening chronic condition can have a substantial impact on family function, which can impact parent–child interaction and neurodevelopmental outcome. At 3 months of age, infant negative mood and difficulty to soothe are predictive of higher parenting stress and are more common in infants with single-ventricle physiology.[21]

Four to Five Years of Age

At the age of school entry, full-scale intelligence quotient (IQ) scores typically remain in the average range (89-97 ± 7-21) on the Wechsler Preschool and Primary Scale of Intelligence–Third Edition and other intelligence tests.[23,24] Children with tetralogy of Fallot tend to have a higher IQ than those with HLHS, although both are within the average range (111 versus 97, respectively; McCarthy Scales of Children's Abilities).[25] Despite mean IQs in the average range, approximately 20% to 33% of children have IQs greater than 1 SD below the mean, and approximately 11% have IQs greater than 2 SD below the mean.[24,26]

Approximately 25% of 4 to 5 year olds score greater than 1 SD below the mean and 10% score greater than 2 SD below the mean on the total language score of the Preschool Language Scale 4, indicating moderate and severe language impairment, respectively.[26] Mean scores on tests of single-word receptive and expressive vocabulary tend to be similar to population means,[24,25] with better scores in TGA compared with HLHS.[25] However, more complex language productions, such as narratives, which require memory and organization as well as language skills, are deficient compared with control norms in greater than 50% of 4 year olds.[19] The narratives of preschoolers with cCHD are characterized by shorter length and descriptive depth. They contain less information and fewer language devices related to evaluation (eg, "he *wanted* to"), qualification (eg, "he *almost* fell"), and style (eg, repetition for emphasis). Narrative competency may be especially relevant because it can be deficient even when earlier language morphology and syntax were not and because it may be particularly important for socializing, comprehension, and literacy.[18,19]

At 4 to 5 years of age, the relatively high rate of neurologic abnormalities and gross and fine motor delays in children with cCHD persists. Mean Peabody gross motor quotients are 83 ± 12, with 49% scoring below 78 (1.5 SD below the mean), indicating significant delay. The same group has a mean fine motor quotient of 86 ± 16, with 39% scoring less than 78.[27] Motor findings at 12 to 18 months are strongly predictive of findings at 4 to 5 years of age,[17,27] suggesting that motor delays do not "catch up" over this time period.

Fine motor, visual–spatial, and visual–motor integration skills take on increased significance as children are expected to participate in more complex play activities; to increase independence in eating, grooming, and dressing; and to develop writing skills. On the Beery-Buktenica Developmental Test of Visual Motor Integration (Beery VMI) and other tests of visual–motor ability, several cohorts of preschoolers with cCHD have mean fine motor and visual–motor scores in the mid-80s to high 90s (range, 69-135). Between 12% and 30% scored greater than 1 SD below the population mean (moderate impairment), whereas 9% to 12% scored greater than 2 SD below the population mean (severe impairment).[23,25]

Executive functions are the collection of metacognitive abilities that allow humans to persist to accomplish goal-directed behavior. They include working memory (the ability to hold information in mind while analyzing it or completing a related task); behavioral inhibition (the ability to avoid distraction or impulsive reacting that interferes with accomplishing a task); the regulation of attention and cognitive effort (both the ability to persist when appropriate and to shift when appropriate); the abilities to organize, plan, and strategize (use previous experience to guide future behavior); and the ability to monitor one's performance of all of these skills to adapt to changing demands in "real time." Executive functions appear to be based in the frontal lobe, particularly the prefrontal cortex, and its connections to other brain regions. They continue to develop throughout childhood and into young adulthood, as does the frontal lobe. This uniquely protracted period of brain development makes the prefrontal cortex and executive functions uniquely vulnerable to a wide variety of conditions that adversely affect brain function. On the "statue"

subtest of the NEPSY (Developmental Neuropsychological Assessment), which measures motor control and behavioral inhibition, 33% of children with cCHD are moderately impaired and 11% are severely impaired.[26]

Parent- and/or teacher-completed behavior rating scales provide information about internalizing (anxiety, depressive symptoms) and externalizing (hyperactivity, aggression) symptoms, attention, learning, and social problems, as well as adaptive behaviors. Nineteen to 30% of subjects show scores greater than the 80th percentile for attention problems and/or impulsivity on an attention-deficit hyperactivity disorder (ADHD)–specific rating scale[23,26] compared to approximately 4% to 7% in the general population. Over 30% and 15% scored in the "at risk" or abnormal range on internalizing and externalizing problems, respectively, on the Child Behavior Checklist.[24] Children with HLHS appear to have a greater risk for attention and externalizing disorders than do children with TGA.[28] Measures of social function are lower than population norms at this age in some groups or on some measures,[26] but not others.[23,28]

Functional outcomes have been measured with the WeeFIM and Vineland Adaptive Behavior Scales (VABS), The Child Health Questionnaire (CHQ), and the Parenting Stress Index. WeeFIM mean scores are in the low average range for self-care and cognition and average for mobility. Over 20% of the study group had a standard score of less than 75 for independence in age-level self-care and cognition. Parent report on the VABS shows low average standard scores, with 10% to 17% showing significant problems with socialization, communication, daily living skills, and/or adaptive behavior.[24] On the CHQ, mean scores are within the normal range; however, parents have concerns about general health (35%), mental health (25%), attention (>30%), speech and/or learning (>20%), developmental delay (15%), anxiety (13%), and behavior problems (13%). Just under half endorse parenting stress that falls outside the normal range, primarily related to difficult child characteristics, such as mood. Thirty-three to 35% of parents show defensive responding on the Parenting Stress Index,[26] indicating that child problems and parent stress may be underreported.

School-Age Children and Adolescents

Some studies are limited to either school-age children or adolescents, but most include an age range that encompasses both; thus, these age groups will be discussed together but identified separately when relevant. Older adolescents and young adults may show outcomes that are not predictive of those expected for today's infants due to significant changes in medical and surgical management.

Cognition continues in the normal range, although it is lower than population means or controls.[29-31] Children with HLHS continue to have lower mean IQs than other diagnostic groups.[32,33] Across studies, a more substantial adverse effect on performance than verbal IQ is typical.[29-34] In contrast, children with acyanotic CHD do not differ from controls on the Wechsler Abbreviated Scale of Intelligence screening total IQ measure.[1]

Abnormal neurologic examination findings also persist and are consistently associated with poorer neurodevelopmental performance. Approximately 30% of school-age children and teens with either TGA or total anomalous pulmonary venous return (TAPVR) have abnormal neurologic examinations with either focal findings or diffuse abnormalities of tone (versus 5% expected).[27,34,35] Twenty-eight percent of a group with TAPVR[33] and 13% of a group with HLHS[34] have microcephaly. Head circumferences that are smaller than controls or population means continue to be noted across studies.[29,30] Twenty-one percent of teens with a variety of types of cCHD (excluding HLHS) have brain magnetic resonance imaging abnormalities consistent with hypoxic-ischemic injury in the neonatal period. In contrast to the focal white matter injury commonly seen before and after neonatal cardiac surgery, the findings in this group are primarily more diffuse white matter volume loss, an expected chronic change with remodeling after an acute lesion.[36]

Fine and gross motor performance, including manual dexterity, balance, and total motor skills, are below average.[30] Children with a variety of diagnoses who required multiple operations in the first year have a 5- to 11-fold increased risk of motor impairment.[37] In the Boston Circulatory Arrest Trial, motor skill is the one area in which children with dextro-TGA after an arterial switch with total circulatory arrest (compared with low-flow cardiopulmonary bypass) consistently perform more poorly up to 8 years of age.[29]

Teachers report problems with motor aspects of speech, expressive language, and learning problems more frequently in subjects with TGA than controls.[30] Using an in depth battery of tests assessing receptive and expressive language, among children with TGA, higher order language skills, motor aspects of speech, and phonologic awareness are weaker than what would be expected in the general population.[29] School-age children with tetralogy of Fallot have similar findings.[38] Language skill is an important prerequisite for adequate learning, and language deficits are important risk factors for learning disability (academic underachievement compared with expectations based on IQ). When compared with siblings, children with TGA score lower on measures of early academic achievement, with significant differences on the Woodcock-Johnson letter-word

identification subtest. Thirty-one percent of preschoolers have deficient skill acquisition, placing them at risk for a learning disability, and over 30% of school-age children/teens meet criteria for a learning disability (significant discrepancy between IQ and achievement).[39]

Perceptual processing, fine motor skills, and visual–motor integration are required for efficient and accurate completion of activities of daily living and academic tasks. In a group of children and adolescents with acyanotic CHD, visual–motor integration as measured by the Beery VMI did not differ from controls, did not differ before and after surgery, and did not differ whether or not cardiopulmonary bypass was used.[1] However, children with TGA, while still technically performing within the normal range, had a mean score in the 25th percentile rather than 50th percentile on this test.[29] Among children with TAPVR, visual–motor integration on the Beery VMI and Grooved Pegboard Test with the dominant hand is also significantly lower than population means (89.5 ± 16 and -1.9 ± 2.3, z score). Eight year olds also have twice the expected rate of low scores (52%; for poor organization) on the Rey-Osterrieth Complex Figure Test due to poor visual–perceptual skills.[40]

Social cognition (the ability to accurately interpret and respond to social information) can be compromised in children with language, perceptual, attention, and/or executive deficits. Although most widely studied in the context of autism, it has been shown to be an issue for children with a variety of neurodevelopmental conditions. Several factors appear to contribute to deficient social cognition, including difficulty with recognition of facial expression of emotion, limited awareness of one's own internal emotional state, and deficient theory of mind—the ability to deduce what another person knows and feels. Several studies indicate that children with cCHD have social difficulties measured by parent and/or teacher rating scales.[41-44] Direct assessment indicates that school-age children have deficits in social cognition on tests assessing their abilities to infer the beliefs of characters in a story,[45] sufficiently orient the listener in oral and written narratives, and use symbolic language and play scenarios.[18] Teens are being given specific self-report questionnaires about autism symptoms, empathy, overly systematic behavior, and emotional self-awareness and tasks related to recognition of facial emotion in ongoing follow-up of the Boston Circulatory Arrest Trial.[18] These characteristics may explain parent- and teacher-endorsed social difficulties.

Standardized measures of memory are available for school-age children and adolescents and have been evaluated in several cohorts with variable results. Children with TGA and TAPVR performed similarly to controls or population means on general memory assessments[34] in some studies, but another group of children with TGA performed approximately 1 SD lower than population means on several specific memory tests, with weakest performance on design (visual) memory.[29]

Higher scores on measures of attention problems are among the most consistent findings in children and adolescents. Both parent and teacher rating scales commonly used to assess attention problems demonstrate a higher rate of such problems than expected from population norms[29,46] or a control group.[44] Furthermore, even when ratings are within the normal range, specific laboratory tests of sustained and divided attention[34]; alerting, orienting, and executive control[47]; and measures of errors of omission (inattention), errors of commission (impulsive responding), and response time[29] indicate performance that is worse than population means.

Ratings for behavior problems encompassing both internalizing and externalizing domains are higher for subjects than controls, and controls are rated higher for behavioral competence on broad behavior rating scales.[29-31,43] In 8 year olds with TGA, 20% have scores in the clinical range for total behavior problems according to both parents and teachers.[41]

Functional measures tend to show increasing problems with age, although different outcome measures may limit comparisons. For example, children 3 to 8 years of age with HLHS have Vineland Adaptive Behavior subscale means below 100, but within the average range,[32] whereas an older group of patients with HLHS (mean age of 9 years) have significant fine motor (48%), gross motor (39%), and speech (30%) limitations. Seventeen percent of this group has cerebral palsy, 32% are diagnosed with a learning disability, and 18% have a global intellectual disability (mental retardation).[33] It is important to point out that this "historical" cohort of children reported in 2000 were some of the first survivors with HLHS; current results are much more reassuring.[16] In children with TGA, the rate of identified developmental impairment increases from 26% at 5 years to 55% at 8 to 14 years,[35] and approximately 30% are diagnosed with a learning disability.[39] Approximately 50% of children with mixed diagnoses or TAPVR are also found to have 1 or more areas of developmental dysfunction at late follow-up.[34,35] Thirty to 50% of children are receiving special education services.[33,46] Parents of children with a variety of cardiac diagnoses report more school problems in general, lower academic scores, and a higher frequency of grade retention than controls.[44] Despite these functional impairments and the prominent parenting stress identified in families of children with cCHD, quality-of-life measures tend to be average or better by parent[33,41] and teen self-report.[40] This may signify parental defensive responding or a heightened appreciation for the health of oneself or one's children.

Summary

Approximately half of children operated on in infancy for CHD will have at least 1 area of developmental deficit.[34,35] Those with single-ventricle diagnoses are at greater risk than those who undergo biventricular repair. Those with "cyanotic CHD" seem to be at greater risk than those with "acyanotic CHD." Abnormal findings on neurologic examination tend to persist and are associated with developmental risk. The most common developmental findings in infancy and the preschool period are feeding disorder and gross motor, fine motor, and expressive language delays. In the school-age population, visual–perceptual–motor, speech and complex language, executive, attention, behavioral, and social deficits emerge, setting the stage for future increased psychiatric morbidity and decreased adaptive functioning (Table 11-2).

Although some children with cCHD and developmental deficits will meet criteria for specific clinical diagnoses such as ADHD, expressive language disorder, apraxia of speech, phonologic disorder, developmental coordination disorder, and nonverbal learning disability (Table 11-3), resources in these areas may still be helpful for those children who "approximate," "fall just short of," or "fall between" diagnostic categories. Treating symptoms that cause impairment rather than "labels" should be the focus of attention. Although the most common deficits in this group are described as "high-prevalence, low-severity," this is a misnomer. Any one of these disabilities occurring to a significant degree or several co-occurring in the same individual (not uncommon) can have a profound effect on childhood functioning, adult outcome, and quality of life for the individual and his or her family. Given the cognitive and imaging findings described previously, children with cCHD are also more likely than controls to have intellectual disability and cerebral palsy. Given their risk for communicative, social cognition, and executive deficits, they may also be at higher risk for autism spectrum diagnoses, although epidemiologic research is lacking.

TREATMENT

Early intervention services are present throughout the United States as a result of federal legislation (the Education of the Handicapped Act Amendments of 1986, PL 99-457). Initially designed for children with disabilities, subsequent modifications (Individuals with Disabilities Education Act [IDEA] 1997; 2004 re-authorization, PL 108-446, Part C, Infants and Toddlers with Disabilities) extended services to children from birth, including those "at risk" for disabilities as a result of medical or environmental risk factors. A major congenital anomaly, such as cCHD, constitutes a risk factor for developmental delay, which allows referral/monitoring prior to the diagnosis of

The Trajectory of Developmental Deficits in Children with Complex Congenital Heart Disease

Infants and toddlers	▪ Difficult to soothe
	▪ Decreased prone skills
	▪ Increased or decreased muscle tone
	▪ Delayed motor milestones
	▪ Less active than peers
	▪ Delayed fine motor skills
	▪ Decreased play skills
	▪ Poorly coordinated suck/swallow
	▪ Difficulty with safe swallowing of thin liquids or solids
	▪ Decreased expressive language
Preschool children	▪ Increased incidence of internalizing (anxiety, depression) and externalizing (hyperactivity, impulsivity, disruptive) behavior problems (inflexibility, tantrums)
	▪ Decreased coordination and balance
	▪ Difficulty with fine motor/adaptive skills (feeding, dressing, prewriting)
	▪ Reduced intelligibility of speech/apraxia of speech
	▪ Delays in visual–perceptual–motor skills (puzzles, drawing shapes)
	▪ Over- or undersensitivity to sensory input, decreased body-in-space awareness
	▪ Slightly below average cognition
School-age children	▪ Difficulty sustaining attention and regulating activity level and emotions
	▪ Increased incidence of internalizing (anxiety, depression) and externalizing (hyperactivity, impulsivity, disruptive) behavior problems (inflexibility, tantrums)
	▪ Decreased coordination and balance
	▪ Difficulty with fine motor/adaptive skills (writing, grooming, tying shoes)
	▪ Reduced intelligibility and complexity of speech
	▪ Apraxia of speech
	▪ Decreased writing, note taking, copying skills
	▪ Executive function problems with sequencing, following directions, organizing, and planning
	▪ Adaptive and social deficits
Teens and young adults	▪ Increased internalizing and externalizing behaviors
	▪ May self-limit activities due to fatigue, speed, attention
	▪ Early language deficits impact thinking, reading, writing
	▪ Difficulties more likely in math and writing
	▪ Executive function problems with self-regulation, processing speed, and higher order thinking
	▪ Problems with social cognition and theory of mind
	▪ Strained interpersonal relationships
	▪ Difficulty with independence in schoolwork and activities of daily living

a specific delay. Key components of this program include a system to identify children at risk, a comprehensive and multidisciplinary assessment, the development of an Individualized Family Service Plan, service coordination, and procedural safeguards. Services provided may include therapies (occupation, physical, speech, and language), psychological services, family training, counseling, home visits, medical services for diagnostic purposes, social work services, assistive technology, and care coordination. States may modify specifics about service provision (eg, the degree of delay necessary for eligibility for services). In some cases, when children are delayed but not sufficiently to qualify for services, consultation with the relevant specialist and possible ongoing treatment may be covered by private or public insurance or may be

paid for "out-of-pocket." In any case, it is important for a therapist to provide "carry-over" activities to be practiced on a daily basis at home.

To date, there has been little study of the effects of early intervention on infants and children with cCHD. Interventional trials aimed at reducing maternal stress have shown promise in improving both maternal and infant outcomes.[48] More extensive studies do exist for children at risk due to poverty or prematurity or those with specific diagnoses. These studies tend to show that (1) children at risk due to poverty are most likely to derive benefit from early intervention[49]; (2) cognitive outcomes are more likely than motor outcomes to improve, regardless of the type of intervention[50,51]; and (3) interventions that involve parent training such that

Relevant Clinical Diagnoses for Some Children with Complex Congenital Heart Disease

Developmental coordination disorder	Deficits in fine and/or gross motor coordination sufficient to interfere with activities of daily living in the absence of focal neurologic signs or abnormalities of tone, posture, or reflexes that would signify cerebral palsy
Receptive and/or expressive language disorder	Deficits in the age-appropriate understanding and/or use of language not explained by a global intellectual disability
Apraxia of speech	Deficits in expressive language due to deficits in motor planning and coordination within the oral–motor system
Dyspraxia/apraxia	Deficits in fine and/or gross motor skills related to general deficits in motor planning (often co-occurs with apraxia of speech)
Attention-deficit hyperactivity disorder (ADHD)	Age-inappropriate levels of inattention, distractibility, and/or hyperactivity/impulsivity that are functionally impairing in multiple settings and not due to a differently treatable cause (eg, hearing loss)
Oppositional defiant disorder	Inflexibility leading to oppositional and defiant behavior that is functionally impairing
Specific learning disability	A deficit in reading, math, listening, writing, or spelling unexpected for cognitive ability or grade level, not due to a sensory deficit, psychosocial deprivation, or lack of educational exposure
Nonverbal learning disability	A learning disability characterized by relative deficits in performance intelligence quotient (IQ), perceptual skills, math, writing, social cognition, and inferential thinking
Executive function disorder	An age-inappropriate deficit in one or more executive functions (see text) in the absence of full characteristics for another disorder in which executive deficits are common such as ADHD, high-functioning autism, or depression
Static encephalopathy	Sometimes used for one or more of the above diagnoses or symptoms of an incomplete diagnosis, in the setting of a known brain insult (eg, "static encephalopathy with symptoms of ADHD and apraxia"). Serves to highlight the underlying neurologic etiology.
Intellectual disability	IQ <70 associated with adaptive skill deficits. (Previously called mental retardation). May be mild (55-69), moderate (40-54), severe (25-39), or profound (>25).
Cerebral palsy	Motor disability characterized by abnormalities of movement, muscle tone, and/or posture due to a static neurologic insult in the developmental period
Autism spectrum disorder	Anticipated DSM-5 condition (in place of current pervasive developmental disorders) of significant social and communicative deficits with repetitive behaviors and/or restricted interests
Social communication disorder	Anticipated DSM-5 condition of significant social and communicative deficits without repetitive behaviors and/or restricted interests

Data from American Psychiatric Association. *Diagnostic and Statistical Manual of Mental Disorders.* 4th ed., Text Revision, 2000 (DSM-IV-TR). Arlington, VA: American Psychiatric Association, 2000. DSM-5 publication anticipated in 2013.

parents have a significant role in the provision of therapy are most effective.[52,53]

Upon reaching 3 years of age, the responsibility for the provision of special education services is assumed by the child's school district. IDEA 2004 (PL 108-446, Part B) also mandates a free and appropriate public education for all children with disabilities from ages 3 to 21 in the least restrictive environment. Special education may include specially designed instruction by a qualified special education teacher, accommodations and modifications to the regular curriculum, therapies, paraprofessional support (ie, a personal assistant or a job coach), consultation by a special education teacher to the regular education teacher, and related services. IDEA recognizes specific disabilities including intellectual disability, hearing and vision impairments, speech and language impairments, emotional disorders, orthopedic impairments, traumatic brain injury, autism, specific learning disabilities, and a general category of "other health impairment." It does not recognize ADHD, although some states and school districts will include it in the "other health impairment" category. The cornerstone of special education is the student's Individualized Education Plan (IEP). The process of assessment, the inclusion of specific personnel including parents and student, the development of goals, progress monitoring and IEP revision, transition to adulthood, and the processes for handling disagreements are clearly delineated in legislation pertaining to special education.

Specialized instruction may include academic, functional, and behavioral subjects and vocational and social skills. In addition, the teaching of specific strategies for learning, remembering, and responding to educational material is also considered specialized instruction. A comprehensive assessment, not diagnosis per se, determines a student's eligibility for specialized instruction and related services. Related services may include therapies, therapeutic recreation, and services related to audiology, vision, mobility, rehabilitation, social work, counseling, and medical/nursing support.

Some students will not require specialized instruction but will require accommodations and/or modifications that allow them to effectively access the regular curriculum. Federal legislation also provides for these supports to students with disabilities under Section 504 of the Rehabilitation Act of 1973 (PL 93-112) and the Americans with Disabilities Act of 1990 (PL 101-336). A "504 Plan" or "Chapter 15 Agreement" is a legal document similar to, but far less formal and regulated than, an IEP. Common types of accommodations/modifications include allowing additional time on tests, making adjustments to the volume of assigned material, providing assistance or feedback with organizational tasks, and developing a cooperative home–school communication system to work on academic and/or behavioral goals.

Although federally mandated, the federal government does not regulate all aspects of special education. States and individual school districts have substantial discretion as to when and how services are provided. It is also important to note that while many aspects of assessment, diagnosis, and service provision are clearly delineated in federal legislation, there is plenty of wording that leaves room for controversy and confusion. Schools are required to provide services deemed "necessary" (not "optimal"). Supports are required when a disability "substantially" limits 1 or more "major life activities." It is important, in negotiating the complex world of educating a child with special needs, for parents to have skills to work collaboratively with school personnel and to understand federal, state, and school district legislation.

Another source of controversy about instruction pertaining to the "high-prevalence, low-severity" disabilities is a relative lack of proven educational interventions for areas other than reading. Well-researched instructional strategies are known to effectively improve both reading skill and relevant brain function in disabled readers.[54] In contrast, although psychosocial and pharmacologic treatments for ADHD have been sufficiently studied to be included in evidence-based professional practice guidelines, studies of how to actually teach improved focus, working memory, and other executive functions are in their infancy.[55]

Pediatricians have an important role to play in assisting families to optimize their child's developmental outcome. Assessing milestones and providing suggestions for activities to support their development, identifying eligible children and referring for early intervention, recognizing and addressing modifiable risk factors, understanding the developmental "trajectory" of the "high-prevalence, low-severity" disabilities (Table 11-2), advocating for appropriate intervention, keeping up with relevant developments in intervention and service provision, and supporting family education and interpersonal functioning are all important components of treatment in primary care. Examples of addressing risk factors might include aggressively addressing undernutrition. Another way to address risk would be to support behavioral counseling to improve dysfunctional parent–child interaction, a particular risk in families with a child with birth defects and developmental delay. An example of promoting intervention might be to encourage families to take advantage of knowledge and resources currently available for children without cCHD because the same deficits have been recognized in children without cCHD for many years (see Appendix 11-2). Physicians must also provide a plan for developmental follow-up. Together, researchers and clinicians have the potential to make a significant impact on the developmental outcome of children with cCHD.

Clinical Pearls

- Complex forms of CHD impact fetal circulation resulting in alterations in expected brain growth and development.
- Alterations in fetal brain development predispose infants with cCHD to brain injury, particularly white matter injury (periventricular leukomalacia), even before heart surgery.
- Infants with cCHD requiring intervention in the first year of life are at high risk for neurodevelopmental disorders that may be underdiagnosed and undertreated if delays in skill acquisition are attributed to recently having undergone surgery.
- Attention problems, executive dysfunction, and perceptual–motor and visual–spatial memory deficits are most common and result in academic underachievement.
- Developmental and learning disorders are common long-term sequelae of cCHD and increase the risk for mental health disorders and limited functional independence in teens and adults.

REFERENCES

1. Quartermain MD, Ittenbach RF, Flynn TB, et al. Neuropsychological status in children after repair of acyanotic congenital heart disease. *Pediatrics*. 2010;126:e351-e359.

2. Ballweg JA, Wernovsky G, Gaynor JW. Neurodevelopmental outcomes following congenital heart surgery. *Pediatr Cardiol*. 2007;28:126-133.

3. Limperopoulos C, Tworetzky W, McElhinney DB, et al. Brain volume and metabolism in fetuses with congenital heart disease: evaluation with quantitative magnetic resonance imaging and spectroscopy. *Circulation*. 2010;121:26-33.

4. Washington Smoak I, Byrd NA, Abu-Issa R, et al. Sonic hedgehog is required for cardiac outflow tract and neural crest cell development. *Dev Biol*. 2005;283:357-372.

5. Srivastava D. Making or breaking the heart: from lineage determination to morphogenesis. *Cell*. 2006;126:1037-1048.

6. Hoch RV, Rubenstein JL, Pleasure S. Genes and signaling events that establish regional patterning of the mammalian forebrain. *Semin Cell Dev Biol*. 2009;20:378-386.

7. Boni A, Urbanek K, Nascimbene A, et al. Notch1 regulates the fate of cardiac progenitor cells. *Proc Natl Acad Sci USA*. 2008;105:15529-15534.

8. Licht DJ, Shera DM, Clancy RR, et al. Brain maturation is delayed in infants with complex congenital heart defects. *J Thorac Cardiovasc Surg*. 2009;137:529-536.

9. Miller SP, McQuillen PS, Hamrick S, et al. Abnormal brain development in infants with congenital heart disease. *N Engl J Med*. 2007;357:1928-1938.

10. Shillingford AJ, Ittenbach RF, Marino BS, et al. Aortic morphometry and microcephaly in hypoplastic left heart syndrome. *Cardiol Young*. 2007;17:189-195.

11. Fuller S, Nord AS, Gerdes M, et al. Predictors of impaired neurodevelopmental outcomes at one year of age after infant cardiac surgery. *Eur J Cardiothorac Surg*. 2009;36:40-48.

12. Gaynor JW, Wernovsky G, Jarvik GP, et al. Patient characteristics are important determinants of neurodevelopmental outcome at one year of age after neonatal and infant cardiac surgery. *J Thorac Cardiovasc Surg*. 2007;133:1344-1353.

13. Hoskoppal A, Roberts H, Kugler J, et al. Neurodevelopmental outcomes in infants after surgery for congenital heart disease: a comparison of single-ventricle vs. two-ventricle physiology. *Congenit Heart Dis*. 2010;5:90-95.

14. Kaltman JR, Jarvik GP, Bernbaum J, et al. Neurodevelopmental outcome after early repair of a ventricular septal defect with or without aortic arch obstruction. *J Thorac Cardiovasc Surg*. 2006;131:792-798.

15. Matsuzaki T, Matsui M, Ichida F, et al. Neurodevelopment in 1-year-old Japanese infants after congenital heart surgery. *Pediatr Int*. 2010;52:420-427.

16. Tabbutt S, Nord AS, Jarvik GP, et al. Neurodevelopmental outcomes after staged palliation for hypoplastic left heart syndrome. *Pediatrics*. 2008;121:476-483.

17. Limperopoulos C, Majnemer A, Shevell MI, et al. Predictors of developmental disabilities after open heart surgery in young children with congenital heart defects. *J Pediatr*. 2002;141:51-58.

18. Bellinger DC. Are children with congenital heart malformations at increased risk of deficits in social cognition? *Cardiol Young*. 2008;18:3-9.

19. Hemphill L, Uccelli P, Winner K, et al. Narrative discourse in young children with histories of early corrective heart surgery. *J Speech Lang Hear Res*. 2002;45:318-331.

20. Limperopoulos C, Majnemer A, Shevell MI, et al. Functional limitations in young children with congenital heart defects after cardiac surgery. *Pediatrics*. 2001;108:1325-1331.

21. Torowicz D, Irving SY, Hanlon AL, et al. Infant temperament and parental stress in 3-month-old infants after surgery for complex congenital heart disease. *J Dev Behav Pediatr*. 2010;31:202-208.

22. Alton GY, Rempel GR, Robertson CM, et al. Functional outcomes after neonatal open cardiac surgery: comparison of survivors of the Norwood staged procedure and the arterial switch operation. *Cardiol Young*. 2010;20:668-675.

23. Fuller S, Rajagopalan R, Jarvik GP, et al. Deep hypothermic circulatory arrest does not impair neurodevelopmental outcome in school-age children after infant cardiac surgery. *Ann Thorac Surg*. 2010;90:1985-1995.

24. Majnemer A, Limperopoulos C, Shevell M, et al. Developmental and functional outcomes at school entry in children with congenital heart defects. *J Pediatr*. 2008;153:55-60.

25. Brosig CL, Musatto KA, Kuhn EM, et al. Neurodevelopmental outcome in preschool survivors of complex congenital heart disease: implications for clinical practice. *J Pediatr Health Care*. 2007;21:3-12.

26. Gaynor JW, Nord AS, Wernovsky G, et al. Apolipoprotein E genotype modifies the risk of behavior problems after infant cardiac surgery. *Pediatrics*. 2009;124:241-250.

27. Majnemer A, Limperopoulos C, Shevell M, et al. Long-term neuromotor outcome at school entry of infants with congenital heart defects requiring open-heart surgery. *J Pediatr*. 2006;148:72-77.

28. Brosig CL, Mussatto KA, Kuhn EM, et al. Psychosocial outcomes for preschool children and families after surgery for complex congenital heart disease. *Pediatr Cardiol*. 2007;28:255-262.

29. Bellinger DC, Wypij D, duPlessis AJ, et al. Neurodevelopmental status at eight years of age in children with dextro-transposition of the great arteries: the Boston Circulatory Arrest Trial. *J Thorac Cardiovasc Surg*. 2003;126:1385-1396.

30. Karl TR, Hall S, Ford G, et al. Arterial switch with full-flow cardiopulmonary bypass and limited circulatory arrest: neurodevelopmental outcome. *J Thorac Cardiovasc Surg*. 2004;127:213-222.

31. Karsdorp PA, Everaerd W, Kindt M, et al. Psychological and cognitive functioning in children and adolescents with congenital heart disease: a meta-analysis. *J Pediatr Psychol*. 2007;32:527-541.

32. Goldberg CS, Schwartz EM, Brunberg JA, et al. Neurodevelopmental outcome of patients after the Fontan operation: a comparison between children with hypoplastic left heart syndrome and other functional single ventricle lesions. *J Pediatr*. 2000;137:646-652.

33. Mahle WT, Clancy RF, Moss EM, et al. Neurodevelopmental outcome and lifestyle assessment in school-aged and adolescent children with hypoplastic left heart syndrome. *Pediatrics*. 2000;105:1082-1089.

34. Kirshbom PM, Flynn TB, Clancy RR, et al. Late neurodevelopmental outcome after repair of total anomalous

pulmonary venous connection. *J Thorac Cardiovasc Surg.* 2005;129:1091-1097.

35. Hovels-Gurich HH, Seghaye MC, Schnitker R, et al. Long-term neurodevelopmental outcomes in school-aged children after neonatal arterial switch operation. *J Thorac Cardiovasc Surg.* 2002;124:448-458.

36. von Rhein M, Scheer I, Loenneker T, et al. Structural brain lesions in adolescents with congenital heart disease. *J Pediatr.* 2011;158:984-989.

37. Holm I, Fredriksen PM, Fosdahl MA, et al. Impaired motor competence in school-aged children with complex congenial heart disease. *Arch Pediatr Adolesc Med.* 2007;161:945-950.

38. Hovels-Gurich HH, Bauer SS, Schnitker R, et al. Long-term outcome of speech and language in children after corrective surgery for cyanotic or acyanotic cardiac defects in infancy. *Eur J Paediatr Neurol.* 2008;12:378-386.

39. Williams WG, McCrindle BW, Ashburn DA, et al.; and the Congenital Heart Surgeons Society. Outcomes of 829 neonates with complete transposition of the great arteries 12-17 years after repair. *Eur J Cardiothorac Surg.* 2003;24:1-10.

40. Bellinger DC, Bernstein JH, Kirkwood MW, et al. Visual spatial skills in children after open heart surgery. *J Dev Behav Pediatr.* 2003;24:169-179.

41. Bellinger DC, Newburger JW, Wypij D, et al. Behavior at eight years in children with surgically corrected transposition: the Boston Circulatory Arrest Trial. *Cardiol Young.* 2009;19:86-97.

42. Culbert EL, Ashburn DA, Cullen-Dean G, et al.; and the Congenital Heart Surgeons Society. Quality of life of children after repair of transposition of the great arteries. *Circulation.* 2003;108:857-862.

43. Hovels-Gurich HH, Konrad K, Wiesner M, et al. Long term behavioral outcome after neonatal arterial switch operation for transposition of the great arteries. *Arch Dis Child.* 2002;87:506-510.

44. Miatton M, De Wolf D, Francois K, et al. Behavior and self-perception in children with surgically corrected congenital heart disease. *J Dev Behav Pediatr.* 2007;28:294-301.

45. Calderon J, Bonnet D, Courtin C, et al. Executive function and theory of mind in school-aged children after neonatal corrective cardiac surgery for transposition of the great arteries. *Dev Med Child Neurol.* 2010;52:1139-1144.

46. Shillingford AJ, Glanzman MM, Ittenbach RF, et al. Inattention, hyperactivity, and school performance in a population of school-age children with complex congenital heart disease. *Pediatrics.* 2008;121:e759-e767.

47. Hovels-Gurich HH, Konrad K, Skorzenski D, et al. Attentional dysfunction in children after corrective cardiac surgery in infancy. *Ann Thorac Surg.* 2007;83:1425-1430.

48. McCusker CG, Doherty NN, Molloy B, et al. A controlled trial of early interventions to promote maternal adjustment and development in infants born with severe congenital heart disease. *Child Care Health Dev.* 2010;36:110-117.

49. Gray R, McCormick MC. Early childhood intervention programs in the US: recent advances and future recommendations. *J Prim Prev.* 2005;26:259-275.

50. Nordhov SM, Ronning JA, Dahl LB, et al. Early intervention improves cognitive outcomes for preterm infants: randomized controlled trial. *Pediatrics.* 2010;126:e1088-e1094.

51. Spittle AJ, Orton J, Doyle LW, et al. Early developmental intervention programs post hospital discharge to prevent motor and cognitive impairments in preterm infants. *Cochrane Database Syst Rev.* 2007;2:CD005495.

52. McConachie H, Diggle T. Parent implemented early intervention for young children with autism spectrum disorder: a systematic review. *J Eval Clin Pract.* 2007;13:120-129.

53. Spittle AJ, Anderson PJ, Lee KJ, et al. Preventative care at home for very preterm improves infant and caregiver outcomes at 2 years. *Pediatrics.* 2010;126:e171-e178.

54. Shaywitz SE, Morris R, Shaywitz BA. The education of dyslexic children from childhood to young adulthood. *Ann Rev Psychol.* 2008;59:451-475.

55. Blair C, Diamond A. Biological processes in prevention and intervention: the promotion of self-regulation as a means of preventing school failure. *Dev Psychopathol.* 2008;20:899-911.

Commonly Used Neurodevelopmental Assessment Tools

Bayley Scales of Infant Development (edition III current; edition II used in reported studies)	Cognitive test for infants 1-42 months of age comprised of mental (perceptual, memory, learning, language, problem solving) and motor (gross and fine motor skills, dynamic and postural control, praxis and stereognosis) development scales.[a]
Wechsler Preschool and Primary Scale of Intelligence (3rd edition) (WPPSI)	Test of intelligence for ages 3.5-7 years with verbal and performance standard scores comprised of 12 subscales, combined to provide a full-scale intelligence quotient (IQ).[b]
Wechsler Abbreviated Scale of Intelligence (WASI)	Test of intelligence for ages 6-89.11 years using either 1 or 2 verbal and performance subtests to obtain a verbal, performance, and full-scale IQ estimate.[c]
Woodcock-Johnson Test of Achievement (edition III)	Test of academic achievement for ages 2-90+ in areas paralleling IDEA: oral expression, listening comprehension, written expression, basic reading, reading comprehension, reading fluency, math calculations, and math reasoning.[d]
NEPSY-II (Developmental Neuropsychological Assessment)	A test of neuropsychological function for ages 3-16 comprised of 36 subtests in 6 domains: executive function and attention, language, memory and learning, sensorimotor, visual–spatial processing, and social perception. The statue subtest measures motor persistence and inhibition in children ages 3-6.[e]
Peabody Developmental Motor Scales	An assessment for ages birth to 5 years measuring reflexes, stationary and locomotor skills, object manipulation, grasping, and visual–motor integration, providing gross motor, fine motor, and total motor quotients.[f]
Movement ABC	An assessment of movement skill, manual dexterity, ball skills, and static and dynamic balance for ages 3-16.11.[g]
Beery-Buktenica Test of Visual Motor Integration (Beery VMI)	A pencil and paper test of copying increasingly complex shapes to screen for visual–perceptual–motor deficits in ages 2 through adult.[h]
Grooved Pegboard Test	A manual dexterity test for ages 5 to adult that requires more visual–motor coordination than most pegboards due to the shape of the pegs and grooves. It is completed in order with the dominant hand and then the nondominant hand. It is scored for total time to completion, number of "drops," and number of correctly inserted pegs.[i]
Rey-Osterrieth Complex Figure Test	A test of visual–perceptual–constructional skill, visual memory, and executive skills for ages 5 through adult using a specific complex figure. It is first copied, and then reproduced from memory without the examinee knowing this in advance. Scaled scores are provided from a 36-point scoring system based on 18 design elements. Preschool Language Scale-IVA test of receptive and expressive language for children from birth to 6.11 years, with additional items that target attention and social interaction in the younger age range and phonologic awareness in the older age range.[j]
Achenbach Child Behavior Checklist	A broad behavior rating scale in the Achenbach System of Empirically Based Assessment (ASEBA). This specific product provides normed, parent-rated information on 20 areas of behavior issues and competencies in children ages 1½ to 18, as well as DSM-oriented scales. There are corresponding teacher and self-report formats.[k]
Behavior Assessment System for Children–2	Another broad behavior rating scale system providing normed parent and teacher ratings in 16 problem behavior and competency areas for children ages 2 to 21.11 and self-report measures from age 6.[l]
WeeFIM-II (Functional Independence Measure for Children)	A functional independence measure scored by observation for children ages 6 months to 7 years. It is based on 18 items in 3 domains: self-care, mobility, and cognition.[m]
Vineland Adaptive Behavior Scale-II	An adaptive behavior rating or interview for parents/caregivers of individuals from birth to adulthood and for teachers of individuals ages 3-21 comprised of 5 domains, each with 2-3 subdomains (communication, daily living skills, socialization, motor skills, and maladaptive behavior index). Widely used in conjunction with an IQ test to support a diagnosis of intellectual disability.[n]

(Continued)

Commonly Used Neurodevelopmental Assessment Tools (Continued)

Parenting Stress Index	A 101-item parent self-report rating designed to identify risk for dysfunctional parent–child interaction with children ages 3 months to 10 years. It is comprised of questions related to 6 child domains (distractibility/hyperactivity, adaptability, reinforces parent, demandingness, mood, acceptability) and 7 parent domains (competence, social isolation, attachment to child, health, role restriction, depression, spouse). There is a separate questionnaire for parents of adolescents.[o]

DSM, Diagnostic and Statistical Manual of Mental Disorders.
[a] Nancy Bayley, The Psychological Corporation, www.pearsonassessments.com.
[b] David Wechsler, Harcourt Assessment, www.pearsonassessments.com.
[c] David Wechsler, The Psychological Corporation, www.pearsonassessments.com.
[d] Richard W. Woodcock, Kevin S. McGrew, Nancy Mather, Riverside Publishing, www.riversidepublishing.com.
[e] Marit Korkman, Ursula Kirk, Sally Kemp, The Psychological Corporation, www.pearsonassessments.com.
[f] M. Ronda Fogio, Rebecca R. Fewell, Pro-Ed, Inc., www.proedinc.com.
[g] Sheila E. Henderson, David A. Sugden, Anna Barnett, Pearson, www.pearsonassessments.com.
[h] Keith E. Beery, Natasha A. Beery, Norman A. Buktenica, The Psychological Corporation, www.pearsonassessments.com.
[i] Dr. Ronald L. Trites, Lafayette Instruments, www.lafayetteinstruments.com.
[j] Rey-Osterreith – Andre Rey, Paul-Alexandre Osterreith, Pyschological Assessment Resources, www.parinc.com.
[k] Dr. Thomas Achenbach, ASEBA (Achenbach System of Empirically Based Assessment), www.aseba.org.
[l] Kimberly Vannest, Cecil R. Reynolds, Randy Kamphaus, The Psychological Corporation, www.pearsonassessments.com.
[m] Carl V. Granger, Margaret A. McCabe, Uniform Data System for Medical Rehab, www.udsmr.org.
[n] Sara S. Sparrow, Domenic V. Cicchetti, David A. Balla, The Psychological Corporation, www.pearsonassessments.org.
[o] Richard R. Abidin, Psychological Assessment Resources, www.parinc.com.

Resources for Parents and Clinicians

Educational Law
www.ed.gov/osers (Office of Special Education and Rehabilitation Services; also check individual state Offices of Special Education)
www.idea.ed.gov (Official IDEA website)
www.wrightslaw.com

General Information About Education/Disabilities
www.greatschools.org
www.schwabfoundation.org

Information About Specific Conditions
www.nimh.nih.gov (National Institutes of Mental Health)
www.asha.org (American Speech and Hearing Association)
www.apraxia-kids.org (Apraxia of Speech)
www.dyspraxiafoundation.org (Dyspraxia)
www.ldanatl.org (Learning Disabilities Association of America)
www.interdys.org (International Dyslexia Association)
www.ncld.org (National Center for Learning Disabilities)
www.ldonline.org (Learning Disability)
www.nldontheweb.org (Nonverbal Learning Disability)
www.aspergersyndrome.org (Asperger Syndrome)
www.chadd.org (Attention-Deficit Hyperactivity Disorder)
www.autismspeaks.org (Autism)
www.ucp.org (United Cerebral Palsy)
www.22qCentral.org (Velocardiofacial Syndrome)
www.thearc.org (Intellectual and Developmental Disabilities)

CHAPTER 12

Cardiac Arrhythmias

Akash Patel, William Bonney and Maully Shah

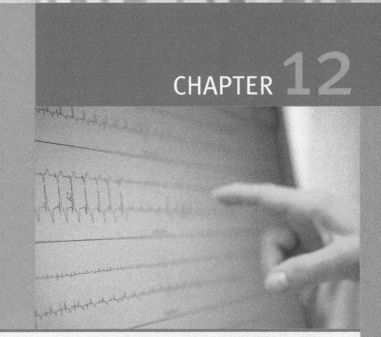

INTRODUCTION

Cardiac arrhythmias are due to abnormalities in the heart rhythm or conduction that can range in clinical significance from benign to life threatening. The frequency with which these occur varies with age and comorbid conditions, and true cardiac arrhythmias are rare in young people. It is important for the clinician to identify the arrhythmia and determine whether further evaluation or treatment is required. In general, the principle of treatment in this population is to minimize or alleviate symptoms, reduce associated risks (ie, cardiac dysfunction), prevent hemodynamic compromise, and/ or prevent mortality.

Proper identification of cardiac arrhythmias in the young requires a clear understanding of the normal physiologic changes in heart rate that occur with age and activity. It is also important to understand the average expected resting heart rate for a given age (Table 12-1).[1,2] Identification of clinically relevant arrhythmias requires assessment of the patient's heart rate, a basic understanding of electrocardiogram interpretation in the context of the patient's age, a focused clinical history, and awareness of the patient's current hemodynamic state. This provides a framework for appropriate evaluation and management.

This chapter will outline basic pediatric arrhythmias and focus on several important cardiac conditions that may result in malignant arrhythmias or syncope. Each cardiac arrhythmia will be described based on electrocardiographic findings, causes, clinical features, and management options.[2-6]

BRADYARRHYTHMIAS

Sinus Bradycardia

Definition

A slow heart rate that is below the lower limits of normal for age but regular and originating from the sinus node. This is characterized by (1) a P wave preceding every QRS complex with a normal PR interval and (2) a normal P-wave morphology and axis (upright/positive in leads I and aVF).

Causes

Sinus bradycardia can be due to increased parasympathetic (vagal) tone as seen in well-conditioned athletes; withdrawal of sympathetic tone as seen during sleep and obstructive sleep apnea; drugs such as sedatives, parasympathomimetics, sympatholytics, and many antiarrhythmics agents; increased intracranial pressure; hypothyroidism; hypothermia; prolonged hypoxia; or sinus node dysfunction.

Clinical features

Most patients with sinus bradycardia are asymptomatic. However, symptoms of bradycardia include lightheadedness, dizziness, fatigue, exercise intolerance, presyncope, or syncope.

Management

Generally, no therapy is required, but in symptomatic patients, the primary management is to diagnose and treat the underlying cause. In rare cases of symptomatic

Normal Heart Rate Range Based on Age

Age Group	Average Heart Rate	Normal Heart Rate Range
Birth-6 months	145	95-180
6 months-1 year	135	110-170
1-3 years	120	90-150
3-5 years	110	65-135
5-12 years	85	60-110
12-adult	80	60-100

Data from Park MK. Pediatric Cardiology for Practitioners. 4th ed. St. Louis, MO: Mosby, 2002; and Davignon A, Rautaharju P, Boisselle E, et al. Normal ECG standards for infants and children. Pediatr Cardiol. 1979;1:123-131.

bradycardia with or without sinus pauses, patients may require short-term treatment with atropine (a vagolytic) or long-term treatment with a permanent atrial pacemaker to increase the atrial heart rate.

Junctional Bradycardia (Figure 12-1)

Definition

A slow heart rhythm, below the lower limits of normal for age, that originates from the atrioventricular (AV) junction. This is characterized by (1) a regular, narrow QRS rhythm with no P waves preceding the QRS complexes and (2) P waves that are totally absent, unrelated to the QRS complexes, or inverted and following QRS complexes.

Causes

Junctional bradycardia is often benign and due to excessive vagal tone in a structurally normal heart. Other causes include increased intracranial pressure, sequelae of cardiac surgery, sinus node dysfunction, and digitalis toxicity.

Clinical features

As with sinus bradycardia, most patients are asymptomatic, but symptoms of bradycardia may occur.

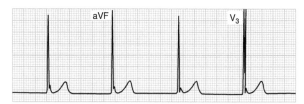

FIGURE 12-1 ■ Junctional bradycardia.

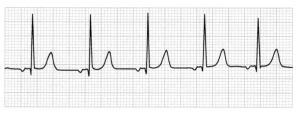

FIGURE 12-2 ■ Ectopic atrial rhythm.

Management

Generally, no therapy is required, but as with sinus bradycardia, atropine and/or pacemaker therapy may be needed in symptomatic patients.

Ectopic Atrial Rhythm (Figure 12-2)

Definition

A slow to low-normal heart rate that is below or at the lower limits of normal for agethat originates from a nonsinus location in the atrium. This is characterized by (1) a regular rhythm with P waves preceding every QRS complex and a normal PR interval and (2) an abnormal P-wave morphology and axis (ie, P waves are not upright in leads I and aVF). Commonly, low right atrial rhythmsshowan upright/positive P wave in lead I and inverted/negative P wave in lead aVF.

Causes

Ectopic atrial rhythm is often benign but can also occur in the setting of sinus node dysfunction.

Clinical features

As with sinus bradycardia, most patients are asymptomatic, but symptoms of bradycardia may occur.

Management

Generally, no therapy is required, but as with sinus bradycardia, atropine and/or pacemaker therapy may be needed in symptomatic patients.

Wandering Atrial Pacemaker (Figure 12-3)

Definition

A slow to normal heart rhythm that originates from 2 alternating sites in the atrium. Most commonly, low

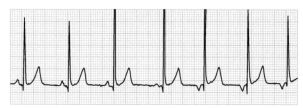

FIGURE 12-3 ■ Wandering atrial pacemaker.

atrial rhythm may alternate with sinus rhythm to produce this effect. This is characterized by (1) a P wave occurring before every QRS complex and (2) a gradual or abrupt change in the P-wave morphology and axis, which may result in a change in the PR interval.

Causes

Wandering atrial pacemaker is a benign finding due to alterations in vagal tone. Increases in vagal tone may result in suppression of sinus node function shifting the site of the natural atrial pacemaker to another focus in the atrium that has inherent automaticity.

Clinical features

Patients are asymptomatic with no clinical manifestations related to the wandering location of atrial activity.

Management

No therapy is required.

Premature Atrial Contractions (Figure 12-4)

Definition

A premature beat originating from a nonsinus location in the atrium. This is characterized by (1) a P wave occurring prematurely that is usually followed by a QRS, (2) an abnormal P-wave morphology, and (3) a PR interval that is usually prolonged. If the P wave occurs early enough, there may be AV block.

Causes

Premature atrial contractions (PACs) are usually idiopathic and not associated with any heart disease. However, causes should be considered and include electrolyte derangements, fever, hyperthyroidism, drug toxicity, infection, and foreign body in the atrium (ie, catheter or wire).

Clinical features

Patients are usually asymptomatic. Occasionally, PACs produce palpitations.

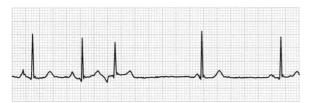
FIGURE 12-4 ■ Premature atrial contractions.

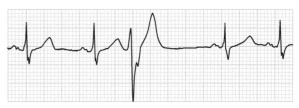
FIGURE 12-5 ■ Premature ventricular contractions.

Management

No therapy is required. In rare cases when patients are clearly symptomatic, β-blocker therapy may be used.

Premature Ventricular Contractions (Figure 12-5)

Definition

A premature beat originating from the ventricle. This is characterized by a wide QRS beat occurring prematurely. The premature ventricular contraction (PVC) may or may not perturb the normal atrial rhythm.

Causes

PVCs are usually idiopathic and not associated with any heart disease. Benign PVCs are usually suppressed during exercise, and PVCs that increase in frequency with activity are more ominous. However, causes should be considered and include electrolyte derangements, fever, hyperthyroidism, drug toxicity, infection, or foreign bodies in the ventricle (ie, catheter or wire).

Clinical features

Patients are usually asymptomatic. Occasionally PVCs produce palpitations.

Management

No therapy is required. Although most PVCs are benign, the incidence of underlying heart disease is slightly more than with PACs. Echocardiography is usually advised to assess for underlying structural heart disease or cardiomyopathy. In rare cases when patients are clearly symptomatic, β-blocker therapy may be used.

Heart Block, First Degree (Figure 12-6)

Definition

First-degree heart block is a sinus rhythm with prolonged conduction from the atrium to the ventricle. This is characterized by (1) a P wave preceding every QRS complex, (2) a QRS complex following every P wave, and (3) a PR interval greater than the upper limits of normal. A PR interval of greater than 200 ms is considered first-degree heart block in adults. However, the PR interval is age and heart rate dependent, with shorter PR intervals for

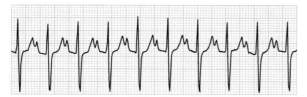

FIGURE 12-6 ■ Heart block, first degree.

younger age and faster heart rates. A PR interval greater than 120 ms for an infant, 150 ms for a toddler, and 180 ms for a young child is considered prolonged for heart rates below 100 beats per minute (bpm).

Causes

The PR interval will be prolonged if there is delayed conduction above the AV node, through the AV node, or below the AV node in the His-Purkinje system. Causes include inflammatory processes (ie, Lyme myocarditis), congenital heart defects (ie, Ebstein anomaly), medication exposure (ie, digitalis toxicity), postsurgical injury to the native conduction system, and increased vagal tone in anotherwise healthy child.

Clinical features

First-degree block typically does not result in symptoms but can progress to more advanced heart block that could result in symptomatic bradycardia.

Management

Assessment of secondary causes should be identified to allow for appropriate treatment, which may result in resolution of the first-degree block (ie, treatment of digitalis toxicity or treatment of Lyme myocarditis with appropriate antibiotics).

Heart Block,Second Degree (Mobitz Type I) (Figure 12-7)

Definition

Sinus rhythm with progressive prolongation of conduction from the sinus node to the ventricle until the sinus impulse is blocked from conducting to the ventricle. This is characterized by progressive prolongation of the PR

interval until there is a P wave that is not followed by a QRS. The PR interval of the next beat is short, and the cycle may repeat. Progressive delay in conduction with eventual block is referred to as Wenckebach phenomenon.

Causes

Mobitz I block usually occurs within the compact AV node and is typically a benign finding that occurs in healthy patients, especially well-conditioned athletes with increased vagal tone. Additional causes include inflammatory processes such as myocarditis, medication exposure such as digitalis toxicity, and postsurgical injury to the conduction system.

Clinical features

Mobitz I block typically does not result in symptoms or progress to more advanced heart block.

Management

Generally, no therapy is required.

Heart Block,Second Degree (Mobitz Type II) (Figure 12-8)

Definition

Second-degree heart block is a sinus rhythm with intermittent "all or none" conduction to the ventricle and no alteration in the preceding PR interval. This is characterized by intermittent P waves that are not followed by a QRS and without prolongation in the PR interval of the preceding conducted beats.

Causes

The causes of Mobitz II block are similar to the causes of Mobitz I block; however, Mobitz II block typically occurs below the AV node at the level of the His bundle. This is more ominous and may progress to complete heart block.

Clinical features

Mobitz II block usually does not produce symptoms unless there are significant pauses or bradycardia. It may progress to more advanced heart block.

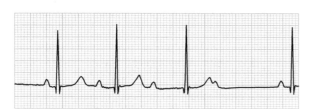

FIGURE 12-7 ■ Heart block, second degree (Mobitz type I).

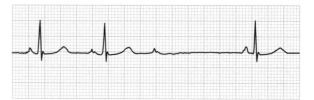

FIGURE 12-8 ■ Heart block, second degree (Mobitz type II).

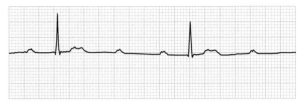

FIGURE 12-9 ■ Heart block, high grade.

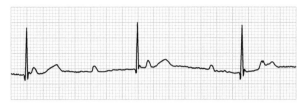

FIGURE 12-10 ■ Heart block, third degree.

Management

Assessment of secondary causes should be identified to allow for appropriate treatment, which may result in resolution of the second-degree block. Pacemaker therapy may be required for symptomatic bradycardia or symptomatic pauses due to intermittent loss of ventricular activation.

Heart Block, High Grade (Figure 12-9)

Definition

High-grade AV block is characterized by several consecutive nonconducted P waves occurring in a row. Conduction may occur with every third or fourth beat.

Causes

High-grade AV block, like Mobitz II block, typically occurs below the AV node at the level of the His bundle. Causes include postsurgical injury, myocarditis, drug toxicity, and congenital heart block.

Clinical features

Symptoms depend on the rate and reliability of the ventricular heart rate. Patients with significant bradycardia or sinus pauses can have symptoms that include lightheadedness, dizziness, fatigue, exercise intolerance, presyncope, or syncope.

Management

Management includes assessment for secondary causes and appropriate treatment. Pacemaker therapy may be required for symptomatic bradycardia or symptomatic pauses due to intermittent loss of ventricular activation.

Heart Block, Third Degree (Figure 12-10)

Definition

Third-degree heart block is defined as blocked conduction in the AV node or His-Purkinje system, resulting in independent atrial and ventricular rhythms. This is characterized by (1) a regular ventricular rhythm with regular QRS complexes that are not related to the P waves and (2) a ventricular rate that is slower than the atrial rate (ie, more p waves than QRS complexes). The QRS complex can be narrow or wide depending whether the escape rhythm originates from the AV junction or the ventricle.

Causes

Third-degree AV block can be congenital or acquired. Fetal exposure to maternal autoantibodies related to lupus or Sjögren syndrome is the most common cause of congenital complete heart block. Over half of congenital heart block cases are "idiopathic" and do not have any specific identifiable cause. Complete heart block can occur in the setting of congenital heart disease, especially congenitally corrected transposition of the great vessels. Acquired complete heart block occurs in conditions that injure the AV node, including myocarditis, Lyme carditis, rheumatic fever, cardiomyopathies, cardiac tumors, drug toxicity (ie, calcium channel blockers or digoxin), myocardial infarction, or direct trauma as a complication of cardiac surgery.

Clinical features

Symptoms depend on the rate and reliability of the ventricular heart rate. Surprisingly, many children with congenital heart block are completely asymptomatic despite heart rates that are well below the "lower limits" for age. Patient with significant bradycardia or sinus pauses may experience lightheadedness, dizziness, fatigue, exercise intolerance, presyncope, or syncope. In very rare cases, prolonged asystolic pauses may precipitate ventricular fibrillation and sudden death.

Management

Assessment for secondary causes and appropriate treatment is paramount. Short-term management of complete heart block that results in low cardiac output and associated symptoms is focused on increasing the effective ventricular rate. This may be accomplished with medications like atropine, isoproterenol, or epinephrine. Temporary transvenous or transcutaneous pacing is indicated for symptomatic patients when medications fail. Permanent pacemaker therapy may be required for children with symptomatic bradycardia or prolonged sinus pauses.

TACHYARRHYTHMIAS

Supraventricular Tachycardias

Supraventricular tachycardia (SVT) is the most common tachyarrhythmia in infants and children after sinus tachycardia. SVT is a broad term that describes any arrhythmia originating from above the AV node or ventricles. The term is often synonymous with paroxysmal SVT of which AV nodal re-entrant tachycardia (AVNRT) and atrioventricular re-entrant tachycardia (AVRT), more specifically orthodromic re-entrant tachycardia, compose more than 90% of SVTs encountered in children and infants.[7,8] Other less common forms of SVT in children include ectopic atrial tachycardias, atrial fibrillation, atrial flutter, and other rare SVTs.

Sinus Tachycardia

Definition

Although not a true supraventricular "arrhythmia," sinus tachycardia is defined as a rapid heart rate, above the upper limits of normal for age (Table 12-1), originating from the sinus node. This is characterized by (1) a regular, narrow QRS rhythm; (2) a P wave that precedes every QRS complex with a normal PR interval; and (3) normal P-wave morphology and axis (upright/positive in leads I and aVF). The heart rates tend to be below 200 bpm, but some infants and small children may be able to generate sinus rates up to 230 bpm.

Causes

Sinus tachycardia can be a result of increased sympathetic tone; withdrawal of parasympathetic tone; endogenous catecholamines in the setting of fever, pain, fear, distress, or dehydration; exogenous catecholamines like epinephrine, norepinephrine, and β-agonists (ie, albuterol); and dehydration. In addition, metabolic disorders that increase the body's metabolic state such as hyperthyroidism or brain injury that results in dysregulation of the autonomic nervous system can result in tachycardia. Finally, compensatory sinus tachycardia can be seen in cardiac dysfunction to maintain cardiac output.

Clinical features

Sinus tachycardia usually presents with a gradual increase in heart rate that may or may not cause symptoms of palpitations. It is important to consider the underlying cause because sinus tachycardia is rarely an isolated finding.

Management

Generally, no antiarrhythmic therapy is required. Primary therapy should be focused on the diagnosis and treatment of the underlying cause. Use of antiarrhythmics to reduce heart rate should be avoided because it may counteract the normal physiologic response, which is preserving adequate cardiac output.

Paroxysmal Supraventricular Tachycardia (Figure 12-11)

Definition

"Paroxysmal" SVT is a term that describes several different types of re-entrant SVT that occur in episodes or paroxysms. These arrhythmias are characterized by (1) a regular tachycardia, usually with narrow QRS that starts and stops abruptly (the rate is almost always >200 bpm); (2) inverted "retrograde" P waves that may follow the QRS and appear on the tail end of the QRS complex or within the T wave; and (3) sustained tachycardia episodes that terminate with vagal maneuvers, adenosine, or spontaneous AV block. Occasionally, there is a transient bundle-branch block that produces a regular wide QRS rhythm referred to as aberration.

Causes

The 2 most common types of paroxysmal SVT are AVRT and AVNRT. "Orthodromic" AVRT is the most common type that propagates from the atrium to the ventricle through the AV node and returns to the atrium using an accessory pathway. Approximately one third of patients with an accessory pathway have a Wolff-Parkinson-White (WPW) syndrome pattern during sinus rhythm (see later discussion of WPW). In AVNRT, the re-entry loop circles the AV node and involves 2 AV nodal extensions or pathways.

Clinical features

Paroxysmal SVT usually causes palpitations, and patients are usually relatively stable during tachycardia. Rarely, patients will present with shock if they have underlying heart disease or prolonged tachycardia. Young children who are unable to specify the sensation of palpitations may say that they are having chest pain. This arrhythmia rarely causes syncope and collapse and is not a cause of sudden cardiac death. Infants who are unable to communicate the sensation of palpitations will be relatively

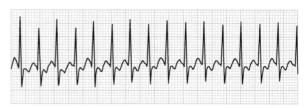

FIGURE 12-11 ■ Paroxysmal supraventricular tachycardia.

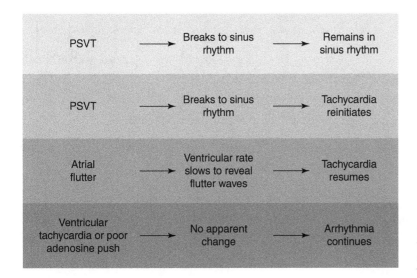

FIGURE 12-12 ■ Potential responses of adenosine for various tachyarrhythmias. PSVT, paroxysmal supraventricular tachycardia.

asymptomatic unless the arrhythmia persists for several hours. After 12 to 24 hours of sustained tachycardia, an untreated infant may develop a tachycardia-induced cardiomyopathy and signs and symptoms of heart failure with poor feeding, tachypnea, and lethargy.

Management

The rare cases of unstable SVT should be terminated with synchronized direct current (DC) cardioversion using an energy dose of 0. 5 to 2 J/kg. However, most sustained SVT can be terminated with adenosine given as a rapid intravenous push (Figure 12-12). Vagal maneuvers will also terminate SVT, although they are not as reliable as adenosine (Table 12-2). Patients with nonsustained, infrequent SVT episodes may be managed without daily antiarrhythmic medications. Patients with significant

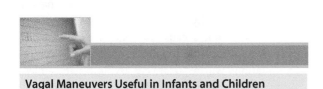

Vagal Maneuvers Useful in Infants and Children

List of Vagal Maneuvers in Children

- Diving reflex
  Immersion of face in cold water
  Ice bag over mouth and nose
- Valsalva maneuvers
  Forced exhalation against a thumb in a closed mouth
  Bearing down
- Carotid sinus massage
- Stimulation of gag reflex with a tongue depressor
- Deep inspiration followed by breath holding
- Coughing
- Brief hand stand
- Gentle rectal stimulation

symptoms or sustained SVT requiring adenosine are likely to have recurrent episodes, and most can be managed with antiarrhythmic medications (digoxin and/or β-blockers).

Catheter ablation is an alternative to pharmacologic therapy in older children that offers a more definitive cure with a 95% success rate and less than 1% complication rate. The risks of catheter ablation increase for younger children and infants, and in those populations, ablation is reserved for incessant SVT refractory to medical therapy.

Wolff-Parkinson-White Syndrome and Associated Arrhythmias (Figure 12-13)

Definition

Accessory AV pathways that allow extra nodal conduction from the atrium to the ventricle produce a WPW pattern on the electrocardiogram during sinus rhythm. This is characterized by (1) a short PR interval, (2) a widened QRS pattern with an initial QRS upstroke or "delta wave," and (3) a predisposition to a variety of arrhythmias including the following:

- AVRT: As indicated earlier, WPW pathways that are capable of conduction in both directions predispose the patient to paroxysmal SVT. The management of

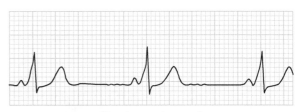

FIGURE 12-13 ■ Wolff-Parkinson-White syndrome.

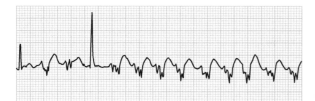

FIGURE 12-14 ■ Atrial fibrillation in the setting of Wolff-Parkinson-White syndrome.

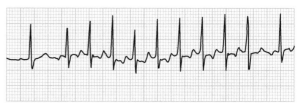

FIGURE 12-15 ■ Ectopic atrial tachycardia.

SVT episodes in patients with WPW is nearly identical to patients with "concealed" accessory pathways.

■ "Antidromic" reciprocating tachycardia: In this rare form of AVRT, conduction propagates from the atrium to the ventricle using the accessory pathway and returns to the atrium via the AV node. This type of tachycardia can also be terminated with adenosine and vagal maneuvers.

■ Atrial fibrillation: Individuals with WPW are predisposed to this disorganized atrial arrhythmia (see later section for a full description of atrial fibrillation), which occurs much less often than AVRT. In very rare cases of rapid accessory pathway conduction, atrial fibrillation can provoke episodes of ventricular fibrillation and sudden cardiac death (Figure 12-14).

Causes

WPW is caused by the presence of accessory cardiac conduction tissues that connect the atrium to the ventricle, bypassing the AV node. Usually these pathways are present from birth, although arrhythmias may not occur until the second decade of life.

Clinical features

In patients with WPW, AVRT and atrial fibrillation episodes are clinically similar to those arrhythmias in patients without WPW. Palpitations that start and stop abruptly are common. Very rarely, rapid atrial fibrillation can be associated with syncope, collapse, and sudden cardiac death.

Management

Paroxysmal SVT episodes are managed with medications and/or catheter ablation, as in patients without WPW.

Ectopic Atrial Tachycardia (Figure 12-15)

Definition

Ectopic atrial tachycardia is a rapid heart rate, above the upper limits of normal for age, that originates from a nonsinus site in the right or left atrium. This is characterized by (1) a P wave that precedes every QRS complex, (2) a P-wave morphology that is distinctly different from the sinus morphology, (3) a P-to-P interval that may be irregular, and (4) intermittent AV block that may occur at the most rapid atrial rates. In addition, there may be evidence of first-degree and second-degree AV block without interruption of the tachycardia.

Causes

Ectopic atrial tachycardia often occurs in nonsustained bursts with an abrupt onset and termination. Sustained episodes may show a gradual increase in the heart rate and gradual decrease before termination. The ectopic foci typically are located in the atrial appendages, in pulmonary vein ostia, along the crista terminalis, or at sites adjacent to surgical suture lines in the atria as a result of previous cardiac surgery. In addition, there can be local atrial irritation caused by the presence of intracardiac lines (ie, a peripherally inserted central line ending in the right atrium).

Clinical features

Patients with ectopic atrial tachycardia usually have palpitations. Young children who are unable to specify the sensation of palpitations may say that they are having chest pain. This arrhythmia rarely causes syncope and collapse and is not a cause of sudden cardiac death. Infants who are unable to communicate the sensation of palpitations will be relatively asymptomatic unless the arrhythmia persists for several hours. After 12 to 24 hours of sustained tachycardia, an untreated infant may develop a tachycardia-induced cardiomyopathy with poor feeding, tachypnea, and lethargy. All of these symptoms will reverse once the heart rate is controlled.

Management

Treatment of ectopic atrial tachycardia includes rate and rhythm control. Rate-controlling agents that limit AV nodal conduction include digoxin, β-blockers, and calcium channel blockers. Rhythm-controlling agents that suppress ectopic automaticity and restore sinus rhythm include β-blockers, procainamide, flecainide, sotalol, and amiodarone. Catheter ablation can permanently cure this arrhythmia and is indicated in older children with sustained tachycardia or in younger children and infants with severe, incessant tachycardia refractory to antiarrhythmic medications.

Atrial Flutter (Figure 12-16)

Definition

Atrial flutter is a re-entrant arrhythmia in the atrium that results in a rapid atrial rate, usually 300 to 400 bpm. The ventricular rate depends on AV nodal conduction. Typically, there is 2:1 AV block resulting in ventricular rates of 150 to 200 bpm. The ventricular rhythm may be irregular in the setting of variable AV block (ie, alternating 2:1, 3:1, or 4:1 conduction). Atrial flutter is characterized by (1) "flutter" waves (abnormal P waves) classically with a "sawtooth" configuration in the inferior leads (II, III, and aVF), (2) a regular atrial rate (ie, constant intervals between flutter waves), and (3) usually a regular ventricular rate with constant 2:1 AV conduction.

Causes

Atrial flutter is most often seen in 2 distinct pediatric groups: newborns with structurally normal hearts and patients who have had surgery to repair congenital heart disease. Neonatal atrial flutter is similar to the "typical" atrial flutter that occurs in adults and depends on a region of slow conduction between the tricuspid valve and the inferior vena cava. Postoperative atrial flutter depends on anatomic barriers and surgical scars that create regions of slow conduction allowing atrial re-entry. This is often called intra-atrial re-entrant tachycardia (IART). The atrial rate in neonatal flutter is usually 350 to 500 bpm, whereas IART rates are slower (150-250 bpm).

Clinical features

Symptoms of atrial flutter depend on the ventricular response rate. With AV block and a slow ventricular response rate, patients may be asymptomatic or have subtle complaints like fatigue and exercise intolerance. With rapid AV conduction, patients may have palpitations, light headedness, or rarely syncope.

Management

Neonatal atrial flutter is usually well tolerated. The ventricular rate can be controlled with antiarrhythmic medications, and atrial flutter can be terminated with transesophageal pacing or synchronized cardioversion. Often the arrhythmia will terminate spontaneously within 24 hours. Once the arrhythmia terminates, recurrence is rare and additional antiarrhythmic therapy is not needed.

In older patients with typical atrial flutter or postsurgical IART, elective cardioversion is usually performed if the arrhythmia does not self-terminate within 12 to 24 hours. Prolonged atrial flutter may lead to thrombus formation in the atrial appendage. When atrial flutter has persisted beyond 24-48 hours, transesophageal echocardiography is usually necessary to rule out thrombus prior to elective cardioversion. In contrast to neonatal flutter, IART recurrence is common. Maintenance antiarrhythmic therapy including β-blockers, calcium channel blockers, amiodarone, or sotalol may be necessary. Catheter ablation is an alternative to pharmacologic therapy, which may be curative. Typically, ablation is reserved for older children and adults with atrial flutter or IART.

Atrial Fibrillation (Figure 2-17)

Definition

Atrial fibrillation is a chaotic arrhythmia in the atrium that results in a fast atrial rate of approximately 300 to 600 bpm and variable ventricular rates depending on the conduction down the AV node. Atrial fibrillation is characterized by (1) f waves (ie, abnormal p waves) with varying rates and morphologies and (2) an irregularly irregular ventricular response with typically a narrow QRS complex.

Causes

Atrial fibrillation is seen in adolescents with structurally normal hearts or in patients with cardiomyopathies, with WPW, or who have undergone congenital heart surgery. The mechanism of atrial fibrillation is multifactorial and requires both an initiating event, such as a premature atrial complex, and a susceptible substrate. Factors that contribute to this include alterations in adrenergic and hemodynamic status, atrial inflammation or scar, underlying cardiac disease, and neurohormonal and metabolic alterations.

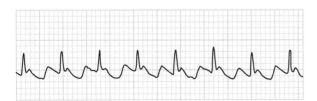

FIGURE 12-16 ■ Atrial flutter.

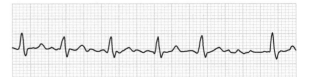

FIGURE 12-17 ■ Atrial fibrillation.

Clinical features

Symptoms of atrial fibrillation depend on the ventricular response rate as with atrial flutter. Therefore, if AV block and a slow ventricular response rate are present, patients may often be asymptomatic or complain of fatigue and exercise intolerance. If the ventricular response is fast, patients may complain of palpitations, inappropriate tachycardia, presyncope, or syncope.

Management

Atrial fibrillation is often well tolerated without significant hemodynamic instability, so management includes observation, medications, or synchronized cardioversion. Potential medications such as digoxin, calcium channel blocker, or β-blockers can be used to slow the AV nodal conduction to allow for time for the arrhythmia to spontaneously self-convert. In addition, attempts at medical cardioversion from fibrillation to sinus rhythm may occur with the use of procainamide, amiodarone, or ibutilide when electrical cardioversion fails or is contraindicated. Finally, synchronized cardioversion can be performed in a controlled setting with appropriate sedation and supervision. However, this should not be undertaken if the arrhythmia has been present for more than 48 hours due to concern for thrombus formation in the heart. If there is concern for intracardiac thrombus, anticoagulation should be initiated with warfarin, and cardioversion should be delayed for 3 to 4 weeks. If the cardioversion cannot be delayed, then heparin should be initiated, and a screening transesophageal echocardiogram should be performed to rule out thrombi before electrical cardioversion. Once the arrhythmia is terminated, recurrence is rare unless there is underlying heart disease. If there is recurrence, then chronic management with rate- or rhythm-controlling medications should be considered, as well as some form of anticoagulation.

In the setting of atrial fibrillation and WPW, there is concern for rapid conduction of the atrial tachyarrhythmias to the ventricle via the accessory pathway, which may result in ventricular fibrillation and sudden death. In this setting, treatment should be catheter ablation of the accessory pathway.

Ventricular Tachycardias

Ventricular tachyarrhythmias are an uncommon form of tachycardia in infants and children. Ventricular tachyarrhythmias include any arrhythmia originating from below the AV node and in either ventricle. Ventricular tachyarrhythmia is often thought of as a life-threatening arrhythmia because older adults with cardiac disease such as coronary artery disease and/or heart failure typically do not tolerate the arrhythmia. In pediatric patients, nonsustained ventricular arrhythmias typically occur in children with structurally normal hearts, and

therefore, the arrhythmia is often well tolerated and may have a similar clinical presentation to SVT unless there is underlying heart disease. Sustained ventricular arrhythmias occur more frequently in the setting of structural heart disease or inherited channelopathies. The most common form is monomorphic ventricular tachycardia, with rare forms being torsade de pointes, polymorphic ventricular tachycardia, and ventricular fibrillation.

Monomorphic Ventricular Tachycardia (Figure 12-18)

Definition

Monomorphic ventricular tachycardia is defined as a fast heart rate that is at or above the upper limits of normal for age with sudden onset and that is a regular rhythm originating from ventricle. This is characterized by (1) a wide QRS complex tachycardia and (2) no visible P waves or P waves with clear ventriculoatrial disassociation (ie, the atrial rate is slower than the ventricular rate). Ventricular tachycardia can be difficult to differentiate from SVT with aberrancy, functional bundle-branch block at fast heart rates, or baseline bundle-branch block.

Causes

Ventricular tachycardia may be idiopathic in origin, but other conditions must be considered. It may occur in cardiomyopathies such as dilated or hypertrophic cardiomyopathy, inflammatory disease such as myocarditis, infiltrative diseases such as arrhythmogenic right ventricular dysplasia, cardiac tumors, false left ventricular tendons, or congenital heart disease such as tetralogy of Fallot after repair or left-sided obstructive lesions such as aortic stenosis.

Clinical features

The symptoms of ventricular tachycardia depend on the ventricular response rate. Therefore, patients with ventricular tachycardia may be asymptomatic or present with sudden death. If the rates are fast, then patients may complain of palpitations, inappropriate tachycardia, presyncope, or syncope. In addition, the underlying disease state including cardiac function and/or congenital heart disease may contribute to how well the ventricular tachycardia is hemodynamically tolerated.

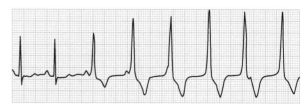

FIGURE 12-18 ■ Monomorphic ventricular tachycardia.

Management

Treatment, as with most arrhythmias, is based on the hemodynamic status of the patient. A hemodynamically stable patient may benefit from acute pharmacologic therapy. This includes correction of electrolyte abnormalities and/or use of antiarrhythmic medications that affect the ventricular myocytes such as intravenous lidocaine, procainamide, β-blockers, and/or amiodarone. If the patient is hemodynamically unstable, DC cardioversion with 0. 5 to 2 J/kg is the treatment of choice. Long-term therapy includes use of antiarrhythmic medications such as β-blockers, amiodarone, sotalol, and verapamil in certain situations to suppress the arrhythmia. In older children and young adults with stable symptomatic monomorphic ventricular tachycardia, catheter ablation is an alternative treatment strategy that provides a more definitive cure. Patients with unstable ventricular tachycardia or stable ventricular tachycardia in the setting of certain underlying diseases such as hypertrophic cardiomyopathy often require an implantable cardioverter-defibrillator (ICD) to prevent sudden death.

Ventricular Fibrillation (Figure 12-19)

Definition

Ventricular fibrillation is a fast irregular heart rhythm that originates from ventricle. This is characterized by very abnormal QRS complexes with varying size and morphology with no discernible atrial activity.

Causes

Ventricular fibrillation is a terminal and life-threatening arrhythmia that results in inadequate circulation. Etiologies for this rhythm include severe hypoxia, hyperkalemia, drug overdose (eg, digoxin, anesthetics), myocarditis, myocardial infarction, degeneration of ventricular tachycardia, or atrial fibrillation with rapid conduction via an accessory pathway to the ventricle.

Clinical features

Ventricular fibrillation presents with a pulseless rhythm and cardiac arrest or sudden death.

Management

Treatment requires immediate cardiopulmonary resuscitation and immediate defibrillation at 2 J/kg.

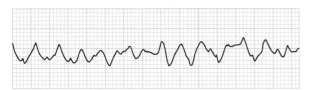

FIGURE 12-19 ■ Ventricular fibrillation.

Polymorphic Ventricular Tachycardia (Figure 12-20)

Definition

Polymorphic ventricular tachycardia is a fast irregular heart rhythm that originates from the ventricle. It is a characterized by (1) a wide QRS complex tachycardia with multiple differing morphologies and (2) no visible P waves or P waves with clear ventriculoatrial disassociation (ie, the atrial rate is slower than the ventricular rate).

Causes

Polymorphic ventricular tachycardia occurs in the setting of a prolonged QT interval due to drugs or an inherited genetic ion channelopathy, which results in the ability for abnormal myocardial depolarization to occur, resulting in this potentially life-threatening arrhythmia. Other causes include drug overdose (ie, digoxin), coronary artery disease/anomalies, and inherited conditions such as catecholamine-induced polymorphic ventricular tachycardia.

Clinical features

Symptoms can vary from life threatening to benign based on the duration of the arrhythmia. Often, episodes are nonsustained, and symptoms may include palpitations, presyncope, or syncope. In addition, this arrhythmia may degenerate into ventricular fibrillation.

Management

Treatment requires immediate cardiopulmonary resuscitation and defibrillation at 2 J/kg if unstable with evidence of ineffective circulation. If patients are conscious and hemodynamically stable, then medications can be tried. This includes treating reversible causes for the ventricular tachycardia such as digoxin overdose or coronary ischemia. In addition, use of intravenous magnesium sulfate (50 mg/kg to up to 2 g) can be used to shorten the QT interval if prolongation of the QT interval is the suspected etiology of the arrhythmia. Additionally, similar antiarrhythmics for ventricular tachycardia can be used for both acute and long-term management. If the episodes are life threatening, then the use of an ICD is indicated.

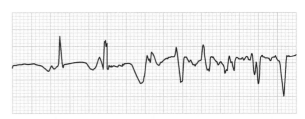

FIGURE 12-20 ■ Polymorphic ventricular tachycardia.

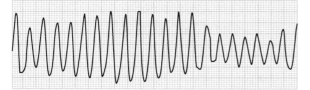

FIGURE 12-21 ■ Torsade de pointes.

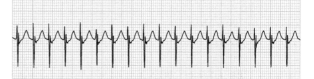

FIGURE 12-22 ■ Junctional ectopic tachycardia.

Torsade de Pointes (Figure 12-21)

Definition

Torsade de pointes is a rapid irregular heart rhythm that originates from the ventricle and is a distinct form of polymorphic ventricular tachycardia. It is characterized by (1) a wide QRS tachycardia with characteristic pattern of positive and negative oscillation of the QRS complex direction around the isoelectric baseline, or "twisting of the points"; (2) no visible P waves or P waves with clear ventriculoatrial disassociation (ie, the atrial rate is slower than the ventricular rate); (3) paroxysmal episodes; and (4) occurrence in the setting of prolonged QT interval.

Causes

Torsade de pointes commonly occurs as a pause-dependent arrhythmia. It is usually initiated by a premature ventricular complex that occurs during a vulnerable period of ventricular repolarization ("R on T phenomenon"). The arrhythmia should raise concern for congenital or acquired long QT syndrome. Causes of acquired long QT syndrome should be investigated including electrolyte derangements and drugs that prolong the QT interval.

Clinical features

Depending on the duration of the torsade de pointes, patients may have no symptoms, syncope, or even sudden cardiac death. The symptoms of torsade de pointes mirror those of polymorphic ventricular tachycardia.

Management

Reversible causes of QT prolongation should be initially treated, including withdrawal of QT-prolonging drugs and correction of metabolic derangements. Pharmacologic therapy should include magnesium supplementation, β-blockers, and/or lidocaine. In addition, isoproterenol and/or pacing will increase the heart rate and shorten myocardial repolarization, decreasing the chance of initiating a pause-dependent arrhythmia.

Junctional Ectopic Tachycardia (Figure 12-22)

Definition

Junctional ectopic tachycardia (JET) is a rapid heart rate that exceeds the sinus rate and originates from the AV junction, usually the AV node or His-Purkinje system just below the level of the AV node. Similar to ectopic atrial tachycardia, JET is an automatic arrhythmia that responds to endogenous and exogenous catecholamines. JET is characterized by (1) narrow QRS tachycardia, usually at rates of ≥160 bpm; (2) no P wave preceding the QRS and inverted P waves that may follow the QRS complex; (3) and occurrence as a sustained, regular rhythm or in short bursts with irregular rhythm. Occasionally, a sinus beat will conduct through the AV node during an episode of JET, which causes a brief irregularity in the rhythm known as a sinus capture beat.

Causes

JET is caused by an enhanced automaticity within the region of the AV node and proximal His bundle. In the pediatric population, JET is most often seen in the 24 hours following surgery to correct congenital heart disease. JET has been seen following nearly all types of congenital heart surgery but occurs most commonly after repair of a large ventricular septal defect, either in isolation or in the setting of tetralogy of Fallot or complete AV canal defect. Outside of the postoperative setting, JET is rare but may occur in a familial form known as "congenital JET," which usually presents in infancy or in utero.

Clinical features

Congenital JET commonly presents with heart failure and is associated with elevated heart rates. There is an incidence of sudden death in patients with the congenital form of JET. Postoperative JET is typically transient and lasts up to 96 hours. During this time period, the patient can have significant hemodynamic compromise due to diminished cardiac function after cardiopulmonary bypass, tachycardia, and loss of AV synchrony.

Management

The goal of treatment for JET is to slow the ventricular rate and decrease automaticity. In the postoperative setting, nonpharmacologic measures such as controlling fever and pain, weaning inotropic support, cooling to induce mild hypothermia, and sedating and paralyzing can be used to reduce endogenous catecholamines. In addition, atrial pacing with temporary epicardial pacing wires at a rate that exceeds the JET rate will re-establish AV synchrony and may improve hemodynamics. Pharmacologic treatments for JET include procainamide and amiodarone. The majority of patients with congenital or postoperative JET can eventually be weaned from antiarrhythmic medications because the rhythm usually resolves with time. In rare circumstances, catheter ablation may be performed, although there is a substantial risk of iatrogenic heart block with ablation near the AV node.

SYNCOPE: BENIGN VERSUS MALIGNANT

Syncope is a transient loss of consciousness due to a variety of cardiac, noncardiac, and/or neurocardiogenic etiologies. Cardiac arrhythmias, which are either too fast or too slow, can result in decreased cardiac output and diminished cerebral perfusion, resulting in malignant syncope. Most cardiac arrhythmias are well tolerated in children but depend on the rate and type of the arrhythmia, presence or absence of structural heart disease, and cardiac function.

A thorough history, physical, and baseline electrocardiogram are important in differentiating between malignant and benign syncope. Red flags that suggest malignant syncope include the following:

- Sudden onset without warning
- Association with palpitations or chest pain
- Occurrence during exertion
- Lack of a prodrome such as dizziness, diaphoresis, or nausea

- Association with trauma or seizures
- Recurrent syncope
- Family history of sudden death, cardiomyopathy, or channelopathy
- Abnormal physical examination (eg, heart murmur)
- Abnormal electrocardiogram

Diseases associated with malignant syncope and sudden death are listed in Figure 12-23.[9] With those diseases being considered, if the evaluation is normal, the patient can be reassured that syncope is a common occurrence and additional diagnostic testing is unnecessary.

CONDITIONS ASSOCIATED WITH MALIGNANT ARRHYTHMIA AND SUDDEN DEATH

Hypertrophic Cardiomyopathy

Diagnosis

Hypertrophic cardiomyopathy is characterized by thickening of the ventricular myocardium in the absence of other cardiac or systemic conditions that may result in ventricular hypertrophy. The myocardial cells often have a disorganized arrangement. This leads to impaired ventricular filling and left ventricular outflow tract obstruction. Patients may be asymptomatic but can present with chest pain, palpitations, dizziness, syncope (especially during or just after exercise), heart failure symptoms, arrhythmias, or sudden death.[10]

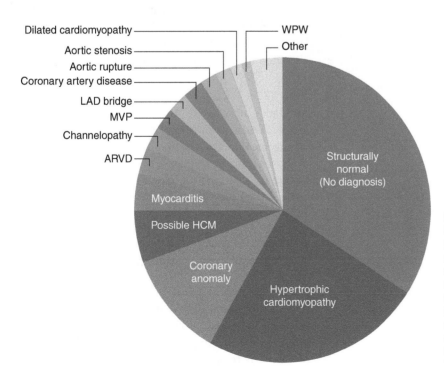

FIGURE 12-23 ■ Cardiac causes of sudden death in young athletes. ARVD, arrhythmogenic right ventricular dysplasia; HCM, hypertrophic cardiomyopathy; LAD bridge, left anterior descending myocardial bridge; MVP, mitral valve prolapse; WPW, Wolff-Parkinson-White syndrome. (*Adapted with permission from Maron BJ, Doerer JJ, Haas TS, et al. Sudden deaths in young competitive athletes: analysis of 1866 deaths in the United States 1980-2006. Circulation. 2009;119:1085-1092.*)

Arrhythmias

A variety of arrhythmias have been identified including atrial fibrillation, atrial flutter, ventricular tachycardia, and ventricular fibrillation. Nonsustained ventricular tachycardia is infrequently seen in children but more often seen in adolescents or young adults. In addition, 2 inherited forms of hypertrophic cardiomyopathy, Danon disease and a mutation in the *PRKAG2* gene, are associated with the presence of accessory pathways and place these patients at risk for AVRT.[10]

Management

Arrhythmia management is independent of the treatment for left ventricular outflow tract obstruction and hypertrophy and starts with antiarrhythmic medication, typically β-blockers or calcium channel blockers. In addition, the risk of sudden death can be as high as 3% per year, and certain high-risk patients with hypertrophic cardiomyopathy should undergo ICD implantation to prevent sudden death.[10,11] Specific risk factors are a family history of premature sudden death, previous cardiac arrest, unexplained syncope, left ventricular thickness of greater than 3 cm, abnormal blood pressure response during exercise, and ventricular tachycardia.[10,12]

Long QT Syndrome (Figure 12-24)

Diagnosis

Long QT syndrome (LQTS) is an inherited condition that results in prolongation of the QT interval, abnormal T waves, and predisposition to polymorphic ventricular tachycardia, particularly torsade de pointes. Diagnosis is made based on a combination of family history, degree of corrected QT interval prolongation typically greater than 460 ms, and genetic testing. The 3 most common forms of LQTS are LQT1, which is caused by a mutation in the *KCNQ1* gene coding for an IKs potassium channel; LQT2, which is caused by a mutation in the *KCNH2* gene coding for an IKr potassium channel; and LQT3, which is caused by a mutation in the *SCN5A* gene coding for a sodium channel. These mutations result in abnormal QT prolongation and delayed ventricular repolarization, increasing the risk of ventricular arrhythmias.[13–15]

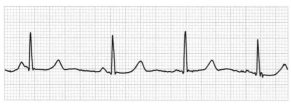

FIGURE 12-24 ■ Long QT syndrome.

Arrhythmias

Polymorphic ventricular tachycardia, particularly torsade de pointes, may be self-limited or may degenerate to ventricular fibrillation and cardiac arrest. The phenotypic presentation of LQTS often depends on the genotype, and the overall lifetime risk of sudden death is about 4%.[14]

Management

Most patients with LQTS can be managed with β-blocker therapy alone. ICD implant is indicated in certain high-risk patients, particularly patients who continue to have syncope and/or torsade despite β-blocker therapy.[16] It is important for these patients to avoid medications that prolong the QT interval and to avoid specific triggers like exercise and swimming that may provoke arrhythmias.[16,17]

Catecholaminergic Polymorphic Ventricular Tachycardia

Diagnosis

Catecholaminergic polymorphic ventricular tachycardia (CPVT) is a genetic condition associated with polymorphic ventricular tachycardia during increased adrenergic states (eg, exercise).[18] The genetic causes include a mutation in the *RYR2* or *CASQ2* genes associated with calcium regulation, which leads to destabilization of the ventricular myocardium.[19]

Arrhythmias

Isolated premature ventricular ectopy to polymorphic ventricular tachycardia is seen with increased adrenergic state. In addition, patients may present with syncope with exertion or during acute emotional states. One distinct finding seen in CPVT is bidirectional ventricular tachycardia. This is characterized by a beat-to-beat alteration in the QRS axis by 180 degrees.

Management

Avoidance of exercise and activities that result in increased adrenergic stimulation is required. Medical management includes β-blocker therapy. In the instance of aborted sudden death or life-threatening arrhythmias despite adequate pharmacologic management, ICD may be needed for prevention of sudden death.[20]

Arrhythmogenic Right Ventricular Dysplasia/Cardiomyopathy

Diagnosis

Arrhythmogenic right ventricular dysplasia/cardiomyopathy is an autosomal dominant inherited cardiomyopathy due to progressive fibrofatty infiltration of primarily the right ventricular myocardium.[21] This predisposes individuals to ventricular arrhythmias and ventricular dysfunction.

Arrhythmias

Ventricular arrhythmias are commonly seen in this patient population. Presenting symptoms can be absent or can include palpitations, syncope, or even sudden death. The arrhythmia burden also is varied and ranges from isolated ventricular ectopy and nonsustained ventricular tachycardia to life-threatening ventricular tachycardia.

Management

Ventricular arrhythmias may be treated with β-blocker therapy, amiodarone, or sotalol.[22] Catheter ablation has also been used as an adjunctive therapy to eliminate the focus for the ventricular tachycardia. Due to the progressive nature of the disease, however, these may only be temporarily effective. In the setting of aborted sudden death or sustained ventricular tachycardia despite medical therapy, ICD placement is recommended, although the guidelines in pediatrics are less clear.[23]

Brugada Syndrome (Figure 12-25)

Diagnosis

Brugada syndrome is a genetic condition that results in characteristic ST-segment abnormalities in the right-sided precordial leads (V_1-V_3) on electrocardiogram and an increased risk of ventricular arrhythmias and sudden death.[24] The result of the genetic condition is to cause an abnormally functioning ion channel that is important in electrical activation in the myocardium. In approximately 30% of patients, this involves a loss of function of a sodium channel, SCN5A.[25]

Arrhythmias

Patients with Brugada syndrome may manifest ventricular tachycardia, ventricular fibrillation, and in some instances, SVTs including atrial fibrillation. Sudden death typically presents in patients in their 40s and often after a history of previous syncopal episodes.

Management

ICD therapy is used in patients with syncope or aborted cardiac arrest to prevent sudden death. Therapy for

asymptomatic patients who may be at lower risk is not as clear. Quinidine may be used to prevent symptoms and resolve electrocardiographic features of the disease. In addition, fevers, certain anesthetic agents such as propofol, antidepressants, and antipsychotics with sodium channel–blocking effects should be avoided. Patients are not typically restricted from activity because events typically occur during sleep or rest.[25]

Myocarditis

Diagnosis

Myocarditis is myocardial inflammation that results in cardiac muscle cell damage or death. This is caused by infectious etiologies including adenovirus, parvovirus, and enterovirus (ie, coxsackie virus) or inflammatory etiologies including autoimmune disorders such as collagen vascular disease. The result is cardiac dysfunction and/or arrhythmias.

Arrhythmias

Inflammation of the cardiac myocytes can result in a wide variety of conduction disturbances. These can include heart block of varying degrees, atrial arrhythmias, and in particular, life-threatening ventricular arrhythmias.

Management

Primary treatment for myocarditis is supportive care for the cardiac dysfunction and arrhythmias while the process of inflammation resolves. Treatment of underlying infectious or immunologic disorders will often result in reversal of the findings and suppression of arrhythmias. Antiarrhythmic medication may be used during the active disease process to control arrhythmias if needed.

Dilated Cardiomyopathy

Diagnosis

Dilated cardiomyopathy is dilation of the cardiac chambers with diminished ventricular function. This is the most common form of cardiomyopathy and can result from a variety of causes including idiopathic, familial, drug toxicity (eg, anthracyclines), metabolic disorders (eg, thyroid dysfunction), nutritional deficiencies (eg, carnitine) muscular dystrophies, ischemia, inborn errors of metabolisms, immunologic disorders (eg, collagen vascular disease), and infections (eg, human immunodeficiency virus).

Arrhythmias

Patients with dilated cardiomyopathy with progressive ventricular dysfunction and dilation are at increased risk for ventricular arrhythmias. In addition, dilation of the atrial chambers as a consequence of AV valve regurgitation seen with ventricular dilation may predispose patients to atrial arrhythmias such as flutter and fibrillation.

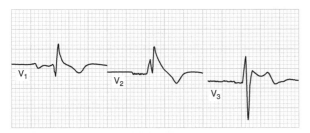

FIGURE 12-25 ▪ Brugada syndrome.

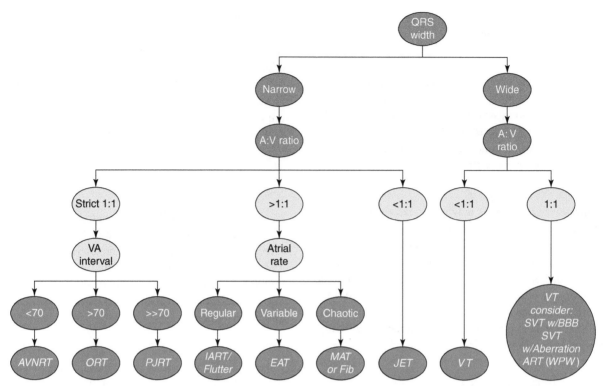

FIGURE 12-26 ■ A practical approach to differentiating tachyarrhythmias. AVNRT, atrioventricular nodal re-entrant tachycardia; BBB, bundle-branch block; EAT, ectopic atrial tachycardia; Fib, fibrillation; IART, intra-atrial re-entrant tachycardia; JET, junctional ectopic tachycardia; MAT, multifocal atrial tachycardia; ORT, orthodromic reciprocating tachycardia; PJRT, permanent junctional reciprocating tachycardia; SVT, supraventricular tachycardia; VT, ventricular tachycardia. (*Adapted with permission from Walsh EP. Clinical approach to diagnosis and acute management of tachycardias in children. In: Walsh EP, Saul JP, Triedman JK, eds.* Cardiac Arrhythmias in Children and Young Adults With Congenital Heart Disease. *Philadelphia, PA: Lippincott Williams & Wilkins, 2001:95-113; and Kaltman H, Shah M. Evaluation of the child with an arrhythmia.* Pediatr Clin North Am. *2004;51:1537-1551.*)

Management

Arrhythmias may be managed with appropriate antiarrhythmic therapy; however, the role of antiarrhythmic therapy in prevention of sudden death in pediatric patients is less certain. Adults with ischemic and nonischemic dilated cardiomyopathy with heart failure and dilated cardiomyopathy have an increased risk of sudden death despite medical therapy and therefore warrant implantation of an ICD for primary prevention.[26] However, the use of ICD in pediatric patients with heart failure and dilated cardiomyopathy is limited due to the low incidence of sudden death (1%-2%) in patients awaiting transplantation.[27] As a result, the role of ICD therapy in pediatrics has mainly been used for secondary prevention.[28,29]

CONCLUSIONS

Arrhythmias in pediatric patients are due to a wide variety of etiologies. Accurate rhythm interpretation, identification of the arrhythmia's etiology, hemodynamic assessment, and comprehension of the mechanisms of bradyarrhythmias and tachyarrhythmias are needed to provide the most appropriate management (Figure 12-26). Treatment includes correcting reversible causes, using appropriate antiarrhythmics, administering electrical cardioversion/defibrillation, catheter ablation, and/or device therapy including pacemakers or ICDs. The appropriate management of arrhythmias using various therapies is paramount to minimize or alleviate symptoms, reduce the risk of cardiac dysfunction, prevent hemodynamic compromise, and/or prevent mortality.

Clinical Pearls

- A 12-lead electrocardiogram is integral to appropriate rhythm diagnosis.
- Bradyarrhythmias that result in symptoms such as exercise intolerance, dizziness, or syncope require further evaluation.
- Administration of adenosine can be useful for diagnosis and treatment of tachyarrhythmias.
- Supraventricular tachycardias are not life threatening in patients with structurally normal hearts.
- A detailed clinical history is important in the evaluation of syncope.
- Arrhythmias or sudden death may be the initial presentation of an underlying pathologic disorder including cardiomyopathies, channelopathies, or structural heart disease.

REFERENCES

1. Davignon A, Rautaharju P, Boisselle E, et al. Normal ECG standards for infants and children. *Pediatr Cardiol.* 1979;1:123-131.

2. Park MK. *Pediatric Cardiology for Practitioners.* 4th ed. St. Louis, MO: Mosby; 2002.

3. Deal BJ, Keane JF, Gillette PC, Garson A Jr. Wolff-Parkinson-White syndrome and supraventricular tachycardia during infancy: management and follow-up. *J Am Coll Cardiol.* 1985;5:130-135.

4. Gillette PC, Garson A, eds. *Clinical Pediatric Arrhythmias.* Philadelphia, PA: W. B. Saunders Company; 1999.

5. Kaltman J, Shah M. Evaluation of the child with an arrhythmia. *Pediatr Clin North Am.* 2004;51;1537-1551.

6. Walsh EP, Saul JP, Triedman JK, eds. *Cardiac Arrhythmias in Children and Young Adults With Congenital Heart Disease.* Philadelphia, PA: Lippincott Williams & Wilkins; 2001.

7. Ko JK, Deal BJ, Strasburger JF, Benson DW Jr. Supraventricular tachycardia mechanisms and their age distribution in pediatric patients. *Am J Cardiol.* 1992; 69:1028-1032.

8. Kugler JD, Danford DA, Houston K, Felix G. Radiofrequency catheter ablation for paroxysmal supraventricular tachycardia in children and adolescents without structural heart disease. Pediatric EP Society, Radiofrequency Catheter Ablation Registry. *Am J Cardiol.* 1997;80:1438-1443.

9. Maron BJ, Doerer JJ, Haas TS, et al. Sudden deaths in young competitive athletes: analysis of 1866 deaths in the United States 1980-2006. *Circulation.* 2009;119:1085-1092.

10. Maron BJ. Hypertrophic cardiomyopathy in childhood. *Pediatr Clin North Am.* 2004;51:1305-1346.

11. Melacini P, Maron BJ, Bobbo F, et al. Evidence that pharmacological strategies lack efficacy for the prevention of sudden death in hypertrophic cardiomyopathy. *Heart.* 2007;93:708-710.

12. Spirito P, Autore C, Rapezzi C, et al. Syncope and risk of sudden death in hypertrophic cardiomyopathy. *Circulation.* 2009;119:1703-1710.

13. Goldenberg I, Horr S, Moss AJ, et al. Risk for life-threatening cardiac events in patients with genotype-confirmed long-QT syndrome and normal-range corrected QT intervals. *J Am Coll Cardiol.* 2011;57:51-59.

14. Schwartz PJ, Priori SG, Spazzolini C, et al. Genotype-phenotype correlation in the long-QT syndrome: gene-specific triggers for life-threatening arrhythmias. *Circulation.* 2001;103:89-95.

15. Ackerman MJ. Genotype-phenotype relationships in congenital long QT syndrome. *J Electrocardiol.* 2005;38 (4 Suppl):64-68.

16. Schwartz PJ. Management of long QT syndrome. *Nat Clin Pract Cardiovasc Med.* 2005;2:346-351.

17. Kannankeril P, Roden DM, Darbar D. Drug-induced long QT syndrome. *Pharmacol Rev.* 2010;62:760-781.

18. Leenhardt A, Lucet V, Denjoy I, et al. Catecholaminergic polymorphic ventricular tachycardia in children. A 7-year follow-up of 21 patients. *Circulation.* 1995;91:1512-1519.

19. Priori SG, Napolitano C, Memmi M, et al. Clinical and molecular characterization of patients with catecholaminergic polymorphic ventricular tachycardia. *Circulation.* 2002;106:69-74.

20. Liu N, Ruan Y, Priori SG. Catecholaminergic polymorphic ventricular tachycardia. *Prog Cardiovasc Dis.* 2009;51:23-30.

21. Marcus FI, McKenna WJ, Sherrill D, et al. Diagnosis of arrhythmogenic right ventricular cardiomyopathy/dysplasia: proposed modification of the task force criteria. *Circulation.* 2010;121:1533-1541.

22. Sen-Chowdhry S, Lowe MD, Sporton SC, McKenna WJ. Arrhythmogenic right ventricular cardiomyopathy: clinical presentation, diagnosis, and management. *Am J Med.* 2004;117:685-695.

23. Zipes DP, Camm AJ, Borggrefe M, et al. ACC/AHA/ESC 2006 guidelines for management of patients with ventricular arrhythmias and the prevention of sudden cardiac death: a report of the American College of Cardiology/American Heart Association Task Force and the European Society of Cardiology Committee for Practice Guidelines (Writing Committee to Develop Guidelines for Management of Patients With Ventricular Arrhythmias and the Prevention of Sudden Cardiac Death). *J Am Coll Cardiol.* 2006;48:e247-e346.

24. Brugada P, Brugada J. Right bundle branch block, persistent ST segment elevation and sudden cardiac death: a distinct clinical and electrocardiographic syndrome. A multicenter report. *J Am Coll Cardiol.* 1992;20:1391-1396.

25. Antzelevitch C, Brugada P, Borggrefe M, et al. Brugada syndrome: report of the second consensus conference: endorsed by the Heart Rhythm Society and the European Heart Rhythm Association. *Circulation.* 2005;111:659-670.

26. Epstein AE, DiMarco JP, Ellenbogen KA, et al. ACC/AHA/HRS 2008 Guidelines for Device-Based Therapy of Cardiac Rhythm Abnormalities: a report of the American College of Cardiology/American Heart Association Task Force on Practice Guidelines (Writing Committee to Revise the ACC/AHA/NASPE 2002 Guideline Update for Implantation of Cardiac Pacemakers and Antiarrhythmia Devices) developed in collaboration with the American Association for Thoracic Surgery and Society of Thoracic Surgeons. *J Am Coll Cardiol.* 2008;51:e1-e62.

27. Rhee EK, Canter CE, Basile S, et al. Sudden death prior to pediatric heart transplantation: would implantable defibrillators improve outcome? *J Heart Lung Transplant.* 2007;26:447-452.

28. Rosenthal D, Chrisant M, Eden E, et al. International Society for Heart and Lung Transplantation: practice guidelines for management of heart failure in children. *J Heart Lung Transplant.* 2008;23:1313-1333.

29. Zipes DP, Camm AJ, Borggrefe M, et al. ACC/AHA/ESC 2006 Guidelines for Management of Patients With Ventricular Arrhythmias and the Prevention of Sudden Cardiac Death: a report of the American College of Cardiology/American Heart Association Task Force and the European Society of Cardiology Committee for Practice Guidelines (writing committee to develop Guidelines for Management of Patients With Ventricular Arrhythmias and the Prevention of Sudden Cardiac Death): developed in collaboration with the European Heart Rhythm Association and the Heart Rhythm Society. *Circulation.* 2006;114:e385-e484.

CHAPTER 13

Heart Failure, Cardiomyopathy, and Pulmonary Hypertension

Kimberly Lin, Thomas Bernadzikowski, Stephen Walker, Brian Hanna and Beth Kaufman

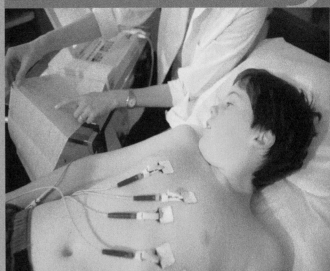

INTRODUCTION

Cardiac physiology in a normal child is an elegant balance requiring many components to work on an interactive basis. In children with congenital or acquired heart disease, some of those parts do not function properly from the start; others develop problems with time or under duress. This chapter begins with a discussion of the syndrome of heart failure. The pathophysiology of heart failure is reviewed, followed by the diagnosis and management of left heart failure (including heart transplantation). This is followed by a more detailed discussion of the primary conditions that can lead to heart failure. We explore the diagnosis and management of various forms of cardiomyopathy, a set of intrinsic cardiac muscle disorders with often overlapping phenotypes. Finally, we present the diagnosis and management of right heart failure as a manifestation of pulmonary hypertension.

HEART FAILURE

Definition and Pathophysiology

Heart failure is a clinical syndrome that develops as a final common pathway of diverse cardiac injuries. Symptoms result from an impairment in the heart's ability to adequately relax and/or contract. Historically, heart failure was defined as a pure mechanical or hemodynamic condition that resulted from an inability of the heart to provide enough cardiac output to meet the metabolic demands of the body. Therapy was directed at altering these hemodynamic derangements by increasing cardiac output, typically with medications that increased heart rate and contractility, and by decreasing metabolic demands. However, there has been a paradigm shift in the approach to heart failure in recent years. We now better understand the compensatory neurohormonal mechanisms and complex molecular signaling cascades that are activated in the setting of decreased cardiac output. These mechanisms cause adverse remodeling that perpetuates the cycle of heart failure.

Patients with heart failure have traditionally been categorized by their functional capabilities, using either the New York Heart Association (NYHA) or Ross classification schemes (Table 13-1). In recent years, the American College of Cardiology and American Heart Association have advocated the additional use of a staging system for heart failure that emphasizes the structural condition of the heart as well as the prevention, evolution, and progression of heart failure (Figure 13-1).[1] It is meant to complement the NYHA classification system, which has been used to describe functional limitations rather than structural abnormalities. Stage A and B patients might best be thought of as "pre–heart failure" patients, in that they are at risk for heart failure but have not yet developed symptoms. Whereas in the following section, we will primarily address the assessment and management of stage C and D heart failure in children, the subsequent section will discuss specific cardiomyopathies, which may present at any stage of the heart failure spectrum. Referral to a cardiologist for evaluation and surveillance of a child with any stage of heart failure is recommended.

Functional Classification of Heart Failure in Infants and Children

Class	Patient Symptoms
Ross classification for infants and young children	
Class I	No limitations or symptoms
Class II (mild)	Mild tachypnea or diaphoresis with feeding in infants Dyspnea on exertion in older children No growth failure
Class III (moderate)	Marked tachypnea or diaphoresis with feeding or exertion Prolonged feeding times Growth failure from heart failure
Class IV (severe)	Symptoms at rest including tachypnea, retractions, grunting, or diaphoresis
New York Heart Association classification for older children and adults	
Class I	No limitation of physical activity Ordinary physical activity does not cause undue fatigue, palpitations, or dyspnea
Class II (mild)	Slight limitation of physical activity Comfortable at rest, but ordinary physical activity results in fatigue, palpitations, or dyspnea
Class III (moderate)	Marked limitation of physical activity Comfortable at rest, but less than ordinary activity causes fatigue, palpitations, or dyspnea
Class IV (severe)	Unable to carry out any physical activity without discomfort Symptoms of cardiac insufficiency at rest If any physical activity is undertaken, discomfort is increased

Stage D
Structural heart disease AND
Refractory heart failure
Intensive intervention, heart transplant referral

Stage C
Structural heart disease AND
Current OR prior symptoms of heart failure
LV enlargement or abnormal systolic function

Stage B
Structural heart disease – NO signs or symptoms
LV enlargement (>95th % normal) or abnormal systolic function
(SF <28% or EF <55%)

Stage A
High risk for CM and CHF
NO structural abnormalities or CHF symptoms
Examples: Muscular dystrophy, sarcomere gene mutation carrier, anthracycline exposure

FIGURE 13-1 ■ American College of Cardiology Foundation/American Heart Association 2009 heart failure staging guidelines. CHF, congestive heart failure; CM, cardiomyopathy; EF, ejection fraction; LV, left ventricle; SF, shortening fraction. (*Adapted with permission from Jessup M, Abraham WT, Casey DE, et al. 2009 focused update: ACCF/AHA Guidelines for the Diagnosis and Management of Heart Failure in Adults: a report of the American College of Cardiology Foundation/American Heart Association Task Force on Practice Guidelines: developed in collaboration with the International Society for Heart and Lung Transplantation. Circulation. 2009;119:1977-2016*).

The term "heart failure" has been used broadly to include volume overloaded conditions due to left-to-right shunt lesions with otherwise normal myocardial function. This section, however, will focus specifically on heart failure as the syndrome that occurs as a result of myocardial dysfunction and injury. Here, we discuss the presentation and management of the failing systemic (ie, left) ventricle; later in this chapter, we discuss the approach to the failing pulmonary (ie, right) ventricle in the context of pulmonary hypertension.

Left Heart Failure

Clinical presentation

In the setting of a biventricular circulation, left heart failure can generally be described in 1 of 3 ways: acute decompensation, chronic compensation, and acute-on-chronic decompensation. It is essential for the general pediatrician or emergency room physician to recognize early that a child may be at risk for decompensated heart failure and, subsequently, to assess, categorize, and initiate treatment for this condition when present.

Symptoms of left heart failure in children may be subtle and nonspecific and often vary with the age at presentation. Constitutional symptoms include decreased activity level, decreased appetite, and increased fussiness. Failure to thrive by weight criteria may be masked by fluid retention. Infants are classically diaphoretic and short of breath with feeding, whereas older children may display dyspnea on exertion or easy fatigability. Gastrointestinal symptoms due to decreased intestinal perfusion are common in left heart failure at any age, manifesting as decreased appetite, poor tolerance of feeds, abdominal pain, or nausea and vomiting. Classic "cardiac" symptoms such as chest pain and palpitations occur but are less common in children than in adults with heart failure.

Although one should always look for signs of congestion of both the right- and left-sided circulations, these are also less commonly seen in children with heart failure as compared with adults. Such signs include facial swelling, elevated jugular venous distension, hepatomegaly, ascites, dependent edema, and pulmonary rales. Assessment of vital signs may reveal tachypnea, tachycardia, and hypotension. On cardiac examination, the point of maximal impulse may be laterally displaced and prolonged, and S_3 and S_4 gallops may be present. One should also assess for diminished peripheral pulses and delayed capillary refill.

Diagnostic testing

With respect to ancillary testing, a chest x-ray often shows cardiomegaly and pulmonary congestion. An electrocardiogram (ECG) may reveal an underlying or secondary arrhythmia or show abnormal ventricular voltages and evidence of ischemia including ST-T wave changes. Laboratory studies that can indicate secondary end-organ hypoperfusion include creatinine and liver function tests. B-type natriuretic peptide (BNP), a hormone released primarily by cardiac ventricular cells in response to elevated filling pressures, can be measured in the blood as well. Although BNP and cardiac enzymes, including troponin I, troponin T, and CK-MB, may be helpful in certain circumstances, their full utility in pediatric heart failure is still under evaluation.

Suspicion for decompensated left heart failure should prompt early cardiology consultation for further evaluation. Such testing may include echocardiography, to assess ventricular function and anatomy, and cardiac catheterization, for information including hemodynamics, coronary anatomy, and endomyocardial biopsy.

Differential diagnosis

Early differentiation of acute decompensated heart failure from common conditions such as sepsis and an acute abdomen is of paramount importance. Whereas the initial resuscitation of a child with sepsis often includes large intravenous fluid boluses and peripheral vasoconstrictors, this approach could potentially harm a child in cardiogenic shock. If a hypotensive or tachycardic child has a known history of heart disease, or if he or she does not mount the expected response to fluid boluses, decompensated heart failure should be suspected. There are many potential underlying conditions that can lead to left heart failure; see Tables 13-2 to 13-4 for etiologies of the most common cardiomyopathies.

Treatment

Most treatments for an acute decompensation are aimed at the singular goal of supporting cardiac output. Depending on the child's volume status, diuresis may be more helpful than fluid resuscitation by shifting the patient's status on the Frank-Starling curve. When vasoactive medications are needed, our center often uses a combination of milrinone with or without dopamine. Choice of these temporizing agents may vary widely between centers.

Chronic heart failure management, in contrast, is primarily aimed at interrupting the underlying pathophysiologic mechanisms of myocyte dysfunction. The pillars of heart failure management are angiotensin-converting enzyme (ACE) inhibitors, β-blockers, and aldosterone antagonists. Each of these agents attacks a different arm of the sympathetic nervous system or renin-angiotensin-aldosterone axis, whose maladaptive compensatory drive would otherwise promote myocyte hypertrophy and fibrosis in the heart failure patient. Stabilization and improvement of ventricular function by this process of reverse remodeling, coupled with

Etiologies of Dilated Cardiomyopathy

- Intrinsic myopathies
  - Metabolic
  - Mitochondrial
  - Neuromuscular
  - Familial
  - Idiopathic
- Congenital heart disease (a few examples below)
  - Aortic valve stenosis
  - Coarctation of the aorta
  - Volume overload lesions (eg, mitral valve regurgitation)
- Acquired conditions
  - Myocarditis
  - Drug- or toxin-related (eg, oncologic therapy, iron overload)
  - Anemia
  - Severe thyroid abnormalities
- Arrhythmias
  - Tachyarrhythmias (eg, longstanding supraventricular tachycardia)
  - Bradyarrhythmias (eg, congenital heart block)
- Ischemic
  - Early coronary artery disease
  - Coronary anomaly
  - Postoperative

Etiologies of Restrictive Cardiomyopathy

- Idiopathic
- Related to drug or toxin exposure
  - Anthracyclines
  - Mediastinal radiation therapy
  - Methysergide
- Infiltrative disorders
  - Amyloidosis
  - Sarcoidosis
  - Glycogen storage disorders
  - Hemochromatosis
- Endomyocardial
  - Endomyocardial fibrosis (tropical countries)
  - Hypereosinophilic syndrome (Löffler endocarditis)
  - Carcinoid heart disease
  - Metastatic cancers

left ventricular dysfunction. The evidence for use of all of these agents has been largely extrapolated from adult heart failure studies; specific comments on the pediatric data behind their use are available in the International Society of Heart and Lung Transplant Practice Guidelines for Management of Heart Failure in Children.[2] A summary of commonly used heart failure medications can be found in Table 13-5.

Cardiac resynchronization therapy is used frequently in adult patients with heart failure whose QRS duration by ECG and ejection fraction by echocardiogram

improved loading conditions, can often be achieved with the help of these medications.

In addition to these agents of neurohormonal blockade, chronic heart failure management may also include agents such as thiazides and loop diuretics to achieve a euvolemic state. Digoxin, which was once used widely in the field, has now been largely relegated to use at low doses in symptomatic (rather than asymptomatic)

Etiologies of Hypertrophic Cardiomyopathy (HCM)

- Sarcomere gene mutations (familial HCM)
  Examples: β-myosin heavy chain and myosin binding protein C mutations
- Metabolic disorders
  Examples: carnitine deficiency, Pompe disease, Hunter syndrome
- HCM associated with syndromes
  Examples: Noonan syndrome, LEOPARD syndrome, Friedreich ataxia, Beckwith-Wiedemann, various mitochondrial myopathies

Commonly Used Outpatient Heart Failure Medications

Therapeutic Class	Notes
ACE inhibitors (eg, lisinopril, enalapril)	Angiotensin receptor blockers may be used if intolerant to ACE inhibitors
β-blockers (eg, carvedilol, metoprolol)	Titrate carefully in light of negative chronotropic effect
Aldosterone antagonists (eg, spironolactone, eplerenone)	For symptomatic heart failure; may raise potassium levels
Diuretics (eg, furosemide, chlorothiazide)	Use to maintain euvolemic state
Digoxin	No proven survival benefit

ACE, angiotensin-converting enzyme.

meet certain criteria. Its utility in pediatric patients is being increasingly explored. To use cardiac resynchronization therapy, an electrophysiologist implants a pacemaker with a separate lead for each ventricle. The signal to pace each ventricle is timed to maximize cardiac output using ECG and/or echocardiographic guidance.

Mechanical circulatory support

When medical interventions, including inotropic support, are unsuccessful at bringing a child back to a compensated state, mechanical circulatory support may be indicated. For example, extracorporeal membrane oxygenation may be used to temporarily support the circulation as well as the lungs. Due to many issues including the size of the circuit, extracorporeal membrane oxygenation is not a viable long-term solution for cardiac support.

An increasing number of pediatric centers are using ventricular assist devices (VADs) for children with stage D heart failure that is refractory to maximal medical therapy. These devices are placed by a cardiothoracic surgeon in the operating room with the goal of unloading a ventricle and providing reliable cardiac output. A surgically implanted cannula typically pulls blood from the apex of the ventricle into a mechanical pump, which then delivers blood back to the body via a second cannula in the aorta. A similar device can be placed on the right side of the heart if needed, although support of the left heart alone is often adequate. The pump is a portable pneumatic device that is connected to a larger driver. All VADs currently used in the pediatric population are paracorporeal; that is, they sit outside of the body, in close proximity to the patient. The recent development of VADs of various sizes has expanded their use to patients as small as a full-term neonate. Several pediatric centers have also started implanting continuous flow VADs in select patients; largely due to their durability and portability, these are now commonly used in adult patients with heart failure.

The major advantage of VADs is the functionality that they give a patient with end-stage heart. A child can be awake, enterally fed, and participate in an active cardiac rehabilitation program with a properly functioning VAD (Figure 13-2). The most common complications are related to bleeding, thrombosis, and infection. Although many adult patients with heart failure have a VAD placed indefinitely ("destination therapy") or with the explicit goal of myocardial recovery that allows explantation ("bridge to recovery"), the majority of pediatric patients who have a VAD will only have their VAD explanted at the time of heart transplantation ("bridge to transplant").

Transplantation

Heart transplantation may be an option for the child who has progressive heart failure that is unresponsive

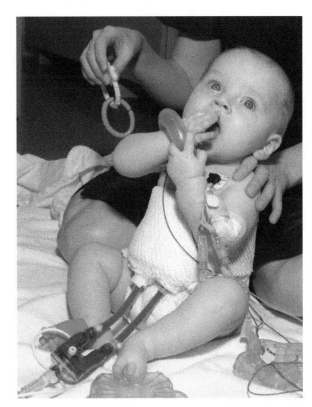

FIGURE 13-2 ■ Ventricular assist device (VAD) patient in action. This infant is on a VAD while awaiting heart transplantation. The VAD pump rests near his feet while he receives physical and occupational therapy. A computerized driver sits in front of him (not seen in this photograph).

to maximal medical therapy.[3] The evaluation of a child for transplantation involves a multidisciplinary team that considers relative morbidity and mortality with and without transplantation, comorbid conditions, and psychosocial support for the child and family. Donor heart allocation in the United States is managed by the United Network for Organ Sharing. A computer-based algorithm takes blood type, waiting time, category of need, size, and distance between the donor and recipient into account when prioritizing who gets an offer for a potential donor heart. Waiting times vary widely for individual patients, centers, and regions. For those who wait for many months, meticulous heart failure management is of paramount importance.

Prognosis

Children with heart failure can survive into adulthood with a good quality of life. Most of these patients, however, should be seen regularly, and for life, by both their primary care physician and a cardiologist. Those who undergo transplantation can expect good outcomes. In 2010, median survival for pediatric heart transplantation recipients was more than 14 years.[4] The majority of transplantation recipients report excellent functional status with respect to physical, cognitive, and psychological well-being.[5,6]

Commonly Used Immunosuppressive Medications in Heart Transplantation Recipients

Medication	Therapeutic Class	Notable Side Effects
Tacrolimus (Prograf, FK-506)	Calcineurin inhibitor	Tremor, diabetes, hypertension, renal insufficiency, pancreatitis
Cyclosporine (Sandimmune, Neoral)	Calcineurin inhibitor	Hirsutism, dental and gingival disease, renal insufficiency, hypertension
Rapamycin (Rapamune, sirolimus)	Antiproliferative	Dermatologic changes, delayed wound healing
Prednisone	Corticosteroid	Multiple, including osteoporosis, GI bleeding, weight gain, hyperglycemia
Mycophenolate mofetil (MMF, CellCept)	Antiproliferative	GI upset, marrow suppression
Azathioprine (Imuran)	Antiproliferative	Marrow suppression, hepatotoxicity

GI, gastrointestinal.

The general pediatrician who sees a patient after heart transplantation should understand that the child has traded the morbidities of heart failure for another set of morbidities. The immunosuppressive medications that work to prevent a recipient from rejecting his or her donor organ add the general risks of infection and malignancy, in addition to adverse side effects specific to each medication (Table 13-6). The following tips may help the primary care physician when caring for posttransplantation patients: (1) call early with concerns about infection or possible rejection; (2) do not administer live virus vaccines without prior discussion with a transplantation specialist; and (3) use care when prescribing other medications, including all antibiotics, because drug–drug interactions may affect the metabolism and effectiveness of immunosuppressive medications. These caveats aside, the care team should always keep in mind that the overall goal of heart transplantation is to give the child as good a quality of life as possible.

CARDIOMYOPATHY

Definition and Epidemiology

Cardiomyopathies are primary heart muscle diseases characterized by abnormally enlarged, thickened, or stiffened myocardium that adversely affect systolic function, diastolic function, or both.[7] Some children with cardiomyopathies maintain lifelong stability. However, the abnormal chambers, walls, or contractility of the affected heart can lead to a progressive or acute loss of effective pump function, serve as substrate for potential arrhythmias, degenerate to congestive heart failure with the potential need for heart transplantation, or result

in sudden cardiac death. This section will discuss primary cardiac muscle disorders as well as those that may occur secondary to certain systemic or toxic exposures. It is worth noting that cardiac dysfunction in children can also result from coronary artery disease, hypertension, valve disease, pulmonary vascular disease, or other structural congenital heart disease.

Cardiomyopathy is the leading reason for heart transplantations and sudden deaths in children, with 100,000 children affected worldwide. The majority of diagnoses are made in infants under the age of 12 months, followed by children 12 to 18 years of age.[8] The 4 main categories of cardiomyopathy representing primary disease of the heart muscle include dilated cardiomyopathy (DCM), hypertrophic cardiomyopathy (HCM), restrictive cardiomyopathy (RCM), and arrhythmogenic right ventricular cardiomyopathy (ARVC). A more recently recognized cardiomyopathy is left ventricular noncompaction (LVNC), which may or may not be associated with other forms of congenital heart disease and other cardiomyopathy phenotypes. There is accumulating evidence that most primary cardiomyopathies have a genetic basis that may occur sporadically or be inherited in families.[9]

Clinical screening with a detailed history, including 3-generation family history for any type of cardiomyopathy, cardiac examination, ECG, and echocardiogram, has been recommended for first-degree family members (siblings, parents, children) of an individual with cardiomyopathy. Serial evaluations every 2 to 3 years during childhood with annual evaluations during puberty, a period of increased likelihood of cardiomyopathy presentation, are recommended, particularly for those with family histories of HCM. Genetic counseling and testing for causative mutations (most commonly in genes of the sarcomere) are available.

Secondary cardiomyopathies associated with other systemic diseases can include inborn errors of metabolism, malformation syndromes, neuromuscular disorders, anthracycline chemotherapy exposure, and other noncardiac conditions. Each type of cardiomyopathy is characterized by a variable and heterogeneous disease process, clinical presentation, management strategy, and prognosis.

Dilated Cardiomyopathy

DCM is characterized by left ventricular dilation and dysfunction, often resulting in diminished cardiac output and secondary congestive heart failure. This is the most common cardiomyopathy, comprising 50% to 60% of children with cardiomyopathy. DCM has a yearly incidence of 0.57 cases per 100,000 and a male predilection.[10] Although the etiology of DCM is idiopathic in more than 60% of cases, DCM may develop due to gene mutations in the myocardial components, as a result of myocarditis or cardiotoxic exposures, or secondary to other systemic disorders such as metabolic, mitochondrial, and neuromuscular disorders (Table 13-2).

Pathogenesis

Myocyte injury, hypertrophy, death, and fibrosis lead to a loss of myocardial contractile function. Regardless of the etiology of DCM, depressed myocardial function stimulates neurohormonal compensatory mechanisms such as the sympathetic nervous system and renin-angiotensin-aldosterone system to attempt to maintain cardiac output in the setting of decreased contractile function. This response, while initially compensatory, perpetuates a pathologic cascade that results in ventricular dilation, fibrosis, and further dysfunction. This process is referred to as cardiac remodeling (see prior section on left heart failure). Associated atrial or ventricular arrhythmias, mitral and/or tricuspid regurgitation, intracavitary thrombi, and hypoperfusion can lead to end-organ damage.

Clinical presentation

The development of DCM can be insidious, as when associated with familial gene mutations or neuromuscular disorders. It may also present as acute decompensated heart failure in the setting of increased cardiac demand such as febrile illness, exercise, or respiratory infections.

Differential diagnosis

When presented with a new diagnosis of DCM, any potentially correctable structural cardiac defects must be excluded before labeling the child with a primary heart muscle disorder. At the top of this list are coronary abnormalities such as anomalous origin of a coronary artery or early-onset atherosclerotic disease (very rare). One should also try to establish the likelihood of an acute inflammatory process (such as myocarditis) and presence of any related systemic disorders, because these may affect the treatment options and prognosis. (Please see the more detailed discussion on myocarditis found in Chapter 14.)

Diagnostic testing

A high suspicion for DCM can be arrived at based on a child's history, clinical presentation, and physical examination. History should be targeted at detecting subtle signs of exercise intolerance, change in level of activity, failure to thrive and feeding difficulty, persistent or recurrent respiratory problems, and underlying skeletal myopathy in addition to standard cardiac symptoms of chest pain, dyspnea with exertion, palpitations, or syncope. A detailed 3-generation family history to detect familial cardiomyopathy should be included. Initial diagnostic evaluation generally includes a chest x-ray (to detect cardiomegaly), ECG, echocardiogram, and laboratory blood tests to assess end-organ function. Cardiac magnetic resonance imaging (MRI), exercise stress testing, ambulatory Holter monitor, and/or cardiac catheterizations are also often performed as part of evaluation and monitoring.

Treatment

Medical therapy is directed at improving underlying heart function, preventing disease progression, managing symptoms of congestive heart failure, and preventing complications such as thrombosis, arrhythmias, or end-organ injury. DCM is the most common reason for heart transplantation in children older than 1 year of age. Please see the prior section on left heart failure for further description of treatment options.

Hypertrophic Cardiomyopathy

HCM is the second most common cardiomyopathy, affecting 40% to 50% of children with cardiomyopathy. It is a heterogeneous and often familial disease of the myocardium. According to the Pediatric Cardiomyopathy Registry, HCM occurs at a rate of 0.47 cases per 100,000 children and is often diagnosed during infancy and adolescence. The results of systematic screening of adult HCM patients have shown that cardiac sarcomere gene mutations are associated with 40% to 60% of cases, which are inherited in an autosomal dominant fashion.[11] HCM is also a part of several genetic syndromes as well as metabolic, neuromuscular, and mitochondrial disorders (Table 13-3). Infants of diabetic mothers may have a clinical and echocardiographic presentation that is mistaken for HCM; however, their ventricular hypertrophy is generally transient, in contrast with that seen in the true HCM patient.

Pathogenesis

HCM is characterized by hypertrophy of the myocardium. This may involve the entire left ventricle, as seen in concentric HCM, or it may be limited to segments of the ventricle such as the intraventricular septum, as seen in asymmetric HCM. The latter condition was formerly referred to as idiopathic hypertrophic subaortic stenosis or hypertrophic obstructive cardiomyopathy. Dynamic outflow tract obstruction occurs secondary to narrowing between the hypertrophied septum and systolic anterior motion of the mitral valve during cardiac contraction. The mitral valve and papillary muscles are often abnormal as part of the HCM phenotype. Systolic function is preserved and typically hyperdynamic, whereas impaired ventricular compliance results in diastolic dysfunction.

The pathologic hypertrophy is most commonly a result of abnormal sarcomere proteins and disorganized myocardial architecture due to genetic defects, or more rarely due to accumulation of abnormal metabolites as in glycogen storage disorders. Abnormal intramural coronary arterioles and associated chronic microvascular ischemia are thought to contribute to myocyte cell death and fibrotic scar formation. This pathology leads to an unstable electrophysiologic substrate susceptible to arrhythmias and possible sudden cardiac death (SCD).[12]

Clinical presentation

The initial presentation of HCM can be as insidious as an abnormal ECG or a newly detected heart murmur or as dramatic as a sudden cardiac arrest. Arrhythmias can occur regardless of the degree of myocardial thickening and left ventricular outflow tract obstruction. A 3-generation pedigree that elicits a family history of cardiomyopathy or unexplained sudden death is essential.

Symptoms of HCM may include easy fatigability, dyspnea, palpitations, dizziness, syncope, or chest pain, particularly with exertion or following exercise. Symptoms in infants may include labored breathing, slow weight gain, diaphoresis, or irritability during feeding. Severe diastolic dysfunction may manifest itself with signs of heart failure such as dyspnea on exertion, orthopnea, resting tachypnea, persistent cough, or abdominal pain and vomiting. Patients with end-stage HCM can develop systolic dysfunction and ventricular dilation.

Although the physical examination in HCM may be entirely normal, a classic presentation includes auscultation of a harsh systolic ejection murmur at the left sternal border or at the apex, which increases in intensity with standing or after exercise. A holosystolic murmur of mitral regurgitation may also be present. The first and second heart sounds are typically normal, but the apical impulse is often prominent and laterally displaced.

Differential diagnosis

In a child with ventricular hypertrophy, it is essential to evaluate for stimulants of ventricular hypertrophy, such as hypertension, and structural causes of left ventricular outflow tract obstruction, including aortic stenosis, subaortic membrane, and coarctation of the aorta. A normal athlete's heart can be mistaken for pathologic HCM; distinguishing between the two may require exercise testing or several months of deconditioning.[13]

Diagnostic testing

The ECG in HCM often demonstrates left ventricular hypertrophy, along with ST-segment changes, T-wave inversions, and abnormal Q waves with diminished or absent R waves in the left precordial leads. Left atrial enlargement may also be seen. The diagnosis of HCM is most commonly made by echocardiogram, with findings that include ventricular hypertrophy (asymmetric or concentric), hyperdynamic systolic function, mitral valve regurgitation, and/or abnormal mitral valve and papillary muscles. Evidence of diastolic dysfunction may also be seen using various echocardiographic techniques (see Chapter 2). In cases with borderline hypertrophy by echocardiogram, cardiac MRI can provide an additional assessment of ventricular muscle thickness, along with detection of fibrosis and infiltrative conditions. Exercise or dobutamine stress echocardiography often reveals dynamic left ventricular outflow tract obstruction, which may or may not be present on resting studies. Sarcomere gene mutation testing is available for idiopathic and familial HCM. If the genotype of the proband is determined, further testing and/or genetic counseling may be indicated for first-degree relatives.

Exercise testing and Holter monitors should be performed annually for ongoing cardiac surveillance and to assess for risk factors for SCD. An abnormal blood pressure response during an exercise stress test or occult arrhythmia detected by Holter monitor may be impetus for further prophylactic interventions in HCM.

Treatment

There are 3 main goals of treatment for HCM: (1) to improve ventricular compliance for those with symptomatic diastolic dysfunction, (2) to minimize and control symptoms related to outflow tract obstruction by slowing the heart rate and decreasing contractility, and (3) to minimize the risk of arrhythmias and SCD. Treatment with medications including β-blockers (eg, propranolol, atenolol) or calcium channel blockers (eg, verapamil) is typically initiated when symptoms are present or in asymptomatic patients with evidence of outflow tract obstruction on diagnostic imaging.

Medical treatment of asymptomatic patients remains a debated topic. Surgical myomectomy may be performed in those with symptoms unresponsive to medical therapy. Implantable cardioverter-defibrillators are often indicated for both primary (if SCD risk factors are present) and secondary prevention of life-threatening arrhythmic events.

Restrictions from competitive sports participation are indicated for children with HCM, and guidelines for participation in recreational sports activities have been developed.[14] Approaches to risk stratification and development of consensus guidelines for preventing SCD in patients with HCM have continued to positively impact patient outcomes.[12]

Restrictive Cardiomyopathy

RCM is a rare form of cardiomyopathy affecting 3% to 5% of children with cardiomyopathy. It is characterized by markedly dilated atria in the setting of impaired ventricular relaxation due to stiff ventricular walls. One or both ventricles may be involved, with generally normal dimensions and normal contractility on presentation. Profound diastolic dysfunction eventually leads to symptoms of right and left heart failure with limited management options that often include listing for transplantation. For potential etiologies of RCM, see Table 13-4.

Pathogenesis

The pathogenesis of RCM is diverse and can be categorized as myocardial or endomyocardial, with myocardial forms further classified as noninfiltrative (eg, idiopathic, familial) or infiltrative (eg, amyloidosis, glycogen storage disease). Endomyocardial biopsies have shown nonspecific changes that include myocardial fibrosis, myocyte hypertrophy, myofibril disarray, increased interstitial connective tissue, and infiltrative and storage materials secondary to amyloidosis, sarcoidosis, hemochromatosis, or glycogen deposits.[15] Pulmonary hypertension develops secondary to elevated ventricular filling pressures that are transmitted to the atria, pulmonary veins, and pulmonary arterial vasculature.

Clinical presentation

Symptoms of RCM are often subtle in children because of slow disease progression. Infants and young children may have a history of irritability, poor feeding, or failure to thrive. Older and more active children may present with exercise intolerance, dyspnea, weakness, wheezing, syncope, palpitations, or chest pain. Atrial arrhythmias related to atrial dilation are common in RCM. Thrombus formation and stroke secondary to stasis and blood pooling in the enlarged atria may also occur. On auscultation, a murmur of atrioventricular valve regurgitation may be present, and gallop rhythms are common.

Differential diagnosis

Most cases of RCM in children are idiopathic, but it is important to evaluate for systemic diseases that can cause secondary restrictive myocardial disease (Table 13-4). Constrictive pericarditis can present with similar signs and symptoms as RCM and should be excluded because it is typically a remediable process.

Diagnostic testing

Chest x-ray may reveal cardiomegaly, atrial enlargement, pulmonary venous congestion, and pleural effusions. ECG commonly shows right and/or left atrial enlargement; it may also demonstrate ST-T wave abnormalities and ventricular hypertrophy. Arrhythmias may be seen including atrial fibrillation and paroxysmal supraventricular tachycardia, and atrioventricular block can be associated with familial RCM. Echocardiography is typically diagnostic for RCM, revealing markedly enlarged atria with normal right and left ventricular dimensions. Left ventricular systolic function is usually normal, thrombi may be present in the atria, and mitral inflow Doppler interrogation demonstrates evidence of diastolic dysfunction. Cardiac MRI allows assessment of cardiac output and can detect fibrosis, scar tissue, and infiltrative conditions in RCM. It may be particularly useful when assessing pericardial thickness if constrictive pericarditis is on the differential diagnosis. Holter monitors and event monitors are useful to monitor for abnormal rhythms, atrial or ventricular ectopy, and conduction disturbances. Cardiac catheterization to measure and serially assess hemodynamics is important for diagnosis and for detection of secondary pulmonary hypertension. Endomyocardial biopsy is generally not useful or necessary.

Treatment

Treatment options for idiopathic RCM are limited to relief of symptoms and provide no evidence-based improvements in outcome. Diuretics can be used to relieve pulmonary or systemic venous congestion but must be used cautiously, as the resulting decrease in end-diastolic pressure can further decrease cardiac output. Even though disease progression may ultimately involve systolic dysfunction, ACE inhibitors are generally avoided as systemic blood pressure would be reduced without augmentation in cardiac output. Anticoagulation with warfarin or the use of antiplatelet agents such as aspirin or dipyridamole may be considered for thromboembolic prophylaxis. Surgical options are limited to heart transplantation, which is the essential treatment for RCM. Risk stratification can be difficult in deciding when to list for transplantation. Some advocate for immediate listing upon diagnosis of RCM to avoid irreversible pulmonary hypertension, although some patients with only mildly elevated pulmonary vascular resistance (PVR) can remain stable and do well for many years. Overall, prognosis in children with RCM is poor, with half of the children dying or undergoing transplantation within 3 years of diagnosis.[16]

Arrhythmogenic Right Ventricular Cardiomyopathy

ARVC is a rare genetic primary disease of the right ventricular myocardium wherein the right ventricle is replaced by fibrous or adipose tissue. It is characterized by ventricular arrhythmias, a thinned and fibrotic right ventricle, fatty infiltration of the right ventricular free wall, and SCD.[17] The left ventricle can be involved but is typically not affected. The etiology is unknown, and 30% of ARVC appears to be familial with both autosomal dominant and autosomal recessive inheritance.[18] The prevalence of ARVC has been estimated at 1:2500 to 1:5000 in northern Italy, although the worldwide incidence of this relatively new entity is unclear. The autosomal recessive form is also known as Naxos disease.[19]

Clinical presentation

The primary presentation of ARVC is usually related to ventricular arrhythmias and conduction abnormalities. The disease is uncommon in children less than 10 years of age and has not been seen in infants. ARVC is often asymptomatic with the first clinical sign being SCD. Patients may have a history of palpitations, syncope, chest pain, dizziness, or symptomatic ventricular arrhythmias.

Diagnostic testing

ECG may show right ventricular hypertrophy, QRS prolongation, right bundle branch block, and inverted T waves in the right precordial leads. A terminal notch in the QRS complex known as an epsilon wave may also be seen. Echocardiogram reveals selective right ventricular dilation and wall motion abnormalities including akinesia or dyskinesia. Cardiac MRI may reveal myocardial fat and right ventricular wall motion abnormalities.

The diagnosis of ARVC is often made at autopsy or upon examination of explanted hearts following orthotopic heart transplantation. A definitive diagnosis requires confirmation of transmural fibrofatty replacement of the right ventricular myocardium. Endomyocardial biopsy is unreliable because fibrofatty lesions may not be present in the area that is sampled.

Treatment

Treatment is focused on control of arrhythmias and prevention of SCD with antiarrhythmic medications and implantable cardioverter-defibrillators.

Left Ventricular Noncompaction

A more recently recognized cardiomyopathy is LVNC. LVNC is characterized by an abnormal spongy appearance of the myocardium with prominent trabeculations and deep recesses that primarily affect the left ventricle. LVNC may occur in isolation or be associated with structural congenital heart disease including septal defects. Because detection of LVNC has improved with increased familiarity with the disease and improved echocardiographic technology, the true incidence is difficult to ascertain. Part of the challenge is the association of LVNC with other cardiomyopathy phenotypes. In an older report on the incidence of cardiomyopathies in Australia, LVNC was the etiology of 9% of childhood cardiomyopathies.[20] The pathogenesis is thought to relate to an arrest or abnormality of fetal cardiac development wherein the myocardium does not undergo its normal transition from a trabeculated to compact state. Similar to many forms of HCM and DCM, LVNC has a genetic etiology.[21] Clinical presentation can vary from congestive heart failure in infancy to asymptomatic incidental findings in adults. LVNC may be accompanied by ventricular dilation and poor systolic function as in DCM, a hypertrophied myocardium that is similar to HCM, or a combined phenotype.

Patients presenting with diminished left ventricular function and dilation are at the highest risk for developing heart failure, death, and need for transplantation.[22] LVNC can be associated with systemic diseases including mitochondrial disorders. For example, Barth syndrome is an X-linked disorder of males caused by a mutation in the G4.5 tafazzin gene that is characterized by LVNC (often with dilated features), skeletal myopathy, cyclic neutropenia, and poor growth.

PULMONARY HYPERTENSION

Definition and Epidemiology

The World Health Organization defines pulmonary hypertension (PH) as a mean pulmonary artery pressure greater than 25 mm Hg at rest and greater than 30 mm Hg during exercise with an elevated PVR. Primary PH is characterized by a progressive loss of pulmonary vessels with a subsequent increase in PVR, ultimately producing right heart failure and death. In severe PH, the body cannot increase pulmonary blood flow to meet increased metabolic demands without symptoms and ultimately right heart failure. Currently, PH is categorized into several diagnostic groups (Table 13-7).[23]

Clinical Classification of Pulmonary Hypertension

- Pulmonary arterial hypertension (PAH)
  - Idiopathic PAH
  - Heritable
    - BMPR2 (bone morphogenetic protein receptor type 2)
    - ALK1 (activin receptor-like kinase type 1), endoglin, with or without hereditary hemorrhagic telangiectasia
    - Unknown
  - Drug- and toxin-induced
  - Associated with
    - Connective tissue diseases
    - Human immunodeficiency virus (HIV) infection
    - Portal hypertension
    - Congenital heart diseases
    - Schistosomiasis
    - Chronic hemolytic anemia
  - Persistent pulmonary hypertension of the newborn
- Pulmonary veno-occlusive disease and/or pulmonary capillary hemangiomatosis
- Pulmonary hypertension due to left heart disease
  - Systolic dysfunction
  - Diastolic dysfunction
  - Valvular disease
- Pulmonary hypertension due to lung diseases and/or hypoxia
  - Chronic obstructive pulmonary disease
  - Interstitial lung disease
  - Other pulmonary diseases: restrictive and obstructive patterns
  - Sleep-disordered breathing
  - Alveolar hypoventilation disorders
  - Chronic exposure to high altitude
  - Developmental abnormalities
- Chronic thromboembolic pulmonary hypertension
- Pulmonary hypertension with unclear multifactorial mechanisms
  - Hematologic disorders: myeloproliferative disorders, splenectomy
  - Systemic disorders: sarcoidosis, pulmonary Langerhans cell histiocytosis, lymphangioleiomyomatosis, neurofibromatosis, vasculitis
  - Metabolic disorders: glycogen storage disease, Gaucher disease, thyroid disorders
  - Others: tumoral obstruction, fibrosing mediastinitis, renal failure on dialysis

Incidence of Pulmonary Hypertension (PH) in Pediatrics

- $1\text{-}2/10^6$ idiopathic PH
  - 6% familial
  - 20% with spontaneous BMPR2 mutations
- 2/1000 newborns in the neonatal intensive care unit
  - Associated mortality of 25%-55%
- 2% of infants following cardiac surgery
- Sickle cell disease
  - 10%-33% between 10 and 21 years of age
  - 50% mortality in the third decade

Pathophysiology

Idiopathic PH is found in both familial and sporadic forms. Familial PH has a high rate of abnormalities mapped to chromosome region 2q32 that result in a defective bone morphogenic protein receptor 2 (BMPR2), a pulmonary vasculature smooth muscle receptor that mediates inhibition of vascular smooth muscle cell proliferation. There is low phenotypic penetrance with asymptomatic obligate carriers. Additional receptors and pathways are also under investigation. Currently, it is believed that genetic defects are not sufficient to cause PH; a second hit or trigger model has been proposed. Viruses, toxins, and drugs (including diet-related pharmaceuticals), and high-flow and/or high-pressure cardiac lesions are the most common culprits.

It is important to understand that the full cardiac output must traverse the lung vasculature; no other capillary bed in the body must adapt to the full range of flows, from rest to maximal exercise, without an increased resistance. The lung is able to accommodate this flow based on vasodilation and recruitment. The pathologic hallmark of end-stage PH is complete occlusion of pulmonary blood vessels with smooth muscle cell proliferation, invasion into the intima, thrombosis, and an abnormal intercellular matrix. With progressive loss of precapillary arterioles, there is an almost logarithmic increase in PVR. However, because of the huge vascular capacitance of the lungs, over 70% of vessels are lost before there is an increase in resting pulmonary arterial pressure and symptoms become evident.

Clinical Presentation

The most common feature of PH, irrespective of etiology, is delayed diagnosis. It is important to recognize that most pediatric patients will present with common complaints that do not reveal the severe limitation in

Although the incidence of idiopathic PH is the same in children and adults, the frequency of secondary causes changes with age (Table 13-8). Children with genetic syndromes such as Down syndrome are predisposed to the development of PH at an early age, particularly those with left-to-right cardiac shunt lesions.

Clinical Findings in Pulmonary Hypertension

Symptoms	Signs
Dyspnea	Low output
Failure to thrive	Venous congestion
Activity intolerance	Active right ventricular impulse
Diaphoresis	Loud P_2: single or paradoxical splitting
Palpitations	Tricuspid regurgitation murmur
Syncope	Pulmonary regurgitation murmur
Chest pain	Cyanosis

cardiopulmonary reserve without a high index of suspicion. The gradual loss of the capacity to increase cardiac output makes the early detection of signs and symptoms difficult (Table 13-9).

Both the symptoms and physical findings in PH can be divided into those associated with either decreased pulmonary blood flow or right heart failure. In the absence of shunt lesions, there is an inability to augment cardiac output with exercise. This can lead to fatigue, chest pain, syncope, or seizures. PH patients may be referred initially to a neurologist with a history of recurrent syncope or seizures. Cyanosis with preserved

cardiac output is seen in the presence of shunt lesions such as an atrial septal defect. With right heart failure, cardiac output and blood pressure fall. Peripheral edema is a rare finding in pediatric heart failure; hepatomegaly and abdominal pain are powerful diagnostic tools. Hemoptysis can cause profound cyanosis and respiratory distress. It can also precipitate a pulmonary hypertensive crisis and death, and thus must be respected as a marker of advanced disease.

Diagnostic Testing

There are no sensitive or specific tests that are diagnostic for PH. Furthermore, no testing has been developed that qualifies as a valid screening test of asymptomatic individuals. Tests that support a clinical suspicion of PH and estimate its severity are listed in Table 13-10. A high degree of suspicion is needed when there is a diagnosis associated with PH. A testing algorithm is presented in Figure 13-3. The backbone of this algorithm is the echocardiogram. However, the clinical sensitivity is limited if there is not sufficient tricuspid regurgitation to estimate right ventricular systolic pressure. Catheterization, or any procedure requiring sedation or anesthesia, is associated with significant risk of morbidity and mortality. A precise plan for sedation or general anesthetic is crucial to prevent a pulmonary hypertensive crisis during the procedure and subsequent recovery. Current national guidelines mandate that the services of specialized PH practitioners be consulted for diagnosis, treatment, and follow-up.

Tests and Findings in Pulmonary Hypertension

Test	Findings
Electrocardiogram (normal in 50%)	Arrhythmias, right atrial enlargement, right axis deviation, right ventricular hypertrophy, ST-segment changes
Chest x-ray (normal in 40%)	Cardiomegaly, increased central pulmonary artery size, decreased distal vasculature
Computed tomography and ventilation-perfusion scan	Evidence of thrombosis, chronic interstitial lung disease
Cardiac magnetic resonance imaging	Right ventricular volume increased, myocardial fibrosis and scarring, calculation of pulmonary and systemic blood flow
Laboratory studies	Complete blood cell count: polycythemia, thrombocytopenia; connective tissue screen; hypercoagulation screen; B-type natriuretic peptide as a marker of right heart failure
Echocardiogram (improved sensitivity with stress versus resting echocardiography)	Right atrial and right ventricular dilation, tricuspid regurgitation estimate of right ventricular pressure, pulmonary regurgitation estimate of pulmonary arterial diastolic pressure, interventricular septal position bowing leftward, pericardial effusion
Catheterization	Direct hemodynamic measurements, assess pulmonary vascular bed reactivity

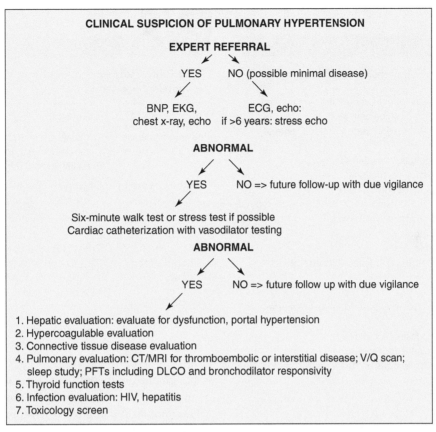

FIGURE 13-3 ■ Algorithm for investigation of suspected pulmonary hypertension. BNP, B-type natriuretic peptide; CT, computed tomography; DLCO, lung diffusion capacity; ECG, electrocardiogram; echo, echocardiography; HIV, human immunodeficiency virus; MRI, magnetic resonance imaging; PFT, pulmonary function test; V/Q, ventilation-perfusion scan.

Treatment

Current long-term treatment algorithms are guided by clinical severity and laboratory results (Table 13-11).[24] Goals of therapy include vasodilation, anticoagulation, preservation of right ventricular function, and inhibition of vascular smooth muscle proliferation. There are 3 main classes of selective pulmonary vasodilators available for off-label use in pediatric PH (Table 13-12). Each comes with a list of warnings and potential adverse effects that necessitates close monitoring by the prescribing PH specialist. Because the long-term prognosis for PH is dependent on stabilization or improvement in hemodynamics, there is an emphasis on both antithrombotic and antimitogenic treatments. In addition to pulmonary vasodilation, all PH-specific pharmaceuticals have theoretic antimitogenic effects on vascular smooth muscle. Prostacyclin analogs are known to have an antiplatelet effect as well.

To date, there have been few patients who have had true disease reversal. However, responders to the above therapeutic classes have a 30- to 60-m improvement in 6-minute walk tests and 5-year survival rates in excess of 50%. Creation of an ASD that allows right-to-left shunting

may be lifesaving in patients with PH and right heart failure. Evaluation for lung transplantation is never an emergent matter, but this may provide a survival benefit for some children with PH. In patients who approach transplantation without other systemic abnormalities, the posttransplantation 5-year survival for pediatric PH patients is 50% to 60% with an improved quality of life.

Acute treatment of right ventricular failure is quite challenging, because neither augmentation of preload nor afterload reduction is a helpful acute maneuver (Table 13-13). Treatment with oxygen and inspired nitric oxide can be lifesaving. The use of nonspecific vasodilators is often limited by their systemic vasodilatory response, and they should be used with extreme caution in hemodynamically labile patients with PH. Inotropic support with dopamine and maintenance of an appropriate ventricular rate with isoproterenol may be successful. Isoproterenol increases heart rate and also decreases PVR; the usual dose is a continuous infusion at a rate of 0.01 to 0.1 μg/kg/min. Inhaled epoprostenol at 30 ng/kg/min, especially in cases with an acute respiratory distress syndrome–like pathophysiology, can improve pulmonary blood flow without risk of hypotension.

Chronic Pulmonary Hypertension Treatment

- Anticongestive therapy for right ventricular dysfunction
  - Nocturnal oxygen use can be beneficial
  - Right ventricular dysfunction frequently limits enteral nutrition
- Anticoagulation should be considered:
  - For all patients with thrombophilia
  - Possibly hold for infants and toddlers
  - INR values of 1.8-2.2 are usual
- Confirmed acute responder to nitric oxide
  - Calcium channel blocker
  - PDE type 5 inhibitor
- Nonresponder to nitric oxide or failed calcium channel blocker therapy
  - NYHA class II-III:
    - PDE type 5 inhibitor and/or endothelin-1 receptor antagonist
  - NYHA class III-IV or failed oral therapy:
    - Prostanoid: Available routes include inhaled, continuous subcutaneous, or intravenous infusion
- Failed prostanoid therapy
  - Combination therapy
  - And/or atrial septostomy
- Prediction of poor 1-year survival or continued symptoms
  - Evaluation for lung transplantation
- Activity limitations
  - Most children already self-limit themselves
  - Isometric exercises/sports are contraindicated
  - Most varsity-level sports are not allowed
  - Early discussion about oxygen therapy during air transport and living at altitude is crucial
- Pulmonary hypertension specialist follow-up
  - Every 3 months
    - ECG, appropriate blood tests (including BNP)
    - Six-minute walk test and/or formal stress testing
    - Echocardiograms for suspected right heart failure, disease staging
  - Cardiac catheterization every 12-24 months for disease staging
  - Emergent visits for acute illness in severely affected children
    - Children who cannot increase oxygen delivery are at most risk of deterioration

BNP, B-type natriuretic peptide; ECG, electrocardiogram; INR, international normalized ratio; NYHA, New York Heart Association; PDE, phosphodiesterase.

Sedative and anesthetic agents such as midazolam and propofol that lower systemic vascular resistance should be used with extreme caution in hemodynamically labile patients with PH. In unstable patients with PH, ketamine is often a better choice because it increases the systemic vascular resistance and helps maintain blood pressure.

Patients with PH may decompensate and sustain a cardiac arrest during sedation or attempted intubation.

Long-Term Treatment Options for Pulmonary Hypertension*

Therapeutic Class	Examples
Phosphodiesterase type 5 inhibitors	Sildenafil (short acting): 6 mg/kg/d; maximum 60 mg/d Tadalafil (long acting): 20-40 mg/d
Endothelin receptor antagonist	Bosentan: nonselective; 5 mg/kg/d; maximum 125 mg twice a day Ambrisentan: selective α-receptor; 5-10 mg/d
Prostacyclin (individualized dosing)	Epoprostenol (intravenous) Treprostinil (intravenous, subcutaneous, or inhaled) Iloprost (inhaled)

Off-label use for pediatrics.

Although anecdotal reports of survival exist, if a ventricular rate and adequate pressure cannot be regained within minutes, it is impossible to supply sufficient oxygen to the brain to avoid profound anoxic injury. We attempt to avoid epinephrine and calcium during the prearrest resuscitation, because both decrease pulmonary blood flow in this disease. Although rapid deployment extracorporeal support is used in our institution for sudden cardiopulmonary arrest, we do not employ extracorporeal cardiopulmonary resuscitation in this population. The only truly successful treatment for cardiopulmonary arrest in the face of PH is avoidance.

Prognosis

In the current era, the 5-year survival rate for PH is 50% to 70%. In the absence of a correctable anatomic lesion, reports of spontaneous remission are rare. PH is a disabling disease that progresses inexorably to death in months to years. All treatment is palliative, and currently there is no cure. Therapeutic interventions are needed to promote vascular remodeling and ensure clinical improvement. The following diagnoses are associated with rapid progression to death in the first year of life: alveolar capillary dysplasia, pulmonary veno-occlusive disease, congenital pulmonary vein stenosis, severe pulmonary hypoplasia, and pulmonary vascular disease associated with congenital heart disease and presenting with cardiovascular collapse in the first year of life. Although PH generally increases the morbidity and mortality of any associated diseases, the prognosis for PH may be better in those cases with a reversible or treatable primary condition.

Emergent Therapy for Pulmonary Hypertensive Crises

- ◼ Goals of emergent care
  - ◼ Decrease PVR
  - ◼ Maintain heart rate (asystole is not reversible)
  - ◼ Improve right ventricular function
  - ◼ Improve oxygen delivery
- ◼ Nitric oxide (40 PPM) and O_2 by nonrebreather mask
  - ◼ Free of side effects
  - ◼ Except will cause pulmonary edema in:
    - ◼ Severe congenital pulmonary vein stenosis
    - ◼ Alveolar capillary dysplasia
- ◼ Inhaled prostacyclin
  - ◼ Continuous epoprostenol often available instead of nitric oxide
  - ◼ Same possible concerns as with nitric oxide
- ◼ Phosphodiesterase inhibitors
  - ◼ Sildenafil: decreases PVR not SVR
  - ◼ Milrinone: decreases SVR not PVR and is not recommended
- ◼ Catecholamines to increase cardiac output
  - ◼ Isoproterenol: maintains HR
  - ◼ Dopamine: maintains right ventricular function
  - ◼ Epinephrine worsens PVR and does not increase cardiac output
- ◼ Antiarrhythmics
  - ◼ Use with caution to maintain CO and SVR
- ◼ Fluid management
  - ◼ Transfusion of RBCs preferred
  - ◼ Large fluid boluses are contraindicated
    - ◼ Will not increase systemic blood pressure
    - ◼ Will cause right ventricular failure

CO, cardiac output; HR, heart rate; PPM, parts per million; PVR, pulmonary vascular resistance; RBCs, red blood cells; SVR, systemic vascular resistance.

Clinical Pearls

- ◼ Chronic heart failure management is primarily aimed at interrupting the underlying pathophysiologic mechanisms of myocyte dysfunction.
- ◼ The majority of transplantation recipients report excellent functional status with respect to physical, cognitive, and psychological well-being.
- ◼ Cardiomyopathy is the leading reason for heart transplantations and sudden deaths in children.
- ◼ The initial presentation of hypertrophic cardiomyopathy can be as insidious as an abnormal electrocardiogram or a new heart murmur or as dramatic as a sudden cardiac arrest.
- ◼ The most common feature of pulmonary hypertension, irrespective of etiology, is delayed diagnosis. It is important to recognize that most pediatric patients will present with common complaints that do not reveal the severe limitation in cardiopulmonary reserve without a high index of suspicion.
- ◼ All treatment for pulmonary hypertension is palliative, and currently there is no cure.

REFERENCES

1. Jessup M, Abraham WT, Casey DE, et al. 2009 focused update: ACCF/AHA Guidelines for the Diagnosis and Management of Heart Failure in Adults: a report of the American College of Cardiology Foundation/American Heart Association Task Force on Practice Guidelines: developed in collaboration with the International Society for Heart and Lung Transplantation. *Circulation.* 2009;119:1977-2016.
2. Rosenthal D, Chrisant MR, Edens E, et al. International Society for Heart and Lung Transplantation: practice guidelines for management of heart failure in children. *J Heart Lung Transplant.* 2004;23:1313-1333.
3. Canter CE, Shaddy RE, Bernstein D, et al. Indications for heart transplantation in pediatric heart disease: a scientific statement from the American Heart Association Council on Cardiovascular Disease in the Young; the Councils on Clinical Cardiology, Cardiovascular Nursing, and Cardiovascular Surgery and Anesthesia; and the Quality of Care and Outcomes Research Interdisciplinary Working Group. *Circulation.* 2007;115:658-676.
4. Kirk R, Edwards LB, Kucheryavaya AY, et al. The Registry of the International Society for Heart and Lung Transplantation: thirteenth official pediatric heart transplantation report–2010. *J Heart Lung Transplant.* 2010;29:1119-1128.
5. DeMaso DR, Douglas Kelley S, Bastardi H, O'Brien P, Blume ED. The longitudinal impact of psychological functioning, medical severity, and family functioning in pediatric heart transplantation. *J Heart Lung Transplant.* 2004;23:473-480.
6. Todaro JF, Fennell EB, Sears SF, Rodrigue JR, Roche AK. Review: cognitive and psychological outcomes in pediatric heart transplantation. *J Pediatr Psychol.* 2000;25:567-576.
7. Elliott P, Andersson B, Arbustini E, et al. Classification of the cardiomyopathies: a position statement from the European Society of Cardiology Working Group on Myocardial and Pericardial Diseases. *Eur Heart J.* 2008;29:270-276.
8. Lipshultz SE, Sleeper LA, Towbin JA, et al. The incidence of pediatric cardiomyopathy in two regions of the United States. *N Engl J Med* 2003;348:1647-1655.
9. Hershberger RE, Lindenfeld J, Mestroni L, Seidman CE, Taylor MR, Towbin JA. Genetic evaluation of cardiomyopathy—a Heart Failure Society of America practice guideline. *J Card Fail.* 2009;15:83-97.
10. Towbin JA, Lowe AM, Colan SD, et al. Incidence, causes, and outcomes of dilated cardiomyopathy in children. *JAMA.* 2006;296:1867-1876.
11. Colan SD, Lipshultz SE, Lowe AM, et al. Epidemiology and cause-specific outcome of hypertrophic cardiomyopathy in children: findings from the Pediatric Cardiomyopathy Registry. *Circulation.* 2007;115:773-781.
12. Maron BJ. Contemporary insights and strategies for risk stratification and prevention of sudden death in hypertrophic cardiomyopathy. *Circulation.* 2010;121:445-456.
13. Petersen SE, Selvanayagam JB, Francis JM, et al. Differentiation of athlete's heart from pathological forms of cardiac hypertrophy by means of geometric indices derived from cardiovascular magnetic resonance. *J Cardiovasc Magn Reson.* 2005;7:551-558.
14. Maron BJ, Chaitman BR, Ackerman MJ, et al. Recommendations for physical activity and recreational sports participation

for young patients with genetic cardiovascular diseases. *Circulation*. 2004;109:2807-16.

15. Mocumbi AO, Yacoub S, Yacoub MH. Neglected tropical cardiomyopathies: II. Endomyocardial fibrosis: myocardial disease. *Heart*. 2008;94:384-390.

16. Russo LM, Webber SA. Idiopathic restrictive cardiomyopathy in children. *Heart*. 2005;91:1199-1202.

17. Sen-Chowdhry S, Lowe MD, Sporton SC, McKenna WJ. Arrhythmogenic right ventricular cardiomyopathy: clinical presentation, diagnosis, and management. *Am J Med*. 2004;117:685-695.

18. Rampazzo A, Nava A, Malacrida S, et al. Mutation in human desmoplakin domain binding to plakoglobin causes a dominant form of arrhythmogenic right ventricular cardiomyopathy. *Am J Hum Genet*. 2002;71:1200-1206.

19. Protonotarios N, Tsatsopoulou A, Anastasakis A, et al. Genotype-phenotype assessment in autosomal recessive arrhythmogenic right ventricular cardiomyopathy (Naxos disease) caused by a deletion in plakoglobin. *J Am Coll Cardiol*. 2001;38:1477-1484.

20. Nugent AW, Daubeney PE, Chondros P, et al.; National Australian Childhood Cardiomyopathy Study. Clinical features and outcomes of childhood hypertrophic cardiomyopathy: results from a national population-based study. *N Engl J Med*. 2003;348:1639-1646.

21. Hoedemaekers YM, Caliskan K, Michels M, et al. The importance of genetic counseling, DNA diagnostics, and cardiologic family screening in left ventricular noncompaction cardiomyopathy. *Circ Cardiovasc Genet*. 2010;3:232-239.

22. Zuckerman WA, Richmond ME, Singh RK, Carroll SJ, Starc TJ, Addonizio LJ. Left-ventricular noncompaction in a pediatric population: predictors of survival. *Pediatr Cardiol*. 2011;32:406-412.

23. Simonneau G, Robbins IM, Beghetti M, et al. Updated clinical classification of pulmonary hypertension. *J Am Coll Cardiol*. 2009;54:S43-S54.

24. Barst RJ, Gibbs JS, Ghofrani HA, et al. Updated evidence-based treatment algorithm in pulmonary arterial hypertension. *J Am Coll Cardiol*. 2009;54:S78-S84.

CHAPTER 14

Acquired Heart Disease

Katherine E. Bates,
Anirban Banerjee and
Marie M. Gleason

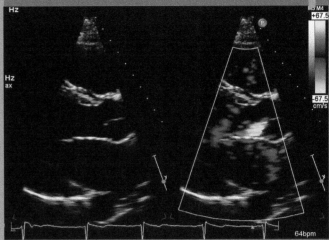

KAWASAKI DISEASE

Introduction

Kawasaki disease is a vasculitis of early childhood that has a propensity for affecting the coronary arteries. It is characterized by a cluster of symptoms and signs, which lead to the diagnosis of Kawasaki disease. It poses a diagnostic quandary for the primary physician because Kawasaki disease often mimics more common childhood illnesses presenting with fever. Moreover, in recent years, Kawasaki disease has presented in an atypical manner, making early diagnosis quite difficult. Therefore, in the present era, a primary care physician should be armed with a high index of suspicion when evaluating a febrile, irritable child. Left untreated, almost 20% to 25% of children with Kawasaki disease may develop aneurysms of coronary arteries. In the United States, the incidence of coronary artery aneurysms decreased to less than 5% after use of intravenous immunoglobulin (IVIG) became more widespread in the 1990s.[1]

Epidemiology

The majority of cases of Kawasaki disease occur between 6 months and 5 years of age. In the United States, the incidence of Kawasaki disease is highest in children of Asian descent (32.5 per 100,000 children under 5 years) and lowest in Caucasians (9.1 per 100,000 children under 5 years). The incidence rates are intermediate in African Americans and Hispanics.[2] Children under 1 year of age have an increased propensity to develop coronary artery aneurysms. Kawasaki disease is prevalent year round but is punctuated by seasonal surges in winter and spring. Recurrences in the same patient

and occurrences in siblings are noted occasionally. The incidence of Kawasaki disease is higher in children of parents who themselves have a past history of Kawasaki disease, which suggests that there may be a genetic predisposition of a child to Kawasaki disease.[3]

Pathogenesis

The hunt for a causative agent of Kawasaki disease has failed to find a definite agent, despite extensive research over the past 4 decades. Nevertheless, the clinical features, the seasonal outbreaks, and other epidemiologic characteristics strongly point toward an infectious agent. However, cultures and serologic tests against bacterial and viral agents have not been able to isolate a causative agent.

Theories

Superantigen theory. In the mid-1990s, superantigens produced by group A *Streptococcus pyogenes* and *Staphylococcus aureus* were implicated as causative agents of Kawasaki disease.[4] In the human body, in response to a conventional antigen, only a limited number of lymphocytes are activated, typically less than 1 cell per 10,000 lymphocytes. In contrast to conventional antigens, superantigens can lead to excessive stimulation of a larger number of lymphocytes (as many as 25% of circulating lymphocytes). This leads to uncoordinated and disproportionate release of inflammatory cytokines from activated T cells. The best characterized superantigens are the staphylococcal enterotoxins and the streptococcal pyrogenic exotoxins that trigger the staphylococcal and streptococcal toxic shock syndromes. Toxic shock syndrome and Kawasaki disease share many common clinical and immunologic features.

Moreover, many Kawasaki disease patients were colonized with *S aureus* producing toxic shock syndrome toxin-1. Therefore, bacterial superantigens were implicated as causative agents of Kawasaki disease. However, more recently, a blinded, randomized, multicenter trial failed to find a statistically significant difference in the recovery of superantigen-producing *S aureus* and *S. pyogenes* in patients with Kawasaki disease.[5] Hence, the superantigen theory cannot fully explain the etiology of Kawasaki disease.

Ribonucleic acid (RNA) virus theory. In acute Kawasaki disease, it has been noted that immunoglobulin A (IgA) plasma cells infiltrate not only the walls of coronary arteries, but also the upper respiratory tract. This is reminiscent of a severe viral respiratory infection, such as influenza. This suggests that the microbe responsible for Kawasaki disease may enter the body via the respiratory tract. Synthetic monoclonal versions of the IgA antibody, found in the walls of the coronary arteries, have now been created in vitro. These synthetic antibodies, in turn, have been used to hunt down the Kawasaki disease–specific antigen found in inclusion bodies in bronchial epithelium and in macrophages.[6] It has been proposed that in children an offending infectious agent enters through the respiratory tract and infects the ciliary bronchial epithelial cells, where it characteristically forms inclusion bodies. These inclusion bodies are characterized by aggregates of viral proteins and RNA. This suggests that the microbe responsible for Kawasaki disease may be a previously unidentified, ubiquitous RNA virus, with limited or no homology to presently known viruses.[7] However, this viral agent will only cause Kawasaki disease in a genetically susceptible host (Figure 14-1). Present data suggest that in Kawasaki disease, IgA antibodies are formed against this unknown viral agent and, therefore, this response is not an autoimmune response. The lack of person-to-person transmission and the rarity of the disease in adults suggest that most humans have possibly experienced asymptomatic infections earlier in life and that there is widespread immunity in the community.

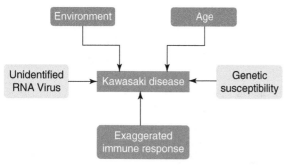

FIGURE 14-1 ■ Kawasaki disease is caused by interplay of multiple factors.

Clinical Presentation

There are no definitive laboratory tests for diagnosing Kawasaki disease, and the disease is often diagnosed by a constellation of clinical symptoms, signs, and some auxiliary laboratory data (eg, platelet count, erythrocyte sedimentation rate). The clinical diagnostic criteria of Kawasaki disease adopted by the American Heart Association (AHA) are outlined in Table 14-1. However, an overriding feature of Kawasaki disease is the high fever and extreme irritability. The latter is quite disproportionate when compared to other childhood febrile illnesses.

In addition to the principal clinical features described earlier, associated clinical characteristics may also be manifested in Kawasaki disease. Children may present with refusal to bear weight on their feet or refusal to move their arms, possibly due to arthralgia of several joints, small and large. The hepatobiliary system may be involved, resulting in hydrops of the gallbladder, hepatomegaly, transient jaundice, and elevated liver enzymes. In fact, hydrops of the gallbladder can be evaluated concurrently during echocardiography and can help clinch the diagnosis in atypical forms of this disease. The patient may also present with gastrointestinal complaints of diarrhea, abdominal pain, and vomiting, rarely masquerading as "acute abdomen." Nonspecific symptoms of vomiting, diarrhea, abdominal pain, and cough that accompany many childhood febrile illnesses also accompany Kawasaki disease, and these symptoms should not dissuade the clinician from thinking of Kawasaki disease.

Atypical Kawasaki disease

In about 15% to 20% of children, especially in infants under 6 months of age, the presentation of Kawasaki disease is atypical. This is also referred to as incomplete Kawasaki disease because only few of the classical signs are manifest. However, the general practitioner needs

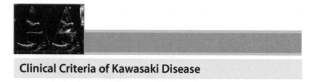

Clinical Criteria of Kawasaki Disease

Fever for 5 days and any 4 of the following 5 clinical manifestations.

1. Bilateral, bulbar conjunctivitis (nonexudative)
2. Diffuse maculopapular rash, especially in diaper area
3. Red, cracked lips; strawberry tongue; erythema of oropharynx
4. Edema of dorsa of hand and feet (Desquamation of fingers and toes is a late feature and not helpful in early stages of illness.)
5. Enlarged, unilateral, cervical lymph node (>1.5 cm)

to remember that the incidence of coronary artery aneurysms is higher in this group of patients, if untreated. Therefore, a high index of suspicion should be maintained when evaluating a febrile child less than 1 year of age. Clinical findings of pharyngitis, presence of bullae in skin, exudative conjunctivitis, and generalized lymphadenopathy often suggest a non-Kawasaki type of illness. It should also be kept in perspective that IVIG treatment before day 5 of Kawasaki disease has not been associated with improved outcomes for coronary artery involvement. In fact, treatment before 5 days of the illness has often necessitated treatment with a second dose of IVIG.

Diagnosis

A scientific statement from the AHA provides us with an algorithm to diagnose atypical (incomplete) Kawasaki disease. A simplified version is depicted in Figure 14-2. Previous studies have shown that children treated after day 10 of illness were 2.8 times more likely to have coronary artery aneurysms than those who were treated earlier. A recent study from Taiwan reported that infants who were less than 6 months old were diagnosed with Kawasaki disease an average of 2 days later than older children; the diagnosis was made beyond 10 days in 50% of these children versus 22% of children who were 6 months old or older.[8]

Recently the AHA algorithm has been applied in a retrospective study from 4 U.S. centers. This study suggested that application of the AHA algorithm would have referred 95% of patients with incomplete Kawasaki disease for IVIG treatment. Only 70% of these patients would have been treated with IVIG infusions if clinicians had relied on fulfillment of the traditional complete case definition.[9]

Diagnostic Tests

The acute-phase reactants, erythrocyte sedimentation rate (ESR) and C-reactive protein (CRP), are virtually always elevated in Kawasaki disease and take about 8 weeks to return to normal. It is important that both are measured (not just 1) because the elevation in ESR and CRP may be variable and discordant in these patients. This is especially important during treatment with IVIG because IVIG itself causes elevation in ESR but does not affect the CRP levels. Therefore, for serial follow-up of the inflammatory response in IVIG-treated Kawasaki disease, CRP levels are preferably monitored, not the ESR. A complete blood cell count, differential, and platelet count are needed. Liver function tests should also be performed. A urine analysis should be sent to evaluate for sterile pyuria. Abdominal ultrasound should be performed to rule out gallbladder hydrops in patients

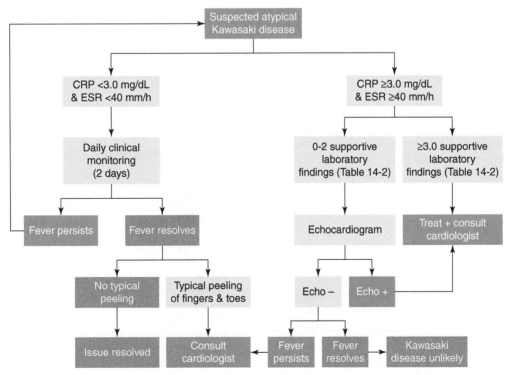

FIGURE 14-2 ■ Simplified algorithm for suspected atypical Kawasaki disease. CRP, C-reactive protein; ESR, erythrocyte sedimentation rate. (*Adapted with permission from Newburger JW, Takahashi M, Gerber MA, et al.; Committee on Rheumatic Fever, Endocarditis and Kawasaki Disease. Diagnosis, treatment, and long-term management of Kawasaki disease: a statement for health professionals from the Committee on Rheumatic Fever, Endocarditis and Kawasaki Disease, Council on Cardiovascular Disease in the Young, American Heart Association. Circulation. 2004;110:2747-2771.*)

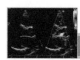

Supportive Laboratory Findings in Kawasaki Disease

WBC count	>15,000/µL
Normocytic, normochromic anemia	Mild anemia
Albumin	<3 g/dL
Alanine transaminase	Elevated
Platelets (after 7 days)	>450,000/µL
Urine leukocytes	>10 leukocytes per high-power field

with gastrointestinal symptoms. A chest x-ray should be performed in febrile patients with respiratory issues; in addition to evaluating the lung parenchyma, one can look for cardiomegaly or effusions. In some patients who present with fever and meningismus, a lumbar puncture with cell count, fluid glucose and protein levels, and fluid culture should be performed. Table 14-2 lists the supportive laboratory findings in Kawasaki disease.

Cardiac testing should include a baseline 12-lead electrocardiogram to assess for ST-segment or T-wave changes and a 2-dimensional and Doppler echocardiogram to assess for pericardial effusion, myocardial function, and valvulitis (aortic or mitral regurgitation) and for complete evaluation of both coronary arteries and their segments. Patients with congestive heart failure symptoms should be on telemetry to evaluate for arrhythmias.

Treatment

Acute therapy

The combined use of IVIG and aspirin has now become the mainstay of treatment of the acute phase of Kawasaki disease (Table 14-3). Randomized clinical trials have established that a single infusion of IVIG in a dose of 2 g/kg, given within 5 to 10 days after the onset of fever in Kawasaki disease, eliminates fever in 85% of children within 36 hours and reduces the risk of coronary artery aneurysms significantly.[10] In the pre-IVIG era, approximately 20% to 25% of patients developed coronary artery aneurysms. However, in the present era of high-dose IVIG therapy, only 5% of children may have coronary artery involvement (some with transient involvement) and 1% develop giant aneurysms (≥ 8 mm). Children who present after 10 days of fever should still be treated with IVIG, if fever is present or signs of inflammation (eg, elevated ESR or CRP) are detected. Approximately 10% to 15% of children with Kawasaki disease do not respond to the initial dose of IVIG and need retreatment. Factors that are associated with resistance to the first dose of IVIG are indicated in Table 14-4.

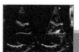

Treatment of Kawasaki Disease During Acute Phase

Initial treatment after diagnosis
- Intravenous immunoglobulin (IVIG): 2 g/kg infusion over 8-10 hours.
- Aspirin:
  - 80-100 mg/kg/d in 4 divided oral doses until patient remains afebrile for 3 days.
  - Thereafter, aspirin dose is lowered to 3-5 mg/kg/d as a single oral dose for 6-8 weeks.
  - Aspirin is discontinued after 6-8 weeks if coronary arteries are normal by echocardiography.

For cases refractory to first dose of IVIG
- Retreatment with IVIG:
  - If fever persists beyond 36 hours after first dose of IVIG.
  - Same dose (2 g/kg infusion).
- Corticosteroids:
  - Generally used after 2 doses of IVIG have failed.
  - Methylprednisone: intravenous pulse therapy, 30 mg/kg once a day up to 3 days.
- More recent therapies:
  - Infliximab (monoclonal antibody against TNF-α); dose: 5 mg/kg infusion over 6 hours.
  - Plasma exchange for 3 consecutive days.
  - Cyclophosphamide

TNF-α, tumor necrosis factor-alpha.

Outpatient Follow up

For straightforward cases without major coronary involvement, echocardiograms are performed at the time of diagnosis and at 2 weeks and 6 to 8 weeks after diagnosis. Therefore, after discharge from the hospital, follow-up visits with a pediatric cardiologist are arranged at those intervals. If the coronary arteries show no involvement, low-dose aspirin therapy is stopped at 6 to 8 weeks or when the inflammatory parameters

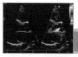

Risk Factors for IVIG Resistance

- Male sex
- Age <4 months
- Cervical lymphadenopathy
- Higher CRP levels
- Absence of conjunctival injection
- Higher total bilirubin and ALT
- Lower albumin levels
- Lower serum Na+ levels
- Early treatment with IVIG (days 2-4 of illness)

ALT, alanine transaminase; CRP, C-reactive protein; IVIG, intravenous immuno-globulin.

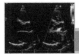

Recent Classification of Coronary Aneurysms¹⁴

Classification	Aneurysm Size
Small to medium	>3 mm to <6 mm
Large	>6 mm to <8 mm
Giant	>8 mm

and platelet count have normalized. In some centers, echocardiograms and follow-ups are also performed at 6 months and 12 months after the diagnosis, at the discretion of the pediatric cardiologist. After 12 months, it is unlikely to see any further coronary artery involvement if the coronary arteries were normal at 6 to 8 weeks.

In patients with coronary artery involvement noted in the acute phase of the illness, the treatment and follow-up vary from a typical, uncomplicated case of Kawasaki disease. The classification of coronary aneurysms is outlined in Table 14-5. A giant coronary aneurysm is depicted in Figure 14-3. The same patient also developed a large pericardial effusion (Figure 14-4). The management of patients with coronary artery involvement follows the risk levels for developing coronary artery thrombosis and myocardial ischemia, proposed by the AHA scientific statement on Kawasaki disease.¹⁰ Such risk stratification may serve as a useful guide in management of these patients. However, patients are variable, and physicians have their own styles. Therefore, the recommendations made for treating coronary artery lesions in Table 14-6, take both the AHA risk stratification¹⁰ and the author's personal experience into account.

Coronary aneurysms that grow rapidly in the acute phase of the disease are at greater risk for thrombosis. These patients should be monitored carefully and treated with β-blockers and a combination of low-dose aspirin

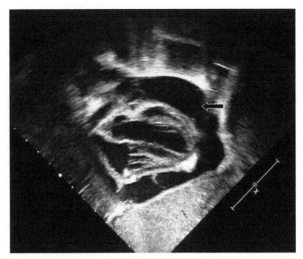

FIGURE 14-4 ■ Large pericardial effusion (black arrow) in patient with Kawasaki disease.

and warfarin. In giant aneurysms, there is often narrowing of the coronary artery segments at either end of the aneurysm. This characteristic is responsible for stasis of the blood flow in the aneurysm, which increases the risk of coronary thrombosis. When multiple aneurysms are arranged in a row (pearl necklace pattern), areas of stenosis and aneurysms alternate with each other. This may result in repeated slowing of blood flow in the coronary arteries. It is postulated that such sluggish blood flow, in combination with an unknown vasculitic process that causes endothelial activation and increased platelet shear stress, may contribute to coronary artery thrombosis.

Thrombotic occlusion of an aneurysmal or stenotic coronary artery is a catastrophic event and the main cause of death in Kawasaki disease. In Japanese children, the greatest risk of suffering a myocardial infarction has been within the first year of the illness. Thrombolytic therapy may be lifesaving in this circumstance. However, the experience of using thrombolytic agents in children is quite meager. Therefore, the guidelines for using thrombolytic agents have been extrapolated from adult clinical trials treating acute coronary syndromes. Thrombolytic agents like streptokinase and tissue plasminogen activator have been used successfully in limited groups of children. Borrowing from the success in adults with acute coronary syndrome, abciximab, a platelet glycoprotein IIb/IIIa receptor inhibitor, has been used with some success in a small number of children.

Noncardiac Issues in Kawasaki Disease

Vaccinations

Patients with Kawasaki disease receiving IVIG treatment should have their measles-mumps-rubella and varicella vaccinations delayed for about a year because the specific antiviral antibody in IVIG may interfere with the

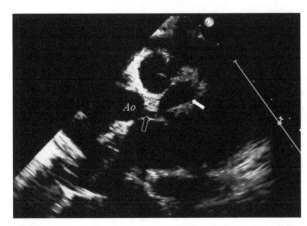

FIGURE 14-3 ■ Giant aneurysm (white arrow) in left anterior descending branch of the left main coronary artery (black arrow). Ao, ascending aorta.

Therapies Aimed at Coronary Artery Lesions

Coronary ectasia	■ Usually transient and resolves spontaneously. ■ Continue low-dose aspirin (3-5 mg/kg/dose once a day) until it resolves. ■ No restriction of physical activity beyond 8 weeks.
Single, small- to medium-sized coronary aneurysm	■ Continue low-dose aspirin (3-5 mg/kg/dose once a day) until it resolves. ■ No restriction of physical activity beyond 8 weeks.
Two or more small- to medium-sized coronary aneurysms in a row ("pearl necklace pattern")	■ Continue low-dose aspirin (3-5 mg/kg/dose once a day). ■ Clopidogrel (1 mg/kg/d as single oral dose up to maximum of 75 mg/d) may be added at discretion of physician. ■ No restriction of physical activity beyond 8 weeks in children <10 years. ■ Sports participation beyond 8 weeks dictated by stress test in older children >10 years old.
Single large coronary aneurysms (>6 mm to <8 mm)	■ β-Blockers are used for rapidly growing large aneurysms, during acute phase of illness. ■ Long-term treatment with low-dose aspirin ± clopidogrel. ■ No restriction of physical activity beyond 8 weeks in children <10 years old. ■ Sports participation beyond 8 weeks dictated by stress test in older children >10 years old. Contact sports discouraged.
Giant coronary aneurysm (>8 mm)	■ β-Blockers during acute phase of illness. ■ Long-term treatment with low-dose aspirin + warfarin, Or ■ Long-term treatment with low-dose aspirin + low-molecular-weight heparin for younger children. ■ Sports participation dictated by stress test in children >10 years old. Contact sports should be avoided in all patients. ■ Low level aerobic activity for all age groups is acceptable with a normal stress test.

immune response to live-virus vaccines. Other vaccinations do not need to be delayed.

Influenza vaccine

Reyes syndrome has not been seen in patients receiving low dose aspirin in recent decades. Nevertheless, children on long-term aspirin should be immunized with yearly influenza vaccine.

Antipyretics

Ibuprofen should be avoided in children taking aspirin because it may interfere with the antiplatelet effects of aspirin.

Infliximab treatment

Newer agents like infliximab, used in IVIG-resistant cases of Kawasaki disease, may cause reactivation of latent tuberculosis infection. This is further complicated by the fact that during acute Kawasaki disease, patients may be anergic and may not respond to skin tests for tuberculosis. In addition, the primary doctor should be aware that acute inflammation at the site of a previous bacillus Calmette-Guérin vaccine is a characteristic feature of Kawasaki disease.

Summary

Kawasaki disease is probably caused by single virus or a group of similar viruses in a small cohort of genetically predisposed children. In these children, the offending infectious agent possibly enters through the respiratory tract and infects the ciliary bronchial epithelial cells, where it characteristically forms cytoplasmic inclusion bodies. It then enters macrophages and is carried in the blood stream to the coronary arteries. An antigen–antibody cascade ensues, which in turn causes destruction of collagen and elastin in the walls of the coronary arteries, resulting in aneurysms. Kawasaki disease should be suspected in young children with persistent, high fever, even if full diagnostic criteria are absent. A high index of suspicion is of paramount importance. Treatment with IVIG reduces the risk of coronary artery aneurysms from 20% to less than 5%. About 10% to 15% of children with Kawasaki disease fail to respond to the initial dose of IVIG. In resistance cases, retreatment with additional doses of IVIG or intravenous methylprednisone may be necessary.

ACUTE RHEUMATIC FEVER

Definitions and Epidemiology

Acute rheumatic fever is the most common cause of acquired heart disease in the world, affecting some 20 million people. It is associated with group A β-hemolytic streptococcal (GAS) (*S. pyogenes*) infections. In decades past, it was a leading cause of cardiovascular death and disability in the United States. The arrival of the antibiotic era led to a remarkable decrease in rheumatic fever in westernized nations, but in less industrialized nations and developing countries, this disease continues to exist and results in significant morbidity and mortality. Cases of rheumatic fever still occur annually in the United States, and the etiology, presenting symptoms, and diagnosis are very important issues for medical personnel to understand. The late-term consequences of untreated rheumatic fever can be serious chronic cardiac disease, which impacts upon lifestyle and longevity. Conversely, the overdiagnosis of this condition has repercussions related to unnecessary long-term antibiotic prophylaxis.

Unlike Kawasaki disease, acute rheumatic fever is a disease more prevalent in school-age children and young adults, generally 5 to 15 years of age. It is not generally seen in children less than 5 years of age. There is no gender preference. There are racial and ethnic differences. The seasonal variation in the United States coincides with GAS infections, particularly in the winter and spring of temperate climates. The incidence is 0.5 to 3 per 100,000 population. In non-Western countries, the incidence is greater than 10 per 100,000 population. There are regions of the world that have a very high incidence of rheumatic fever including sub-Saharan Africa, south central Asia, South America, and the aboriginal populations of Australia and New Zealand. In the United States, there were resurgences in rheumatic fever in several states including Hawaii, Utah, New York, and Pennsylvania in the 1980s. One explanation for these resurgences was that the rheumatogenic strains of GAS had dramatically decreased for several decades after the onset of the antibiotic era. The reappearance of more virulent M-protein serotypes of GAS in recent decades led to recurrent outbreaks of rheumatic fever. There is also an implication of regional variation, because rheumatic fever is less common in the southern United States.[11]

Genetic predisposition appears to play a role in susceptibility to rheumatic fever when exposed to GAS infections. Genetic variation in the *emm* gene that codes for the M protein has been linked to varying manifestations of disease.[12] In the United States, rheumatic fever is more common in Asians and Pacific Islanders compared to Caucasians. Sixty percent (60%) of patients with chorea are female. Rheumatic fever is species specific, occurring only in humans. As such, there is no animal model for this disease.

Pathogenesis

All cases of rheumatic fever are preceded by a Lancefield GAS infection of the upper respiratory tract (ie, tonsillopharyngitis). If the streptococcal infection is untreated, there is risk of developing rheumatic fever

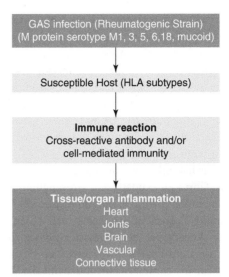

FIGURE 14-5 ■ Proposed mechanism of rheumatic fever pathogenesis. GAS, group A β-hemolytic streptococci; HLA, human leukocyte antigen.

in approximately 3% of cases. If the infection is appropriately treated with antibiotics, then the risk of developing rheumatic fever is markedly diminished.[13] The manifestations of rheumatic fever are not related to direct infection of the tissues by GAS. Rather, there is an autoimmune response, comprising both humoral and cellular mechanisms, implicated in a susceptible host (Figure 14-5). The M protein of the bacterial wall in certain strains of GAS ("rheumatogenic strains") serves as an antigenic stimulus in the host. The susceptible host mounts an autoimmune response to various components of the bacterium (the M protein, the streptococcal carbohydrate, the streptococcal protoplast membrane, and capsule hyaluronidate), which has so-called "antigenic mimicry" with certain tissues in the host. As such, the immune cascade that is meant to eradicate the GAS actually causes inflammation and damage in host organs, including the heart, brain, skin, and joints.

Like Kawasaki disease, the cardiac involvement in rheumatic fever occurs at all levels and should be considered a pancarditis. Clinical manifestations include myocarditis, valvulitis, pericarditis, and conduction abnormalities. The pathognomonic histologic lesion of rheumatic fever is the Aschoff body, described by Aschoff in 1904. These lesions are found only in the myocardium and consist of a perivascular infiltrate of large cells with basophilic cytoplasm and polymorphous nuclei in a rosette pattern around an avascular center of fibrinoid material. It is mostly seen in patients with a chronic myocarditis, often with recurrences of rheumatic fever. The most common cardiac manifestation of rheumatic fever is valvulitis, with inflammation of the endocardium and connective tissues of the heart, including the chordal apparatus. Mitral valve involvement is most common (>80% of patients), followed by aortic valve disease (~20% of patients). Tricuspid valve involvement is uncommon, and pulmonary valve disease is rare. If left unchecked, chronic valvar inflammation can result in thickened, scarred mitral and aortic valves, leading to chronic regurgitation and/or stenosis. In particular, late mitral stenosis due to rheumatic fever is the leading cause of cardiovascular morbidity and mortality in developing countries.

Pericardial inflammation and effusion are due to a serositis. Fibrinous exudates and serosanguinous fluid can be seen. Inflammation of the conduction system can cause varying degrees of atrioventricular block, most commonly first-degree atrioventricular block. Rarely, complete or third-degree atrioventricular block may occur and further compound hemodynamic instability.

Serositis of the synovium is the cause of the migratory arthritis that is the hallmark of rheumatic fever. Vasculitis is the mechanism behind skin manifestations of erythema multiforme and renal and pulmonary symptoms. Central nervous system involvement, such as Sydenham chorea, is also thought to be due to vasculitis of the basal ganglia and cerebellum.

Clinical Presentation

Historically, before the patient presents with symptoms of rheumatic fever, the patient must have experienced a primary GAS infection of the upper respiratory tract. Classically, this manifests as fever, sore throat, painful swallowing, and headache. On examination, there can be pharyngeal erythema with or without exudates, cervical lymphadenopathy, a swollen uvula, and in some cases, a scarlatiniform rash. There may be a history of exposure to others with similar symptoms and known GAS infection. In some cases, patients with rheumatic fever have laboratory evidence of a previous GAS infection but do not have a classic history for an upper respiratory infection. Once the patient has had the exposure to GAS, there is a "latent period" that ranges from 10 to 30 days, averaging 3 weeks, before the symptoms of rheumatic fever appear.

The manifestations of rheumatic fever have been fairly stable over the decades (Table 14-7). Generally, there is some degree of fever present. Approximately 65% to 70% present with migratory arthritis, approximately 50% show some degree of carditis, and only 15% to 20% present with chorea. Erythema multiforme is an uncommon finding. This rash occurs in less than 10% of patients. Subcutaneous nodules are also rare and more likely to occur in patients with chronic inflammation from recurrent rheumatic fever.

Carditis

Carditis is the most serious of the manifestations of rheumatic fever, and it is the most likely cause of morbidity and mortality. The degree of cardiac involvement

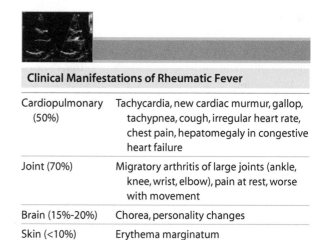

Clinical Manifestations of Rheumatic Fever	
Cardiopulmonary (50%)	Tachycardia, new cardiac murmur, gallop, tachypnea, cough, irregular heart rate, chest pain, hepatomegaly in congestive heart failure
Joint (70%)	Migratory arthritis of large joints (ankle, knee, wrist, elbow), pain at rest, worse with movement
Brain (15%-20%)	Chorea, personality changes
Skin (<10%)	Erythema marginatum

can be quite variable, ranging from only mild valve disease to life-threatening myocarditis and cardiac failure. In the patient with significant carditis and myocardial dysfunction, one may appreciate tachycardia, a gallop rhythm, and new cardiac murmurs. A long systolic murmur of mitral regurgitation may be heard at the lower sternal border and apex. An early high-pitched diastolic murmur of aortic regurgitation may be heard along the left sternal border. Aortic regurgitation is best auscultated with the patient erect and leaning forward. In severe aortic regurgitation, the pulse pressure may be wide and the pulses bounding. An irregular heart rate could be due to ventricular ectopy or second-degree atrioventricular block due to severe myocardial inflammation. In the most severe cases, bradycardia and low cardiac output may be due to third-degree atrioventricular block. The patient with congestive heart failure may show signs of tachypnea, pallor, fatigue, malaise, loss of appetite, and gastrointestinal symptoms such as nausea and vomiting.

Arthritis

Arthritis is the most common presentation of rheumatic fever. It can be transient, asymmetric, and migratory. The joints are painful, warm, red, and swollen. The pain is classically present at rest and worse with motion. The large joints involved are usually the knees and ankles, plus wrists and elbows. The arthritis of rheumatic fever is generally self-limited to 1 to 2 weeks. Classically, the arthritis is very responsive to salicylates (aspirin).

Central nervous system

Chorea is a form of involuntary, purposeless movement. In rheumatic fever, this has been termed Sydenham chorea. In decades past, it was also known as "St. Vitus' dance." It affects 15% to 20% of patients, mostly female, with rheumatic fever. Unlike the cardiac and joint manifestations of rheumatic fever, the central nervous system manifestations have a longer latent period and do not generally appear until 3 or more months after infection with GAS. Clinical signs of cardiac involvement are rare at the time of diagnosis, but late mitral regurgitation has been found in some patients, so they need the same evaluation as patients who present with carditis.

Sydenham chorea most frequently involves the muscles of the face and extremities and is evident when the patient is awake and stressed. It disappears with sleep. Classic manifestations include extension of the arms over the head with pronation of the hands and "milkmaid fingers," where there is irregular contraction of the fingers upon squeezing. The fingers also hyperextend ("spoon") when extended outward. Speech is halting, and handwriting is unsteady. Notably there are significant personality changes with emotional lability, restlessness, and inappropriate behavior. Generally these symptoms resolve after a couple of weeks.

Skin

Erythema marginatum is a rash that is specific to rheumatic fever but rarely seen. There is a red, macular serpiginous border noted around normal skin, about 1 inch in diameter, mostly occurring on the trunk and proximal limbs. It spares the face. It is evanescent and best seen when the patient is warm.

Subcutaneous nodules

Subcutaneous nodules are rarely seen except in patients with chronic rheumatic heart disease. These painless, mobile nodules occur on the extensor surfaces of joints, most commonly the knees, elbows, ankles, and knuckles of the hand. They range in size from 0.5 to 2.0 cm.

Differential Diagnosis

There are a variety of diseases that can mimic some of the clinical symptoms of rheumatic fever. Depending on the organ system involved, the most likely causes are infectious and inflammatory. These are listed in Table 14-8.

Diagnosis

The diagnosis of rheumatic fever is made by gathering information regarding previous exposure to a GAS infection and combining that with current signs, symptoms, and supplemental laboratory findings. The initial criteria were formulated in 1944 by T. Duckett Jones. More recently, the modified Jones criteria[14] were published in 1992 and are summarized in Table 14-9. To make a definitive diagnosis of acute rheumatic fever, the patient must have either 2 major criteria or 1 major and 2 minor criteria, plus evidence of a prior GAS infection.

Accuracy in making the diagnosis of rheumatic fever is important for several reasons. First and foremost is the risk related to underdiagnosis. If mild cases of rheumatic fever are missed and the patient is not given secondary prophylaxis to prevent recurrent disease, then

Differential Diagnosis in Acute Rheumatic Fever

- Juvenile rheumatoid arthritis
- Poststreptococcal reactive arthritis
- Infectious arthritis (septic joint)
- Systemic lupus erythematosus
- Myocarditis (viral, mycoplasmal)
- Dilated cardiomyopathy
- Endocarditis (bacterial)
- Pericarditis (viral, tuberculosis)
- Kawasaki disease
- Degenerative neurologic disease
- Brain tumors

the patient is at risk for repeated bouts of rheumatic fever. Subsequent episodes may include severe carditis with risk for early mortality and long-term morbidity from valvular heart disease. Conversely, some patients may have several elements suggestive of rheumatic fever, but in an effort to avoid missing the diagnosis, they are placed on long-term secondary prophylaxis. As is described in the Treatment section, secondary prophylaxis for rheumatic fever is a long-term commitment. Monthly injections of penicillin are painful,

Modified Jones Criteria for the Diagnosis of Rheumatic Fever—Must Have:
2 Major or 1 Major Plus 2 Minor Criteria and Evidence of a Prior GAS Infection *

Major criteria
- **Carditis:** Mitral regurgitation, aortic regurgitation, myocarditis, pericarditis
  First-, second- or third degree atrioventricular block
- **Arthritis:** Migratory
- **Chorea:** Female predominance
- **Erythema Marginatum:** Evanescent rash
- **Subcutaneous nodules:** With recurrent rheumatic fever

Minor criteria
- Prior history of rheumatic fever
- Arthralgias
- Fever
- Elevated Acute Phase reactants
- Prolonged PR interval

*** positive ASO, anti-DNAase B, antihyaluronidase, antistreptokinase.*
Data from Dajani AS, Ayoub EM, Bierman FZ, et al. Guidelines for the diagnosis of rheumatic fever: Jones criteria, updated 1992. JAMA, Circulation 1992; 268(15):2069-2073.

and there is the expense of long-term medication and cardiac follow-up evaluations. Additionally, if a patient carries the diagnosis of prior rheumatic fever, this could have implications for insurability.

Diagnostic Tests

Diagnosis of GAS infection

There is no specific test that makes the diagnosis of rheumatic fever. In patients who present with fever, sore throat, and malaise, a throat culture should be sent to rule out GAS infection. Rapid antigen detection tests can also be done in the office while awaiting culture results. Of note is the fact that in the winter, up to 15% of asymptomatic school-age children may be GAS carriers.[15] Group C and G streptococcus are common causes of pharyngitis in college students and adults, but these groups are not associated with later onset of rheumatic fever.

Diagnosis of acute rheumatic fever

In patients suspected of having rheumatic fever, the documentation of a GAS infection is mandatory. A throat culture should be sent. Antistreptococcal antibody titers are done to reflect past immunologic exposure. The most common tests are anti–streptolysin O (ASO) and anti–deoxyribonuclease B (anti–DNAase B). The ASO titers peak 3 to 6 weeks after GAS infection. They are elevated in 80% of patients with typical rheumatic fever but in less than 70% of patients with chorea. Anti–DNAase B titers peak 6 to 8 weeks after GAS infection. The elevated titers may persist for several months after infection. In 95% of rheumatic fever patients, there is an elevation in either anti–DNAase B, antistreptokinase, or antihyaluronidase. The streptozyme panel is felt to be less reliable and is not recommended to make the diagnosis of rheumatic fever.

Other blood tests to complete the work-up for rheumatic fever include a complete blood count to evaluate the white blood cell count and look for anemia and an ESR or CRP for inflammation. If there is significant valve leakage and fever, a blood culture may be indicated to rule out infectious endocarditis. In patients presenting with arthritis as the primary clinical symptom, testing for other causes of arthritis should be included, such as an antinuclear antibody, renal profile, urine dip, and microscopic analyses. If the patient has significant joint findings and the diagnosis is unclear, then arthroscopy and sampling of the synovial fluid for infection or other diagnostic criteria many be indicated.

Patients with chorea should have a neurologic consultation performed. To rule out other causes of movement disorders, cranial imaging with magnetic resonance imaging (MRI) may be indicated.

In all patients, evaluation for carditis should be performed, even if there is no overt evidence of cardiac

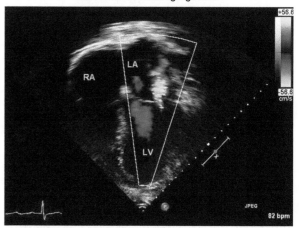

Rheumatic mitral regurgitation

FIGURE 14-6 ■ Two-dimensional and color Doppler echocardiogram (apical view). The blue jet in the left atrium (LA) shows the trajectory and size of the mitral regurgitation jet. LV, left ventricle; RA, right atrium.

involvement. A 12-lead electrocardiogram (ECG) should be performed to look for atrioventricular block and T-wave abnormalities and to define any ectopy if present. A chest x-ray is indicated for any symptomatic patient with tachycardia and/or tachypnea to evaluate for cardiomegaly and pulmonary edema.

A 2-dimensional and Doppler echocardiogram is a mandatory part of the work-up for rheumatic fever (Figure 14-6). In addition to those clinically obvious patients with cardiac signs or symptoms, it should be used to evaluate patients who present with only joint or central nervous system symptoms. Recent studies have shown that documentation of subclinical cardiac involvement is important in not only making the appropriate diagnosis of rheumatic fever and its treatment, but also confirming that cardiac follow-up is required.[16] Findings of mild mitral or aortic valve leakage, without an underlying anatomic cause for such, will increase the detection of patients with rheumatic fever and lead to appropriate treatment and future prevention. The algorithm for evaluating patients for rheumatic fever is summarized in Figure 14-7.

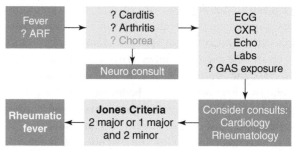

FIGURE 14-7 ■ Algorithm for the diagnosis of rheumatic fever. ARF, acute rheumatic fever; CXR, chest x-ray; ECG, electrocardiogram; Echo, echocardiogram; GAS, group A β-hemolytic streptococci.

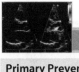

Primary Prevention of Rheumatic Fever (GAS Therapy)*			
	Medication	Dose	Duration
Intramuscular	Benzathine penicillin G	<27 kg: 600,000 units >27 kg: 1.2 million units	Once
Oral	Penicillin V	<27 kg: 250 mg 2-3 times a day	10 days
		>27 kg + adults: 500 mg 2-3 times a day	10 days
	Amoxicillin	50 mg/kg once a day (maximum, 1 g)	10 days
Penicillin allergic	Narrow-spectrum cephalosporin	Variable	10 days
	Clindamycin	20 mg/kg divided in 3 doses (maximum, 1.8 g/d)	10 days
	Azithromycin	12 mg/kg once a day (maximum, 500 mg)	5 days

*Do not use sulfonamides, tetracycline or flouroquinolones in primary prevention.

Treatment

Primary prevention

To prevent rheumatic fever, one must recognize and treat upper respiratory GAS infections, so-called "primary prevention." Skin infections with GAS are not associated with rheumatic fever, except in aboriginal populations of New Zealand. Primary prevention of rheumatic fever is aimed at eradicating an underlying GAS infection. In children with rheumatic fever, other household contacts should undergo a throat swab to check for GAS and treat those who are positive for GAS. The mode of treatment will depend on the patient and compliance.

Intramuscular benzathine penicillin G and oral penicillin V or amoxicillin are the recommended drugs because GAS is not penicillin resistant (Table 14-10). Failure to eradicate GAS from the throat occurs less often if the intramuscular route is used.[17] In patients with a penicillin allergy, oral cephalosporins may be used. For patients who cannot take cephalosporins, clindamycin is the drug of choice, because clindamycin resistance in GAS is rare. Tetracycline and sulfonamide antibiotics should not be used to eradicate GAS due to higher prevalence of resistant strains.

Acute Treatment. As part of the initial rheumatic fever episode treatment, the patient will require anti-inflammatory medication, generally aspirin, until the acute-phase reactants (ESR and CRP) normalize. Serum salicylate levels should be followed to avoid toxicity. Salicylate levels should not exceed 30 mg/dL. The duration of salicylate therapy can range from 2 to 8 weeks depending on the tissues involved. Patients with cardiac involvement are treated longer (4-8 weeks). Anti-inflammatory agents should be tapered off over 2 to 3 weeks to avoid rebound inflammation. Restricted physical activity is also recommended during this period of recuperation, depending on the degree of cardiac inflammation.

Carditis therapy. In mild cases of rheumatic carditis, the mitral valve and aortic valve regurgitation generally improves with time, with minimal, if any, residual valvular disease (Figure 14-8). More severe cases of carditis will require supportive care in the hospital. This should include telemetry monitoring of the cardiac rhythm. Mild to moderate carditis is treated with aspirin at doses of 80 to 100 mg/kg/d. Congestive heart failure and severe valve regurgitation require treatment with inotropic agents, diuretics, and afterload reducing agents (angiotensin-converting enzyme inhibitors and angiotensin receptor blockers). High-dose intravenous pulsed steroids are used in severe valve regurgitation, heart failure, and atrioventricular block. If high-degree atrioventricular block compromises heart rate and cardiac output, then temporary transvenous pacing may be required.

Surgical intervention for cardiac disease. Fortunately, not all patients with rheumatic carditis have enough residual valve disease to require surgical intervention. Patients with residual mitral and/or aortic valve regurgitation may require long-term treatment with afterload-reducing agents, such as angiotensin-converting enzyme inhibitors, diuretics, and digoxin. Medical therapy buys time to allow for spontaneous improvement and resolution of carditis, because most valve leakage improves with time and medication. However, for patients with severe valve disease, there are 2 time frames in which surgery may be necessary: early and late after the episode.

Early intervention. If a patient has hemodynamic instability due to severe mitral and aortic valve regurgitation,

Rheumatic aortic regurgitation-at presentation

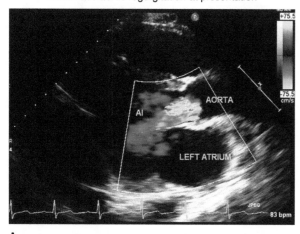

Rheumatic aortic regurgitation-one year later

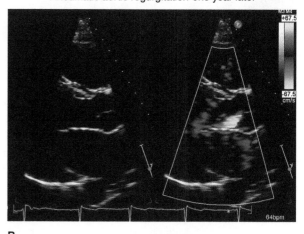

A

B

FIGURE 14-8 ■ A. Rheumatic aortic regurgitation at presentation (parasternal long axis echocardiogram). Color Doppler shows a broad jet of aortic regurgitation going backwards from the aorta into the left ventricle. AI, aortic insufficiency. **B.** Rheumatic aortic regurgitation 1 year later. Note that the size and width of the color Doppler jet is significantly less, indicating spontaneous improvement in valve leakage.

despite medical management, within the first few weeks of the onset of rheumatic fever, then surgical intervention may be needed to avoid mortality. The risks of surgery earlier in the course of the disease are higher due to persistent cardiac inflammation at the valve and myocardial levels. This impacts upon surgical complication rate, cardiac function, and success of valve surgery. In fact, attempts to repair versus replace leaking valves early in the course of the disease are often unsuccessful due to this issue. As such, early in the course of disease, prosthetic valve replacement is often the preferred choice.

Late intervention. After all cardiac inflammation has resolved and medical management has been exhausted, then cardiac valve surgery may be required months or years after the onset of rheumatic fever. When there is no active cardiac inflammation, then attempts to repair the mitral valve (valvuloplasty, annuloplasty) have a higher degree of success. In children, any effort to repair versus replace a valve is preferred to avoid long-term anticoagulation. Bioprosthetic valves may be used in the aortic position, but if the patient prefers a valve with longer durability, then a mechanical valve replacement can be performed.

Late mitral stenosis is a common sequela of rheumatic fever around the world, especially related to recurrent episodes of rheumatic fever. Although this is usually treated by a surgical valve replacement, there are interventional cardiac catheterization techniques available to balloon dilate the mitral valve in an attempt to reduce the valve gradient and avoid a surgical valve replacement.

Arthritis therapy. The joint inflammation in rheumatic fever generally resolves within a couple of weeks of diagnosis. Because these patients are responsive to aspirin, initial dosing of 50 to 75 mg/kg/d is commonly used with good relief of fever and joint symptoms. If needed, the dose can be increased to 100 mg/kg/d to get relief. Some people prefer nonsteroidal anti-inflammatory drugs for the treatment of arthritis. Anti-inflammatory agents and restricted activity should be used for 2 weeks after diagnosis to allow for appropriate resolution of inflammation. They can then be tapered off over 2 to 3 weeks.

Chorea therapy. Patients with chorea get the same primary prophylaxis to eradicate any residual GAS despite the absence of positive laboratory findings in most cases. The choreiform movements may require medical treatment at the discretion of the neurologist. Medications that have been used include haloperidol, phenobarbital, and valproic acid. Anti-inflammatory medications are not indicated in chorea.

Secondary prevention

The goal of secondary prevention is to prevent recurrent episodes of rheumatic fever by preventing recurrent GAS infections. A person with rheumatic fever is susceptible to recurrent episodes, and the manifestations of subsequent episodes may include more serious cardiovascular involvement. This requires continuous antimicrobial prophylaxis for a protracted period of time after the initial episode of rheumatic fever (Table 14-11). The duration of therapy can be modified from the standard recommendations if there is significant cardiac involvement and a likelihood of increased exposure to GAS, such as in parents of young children, teachers, medical personnel, military recruits, or those living in crowded conditions. Prophylaxis should occur indefinitely after valve surgery or replacement.

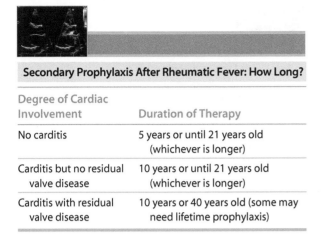

Secondary Prophylaxis After Rheumatic Fever: How Long?

Degree of Cardiac Involvement	Duration of Therapy
No carditis	5 years or until 21 years old (whichever is longer)
Carditis but no residual valve disease	10 years or until 21 years old (whichever is longer)
Carditis with residual valve disease	10 years or 40 years old (some may need lifetime prophylaxis)

The recommended therapy is injection of intramuscular benzathine penicillin G every 4 weeks. This confers the highest protection against recurrent rheumatic fever, but the negatives include discomfort and inconvenience to the patient, which can impact upon compliance. Successful oral prophylaxis requires strict patient compliance and frequent reminders by medical caregivers of the hazards of noncompliance. The recommended oral agent is penicillin V. Children and adults take 250 mg twice a day (Table 14-12). For penicillin-allergic patients, the recommended medication is sulfadiazine or sulfisoxazole as a prophylactic agent. Dosing is 0.5 g daily for weight less than 27 kg and 1.0 g daily for weight greater than 27 kg. However, the use of a sulfonamide in late pregnancy is contraindicated due to transplacental passage and potential adverse affects on the fetus.

The primary care practitioner has a very important role in secondary prophylaxis. In most cases where intramuscular monthly penicillin therapy is being followed, this occurs in the primary care physician's office. If the patient opts to take daily oral antibiotic prophylaxis, those prescriptions are usually procured through the primary care physician. It is the role of the primary care doctor to continuously emphasize to the patient and their family that strict compliance with secondary prophylaxis is critical to the patient's long-term well-being. Ideally, some method of monitoring patient compliance should be in place.

Bacterial endocarditis prophylaxis. The most recent guidelines of the AHA in 2007 no longer require antibiotic prophylaxis for patients with rheumatic heart disease, unless there has been a valve replacement or valve surgery. In these situations, the AHA recommendations should be followed using an alternative medication to the prophylactic penicillin. This is due to the fact that α-hemolytic streptococci found in normal oral flora can become resistant to penicillin over the long term.

Rheumatic fever prevention: vaccines. Although not currently available for use, it is important to know that there is active research in the development of multivalent vaccines against rheumatic fever ongoing in the United States.[18] These vaccines target M proteins from strains of rheumatogenic GAS, and antibodies to these proteins are included in a multivalent vaccine. Much like an influenza vaccine, the challenges in rheumatic fever vaccine development include the fact that regional differences exist in the M proteins. The most virulent GAS strains also can vary from year to year. As such, vaccines may have only regional applications.

In the larger scheme, vaccination against rheumatic fever would be a major breakthrough in improving cardiac health worldwide. Due to strain variations between developing nations, the creation of vaccines would have to be targeted to region-specific M proteins. If this is successful in the future, then the incidence of chronic rheumatic heart disease around the world could significantly decrease, thus improving longevity, returning people to the work force, and eliminating the financial strains associated with the care of these patients.

MYOCARDITIS

Definition and Epidemiology

Myocarditis, an inflammation of the muscular walls of the heart, is a rare disease in pediatrics that remains an important cause of sudden death. Although its annual incidence is estimated to be 1 in 100,000, it may account for up to 12% of sudden cardiac deaths in children.[19]

Secondary Prevention of Rheumatic Fever

Route	Medication	Dose
Intramuscular	Benzathine penicillin G	<27 kg: 600,000 units every 4 weeks >27 kg: 1.2 million units every 4 weeks
Oral	Penicillin V	250 mg twice a day
	Sulfadiazine	<27 kg: 0.5 g daily >27 kg: 1.0 g daily
Penicillin allergic	Macrolide (ie, erythromycin ethyl succinate)	250 mg twice a day

Pathogenesis

Although there are many causes of myocarditis, most pediatric cases in the United States are thought to be due to viral processes. Regardless of the etiology, the pathophysiology involves invasion of the myocardium by inflammatory cells that may be accompanied by cardiomyocyte necrosis. In infectious processes, myocytes can be destroyed either directly by the microorganism or by the host's immune response. Depending on the inflammatory response, acute myocarditis may progress to a dilated cardiomyopathy, as myocytes are replaced by fibrotic tissue.

Clinical Presentation

Myocarditis is often misdiagnosed because its presentation takes many forms (Table 14-13). Acute fulminant myocarditis can present with cardiovascular collapse; however, presentations of less severe forms of myocarditis can be subtle. Older children and adolescents may present with nonspecific respiratory or gastrointestinal complaints and are frequently misdiagnosed, requiring multiple visits before proper diagnosis.[20] In contrast, infants may present with poor feeding, lethargy, and fever.

Differential Diagnosis

The differential diagnosis of myocarditis is listed in Table 14-14.

Myocarditis Symptoms and Signs

Symptoms
- Shortness of breath
- Vomiting
- Poor feeding
- Fever
- Lethargy
- Malaise
- Chest pain
- Abdominal pain
- Diaphoresis
- Palpitations
- Rashes
- Exercise intolerance

Signs
- Tachypnea
- Tachycardia
- Hepatomegaly
- Respiratory distress
- Gallop rhythm
- Pallor
- Jugular venous distension
- Pulmonary rales

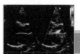

Myocarditis Differential Diagnosis

Common conditions
- Sepsis
- Meningitis
- Pneumonia
- Gastroenteritis
- Bronchiolitis

Rare conditions
- Dilated cardiomyopathy
- Undiagnosed congenital heart disease

Diagnosis

See the algorithm for the diagnosis of myocarditis in Figure 14-9.

Diagnostic Tests

Following a history and physical examination, an ECG and chest x-ray should be obtained because they are frequently abnormal in myocarditis. ECG abnormalities have been identified in up to 100% of cases in some series[20] and include sinus tachycardia, ST-segment elevation (Figure 14-10), abnormal axis deviation, and ventricular hypertrophy. Other ECG abnormalities include T-wave inversions and atrioventricular block. Lyme carditis, in particular, is associated with complete heart block or atrioventricular dissociation. Chest radiographs can show cardiomegaly, pleural fluid, or increased pulmonary vascular markings.

Laboratory studies provide further evidence of cardiac involvement. Elevated troponin levels have been shown to be both sensitive and specific for myocarditis in children.[21] Elevated CRP and ESR are seen. For children presenting with congestive heart failure, it may be difficult to determine if their symptoms are due to a current infectious myocarditis or an undiagnosed chronic dilated cardiomyopathy. Viral studies may therefore be important, although etiologic agents are frequently not identified. Table 14-15 lists viral testing that may be helpful in patient management, depending on availability. In a nonimmunized patient, assays for viruses such as varicella, mumps, measles, and rubella should also be sent.

Cardiac imaging is generally used to confirm the diagnosis of myocarditis. Two-dimensional and Doppler echocardiography should be obtained early in the diagnostic evaluation. Transthoracic echocardiography is often sufficient to characterize the degree of cardiac dysfunction, valve insufficiency, and

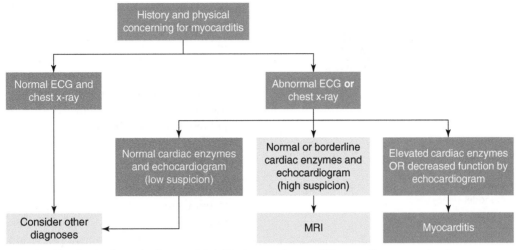

FIGURE 14-9 ■ Algorithm for the diagnosis of myocarditis. ECG, electrocardiogram; MRI, magnetic resonance imaging.

the presence of effusions and note any wall motion abnormalities. Transthoracic echocardiography may be abnormal in up to 98% of cases.[20] Although not universally available, cardiac MRI is a valuable tool in the diagnosis of myocarditis. Because it visualizes the entire myocardium, MRI can demonstrate and quantify myocardial involvement, which can be patchy and subtle in some instances. The use of cardiac MRI has increased because the noninvasive advantage of MRI, combined with good information, outweighs the risks and relative insensitivity of invasive endomyocardial biopsy.[22]

Treatment

Supportive care remains the primary treatment for myocarditis. Patients may require inotropic agents, diuresis, afterload reduction, mechanical ventilation, temporary pacemaker support, or extracorporeal membrane oxygenation in the acute phase depending on their symptoms. Bed rest is recommended during the acute phase because exercise is thought to worsen damage caused by myocarditis. Patients should not participate in vigorous physical activity for 6 months following the diagnosis of myocarditis.

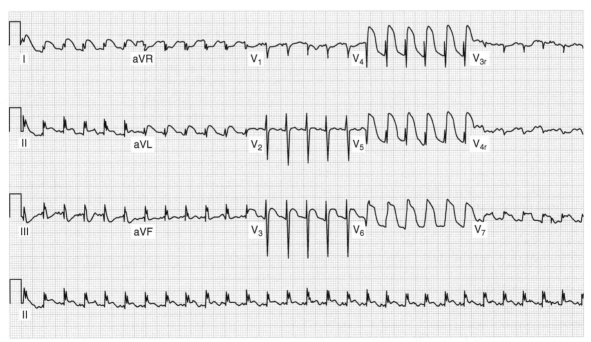

FIGURE 14-10 ■ Twelve-lead electrocardiogram in a patient with fulminant myocarditis, showing diffuse ST-segment elevations in multiple leads.

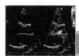

Laboratory Studies to Complete Viral Work-Up

■ Parvovirus B19
■ Enteroviruses
■ Adenovirus
■ Cytomegalovirus
■ Human herpesvirus-6
■ Influenza A
■ Respiratory syncytial virus
■ Human immunodeficiency virus
■ Epstein-Barr virus
■ Norovirus

Interventions to improve long-term cardiac function remain more controversial and are aimed at altering the immune response. Some small pediatric studies have shown improved survival and cardiac function with IVIG treatment.[23] Based on these studies, treatment with IVIG 2 g/kg over less than 24 hours has become the standard of practice in many centers. Further work in the utility of steroids and other immunosuppressive agents is warranted.

Prognosis

Outcomes following myocarditis are incompletely understood, in large part because it is underdiagnosed. Some children regain normal cardiac function, whereas others die in the acute phase. Others have slowly progressive cardiac failure and dilated cardiomyopathy, ultimately requiring cardiac transplantation. Some patients with acute myocarditis who receive rapid treatment may have a favorable prognosis despite the severity of their presentation.

PERICARDITIS

Definition and Epidemiology

The pericardium consists of the visceral pericardium, a single layer of cells overlying the epicardium, and the parietal pericardium, a fibrous sac that surrounds the heart and proximal great vessels. These 2 layers are separated by a potential space that normally contains a small amount of pericardial fluid.[24] Acute pericarditis, or inflammation of the pericardium, can occur with or without a pericardial effusion. It may be an isolated condition or associated with systemic disease. Cardiac tamponade occurs when pericardial fluid accumulates to the point where it exerts pressure on cardiac chambers and alters cardiac filling, ultimately resulting in

increased venous pressures and impaired cardiac output. Chronic pericarditis is defined as pericarditis persisting for greater than 3 months. Recurrent pericarditis can be intermittent or incessant (ie, symptoms recur as soon as treatment is discontinued). Constrictive pericarditis occurs when a scarred, thickened, and often calcified pericardium limits cardiac filling, resulting in equalization of resting pressure in all 4 cardiac chambers.[25]

Pathogenesis

Acute pericarditis is typically idiopathic or caused by a virus, but there are other potential infectious and noninfectious etiologies (Table 14-16). Inflammatory disease, congestive heart failure, and radiation may result in chronic pericarditis. Recurrent pericarditis is seen with rheumatic disease and after open-heart surgery. Constrictive pericarditis is typically secondary to longstanding pericardial inflammation.

Clinical Presentation

Chest pain is the primary complaint for most patients with pericarditis. The pain is retrosternal, sharp, and typically worse with inspiration or lying supine. It may improve when the patient leans forward. Patients may have a history of an upper respiratory tract infection and may be febrile. Patients with purulent pericarditis generally have high fever, tachycardia, chest pain, and dyspnea. Physical examination often reveals a pericardial friction rub, which is a high-pitched, scratchy sound (Table 14-17).

Cardiac tamponade can present as cardiogenic shock or pulseless electrical activity and should be considered during any resuscitation. Anxiety, dyspnea, and chest pain are often seen in patients with early tamponade. Jugular venous distension is usually apparent, reflecting increased venous pressures. Heart sounds may be soft or muffled, particularly if the pericardial effusion is large. The hallmark sign of tamponade is "pulsus paradoxus," defined as a greater than 10 mm Hg drop in systolic blood pressure during inspiration. In tamponade physiology, left ventricular filling is decreased due to decreased right ventricular filling, especially during inspiration, and results in decreased output (lower systolic blood pressure) during inspiration.

Differential Diagnosis

The differential diagnosis of pericarditis is listed in Table 14-18.

Diagnosis

See the algorithm for the diagnosis of pericarditis in Figure 14-11.

Etiologies of Pericarditis

Acute

Infectious

Bacterial
   Staphylococcus aureus, Haemophilus influenza B, Strepto-coccus pneumoniae, Neisseria meningitides, Pseudomonas aeruginosa, Salmonella species, Neisseria gonorrhoeae, Campylobacter fetus

Viral
   Parvovirus, coxsackie virus, echovirus, adenovirus, influenza, mumps, varicella, Epstein-Barr virus, human immunodeficiency virus

Other
   Tuberculosis
   Fungal (*Candida, Aspergillus,* etc)
   Protozoa (*Entamoeba histolytica, Toxoplasma gondii*), *Rickettsia*

Noninfectious

Rheumatic disease
   Rheumatic fever
   Juvenile rheumatoid arthritis
   Systemic lupus erythematosus
Kawasaki disease
Drug-induced: hydralazine, isoniazid, procainamide
Postpericardiotomy
Uremic
Hypothyroidism
Radiation

Chronic

Inflammatory disease
Congestive heart disease
Radiation

Recurrent

Rheumatic disease
Postpericardiotomy

Constrictive

Infectious
Connective tissue disorders
Neoplastic disorders
   Intrapericardial tumor
   Metastatic disease
Radiation
Trauma
Metabolic syndromes (↓ hyperthyroidism)
Genetic syndromes

Diagnostic Tests

Following the physical examination, an ECG should be obtained. ECG changes in pericarditis may include diffuse ST-segment elevation, PR-segment depression, and T-wave inversions (Figure 14-12). Additionally the ECG

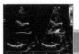

Pericarditis Signs and Symptoms

Pericarditis	Tamponade
Fever	Muffled heart sounds
Tachycardia	Anxiety
Dyspnea	Dyspnea
Chest Pain	Jugular venous distention
Friction Rub	Pulsus paradoxus

may have low voltages throughout. Patients with cardiac tamponade may exhibit electrical alternans, or fluctuating QRS amplitude or axis, caused by the shifting of the heart within a large pericardial effusion.[25]

In terms of imaging, the first test performed in a stable patient should be a chest x-ray. Cardiomegaly due to increased pericardial fluid may be evident with pericarditis or cardiac tamponade. Other diseases in the differential diagnosis, such as pneumonia, can be diagnosed by x-ray. An echocardiogram is the test of choice to delineate a pericardial effusion and evaluate cardiac function (Figure 14-13).[26] Transthoracic echocardiography is generally sufficient to rule out significant pericardial effusions unless the patient has poor acoustic windows. Suspicion for purulent pericarditis may be raised if stranding is seen within the pericardial effusion by echocardiogram. Given the potentially grave consequences of cardiac tamponade, echocardiography should be performed expeditiously and before other testing in an unstable patient with possible tamponade. In patients with a large pericardial effusion, collapse of the right atrium or ventricle during diastole on echocardiography suggests tamponade physiology. Doppler interrogation of tricuspid and mitral inflows can show variable inflow velocities consistent with pulsus paradoxus. If the echocardiogram is concerning for constrictive pericarditis, further imaging with computed tomography or MRI is warranted.

Differential Diagnosis of Pericarditis

Common Conditions
■ Pneumonia
■ Costochondritis
■ Musculoskeletal chest pain

Rare Conditions
■ Myocarditis
■ Pulmonary embolism
■ Myocardial infarction

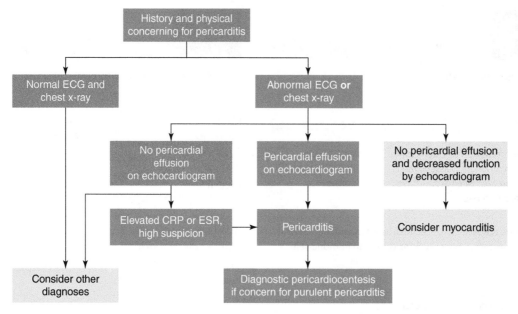

FIGURE 14-11 ■ Algorithm for the diagnosis of pericarditis. CRP, C-reactive protein; ECG, electrocardiogram; ESR, erythrocyte sedimentation rate.

Classic cases of acute pericarditis with a viral pro-drome may require no laboratory testing. In cases where the diagnosis is unclear, ESR and CRP should be obtained to confirm an inflammatory process. Cardiac enzymes (troponin, MB isozyme of creatine phosphokinase) should be obtained if there is concern for myocardi-tis because myocarditis and pericarditis often overlap. Further laboratory testing should be guided by clinical suspicion for nonviral etiologies. Diagnostic pericardio-

centesis, using either echocardiography or fluoroscopic guidance, should be performed if there is a concern for purulent pericarditis; fluid should be sent for cell counts and bacterial culture.

Treatment

Most acute pericarditis of viral or idiopathic origin is self-limited and can be treated in the outpatient setting.

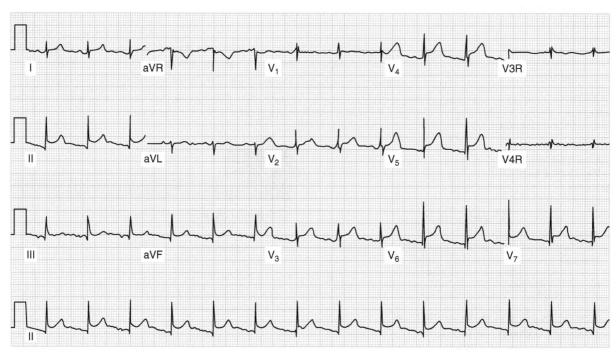

FIGURE 14-12 ■ Twelve-lead electrocardiogram showing ST-segment elevations in a stable outpatient with mild pericarditis and chest pain.

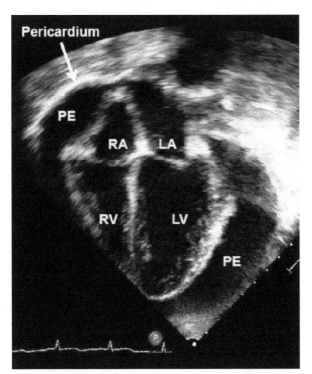

FIGURE 14-13 ■ Transthoracic echocardiogram (apical 4-chamber view) showing a large pericardial effusion in a 13-year-old girl who presented with chest pain and fever. LA, left atrium; LV, left ventricle; PE, pericardial effusion; RA, right atrium; RV, right ventricle.

The mainstays for treatment of acute pericarditis in children are nonsteroidal anti-inflammatory drugs such as ibuprofen. They should be administered at appropriate anti-inflammatory doses (Table 14-19). Refractory cases may require steroid treatment or use of other agents such as colchicine. Patients should be monitored closely for the development of tamponade. Physical activity should be restricted until the patient is asymptomatic and any pericardial effusion has resolved. Pericardiocentesis may be required for large pericardial effusions that cause cardiac tamponade or effusions that are not responsive to medical therapy. Other surgical options, such as creation of pericardial window or pericardiectomy, are reserved for refractory cases and are uncommonly used in children. Pericardiectomy may be necessary for extensive scarring associated with purulent pericarditis.

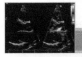

Medications to Treat Pericarditis	
Ibuprofen	10 mg/kg/dose orally every 6 hours
Prednisone	1-2 mg/kg/d divided every 12 hours with a taper
Colchicine	0.6 mg twice a day

In cases of cardiac tamponade, pericardiocentesis should be performed expeditiously. A pericardial drain is often left in place to allow for drainage of reaccumulated fluid. Volume resuscitation may be of some benefit while awaiting the procedure. Inotropic agents are relatively contraindicated given that increasing tachycardia can further compromise the already impaired cardiac filling. Mechanical ventilation with high positive airway pressure in a patient with tamponade may cause hypotension because increased intrathoracic pressure further limits cardiac filling.

ENDOCARDITIS

Definitions and Epidemiology

Although endocarditis is an uncommon disease in children, it causes significant morbidity and mortality. Endocarditis is a microbial infection of the endothelial surfaces of the heart. Infective endocarditis most commonly affects native or prosthetic heart valves but can also affect atrial or ventricular septal defects or foreign intravascular devices, such as intracardiac patches, prosthetic shunts, or intravenous catheters. The epidemiology of infective endocarditis continues to shift. Children without pre-existing heart disease now represent over half of infective endocarditis cases. Of those children with pre-existing heart disease, 81% have congenital heart disease, whereas only 5% have rheumatic heart disease. The incidence of endocarditis by age has bimodal peaks in infancy and late adolescence (17-20 years).[27]

Pathogenesis

The typical sequence of endocarditis pathogenesis begins with damage to the endothelial lining of the heart, followed by formation of a nonbacterial thrombus at the site. Endothelial damage often occurs at a site of turbulent blood flow, such as flow across a narrowed orifice. An episode of transient bacteremia or fungemia results in adherence of bacteria or fungi to the thrombus. Bacteremia may spread from a focal infection, following a dental procedure, or after such daily activities as chewing and brushing teeth. The microorganisms stimulate further deposition of fibrin and platelets and continue to proliferate within the vegetation.

Etiologic agents for infective endocarditis are listed in Table 14-20. Although α-hemolytic streptococci have traditionally been the most common infecting organisms, *S aureus* was found to be the most commonly identified organism in a recent series of pediatric patients, accounting for 57% of cases that specified organisms.[27] Some groups of patients are more vulnerable to specific organisms. Prosthetic valves are generally affected by

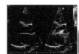
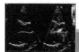

Etiologic Agents of Infective Endocarditis

- Streptococci
  - α-Hemolytic
  - β-Hemolytic
  - Enterococci
  - Pneumococci
  - Other
- Staphylococci
  - *Staphylococcus aureus*
  - Coagulase-negative
- Gram-negative agents
  - Enterics
  - *Pseudomonas* species
  - HACEK
  - *Neisseria* species
- Fungi
  - *Candida* species
  - Other

HACEK, Haemophilus, Actinobacillus, Cardiobacterium, Eikenella, Kingella.

Endocarditis Symptoms and Signs

Symptoms
- Fever
- Myalgia
- Arthralgia
- Headache
- Malaise
- Decreased appetite

Signs
- Heart murmur (new or changing)
- Petechiae
- Splenomegaly
- Neurologic findings
- Osler nodes
- Janeway lesions
- Roth spots
- Splinter hemorrhages

S aureus or coagulase-negative staphylococci. Neonates and immunocompromised patients are at increased risk for gram-negative bacterial and fungal infective endocarditis. Of note, 5% to 10% of endocarditis cases are culture negative.[28]

Clinical Presentation

Endocarditis often presents with nonspecific, generalized symptoms (Table 14-21). Fever is the most common presenting sign, but its pattern differs based on the causative organism. Infections caused by α-hemolytic streptococci often produce low-grade temperatures (<39°C), whereas *S aureus* infections frequently are associated with high, spiking temperatures above 40°C. Patients with subacute infective endocarditis may complain of slowly progressive, nonspecific symptoms such as myalgia, arthralgia, headache, and malaise. In contrast, patients with an acute endocarditis present with high fevers and systemic illness. Neonates may be particularly difficult to diagnose, but endocarditis should be considered in those with systemic hypotension or focal neurologic findings. Because of the nonspecificity of its presentation, clinicians should maintain a high suspicion for endocarditis in any child with underlying heart disease who presents with an unusual or febrile illness.

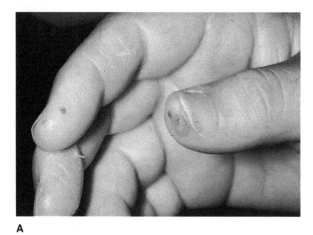
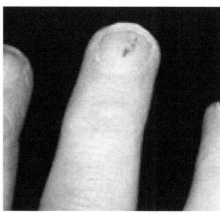

FIGURE 14-14 ■ Peripheral findings of infective endocarditis. **A.** An Osler node is seen on the tips of the thumb and index finger. (*Reproduced with permission from Fuster V, Walsh RA, Harrington RA*. Hurst's the Heart. *13th ed. New York, NY: McGraw-Hill; 2011.*) **B.** Splinter hemorrhages are seen in the nail bed. (Image contributed by Richard P. Usatine, MD.)

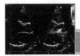

Endocarditis Differential Diagnosis

Common Conditions
- Sepsis
- Influenza
- Mononucleosis

Rare Conditions
- Meningitis

The physical examination may further increase suspicion for infective endocarditis. New or changing murmurs can be appreciated; serial examinations are particularly important for children with pre-existing murmurs to detect interval changes. Petechiae or splenomegaly may be evident. The classic noncardiac physical signs (Osler nodes, Janeway lesions, Roth spots, and splinter hemorrhages; Fig. 14-14) are less common in children. Focal neurologic signs such as seizures or hemiparesis may indicate embolic phenomena from left-sided vegetations.

Differential Diagnosis

The differential diagnosis of infective endocarditis is listed in Table 14-22.

Diagnosis

Given the broad spectrum of findings in the clinical presentation of endocarditis, making the diagnosis can often be difficult. The modified Duke criteria serve as a clinical guide to categorize patients into "definite," "possible," and "rejected" endocarditis (Tables 14-23 and 14-24).[29] In addition to a careful physical examination, the modified Duke criteria require multiple blood cultures and echocardiography for diagnosis.

Diagnostic Tests

Positive peripheral blood cultures are a major criteria for endocarditis under the modified Duke criteria. The

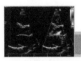

Term Definitions for Modified Duke Criteria for Infective Endocarditis (IE) Diagnosis

Major criteria
- Blood culture positive for IE
  Typical microorganisms consistent with IE from 2 separate blood cultures:
    Viridians streptococci, *Streptococcus bovis*, HACEK group, *Staphylococcus aureus*; or
    Community-acquired enterococci, in the absence of a primary focus; or
  Microorganisms consistent with IE from persistently positive blood cultures, defined as
    At least 2 positive cultures of blood samples drawn ≥12 hours apart; or
    All of 3 or a majority of ≥ 4 separate cultures of blood (with first and last sample drawn at least 1 hour apart)
  Single positive blood culture for *Coxiella burnetii* or antiphase I IgG antibody titer >1:800
- Evidence of endocardial involvement
- Echocardiogram positive for IE (TEE recommended in patients with prosthetic valves, rated at least "possible IE" by clinical criteria, or complicated IE [ie, paravalvular abscess]; TTE as first test in other patients), defined as follows:
  - Oscillating intracardiac mass on valve or supporting structures, in the path of regurgitant jets, or on implanted material in the absence of an alternative anatomic explanation;
  - Abscess;
  - New partial dehiscence of prosthetic valve
- New valvular regurgitation (worsening or changing of pre-existing murmur not sufficient)

Minor criteria
- Predisposing heart condition or injection drug use
- Fever, temperature ≥38°C
- Vascular phenomena, major arterial emboli, septic pulmonary infarcts, mycotic aneurysm, intracranial hemorrhage, conjunctival hemorrhages, and Janeway lesions
- Immunologic phenomena: glomerulonephritis, Osler nodes, Roth spots, and rheumatoid factor
- Microbiologic evidence: positive blood culture but does not meet a major criterion as noted above* or serologic evidence of active infection with organism consistent with IE

HACEK, Haemophilus, Actinobacillus, Cardiobacterium, Eikenella, Kingella; IgE, immunoglobulin E; TEE, transesophageal echocardiography; TTE, transthoracic echocardiography.
Excludes single positive cultures for coagulase-negative staphylococci and organisms that do not cause IE.
Adapted with permission from Li JS, Sexton DJ, Mick N, et al. Proposed modifications to the Duke criteria for the diagnosis of infective endocarditis. Clin Infect Dis. 2000;30:633-638.

Definition of Infective Endocarditis According to the Modified Duke Criteria

Definite infective endocarditis

Pathologic criteria

■ Microorganisms demonstrated by culture or histologic examination of a vegetation, a vegetation that has embolized, or an intracardiac abscess specimen; or

■ Pathologic lesions; vegetation or intracardiac abscess confirmed by histologic examination showing active endocarditis

Clinical criteria (see Table 14-23)

■ 2 major criteria; or

■ 1 major criterion and 3 minor criteria; or

■ 5 minor criteria

Possible infective endocarditis

■ 1 major criterion and 1 minor criterion; or

■ 3 minor criteria

Rejected

■ Firm alternate diagnosis explaining evidence of infective endocarditis; or

■ Resolution of infective endocarditis syndrome with antibiotic therapy for ≤4 days; or

■ No pathologic evidence of infective endocarditis at surgery or autopsy, with antibiotic therapy for ≤4 days; or

■ Does not meet criteria for possible infective endocarditis, as above

Adapted with permission from Li JS, Sexton DJ, Mick N, et al. Proposed modifications to the Duke criteria for the diagnosis of infective endocarditis. Clin Infect Dis. 2000;30:633-638.

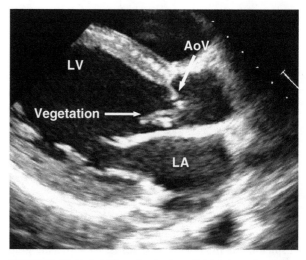

FIGURE 14-15 ■ Two-dimensional echocardiogram (parasternal long axis) showing a large vegetation (arrow) attached to the underside of the closed aortic valve. During the cardiac cycle, this vegetation can prolapse across the aortic valve and result in systemic emboli to the brain or other vital organs.

traditional practice has been to obtain 3 blood cultures at different times from different venipuncture sites within 24 hours. However, this should be adjusted based on patient condition and the index of suspicion for endocarditis. Additional sets may be obtained on day 2 if all cultures remain negative. Each aerobic culture should be sent using 1 to 3 mL of blood from infants and 5 to 7 mL of blood from older children. Other laboratory findings include a positive rheumatoid factor, elevated ESR, anemia, and microscopic hematuria. Additional serologies for less common organisms may be warranted based on clinical suspicion and with the guidance of infectious disease specialists.[28]

Echocardiography should be performed early in the diagnostic work-up because it is the primary method for diagnosis. Transthoracic echocardiography is sufficient to identify vegetations in many children (Figure 14-15). Transesophageal echocardiography may be required for assessment of prosthetic valves, complex congenital heart disease, or limited acoustic windows. Transesophageal echocardiography is indicated if the transthoracic echocardiogram is negative but the clinical suspicion for endocarditis is high, and imaging for very small vegetations is indicated. Additionally, if the surface echocardiogram has findings concerning for more complicated disease, such as a paravalvular abscess, then transesophageal echocardiography is indicated.

Treatment

Intravenous antibiotics are the mainstay of infective endocarditis treatment. Prolonged intravenous therapy (2-6 weeks) is required because the microorganisms are embedded within the vegetations. Because the microorganisms have low rates of cell division and metabolism, bactericidal agents are preferred to static agents. While awaiting blood culture results, initial empiric therapy should include both a semisynthetic penicillin (nafcillin, oxacillin, or methicillin) and an aminoglycoside (gentamicin). If methicillin-resistant *S aureus* is suspected, vancomycin should be used in place of the semisynthetic penicillin. Final antibiotic regimens are tailored to the responsible organism sensitivity. Detailed recommendations are available from the AHA.[30] Compliance and close follow-up with serial echocardiograms and repeat labs are essential. Treatment is often multidisciplinary, including cardiology and infectious disease specialists. Completion of antibiotics as an outpatient may be considered for some children.

Surgery, consisting of vegetation excision and valve repair or replacement, may be an important component of endocarditis therapy. Surgical decisions are individualized based on the site of the infection and the patient's clinical course. Patients with impaired hemodynamic status and congestive heart failure have higher endocarditis mortality and therefore may benefit from surgical therapy. Significant embolic events, worsening congestive heart failure, and persistent infection are clear indications for surgery.

Prevention

Recommendations on prevention of infective endocarditis have changed significantly over the years. The most recent guidelines from the AHA task force emphasize the importance of good oral hygiene and access to preventive dental care.[31] It is thought that patients with dental disease may have increased risk of transient bacteremia with routine daily activities such as brushing or flossing teeth. Surgical repair of congenital heart lesions that predispose to endocarditis is another important preventive measure when clinically indicated. The most recent guideline revisions from the AHA on antibiotic prophylaxis for the prevention of endocarditis published in 2007 were a significant departure from previous AHA guidelines. They reflect the task force committee's conclusion that antibiotic prophylaxis prior to procedures is not always effective in preventing infective endocarditis. The current guideline recommends that only those patients with the highest risk of an adverse outcome from infective endocarditis take antibiotic prophylaxis (Table 14-25). Antibiotics are recommended prior to dental procedures involving manipulation of the gingival tissue, the periapical portion of the teeth, or perforation of oral mucosa. Prophylaxis should also be provided prior to any procedures on the respiratory tract or on infected skin, skin structures, or musculoskeletal tissue. Standard regimens are listed in Table 14-26.

Antibiotic Prophylaxis Regimens

Single dose given 30-60 minutes before procedure	
Oral	Amoxicillin 50 mg/kg/dose
Penicillin allergy	Cephalexin* 50 mg/kg/dose
	or
	Clindamycin 20 mg/kg/dose
	or
	Azithromycin or clarithromycin 15 mg/kg/dose

*Or other first- or second-generation cephalosporin. Of note, cephalosporins should not be used in an individual with a history of anaphylaxis, angioedema, or urticaria with penicillins or ampicillin.

Adapted with permission from Wilson W, Taubert KA, Gewitz M, et al. Prevention of infective endocarditis: guidelines from the American Heart Association: a guideline from the American Heart Association Rheumatic Fever, Endocarditis, and Kawasaki Disease Committee, Council on Cardiovascular Disease in the Young, and the Council on Clinical Cardiology, Council on Cardiovascular Surgery and Anesthesia, and the Quality of Care and Outcomes Research Interdisciplinary Working Group. Circulation. 2007;116:1736-1754.

Clinical Pearls

- In febrile preschool children, maintain a high index of suspicion for Kawasaki disease, especially in infants under 1 year of age.
- Patients with Kawasaki disease receiving IVIG treatment should have their measles-mumps-rubella and varicella vaccinations delayed for about a year.
- Rheumatic fever is a disease of older, school-aged children, unlike Kawasaki disease.
- The enforcement of secondary prophylaxis against rheumatic fever is a prime responsibility of the primary care provider in this patient group.
- Myocarditis should be considered in infants with poor feeding and fever and in children or adolescents with respiratory or gastrointestinal symptoms.
- Pericarditis in children is typically caused by a virus and is self-limited.
- Because of its nonspecific presentation, clinicians should maintain a high level of suspicion for infective endocarditis in children with underlying heart disease or with other risk factors, when unusual symptoms or febrile illness are present.
- Under the most recent guidelines from the American Heart Association, antibiotic prophylaxis prior to dental work is recommended only for children with the highest risk of adverse outcomes from infective endocarditis.

Highest Risk Cardiac Conditions: Endocarditis Antibiotic Prophylaxis Recommended

- Prosthetic cardiac valve (bioprosthetic or mechanical)
- Previous episode of infective endocarditis
- Unrepaired cyanotic congenital heart disease (includes palliative shunts and conduits)
- Completely repaired congenital heart defect with prosthetic material or device (surgical or catheter intervention) during first 6 months after procedure
- Repaired CHD with residual defects or adjacent to site of prosthetic patch or device (inhibit endothelialization)
- Cardiac transplantation recipient with cardiac valvulopathy

Adapted with permission from Baddour LM, Wilson WR, Bayer AS, et al. Infective endocarditis: diagnosis, antimicrobial therapy, and management of complications: a statement for healthcare professionals from the Committee on rheumatic fever, endocarditis, and Kawasaki disease, Council on Cardiovascular Disease in the Young, and the Councils on Clinical Cardiology, Stroke, and Cardiovascular Surgery and Anesthesia, American Heart Association: Endorsed by the Infectious Diseases Society of America. Circulation. 2005;111:e394-e434.

REFERENCES

1. Newburger JW, Takahashi M, Beiser AS, et al. A single intravenous infusion of gamma globulin as compared with four infusions in the treatment of acute Kawasaki syndrome. *N Engl J Med.* 1991;324:1633-1639.
2. Holman RC, Curns AT, Belay ED, Steiner CA, Schonberger LB. Kawasaki syndrome hospitalizations in the United States, 1997 and 2000. *Pediatrics.* 2003;112:495-501.

3. Uehara R, Yashiro M, Nakamura Y, Yanagawa H. Kawasaki disease in parents and children. *Acta Paediatr.* 2003;92:694-697.

4. Leung DY, Giorno RC, Kazemi LV, Flynn PA, Busse JB. Evidence for superantigen involvement in cardiovascular injury due to Kawasaki syndrome. *J Immunol.* 1995;155:5018-5021.

5. Leung DYM, Meissner HC, Shulman ST, et al. Prevalence of super antigen-secreting bacteria in patients with Kawasaki disease. *J Pediatr.* 2002;140:742–746.

6. Rowley AH, Baker SC, Shulman ST, et al. Detection of antigen in bronchial epithelium and macrophages in acute Kawasaki disease by use of synthetic antibody. *J Infect Dis.* 2004;190:856-865.

7. Rowley AH, Baker SC, Shulman ST, et al. RNA-containing cytoplasmic inclusion bodies in ciliated bronchial epithelium months to years after acute Kawasaki disease. *PLoS One.* 2008;3:e1582.

8. Chang FY, Hwang B, Chen SJ, Lee PC, Meng CC, Lu JH. Characteristics of Kawasaki disease in infants younger than six months of age. *Pediatr Infect Dis J.* 2006;25:241-244.

9. Yellen ES, Gauvreau K, Takahashi M, et al. Performance of 2004 American Heart Association recommendations for treatment of Kawasaki disease. *Pediatrics.* 2010;125:e234-e241.

10. Newburger JW, Takahashi M, Gerber MA, et al.; Committee on Rheumatic Fever, Endocarditis and Kawasaki Disease. Diagnosis, treatment, and long-term management of Kawasaki disease: a statement for health professionals from the Committee on Rheumatic Fever, Endocarditis and Kawasaki Disease, Council on Cardiovascular Disease in the Young, American Heart Association. *Circulation.* 2004;110:2747-2771.

11. Miyake CY, Gauvreau K, Tani LY, et al. Characteristics of children discharged from hospitals in the United States in 2000 with the diagnosis of acute rheumatic fever. *Pediatrics.* 2007;120:503-508.

12. Smoot JC, Korgenski EK, Daly JA, et al. Molecular analysis of group A streptococcus type *emm* 18 isolates temporally associated with acute rheumatic fever outbreaks in Salt Lake City, Utah. *J Clin Microbiol.* 2002;40:1805-1810.

13. Siegel AC, Johnson EE, Stollerman GH. Controlled studies of streptococcal pharyngitis in a pediatric population, 1. Factors related to the attack rate of rheumatic fever. *N Engl J Med.* 1961;265:559-565.

14. Dajani AS, Ayoub EM, Bierman FZ, et al. Guidelines for the diagnosis of rheumatic fever: Jones criteria, updated 1992. *JAMA Circulation.* 1992;87:302-307.

15. Kaplan EL. The group A streptococcal upper respiratory tract carrier state: an enigma. *J Pediatr.* 1980;97:337-345.

16. Nigel W. Echocardiography and subclinical carditis: guidelines that increase sensitivity for acute rheumatic fever. *Cardiol Young.* 2008;18:565-568.

17. Feinstein AR, Wood HF, Epstein JA, et al. A controlled study of three methods of prophylaxis against streptococcal infection in a population of rheumatic children. II. Results of the first three years of the study, including methods for evaluating the maintenance of oral prophylaxis. *N Engl J Med.* 1959;260:697-702.

18. Kotloff KL, Corretti M, Palmer K, et al. Safety and immunogenicity of a recombinant multivalent group A streptococcal vaccine in healthy adults: phase 1 trial. *JAMA.* 2004;292:709-715.

19. Levine MC, Klugman D, Teach SJ. Update on myocarditis in children. *Curr Opin Pediatr.* 2010;22:278-283.

20. Durani Y, Egan M, Baffa J, et al. Pediatric myocarditis: presenting clinical characteristics. *Am J Emerg Med.* 2009;27:942-947.

21. Soongswang J, Durongpisitkul K, Ratanarapee S, et al. Cardiac troponin T: its role in the diagnosis of clinically suspected acute myocarditis and chronic dilated cardiomyopathy in children. *Pediatr Cardiol.* 2002;23:531-535.

22. Danti M, Sbarbati S, Alsadi N, et al. Cardiac magnetic resonance imaging: diagnostic value and utility in the follow-up of patients with acute myocarditis mimicking myocardial infarction. *Radiol Med.* 2009;114:229-238.

23. Drucker NA, Colan SD, Lewis AB, et al. Gamma-globulin treatment of acute myocarditis in the pediatric population. *Circulation.* 1994;89:252–257.

24. Little WC, Freeman GL. Pericardial disease. *Circulation.* 2006;113;1622-1632.

25. Rheuban KS. Pericardial diseases. In: Allen HD, Driscoll DJ, Shaddy RE, et al., eds. *Moss and Adams' Heart Disease in Infants, Children and Adolescents.* 7th ed. Philadelphia, PA: Lippincott Williams & Wilkins; 2008:1290-1299.

26. Imazio M, Spodick DH, Brucato A, et al. Controversial issues in the management of pericardial diseases. *Circulation.* 2010;121;916-928.

27. Day MD, Gauvreau K, Shulman S, et al. Characteristics of children hospitalized with infective endocarditis. *Circulation.* 2009;119;865-870.

28. Taubert KA, Gewitz M. Infective endocarditis. In: Allen HD, Driscoll DJ, Shaddy RE, et al., eds. *Moss and Adams' Heart Disease in Infants, Children and Adolescents.* 7th ed. Philadelphia, PA: Lippincott Williams & Wilkins; 2008:1299-1312.

29. Li JS, Sexton DJ, Mick N, et al. Proposed modifications to the Duke criteria for the diagnosis of infective endocarditis. *Clin Infect Dis.* 2000;30:633-638.

30. Baddour LM, Wilson WR, Bayer AS, et al. Infective endocarditis: diagnosis, antimicrobial therapy, and management of complications: a statement for healthcare professionals from the Committee on rheumatic fever, endocarditis, and Kawasaki disease, Council on Cardiovascular Disease in the Young, and the Councils on Clinical Cardiology, Stroke, and Cardiovascular Surgery and Anesthesia, American Heart Association: Endorsed by the Infectious Diseases Society of America. *Circulation.* 2005;111:e394-e434.

31. Wilson W, Taubert KA, Gewitz M, et al. Prevention of infective endocarditis: guidelines from the American Heart Association: a guideline from the American Heart Association Rheumatic Fever, Endocarditis, and Kawasaki Disease Committee, Council on Cardiovascular Disease in the Young, and the Council on Clinical Cardiology, Council on Cardiovascular Surgery and Anesthesia, and the Quality of Care and Outcomes Research Interdisciplinary Working Group. *Circulation.* 2007;116:1736-1754.

CHAPTER 15

Preventive Cardiology

Aimee Parnell,
Aaron Dorfman and
Julie Brothers

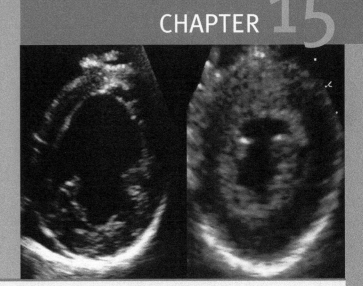

INTRODUCTION

Pediatric preventive cardiology has increased in importance over the past several years due to the increasing number of children with obesity, hypertension, and dyslipidemia. In adults, elevated blood pressure, abdominal obesity, atherogenic dyslipidemia, and elevated plasma glucose levels are collectively known as the metabolic syndrome. The metabolic syndrome is associated with significantly increased risk of developing premature cardiovascular disease. Although there is currently no agreed upon definition of metabolic syndrome in children and adolescents, we do know that the extent of atherosclerotic progression is significantly correlated with several cardiovascular risk factors found in childhood, including elevated total cholesterol and low-density lipoprotein cholesterol, low levels of high-density lipoprotein cholesterol, obesity, high blood pressure, and smoking. Identifying children at a young age is beneficial because it allows for early implementation of dietary and lifestyle changes that may help delay the onset or progression of atherosclerosis. Indeed, in 2011, integrated cardiovascular risk reduction guidelines were published, specifically focusing on the promotion of cardiovascular health in children and adolescents as well as the identification and management of certain cardiovascular risk factors.[1] This chapter will focus on 3 main areas of preventive cardiology: obesity, hypertension, and dyslipidemia.

OBESITY

Definition

Over the past 2 decades, the labels and definitions for overweight and obesity have changed[2] and are demonstrated in Table 15-1. Not included in Table 15-1 are definitions for healthy weight (5th-84th percentile) and underweight (<5th percentile) children. The body mass index (BMI = body weight in kilograms/height in meters squared) category classifications are defined using the 2000 Centers for Disease Control and Prevention growth charts.[2] The BMI value used to plot on the growth curves can be obtained in a variety of ways, including calculators and formulas, nomograms, and tables and wheels. Over the past few years, many practitioners calculate the BMI using personal electronic data assistant programs, smart phone applications, electronic healthcare record software, or Internet calculators. Although most of these applications will provide output in BMI percentiles, in most instances, these values still need to be manually plotted on a curve in order to track trends over time. For children less than 2 years of age, the practitioner should plot weight for height values over time.[3]

Although BMI is a widely used and inexpensive method for assessment of body fat, it does have limitations. These limitations are in some part due to the fact that body fat is typically higher among older individuals as well as females. In the older adolescent population, it can be particularly troublesome because the classification of obese versus overweight may be different using the adult versus pediatric definitions given the same BMI in the same patient. In addition, the scale cannot differentiate between lean muscle mass and fat; therefore, an athletic child who is very muscular may fall into the overweight or obese category when he or she has a larger percentage of muscle mass making up his or her body weight.

Alternative methods for assessing body fat such as skinfold thickness or waist and/or thigh circumferences may be more accurate for assessing overweight and obesity. However, they are more labor intensive and have more subjective variability when making

Body Mass Index Category Recommended Terminology[2,3]		
Body Mass Index (BMI) Category	1994 Recommended Terminology	2007 Recommended Terminology
BMI ≥ 85th and < 95th percentile	At risk for overweight	Overweight
BMI ≥ 95th percentile	Overweight	Obese

measurements. More research is necessary using these methods in the pediatric population before recommending them for use in everyday practice.

Epidemiology

As shown in Figure 15-1, the past 3 decades have seen a dramatic increase in obesity in the United States, with the rate of obesity doubling in adults and the rates among children tripling.[4] According to the statistics reported by the Department of Health and Human Services Expert Committee, obesity prevalence in U.S. children has increased from approximately 5% in 1963 to 1970 to 17% in 2003 to 2004.[3]

Data from the National Health and Nutrition Examination Survey (NHANES) showed significant differences over the past 25 years in prevalence rates of obesity by race, sex, and poverty level (Figure 15-2). For example, minority groups had a significantly higher prevalence of severe obesity than the Caucasian population. Additionally, there were significant differences by poverty–income ratio, with the most affluent (poverty–income ratio >3) demonstrating the lowest prevalence of severe obesity. In select BMI percentiles, there were significant differences by age groups, with the greatest prevalence of high BMI in the older age groups. The prevalence of those with a BMI ≥99th percentile was found to be significantly higher in boys compared with girls.[5] In addition, data from the Early Childhood Longitudinal Study birth cohort demonstrated that the highest prevalence of obesity among 4-year-old children in the United States was in American Indian/Native Alaskan children.[6]

Clinical Presentation

Most children will present with only an elevated BMI noted during routine physical examination. Other children with more extreme obesity may present with a spectrum of physical findings associated with obesity itself and/or secondary to other associated comorbid conditions.

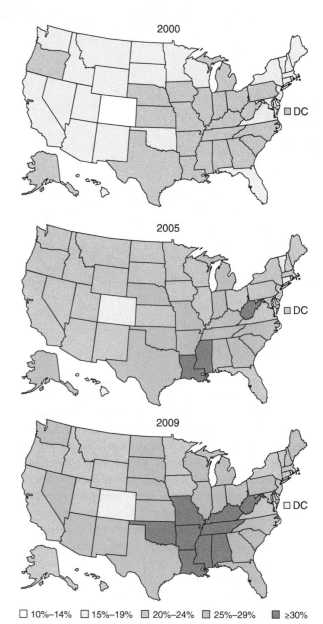

□ 10%–14%　□ 15%–19%　□ 20%–24%　□ 25%–29%　■ ≥30%

FIGURE 15-1 ■ Self-reported prevalence of obesity among adults: Behavioral Risk Factor Surveillance System, United States, 2000, 2005, and 2009. Obesity is defined as body mass index (BMI) ≥ 30.0; BMI was calculated from self-reported weight and height (weight in kilograms divided by height in meters squared). (*From Centers for Disease Control and Prevention. Vital signs: state-specific obesity prevalence among adults—United States, 2009. Available at: http://www.cdc.gov/mmwr/preview/mmwrhtml/mm59e0803a1.htm. Accessed on March 1, 2011.*)

In addition to elevated BMI, some examples of presenting clinical signs on physical examination may include truncal/central adipose deposition, striae, acanthosis nigricans (Figure 15-3), acne, or hirsutism (Figure 15-4).

Screening and Prevention

In the current era of increasing prevalence of childhood obesity, it is essential that primary care providers screen patients for the development of obesity as well as for environmental and genetic risk factors that place them

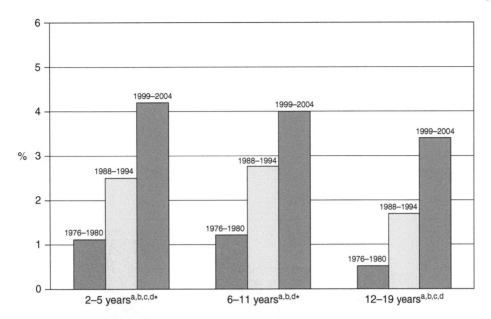

a p < 0.001 for trends from NHANES II to NHANES III to NHANES 1999–2004
b p < 0.001 comparing NHANES II to NHANES 1999–2004
c p < 0.05 comparing NHANES III to NHANES 1999–2004
d p ≤ 0.01 comparing NHANES II to NHANES III
*Estimates for NHANES II based on sample size <30 or relative standard error >30% and
may be unreliable.

A

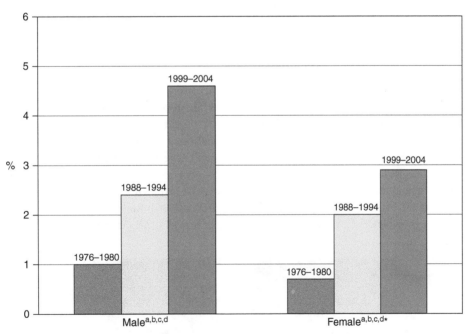

a p < 0.001 for trends from NHANES II to NHANES III to NHANES 1999–2004
b p < 0.001 comparing NHANES II to NHANES 1999–2004
c p = 0.04 comparing NHANES III to NHANES 1999–2004
d p ≤ 0.003 comparing NHANES II to NHANES III
*Estimates for NHANES II females based on sample size <30 or relative standard error >30%
and may be unreliable.

B

FIGURE 15-2 ■ Prevalence of body mass index ≥ 99th percentile among U.S. children ages 2 to 19 years, National Health and Nutrition Examination Survey (NHANES) II (1976-1980), NHANES III (1988-1994), and NHANES 1999–2004, by **(A)** age groupings, **(B)** sex, and **(C)** race/ethnic groups. (*Reprinted, with permission, from Skelton JA, Cook SR, Auinger P, et al. Prevalence and trends of severe obesity among US children and adolescents.* Acad Pediatr. *2009;9:322-329.*)

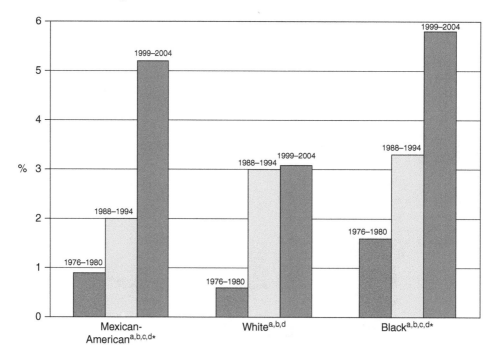

a p < 0.001 for trends from NHANES II to NHANES III to NHANES 1999–2004
b p < 0.001 comparing NHANES II to NHANES 1999–2004
c p < 0.001 comparing NHANES III to NHANES 1999–2004
d p ≤ 0.03 comparing NHANES II to NHANES III
*Estimates for NHANES II Mexican-American and Black based on sample size <30 or relative
standard error >30% and may be unreliable.

C

FIGURE 15-2 ■ (*Continued*)

at a higher risk for developing obesity. The difficulty of behavioral weight-loss therapy and the often life-long struggle with weight maintenance in the obese population or, alternatively, the potential expense and dangers of medication use and surgical treatment highlight the importance of prevention strategies in this population. Primary care providers are accustomed to providing prevention counseling for a number of entities beginning in the newborn period through adolescence; in the face of the

increasing prevalence of childhood obesity, counseling to aid in prevention of obesity should now be included.

In 2007, a report was published regarding the prevention, assessment, and treatment of childhood obesity. The recommendations were subsequently endorsed by many organizations, including the American Academy of Pediatrics. The report emphasizes that obesity prevention should include all children beginning from the time of birth. As shown in Figure 15-5, in addition to

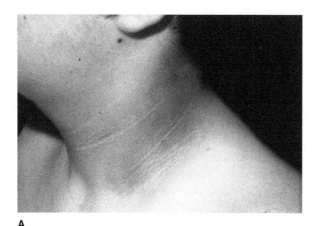

A

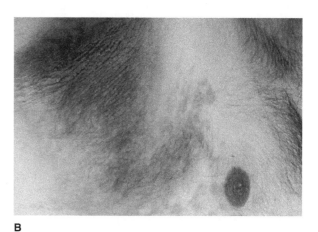

B

FIGURE 15-3 ■ **A.** Acanthosis nigricans demonstrating velvety brownish thickening of the skin with prominent skin creases on the neck in a 12-year-old boy. (*Reprinted, with permission, from Wolff K, Johnson RA. Fitzpatrick's Color Atlas and Synopsis of Clinical Dermatology. 6th ed. New York, NY: McGraw Hill; 2009.*) **B.** Acanthosis nigricans demonstrating typical hyperpigmented axillary plaques with a velvet-like, verrucous surface. (*Reprinted, with permission, from Fauci AS, Kasper DL, Braunwald E, et al. Harrison's Principles of Internal Medicine. 17th ed. New York, NY: McGraw-Hill; 2008.*)

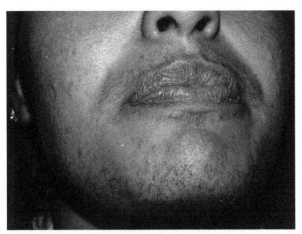

FIGURE 15-4 ■ Adolescent female with slowly progressive generalized hirsutism. (*Reprinted with permission from Zikry KS. Dermatlas. Available at: http://www.dermatlas.org. Accessed October 17, 2011.*)

and physical activity is important for all patients, regardless of the presence of obesity. Providers should counsel patients and their families to adopt and maintain a spectrum of healthy behaviors focused on improving physical activity and eating habits and decreasing sedentary behaviors. Some specific examples include limiting sugar-sweetened beverages, encouraging fruit and vegetable consumption, limiting screen time (including television, video games, computers, and other electronic devices) to less than 2 hours daily, eating breakfast, limiting eating at restaurants, encouraging family meals, and limiting portion sizes. In patients with overweight and obesity, these are opportunities for dietary and activity changes to help with either weight loss or weight stabilization. In those with a normal BMI, at-risk diet and activity behaviors can be identified early to provide counseling and early intervention in efforts to prevent the development of obesity. Because children who have parents and/or siblings who are obese are at a higher risk of developing obesity, those patients should be identified, and the family should be counseled as early as possible. The challenge for the provider is not in the

the routine measurement of height, weight, and growth curves and BMI assessment, additional information should be obtained regarding environment and lifestyle. A detailed history of dietary intake (including beverages)

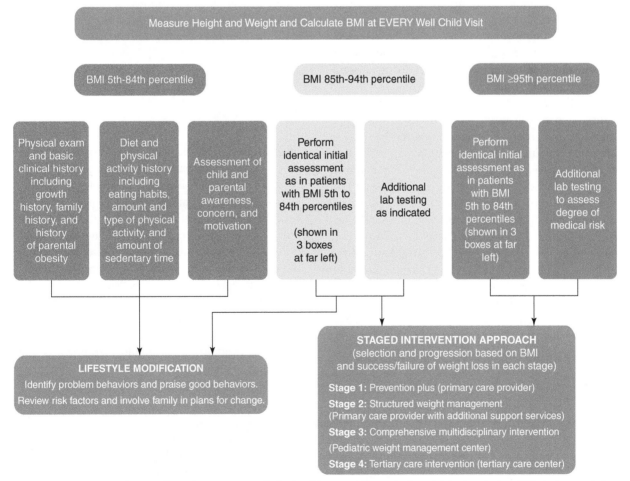

FIGURE 15-5 ■ Universal approach to the assessment of obesity risk, prevention strategies, and treatment plan. BMI, body mass index. (*Adapted with permission from Barlow SE; The Expert Committee. Expert Committee recommendations regarding the prevention, assessment, and treatment of child and adolescent overweight and obesity: summary report.* Pediatrics. *2007;120:S164-S192.*)

provision of this prevention counseling, but rather the process of providing this information and support in such a way as to influence the family to alter behaviors influenced by long-standing traditions, habits, culture, and physical environment. As a guide to implement this plan for prevention, the report also details a 15-minute "Obesity Prevention Protocol."[3]

Diagnosis and Evaluation

According to the 2007 recommendations, a BMI under the 5th percentile is defined as underweight, BMI in the 5th to 84th percentile is defined as a healthy weight, BMI in the 85th to 94th percentile is defined as overweight, and BMI in the 95th percentile or higher is defined as obese.

Children with elevated BMI levels face more than just the risk of persistent or future obesity. A BMI level in the 85th percentile or higher places a child at risk for other medical problems affecting multiple organ systems. An evaluation of these other associated conditions must be included in the evaluation of a child with obesity. Some examples of weight-related problems include sleep disturbances, respiratory problems, gastrointestinal problems, orthopedic issues, psychiatric and nervous system problems, skin problems, and cardiovascular disorders. Table 15-2 illustrates the signs, symptoms, and physical examination findings in children with obesity and the respective possible causes for each.

Although a detailed history and physical examination with an exhaustive review of systems can elicit many of the associated comorbid conditions, there are some conditions that require screening with other modalities, as illustrated in Table 15-3. For example, it is recommended that all children ages 2 years and older with a BMI in the 85th percentile or higher have a fasting lipid panel. In addition, if additional risk factors are identified, liver function tests and a fasting glucose should be evaluated every 2 years beginning at age 10 years. For those with BMI >95th percentile, these tests should be completed every 2 years regardless of additional risk factors. Abnormal elevation of liver enzymes on 2 occasions may indicate the need for further evaluation including the assistance of gastrointestinal specialists. Abnormalities revealed from initial history, review of systems, physical examination, and laboratory testing may prompt further testing to evaluate for additional comorbidities, as outlined in Table 15-3.

Treatment

The goals for treatment of childhood obesity are to improve health and reduce long-term medical complications by introducing permanent healthy lifestyle changes. With more severe obesity, escalation to additional forms of therapy may be indicated. Individual patient characteristics may determine which therapies are likely to be successful. Younger patients and those with lower BMI percentiles should generally change weight more gradually than older patients and those with higher BMI percentiles. In accordance with these principles, a staged approach should be implemented for treatment of obesity in children and adolescents. This approach emphasizes healthy lifestyle changes regarding dietary habits and physical activity to promote slow sustained weight loss and continued practice of these new lifestyle changes. It allows for adjustment of treatment and escalation to other stages in light of differing patient characteristics or failed weight loss after 3 to 6 months in the current stage.[3]

When traditional weight-loss measures are unsuccessful, there are medications and surgical treatment options that are now available; however, these are reserved for only the most severe cases and in the older adolescent and adult population. Although the detailed discussion of these therapies is beyond the scope of this text, consideration for medication and/or bariatric surgery should only be considered after well-documented failure of lifestyle modifications. These patients should be referred to an obesity and/or bariatric medicine specialist for further evaluation and treatment.

HYPERTENSION

Introduction

Hypertension in the pediatric population is an incredibly complex phenomenon, representing the end result of a wide variety of underlying pathologic processes. Although the most common cause of hypertension in childhood is essential hypertension, there are many renal, cardiovascular, endocrine, and metabolic conditions that predispose to or directly cause hypertension. To make the diagnosis, the blood pressure must be measured accurately, which can be challenging due to patient cooperation and proper cuff selection. Furthermore, the diagnosis of hypertension is not constant, with normal blood pressure values changing with age, sex, and height. When the diagnosis is made, initial treatment is often with lifestyle changes followed by medication therapy, usually with the assistance of subspecialty consultation.

Definition

Hypertension in children is classified as prehypertension, stage 1 hypertension, and stage 2 hypertension. These classifications are dependent on the degree of blood pressure elevation relative to normative values for age, sex, and height. Blood pressure should be measured

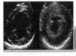

History and Physical Examination Findings Suggestive of Obesity-Related Disorders

System	Review of Systems Findings	Physical Examination Findings	Possible Causes
General symptoms/ physical findings	Weight gain	High BMI percentile, short stature, violaceous striae, hirsutism, acanthosis nigricans, skin inflammation/irritation	Consequences of overweight/ obesity; underlying endocrine disorder
Endocrine	Weight gain, fatigue, coarse dry hair, hair loss, depression, cold intolerance	Goiter, coarse dry hair, hair loss	Hypothyroidism
Endocrine	Polyuria, polydipsia, unexpected weight loss		Type 2 diabetes mellitus
Psychiatric/ behavioral	Anxiety, school avoidance, social isolation		Depression
Neurologic/ ophthalmologic	Severe, recurrent headaches	Papilledema, cranial nerve VI paralysis	Pseudotumor cerebri
Respiratory	Shortness of breath, exercise intolerance	Wheezing, increased work of breathing	Asthma, exercise intolerance
Sleep hygiene	Snoring, apnea, daytime sleepiness, nocturnal enuresis	Tonsillar hypertrophy	Obstructive sleep apnea
Gastrointestinal	Abdominal pain	Abdominal tenderness; hepatomegaly (only in nonalcoholic fatty liver disease [NAFLD])	Gastroesophageal reflux disease, constipation, gallbladder disease, NAFLD
Orthopedic	Hip pain, knee pain, walking pain	Gait disturbances, decreased range of motion of hips, bowing of tibia (only in Blount disease)	Slipped capital femoral epiphysis, musculoskeletal stress from weight, Blount disease
Orthopedic	Foot pain		Musculoskeletal stress from weight
Reproductive	Irregular menses (<9 cycles per year)		Polycystic ovarian syndrome (PCOS)
Reproductive	Primary amenorrhea		PCOS, Prader-Willi syndrome
Reproductive	Early menarche	Advanced Tanner stage for expected age	Premature puberty (males and females)
Reproductive		Apparent micropenis (may be a normal penis buried in fat)	Obesity
Reproductive		Undescended testes	Prader-Willi syndrome
Cardiovascular		Elevated blood pressure	Hypertension

Adapted with permission from Barlow SE; The Expert Committee. Expert Committee recommendations regarding the prevention, assessment, and treatment of child and adolescent overweight and obesity: summary report. Pediatrics. 2007;120:S164-S192.

in a standardized way. According to the American Academy of Pediatrics, patients should be in a seated position for 5 minutes, with both feet on the ground, back supported, and the right arm elevated and supported with the elbow at the level of the heart.[7] A properly sized blood pressure cuff should be selected, with a bladder width of about 40% of the arm circumference midway between the acromion and the olecranon. The bladder length should cover 80% to 100% of the circumference of the arm, as shown in Figure 15-6. Failure to select the proper cuff size for patient size can cause spurious

values to be measured, with cuffs that are too small causing artificially elevated blood pressure and cuffs that are too large causing artificially low blood pressure.

Blood pressure can be determined by either auscultatory measurement or oscillometric devices. The standard method for auscultation is to use a standard sphygmomanometer with the bell of the stethoscope placed over the brachial artery pulse. The systolic blood pressure is defined as the onset of the Korotkoff sounds (K1), and the diastolic blood pressure is defined as the disappearance of Korotkoff sounds (K5). In some

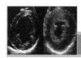

Screening and Additional Testing for Identification of Obesity-Related Disorders

System	Weight-Related Medical Problem	Screening Measure	Additional Testing
Sleep disturbances	Obstructive sleep apnea Obesity hypoventilation syndrome	History and physical examination	Polysomnography
Respiratory	Asthma	History and physical examination	Pulmonary function testing
Gastrointestinal	Nonalcoholic fatty liver disease	ALT and AST	Ultrasound, CT of abdomen, liver biopsy
	Gallstones	History and physical examination	Abdominal ultrasound
Endocrine	Type 2 diabetes	History and physical examination, fasting serum glucose	Evaluation by pediatric endocrinologist
	Polycystic ovarian syndrome	History and physical examination	Reproductive hormone testing; evaluation by pediatric endocrinologist
	Hypothyroidism	History and physical examination; assessment of change in linear height over time	Thyroid function tests
	Primary Cushing syndrome	Physical examination	Cortisol, adrenocorticotropic hormone testing; evaluation by endocrinologist
Nervous system	Pseudotumor cerebri	History and physical examination including ophthalmologic examination	Urgent referral to neurology service
Psychiatric disorders	Depression	History and physical examination	Referral to psychiatrist
Orthopedic disorders	Blount disease	Physical examination	Radiographic evaluation of bilateral lower extremities
	Slipped capital femoral epiphysis	History and physical examination	Radiographic evaluation of bilateral hips (frog-leg views)
Skin conditions	Acanthosis nigricans	Physical examination	No additional testing required unless hyperinsulinemia is suspected

ALT, alanine aminotransferase; AST, aspartate aminotransferase; CT, computed tomography.
Adapted with permission from Barlow SE; The Expert Committee. Expert Committee recommendations regarding the prevention, assessment, and treatment of child and adolescent overweight and obesity: summary report. Pediatrics. 2007;120:S164-S192.

children, Korotkoff sounds may be heard until virtually 0 mm Hg, in which case the diastolic blood pressure is identified at the muffling of sounds (K4). The average of 2 to 3 measurements should be used to determine the blood pressure value.

Although auscultation is considered to be the standard method for measuring blood pressure, many offices and hospital settings use oscillometric devices for rapidly measuring blood pressure. The advantage to these devices is that they are quick and easy to use and they minimize interobserver variability. These devices measure mean blood pressure and then use proprietary algorithms to calculate systolic and diastolic values. The principal uses

for these devices are for serial in-hospital measurements where auscultation would be impractical, outpatient screening of infants and small children where auscultation is very difficult, and screening in an office setting. Blood pressure values greater than the 90th percentile for age, sex, and height should be repeated by auscultation.

Blood pressure should be measured in every child 3 years of age and older at all visits to medical care. In addition, patients younger than 3 years of age meeting specific high-risk criteria should also be screened. These patients include those with a history of prematurity, congenital heart disease, recurrent urinary tract infections, known renal/urologic disease, malignancy, or

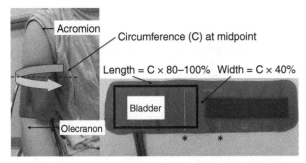

FIGURE 15-6 ■ Blood pressure cuff sizing in children. The bladder width should measure 40% of the arm circumference, measured at the midpoint between the acromion and olecranon. Bladder length should cover 80% to 100% of the arm circumference. Most manufacturers print appropriate lines on the cuffs to aid in cuff selection (*). (*Adapted with permission from National High Blood Pressure Education Program Working Group on Hypertension Control in Children and Adolescents. The fourth report on the diagnosis, evaluation, and treatment of high blood pressure in children and adolescents. Pediatrics. 1996;98:649-658*)

solid organ transplantation. In addition, patients with a systemic disease or taking medications known to elevate the blood pressure should be screened at a young age. Importantly, any measurement of elevated blood pressure should be repeated several times in a single clinic visit and confirmed at follow-up visits. Results are compared to published normative values based on age, sex, and height.[7] Normal values are considered to be less than the 90th percentile and should be repeated at the next medical evaluation. Patients with blood pressure measurements ≥90th percentile and less than the 95th percentile are considered to have prehypertension. In addition, adolescents with a blood pressure greater than 120/80 mm Hg but less than the 95th percentile are also considered to have prehypertension. Hypertension is defined as average systolic or diastolic blood pressure >95th percentile on 3 separate occasions. This can be further subdivided into stage 1 hypertension for blood pressures ranging from the 95th percentile to 5 mm Hg above the 99th percentile and stage 2 hypertension for blood pressures greater than 5 mm Hg above the 99th percentile for age, sex, and height.

Hypertensive urgency or emergency is when patients have severely elevated blood pressure and other risk factors, including symptomatic hypertension, underlying diabetes, or other serious medical conditions. A hypertensive emergency is defined as severe hypertension with evidence of end-organ dysfunction. Hypertensive urgency is defined as severe hypertension without evidence of end-organ dysfunction.[8]

White coat hypertension is defined as an average blood pressure greater than the 95th percentile when measured in the physician's office but consistently less than the 90th percentile when measured in a nonmedical setting. Although initially thought to be harmless, there is some indication that these children may be at higher risk for developing hypertension later in life.

Clinical Presentation

The most common presentation of hypertension is measuring an elevated blood pressure in otherwise well-appearing children during routine medical evaluations. Generally, children who present with symptoms are those with a hypertensive urgency or emergency and who require immediate evaluation. During the initial evaluation, it is important to determine whether primary or secondary hypertension is present because the incidence of secondary hypertension is much higher in children than adults.

Primary hypertension

Previously thought to be a disease of adulthood, primary hypertension is now recognized as a disease of childhood and adolescence. Characteristically, primary hypertension is stage 1 hypertension and is asymptomatic. It is typically found in older children and adolescents with a strong family history of primary hypertension. Younger children with more severe hypertension and without a family history of hypertension are at higher likelihood of having a secondary cause. As with adults, primary hypertension often presents with other comorbidities, including obesity, insulin resistance, hyperlipidemia, and obstructive sleep apnea. Together, these disorders increase the risk for each other and for long-term cardiovascular disease.

Many children with hypertension are found to be overweight, and the current increasing rise in obesity is thought to be a contributing factor to the increasing prevalence of hypertension. There is evidence to show that elevation of blood pressure is related to higher BMI, with the likelihood of having hypertension doubling for each 1-unit increase in the BMI z-score in school-aged children. Other data have shown increases in blood pressure in all age groups with increasing BMI.[9-11]

Secondary hypertension

Compared to primary hypertension, which almost always presents asymptomatically during routine screening, secondary hypertension is far more likely to present with symptoms. These presenting symptoms may either be indications of the underlying disease process or a manifestation of the markedly elevated blood pressure. Cardiac and neurologic indicators of hypertension include headache, stroke, seizure, visual disturbances, chest pain, syncope, and shortness of breath. Although these presenting symptoms are not specific for any particular cause of secondary hypertension, patients presenting with symptoms are at a higher likelihood of having a secondary cause.

Clinical Findings Suggestive of Secondary Hypertension

	Clinical Findings	Potential Etiologies
Vital signs	Tachycardia	Hyperthyroidism, pheochromocytoma
	Blood pressure gradient	Coarctation of the aorta
	Growth delay	Renal disease
	Truncal obesity	Cushing syndrome
Eyes	Retinal changes	Stage 2 hypertension
	Papilledema	Elevated intracranial pressure
Head/neck	Thyromegaly	Hyperthyroidism
	Elfin facies	Williams syndrome
	Webbed neck	Turner syndrome
Skin	Hirsutism	Cushing syndrome
	Café-au-lait spots	Neurofibromatosis
	Adenoma sebaceum	Tuberous sclerosis
	Malar rash	Systemic lupus erythematosus
	Wide-spaced nipples	Turner syndrome
Cardiac	Murmur	Coarctation of the aorta
	Pericardial friction rub	Pericarditis, renal disease with uremia
	Apical heave	Left ventricular hypertrophy
Abdomen	Mass	Malignancy
	Bruit	Renal artery stenosis
	Palpable kidneys	Polycystic kidney disease, hydronephrosis
Genitalia	Ambiguous	Adrenal hyperplasia
Extremities	Joint swelling	Systemic lupus erythematosus
	Muscle weakness	Hyperaldosteronism
	Decreased femoral pulses	Coarctation of the aorta

Adapted with permission from Flynn JT. Evaluation and management of hypertension in childhood. Prog Pediatr Cardiol. 2001;12:177-188.

Some of the clinical signs of secondary causes of hypertension are summarized in Table 15-4. A careful and complete history and physical examination with specific attention for the common and uncommon findings of these underlying processes is vital to making a rapid diagnosis of the underlying cause of the secondary hypertension. Specific attention must be paid to screening for the signs and symptoms of the emergent conditions such as elevated intracranial pressure, coarctation of the aorta, and acute renal failure. In addition, there are numerous genetic syndromes, such as Williams and Turners syndromes, that have very characteristic physical examination findings.

Diagnosis

The diagnosis of hypertension is reliant on the careful measurement of blood pressure using proper technique, which is outlined earlier. All elevated blood pressure measurements should be confirmed on 3 separate occasions. The diagnostic algorithm is summarized in Figure 15-7. Patients with prehypertension and stage 1 hypertension can often be evaluated as outpatients over a time

course of weeks or months. All patients with stage 2 and symptomatic hypertension should be evaluated very rapidly with the degree of urgency directly related to the amount of blood pressure elevation and the severity of the symptoms. Some of these patients may require referral to the emergency department and hospital admission for diagnosis and treatment.

Differential Diagnosis

The differential diagnosis for hypertension is a stepwise process that begins with a healthcare provider recognizing the elevated blood pressure measurement and ultimately leading to a final diagnosis. This process can be summarized as follows:

1. Recognize elevated blood pressure for age, sex, and height.
2. Separate from spurious measurement due to technique.
3. Confirm elevated blood pressure on 3 separate measurements.

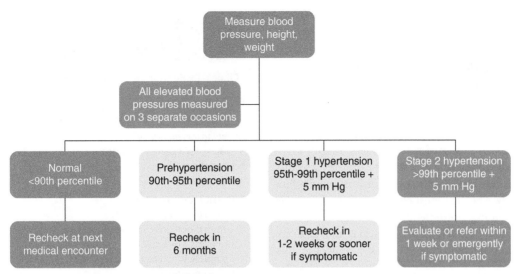

FIGURE 15-7 ▪ Algorithm for initial diagnosis of hypertension in children. (*Adapted with permission from National High Blood Pressure Education Program Working Group on High Blood Pressure in Children and Adolescents. The fourth report on the diagnosis, evaluation, and treatment of high blood pressure in children and adolescents.* Pediatrics. *2004;114:555-576.*)

4. Distinguish primary from secondary hypertension.
5. If secondary, identify underlying cause of hypertension.

The differential diagnosis of hypertension is summarized in Table 15-5. This can further be refined by patient age because the likely causes of secondary hypertension can vary for infants compared to adolescents. Common causes of hypertension at any age include drug-induced, pain-related, and endocrine abnormalities.

Coarctation of the aorta can present at any age, with severe forms generally presenting with cardiovascular collapse in the newborn period and moderate forms presenting with hypertension, murmur, and decreased lower extremity pulses in childhood. Milder cases of coarctation can present at any age and may not be recognized until adulthood. Importantly, all patients with a history of repaired coarctation remain at lifelong risk for hypertension even after complete repair.

In newborns, the most common causes of hypertension are renovascular and include renal artery and

Differential Diagnosis of Hypertension

	Cardiac	Renal	Endocrine and Metabolic	Other
Common	Coarctation	Renal parenchymal disease	Cushing syndrome	Primary hypertension
	Anemia	Reflux nephropathy	Hyperthyroidism	Drug induced
		Obstructive uropathy	Hyperaldosteronism	Pain
		Renal artery stenosis	Insulin resistance	Elevated intracranial pressure
		Renal artery thrombosis		Neurofibromatosis
		Renovascular disease		Collagen vascular disease
		Renal failure		
Uncommon	Patent ductus arteriosus	Congenital renal abnormalities	Liddle syndrome	Pheochromocytoma
	Arteriovenous fistula	Glomerular disease		Wilms tumor
	Turners syndrome	Hemolytic uremic syndrome		Neuroblastoma
	Williams syndrome	Chronic pyelonephritis		Lupus
				Solid organ transplantation

Adapted with permission from Rowan S, Adrogues H, Mathur A, et al. Pediatric hypertension: a review for the primary care provider. Clin Pediatr. *2005;44:289-296.*

vein thrombosis, as well as congenital renal artery steno-sis. Renal artery thrombosis is particularly common in premature infants with indwelling or previous umbilical artery catheters. Other causes that may be directly related to prematurity and often occur in the neonatal intensive care unit are bronchopulmonary dysplasia and intra-ventricular hemorrhage. Patent ductus arteriosus, while commonly associated with low mean and diastolic blood pressures, can be a cause of systolic hypertension.

In childhood, renal parenchymal diseases are most common. These include obstructive uropathy and reflux nephropathy. The next most common are renovascular causes, including fibromuscular dysplasia. Endocrine abnormalities, coarctation of the aorta, and primary hypertension are the other most likely causes in this age group.

In adolescents, the typical causes of hypertension begin to mimic those in adulthood, with primary hyper-tension being the most common cause. This is particu-larly true in teenagers with the common comorbidities of obesity, hyperlipidemia, obstructive sleep apnea, and insulin resistance. Secondary causes of hyperten-sion in adolescents can include many of the common renal, cardiac, and endocrine abnormalities seen both in childhood or adulthood. Other possible causes include medications, such as stimulants for attention-deficit hyperactivity disorder, nonsteroidal anti-inflammatory medications, and oral contraceptive pills. Powerful stimulants such as energy drinks, cocaine, and anabolic steroids must also be considered in this population.[12]

Many specific syndromes and genetic mutations can be associated with hypertension. Turner syndrome is classically associated with bicuspid aortic valve and coarctation of the aorta, and Williams syndrome is typically associated with supravalvar aortic stenosis and branch pulmonary artery stenosis. Both syndromes are also independently associated with hypertension, pre-sumably due to an underlying vasculopathy. In addition, there are several monogenic mutations in the adreno-corticotropic hormone and aldosterone pathways that ultimately result in hypertension. These include familial hyperaldosteronism type 1, Liddle syndrome, types 1 and 2 pseudohypoaldosteronism, congenital adrenal hyper-plasia, and apparent mineralocorticoid excess.[10]

Clinical Evaluation

The role of the clinical evaluation serves several pur-poses, including establishing the diagnosis, screening for comorbidities, testing for common causes, evaluat-ing for end-organ dysfunction, and targeted testing for other abnormalities. Common testing is summarized in Table 15-6. All patients with a new diagnosis of hyper-tension should be screened with basic serum chemis-tries, a complete blood count, urinalysis and culture,

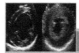

Clinical Evaluation for Hypertension

Confirming diagnosis
- Ambulatory blood pressure monitoring

Screening for comorbidities
- Fasting lipid panel and glucose
- Drug screen
- Sleep study

Testing for common causes
- Serum electrolytes
- Serum blood urea nitrogen, creatinine
- Urinalysis, urine culture
- Complete blood count
- Renal ultrasound

End-organ dysfunction
- Echocardiogram
- Retinal examination

Targeted evaluations, as indicated
- Plasma renin
- Renovascular imaging
- Plasma and urine steroid levels
- Plasma and urine catecholamines
- Genetic testing

Adapted with permission from National High Blood Pressure Education Program Working Group on High Blood Pressure in Children and Adolescents. The fourth report on the diagnosis, evaluation, and treatment of high blood pressure in children and adolescents. Pediatrics. 2004;114:555-576.

renal ultrasound, echocardiogram, and ophthalmic examination. Additional testing can be customized to the individual patient based on history, physical, and the screening evaluations.

A large portion of the morbidity caused over time by hypertension is related to the end-organ damage of the cardiovascular system. In adults, noninvasive mark-ers of end-organ dysfunction, such as urine microalbu-minuria and carotid intimal-medial thickness, have been well established. These markers have not been validated in children and, at the present time, do not provide a reliable way to monitor for end-organ damage. Further-more, many children with hypertension do not manifest retinal changes until adulthood. Echocardiography for evaluation of left ventricular hypertrophy and calcula-tion of left ventricular mass has become the mainstay of monitoring end-organ dysfunction over time in chil-dren (Figure 15-8). From standard 2-dimensional mea-surements of left ventricular wall thickness and cavity size, an estimated left ventricular mass can be calculated. This value is then indexed to patient size for compari-son to normative data and tracking over time. A num-ber of methods for standardizing left ventricular mass exist, but the most commonly used is to index to height

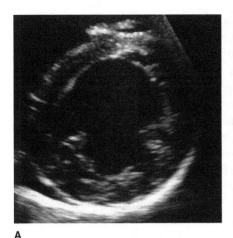
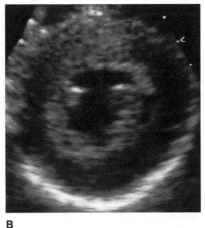

A   B

FIGURE 15-8 ■ Echocardiogram of **(A)** normal left ventricle and **(B)** left ventricular hypertrophy due to severe hypertension.

$(m^{2.7})$. A common cutoff for the presence of left ventricular hypertrophy is 51 $g/m^{2.7}$, which correlates to the 99th percentile in children and adolescents.[7]

Ambulatory blood pressure monitoring

One of the newer tools in the evaluation of hypertension in children is the use of ambulatory blood pressure monitoring. This device, similar in concept to a Holter monitor, is an appropriately sized blood pressure cuff that is connected to a mechanical inflating and recording device. It is worn as an outpatient for a 24-hour period with the device cycling and recording the blood pressure at preset time intervals. This can be most useful for identifying white coat hypertension, as well as monitoring the severity of hypertension and response to treatment. The 2 most standardized data outputs from ambulatory blood pressure monitoring are mean 24-hour systolic blood pressure and blood pressure "load," which is defined as the percentage of daily measurements that fall above the 95th percentile. A systolic blood pressure load greater than 25% is considered abnormal, and a load greater than 50% is severely elevated. The interpretation of clinic blood pressure, mean ambulatory systolic blood pressure, and blood pressure load is summarized in Table 15-7.

Treatment

The primary aim of treatment for hypertension is to reduce long-term morbidity and mortality associated with prolonged elevated blood pressure. With the exception of stage 2 and symptomatic hypertension, the majority of children with hypertension will not experience adverse events until adulthood. Thus, the goals of therapy in the treatment of hypertension in children are to reduce both the measured blood pressure to below the 90th to 95th percentile and the left ventricular mass. In general, lifestyle changes are usually attempted first before starting pharmacotherapy. This may not be true for patients with severe or symptomatic elevations in blood pressure. Reversible causes of secondary hypertension should be treated aggressively.

Interpretation of Ambulatory Blood Pressure Monitoring

	Clinic SBP	Mean Ambulatory SBP	SBP Load
Normal	Normal	Normal	<25%
White coat hypertension	High	Normal	<25%
Prehypertension	High	Normal	25%-50%
Ambulatory hypertension	High	High	25%-50%
Severe hypertension	High	High	>50%

SBP, systolic blood pressure.
NOTE. Normal indicates <95th percentile for age, sex, and height. High indicates >95th percentile for age, sex, and height.
Adapted with permission from Urbina E, Alpert B, Flynn J, et al. Ambulatory blood pressure monitoring in children and adolescents: recommendations for standard assessment. A scientific statement from the American Heart Association Atherosclerosis, Hypertension, and Obesity in Youth Committee of the Council on Cardiovascular Disease in the Young and the Council for High Blood Pressure Research. Hypertension. 2008;52:433-451.

Lifestyle interventions

Because hypertension and obesity are strongly related, all children and adolescents with obesity-related hypertension should first undergo lifestyle modifications to reduce their weight. These changes should include decreasing caloric intake, increasing physical activity, and limiting sedentary activities. Families may require the assistance of a nutritionist to help guide dietary changes. Recreational activities that engage the child and that the whole family can participate in together are recommended. Interventions for obesity are discussed in more detail in the Obesity section. If successful, weight loss has been shown to decrease absolute blood pressure, blood pressure sensitivity to salt, dyslipidemia, and insulin resistance.[7] In many cases, weight loss alone is sufficient to avoid pharmacologic therapy.

In addition to weight loss, dietary intervention is recommended for all individuals with elevated blood pressure. Reduction of daily sodium intake is a mainstay of treatment for hypertension in adults and certainly applies to children as well, despite a lack of convincing evidence. The recommendation for total daily dietary intake of sodium is 1.5 g/d for most children and less for smaller children. Most children eat far more than this, particularly those who consume significant quantities of processed or fast foods. Additional dietary changes that have been suggested to reduce blood pressure are increasing total daily intake of potassium, magnesium, folic acid, fiber, and calcium and decreasing dietary intake of total fats. This can be accomplished by eating more fresh fruits, vegetables, fiber, and nonfat dairy products. Regular physical activity should also be part of a healthy lifestyle and is strongly suggested for nearly all children, especially those with hypertension, obesity, and related conditions. Only patients with severe elevations in blood pressure should be restricted from physical activity until other methods are used to bring the blood pressure into a safe range.

Medications

Pharmacologic intervention in children and adolescents with hypertension is generally reserved for individuals in whom lifestyle modifications have failed and those with secondary hypertension, symptomatic hypertension, end-organ dysfunction, and diabetes. There are a wide variety of medication classes to choose from in the management of hypertension, and unlike treatment of adults, there are few landmark studies to guide the selection process. In general, the principle has been to select a medication class based on the patient's underlying disease process, comorbidities, and contraindications. Long-acting medications with once- or twice-daily dosing regimens are preferred to increase compliance in children who may be reluctant to take medications. A selection of commonly used medications and dosages is shown in Table 15-8. Many practitioners choose to start with an angiotensin-converting enzyme inhibitor, calcium channel blocker, or diuretic. Dosing should start at the lowest possible dose and then be slowly escalated, for a goal blood pressure of less than the 95th percentile in patients with uncomplicated hypertension. For those with diabetes, renal disease, or end-organ dysfunction a goal of less than the 90th percentile should be achieved. If single-drug therapy is ineffective, a second agent from a different class should be added.

Patients on antihypertensive medications should be followed very carefully for blood pressure response to medications with a combination of clinic and ambulatory blood pressure monitoring. In addition, they should be encouraged to maintain lifestyle modifications in diet and physical activity. With these tools and with consultation from specialists in nephrology and cardiology, these patients can often be managed successfully and enjoyably.

DYSLIPIDEMIA

Definition

Dyslipidemia is an abnormality of lipoprotein metabolism resulting in elevated levels of total cholesterol (TC), low-density lipoprotein cholesterol (LDL-C), and/or triglycerides (TGs) or low levels of high-density lipoprotein cholesterol (HDL-C). Cholesterol and TGs are important lipids (or fats) that are either produced by the body or absorbed from food. Cholesterol is a major component of cell membranes, fat-soluble vitamins, and bile; the body also uses cholesterol to make hormones. TGs are necessary to store and provide energy to the body. Because lipids are hydrophobic, they cannot travel in the bloodstream alone; instead, they circulate attached to hydrophilic structures called lipoproteins. Plasma lipoproteins have a polar outer layer that contains specific proteins, called apolipoproteins, which are important in stabilizing the lipoproteins and play important roles in lipoprotein metabolism (Table 15-9).[13] Lipoproteins are classified by size and density (ratio of lipid to protein), and each has a different purpose and is metabolized somewhat differently (Table 15-10).[13]

Pathogenesis

Research has demonstrated that elevated cholesterol can be present from a very young age. Children with dyslipidemia may demonstrate evidence of arterial fatty streaks, which are the first pathologic abnormalities during the progression of atherosclerosis. If dyslipidemia persists, these fatty streaks can progress to fibrous plaques as early

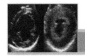

Antihypertensive Medications Commonly Used in Children and Adolescents

Class and Drug	Dose	Interval (no. of daily doses)	Notes (for class)
ACE inhibitor			
Captopril	Initial: 0.3-0.5 mg/kg/dose Max: 6 mg/kg/d or 450 mg/d	3	Contraindicated in pregnancy Contraindicated with renal failure
Enalapril	Initial: 0.1 mg/kg/d Max: 0.5 mg/kg/d or 40 mg/d	1-2	Follow electrolytes
Lisinopril	Initial: 0.07 mg/kg/dose to max 5 mg/dose Max: 0.6 mg/kg/d or 40 mg/d	1	Lisinopril approved for children ≥6 years only
Angiotensin receptor blocker			
Losartan	Initial: 0.7 mg/kg/d to max 50 mg/d Max: 1.4 mg/kg/d or 100 mg/d	1	Same as ACE inhibitors
β-Blocker			
Atenolol	Initial: 0.5-1 mg/kg/d Max: 2 mg/kg/d or 100 mg/d	1-2	Contraindicated in type 1 diabetes
Metoprolol	Initial: 1-2 mg/kg/d Max: 6 mg/kg/d or 200 mg/d	2	Caution in asthma and heart failure
Propranolol	Initial: 0.5-1 mg/kg/d Max: 4 mg/kg/d or 640 mg/d	2-4	Cause bradycardia May limit exercise tolerance
Calcium channel blocker			
Amlodipine	Initial: 2.5-5 mg/d Max: 15 mg/d	1	Children ≥6 years Caution in hepatic failure May cause marked hypotension
Diuretic			
Hydrochlorothiazide	Initial: 1 mg/kg/dose Max: 3 mg/kg/d or 50 mg/d	1	Monitor electrolytes Useful adjunct to other agents
Spironolactone	Initial: 1 mg/kg/d Max: 3.3 mg/kg/d or 100 mg/d	1-2	

ACE, angiotensin-converting enzyme; Max, maximum.
Adapted with permission from National High Blood Pressure Education Program Working Group on High Blood Pressure in Children and Adolescents. The fourth report on the diagnosis, evaluation, and treatment of high blood pressure in children and adolescents. Pediatrics. 2004;114:555-576.

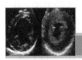

Important Apoproteins and Enzymes in Lipid Metabolism

Apoprotein or Enzyme	Location	Role
A-I	HDL	Main component of HDL
A-II	HDL	Unknown
B100	VLDL, IDL, LDL, Lp(a)	LDL receptor ligand
C-II	Chylomicrons, VLDL, HDL	LPL cofactor
E	Chylomicrons, remnants, VLDL, HDL	LDL receptor ligand
ABCAI	Intracellular	Intracellular cholesterol transport to membranes
CETP	HDL	Mediates transfer of cholesteryl esters from HDL to VLDL
LCAT	HDL	Esterifies free cholesterol for transport within HDL

ABCAI, adenosine triphosphate binding cassette AI; CETP, cholesteryl ester transfer protein; HDL, high-density lipoprotein; IDL, intermediate-density lipoprotein; LCAT, lecithin-cholesterol acyltransferase; LDL, low-density lipoprotein; Lp(a), lipoprotein (a); LPL, lipoprotein lipase; VLDL, very-low-density lipoprotein.
Adapted, with permission, from Stone NJ, Blum CB. Pathophysiology of hyperlipoproteinemias. In: Management of Lipids in Clinical Practice. 6th ed. Caddo, OK: Professional Communications, Inc., 2006:23-53.

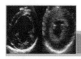

Major Lipoprotein Classes

Name	Size (diameter, nm)	Density (g/mL)	Major Apolipoproteins	Origin	Lipid Composition	Function
Chylomicron	75-300	<1.006	A-I, A-IV, B48, C-I, C-II, C-III, E	Dietary fat	90%-96% triglyceride	Transport dietary fat
Very-low-density lipoprotein (VLDL)	30-80	<1.006	B100, C-I, C-II, C-III, E	Secreted by the liver	60% triglyceride	Transports endogenous triglycerides from liver to fat
Low-density lipoprotein (LDL)	20	1.019-1.063	B100	Breakdown product from VLDL	5% triglyceride, 50% cholesterol	Major carrier of cholesterol
High-density lipoprotein (HDL)	7-10	1.063-1.210	A-I, A-II, C-I, C-II, C-III	Intestine and liver	50% protein, 5% triglyceride, 20% cholesterol	Removes cholesterol from the body

Adapted with permission from Stone NJ, Blum CB. Pathophysiology of hyperlipoproteinemias. In: Management of Lipids in Clinical Practice. 6th ed. Caddo, OK: Professional Communications, Inc., 2006:25.

as adolescence and can increase in number and severity into adulthood. Although no long-term studies have shown a direct relationship between childhood lipid values and adult cardiovascular disease (CVD), studies have demonstrated correlations between lipid levels and the progression of atherosclerosis over time.[14]

Lipoprotein metabolism plays a major role in the development and progression of atherosclerosis. It involves the synthesis, breakdown, and transfer of lipids, notably cholesterol and TG, to and from different locations in the body. There are 2 major pathways of cholesterol synthesis: exogenous and endogenous (Figure 15-9). Not shown in Figure 15-9 is HDL metabolism. HDLs are made by the liver and intestine and are secreted into the circulation with apolipoproteins, unesterified cholesterol, and phospholipid. Nascent HDLs remove cholesterol from peripheral tissues. The unesterified cholesterol in the nascent HDLs is esterified to cholesteryl ester, making mature HDLs, which return cholesterol to the liver for further processing.[13]

Clinical Presentation and Epidemiology

This section highlights the most common genetic dyslipidemias. Most children with the less common, and usually more severe, dyslipidemias should be referred to a lipid specialist (Table 15-11).

Heterozygous familial hypercholesterolemia

Heterozygous familial hypercholesterolemia (HeFH) is an autosomal codominant disorder with a prevalence rate in the general population of 1:500. It is also referred to as type IIa hyperlipoproteinemia (Table 15-12) by the Fredrickson classification system.[15] HeFH is caused by one of several hundred genetic defects in the LDL receptor causing defective or deficient LDL receptors. This leads to decreased hepatic clearance of LDL from the circulation and excess accumulation of LDL particles in the blood. Elevated LDL-C leads to premature atherosclerosis, with at least one half of males and one quarter of females with HeFH developing CVD by the age of 50. Children and adolescents with HeFH demonstrate greater carotid intimal-medial thickness and abnormal brachial artery reactivity—both markers of subclinical atherosclerosis—but usually do not manifest coronary artery disease until adulthood. A rarer condition (~1:1000 people) but with a similar phenotype is familial defective apolipoprotein B100.

Children with HeFH have fasting lipoprotein profiles with TC and LDL-C levels well above the 95th percentile for age and sex. They may have normal or low HDL-C and usually normal TG. Having 1 parent with significantly elevated TC and LDL-C, tendon xanthomas (Figure 15-10), and a family history of premature CVD helps solidify the diagnosis. Children and adolescents with HeFH rarely have tendon xanthomas because these normally develop in early to mid adulthood.

Familial combined hyperlipidemia

Familial combined hyperlipidemia (FCHL) or type IIb hyperlipoproteinemia (Table 15-12) is autosomal dominant and is the most common primary lipid disorder, affecting approximately 1:200 people in the general population. The phenotype often manifests differently

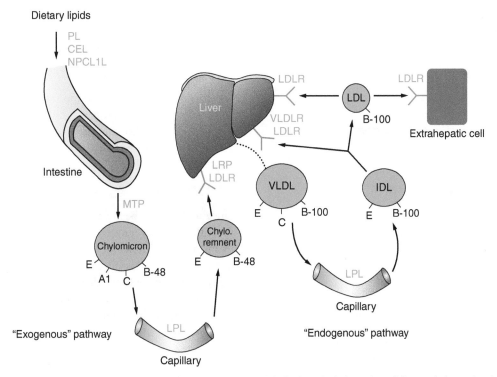

FIGURE 15-9 ■ Lipoprotein metabolism. The exogenous pathway begins with the intestinal absorption of dietary cholesterol and fat. Different intestinal enzymes act on the dietary lipids by combining free fatty acids with glycerol to form triglycerides that are packaged with a small amount of cholesterol, protein, and phospholipids to form chylomicrons. The chylomicrons then enter the circulation and are transported to the peripheral tissues. Apolipoproteins A-I, B48, C-II, and E are added to the chylomicrons as they enter the circulation. The enzyme lipoprotein lipase (LPL) is found in the muscle and adipose tissues where it breaks down the chylomicrons to chylomicron remnants, which are subsequently absorbed by the liver via the low-density lipoprotein (LDL) receptor (LDLR). The endogenous pathway of lipid metabolism begins with the liver producing very-low-density lipoproteins (VLDL) that are acted upon by lipoprotein lipase (LPL) to form LDL. LDLs bind to the LDLR on the liver with apolipoprotein B100 acting as the ligand on the surface of the LDL particle. In the liver, LDL can be converted to bile acids to be subsequently secreted into the intestinal lumen. LDL circulating in the bloodstream can enter macrophages and other tissues, which can result in excess buildup of cholesterol-enriched cells (foam cells) that are a main component of the atherosclerotic process. CEL, carboxyl ester lipase; IDL, intermediate-density lipoprotein; LRP, low-density lipoprotein–related protein; MTP, microsomal triglyceride transfer protein; NPC1L1, Niemann-Pick C1-like 1; PL, pancreatic lipase. (*Reprinted, with permission, from Daniels TF, Killinger KM, Michal JJ, et al. Lipoproteins, cholesterol homeostasis and cardiac health. Int J Biol Sci. 2009;5:474-488.*)

in affected family members, the most common being elevated LDL-C or elevated TG and very-low-density lipoprotein cholesterol (VLDL-C) or elevated LDL-C and VLDL-C. A unifying characteristic with FCHL is elevated plasma apolipoprotein B (apoB) particles relative to the LDL-C levels. FCHL is often seen in conjunction with overweight, insulin resistance, and hypertension.

In general, the diagnosis can be made when one sees a mixed dyslipidemia with elevated TG (200-800 mg/dL), low HDL (<40 mg/dL), and mildly elevated TC levels (200-400 mg/dL) with a family history of hypercholesterolemia or premature CVD. Elevated apoB levels help confirm the diagnosis. Patients with FCHL do not develop tendon xanthomas.

Familial hypertriglyceridemia

Familial hypertriglyceridemia (FHTG) is an autosomal dominant disorder also referred to as type IV hyperlipoproteinemia (Table 15-12). It has a prevalence of approximately 1:500 in the general population. It is

caused by increased VLDL production and/or decreased VLDL catabolism. Type V hyperlipoproteinemia is a more severe form of FHTG where both VLDL and chylomicrons are increased. Increased dietary carbohydrate intake, overweight, insulin resistance, alcohol use, or estrogen therapy can precipitate chylomicronemia because they each increase VLDL production.

Diagnosis of FHTG is usually made by noting increased TG (250-1000 mg/dL), normal or mildly increased TC (<250 mg/dL), and decreased HDL-C. LDL-C is usually normal or low. In some cases, patients may present with eruptive xanthomas (Figure 15-11), although this skin finding is more frequent in adulthood or with the rarer causes of hypertriglyceridemia (Table 15-10). Levels of apoB and the ratio of TC to TG tend to be lower in FHTG than in FCHL.

Familial dysbetalipoproteinemia

Familial dysbetalipoproteinemia (FDBL) is characterized by elevated TC and TG, usually to approximately

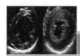

Rare Genetic Causes of Dyslipidemia

Disorders of LDL metabolism
- Homozygous familial hypercholesterolemia
- Autosomal recessive hypercholesterolemia
- Sitosterolemia
- Abetalipoproteinemia
- Familial hypobetalipoproteinemias

Disorders of triglyceride metabolism
- Lipoprotein lipase deficiency
- Defective apolipoprotein C-II
- Defective lipoprotein lipase cofactor
- Hepatic lipase deficiency

Disorders of HDL metabolism
- Low HDL cholesterol levels
    Familial hypoalphalipoproteinemia
    Apolipoprotein A-I deficiency and mutations
    Tangier disease
    Lecithin-cholesterol acyltransferase deficiency
- Elevated HDL cholesterol levels
    Familial hyperalphalipoproteinemia
    Cholesteryl ester transfer protein deficiency

HDL, high-density lipoprotein; LDL, low-density lipoprotein.

equal levels ≥300 mg/dL. It is also known as type III hyperlipoproteinemia (Table 15-12) or familial broad β disease. The disorder is caused by the accumulation of chylomicron and VLDL remnants, known collectively as β-VLDL. The most common form of FDBL is autosomal recessive; however, manifestation of hyperlipidemia occurs in less than 10% of the patients and is almost always delayed until adulthood. In those who do develop hyperlipidemia, the inciting factors may be obesity, hypothyroidism, alcohol use, estrogen deficiency, high-fat diet, or diabetes mellitus.

Elevated lipoprotein (a)

Lipoprotein (a) [Lp(a)] is a lipoprotein consisting of a single copy of apolipoprotein A linked to 1 molecule of LDL. Elevated Lp(a) concentrations have been associated with premature atherosclerosis.

Differential Diagnosis

Once a child has been identified with dyslipidemia, a more thorough evaluation is necessary. A complete family history should include identifying first- and second-degree relatives who have a history of hypercholesterolemia, premature CVD, diabetes mellitus, overweight, and hypertension. It is necessary to evaluate for secondary causes of dyslipidemia, as presented in Table 15-13, the majority of which can be ascertained through a complete history, review of systems, and physical examination. However, additional laboratory studies should be obtained, including liver tests to evaluate for fatty liver or obstructive liver disease, thyroid function tests to rule out hypothyroidism, fasting blood sugar levels to evaluate for diabetes or glucose intolerance, and a urinalysis to evaluate for kidney disease.

Diagnosis

Screening for dyslipidemia

In 2011, new guidelines were recommended for screening children and adolescents for dyslipidemia. The most significant change was the recommendation that all children

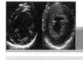

The Fredrickson Classification: Phenotypes of Different Genetic Dyslipidemias 14

Phenotype	Lipoprotein Elevated	Cholesterol	Triglycerides	LDL Cholesterol	HDL Cholesterol	Atherogenicity	Name
I	Chylomicrons	↑-↑↑	↑↑↑↑	↓	↓↓↓	—	FCS
IIa	LDL	↑↑↑	—	↑	↓	+++	FH, FDB
IIb	LDL and VLDL	↑↑-↑↑↑	↑↑	↑	↓	+++	FCHL
III	Chylomicrons and VLDL remnants	↑↑-↑↑↑	↑↑-↑↑↑	↓	—	+++	FDBL
IV	VLDL	— to ↑	↑↑	↓	↓↓	— to ↑	FHTG
V	Chylomicrons and VLDL	↑↑-↑↑↑	↑↑↑↑	↓	↓↓↓	— to ↑	FHTG

FCHL, familial combined hyperlipidemia; FCS, familial chylomicronemia syndrome; FDB, familial dysbetalipoproteinemia; FDBL, familial dysbetalipoproteinemia; FH, familial hypercholesterolemia; FHTG, familial hypertriglyceridemia; HDL, high-density lipoprotein; LDL, low-density lipoprotein; VLDL, very-low-density lipoprotein.

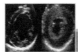

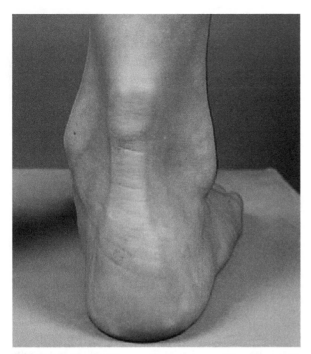

FIGURE 15-10 ■ Tendon xanthoma in an adult patient with heterozygous familial hypercholesterolemia. (*Reprinted, with permission, from White LE. Xanthomatoses and lipoprotein disorders. In: Wolff K, Goldsmith LA, Katz SI, Gilchrest B, Paller AS, Leffell DJ, eds. Fitzpatrick's Dermatology in General Medicine. 7th ed. New York, NY: McGraw-Hill; 2008.*)

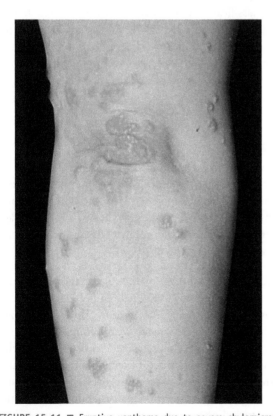

FIGURE 15-11 ■ Eruptive xanthoma due to severe chylomicrone-mia. (*Reprinted, with permission, from White LE. Xanthomatoses and lipoprotein disorders. In: Wolff K, Goldsmith LA, Katz SI, Gilchrest B, Paller AS, Leffell DJ, eds. Fitzpatrick's Dermatology in General Medicine. 7th ed. New York, NY: McGraw-Hill; 2008.*)

Four "D's": Secondary Causes of Dyslipidemia[14]

Diet	High saturated fat
	High calorie
	Excessive carbohydrate
	Excessive alcohol intake
	Anorexia nervosa
Drugs	Oral estrogens
	Oral progestins
	Oral contraceptives
	Anabolic steroids
	Corticosteroids
	Thiazide diuretics
	β-Blockers
	Bile acid–binding resins
	Glucocorticoids
	Protease inhibitors (most)
	Retinoic acid derivatives
	Anticonvulsants
Diseases	Hepatic
	Intrahepatic cholestasis
	Chronic liver disease
	Primary biliary cirrhosis
	Hepatitis (acute or chronic)
	Biliary atresia
	Alagille syndrome
	Renal
	Chronic renal failure
	Nephrotic syndrome
	Hemolytic-uremic syndrome
	Rheumatic
	Systemic lupus erythematosus
	Rheumatoid arthritis
	Cardiac
	Kawasaki disease
	Heart transplantation
	Congenital heart disease
	Storage
	Gaucher disease
	Glycogen storage disease
	Tay-Sachs disease
	Niemann-Pick disease
	Other
	Post cancer therapy
	Klinefelter syndrome
	Progeria
	Burns
Dysmetabolism	Hypothyroidism
	Diabetes, types 1 and 2
	Obesity
	Insulin resistance
	Acute intermittent porphyria
	Hypopituitarism
	Lipodystrophy

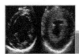

Recommended Conditions/Factors for Screening Children for Dyslipidemia, ages 2-8 years[1]

- Positive family history: a first or second-degree relative with documented CVD (eg, angina pectoris, peripheral or cerebral vascular disease, myocardial infarction, coronary artery disease, or sudden death) by age ≤ 55 years for a male and ≤ 65 years for females
- High risk factor/condition
  - Hypertension requiring drug therapy
  - Cigarette smoking
  - Severe obesity (BMI ≥ 97th percentile)
  - Diabetes (Type I and Type 2)
  - Chronic/end-stage kidney disease/post-renal transplant
  - Post-orthotopic heart transplantation
  - Kawasaki disease, currently with aneurysm
- Moderate risk factor/condition
  - Hypertension (blood pressure > 95th percentile for gender and age) not requiring drug therapy
  - Obesity (BMI ≥ 95th percentile but < 97th percentile)
  - HDL-C < 40 mg/dL
  - Kawasaki disease with regressed aneurysm
  - Chronic inflammatory disease
  - HIV infection
  - Nephrotic syndrome

CVD, cardiovascular disease; BMI, body mass index

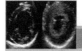

Classification of Cholesterol Levels for Children and Adolescents (in mg/dL)[1,16,19]

Lipid Category	Optimal	Borderline	High	Low
TC	<170	170-199	≥200	
LDL-C	<110	110-129	≥130	
Non–HDL-C	<120	120-144	≥145	
TG				
0-9 yr	<75	75-99	≥100	
10-19 yr	<90	90-129	≥130	
HDL-C	>45	40-45		<40

HDL-C, high-density lipoprotein cholesterol; LDL-C, low-density lipoprotein cholesterol; TC, total cholesterol; TG, triglycerides.

be screened for high cholesterol at least once between the ages of 9 and 11 years, and again between ages 17 and 21 years. This can be done using a fasting lipid profile (FLP) or non-FLP. However, if they have one or more of the conditions outlined in Table 15-14[1,16-18], then initial screening should occur between ages 2-8 years.

How to screen

Ideally, a lipoprotein analysis should be performed after an overnight fast. This should include TC, HDL-C, TG, and a calculated LDL-C. The LDL-C can usually be determined indirectly from the Friedewald formula: LDL-C = TC − (HDL-C + TG/5). As well, the non-HDL-C should be calculated. The practitioner should request that the laboratory measure the LDL-C directly if the TGs are greater than 400 mg/dL because the Friedewald formula is not accurate when TGs are significantly elevated. Values for TC, HDL-C, and non–HDL-C (TC − HDL-C) can be obtained from nonfasting values. If the initial FLP reveals the LDL-C to be "borderline-high" or "high", a repeat analysis should be performed between 2 weeks and 3 months after the first FLP and the average of the two results should be used for further decision making. If the initial screening is a non-FLP and if the non-HDL ≥ 145 mg/dL and/or the HDL< 40 mg/dL, then two FLPs

should be performed, with the average of the two results used for treatment. If the values are within the normal reference range, then the patient can have repeat lipid levels performed in 3 to 5 years.

Classification of cholesterol values

The classification of optimal, borderline, and high lipid levels is found in Table 15-15.[16,19] The cutoff values for "borderline" or "high" levels correspond to the 75th and 95th percentiles, respectively, and cutoff value for "low" corresponds to the 5th percentile.

Treatment

Dietary interventions

In an effort to maintain normal cholesterol levels or to decrease elevated levels, a 2-tiered approach has been advocated. The first approach is for the general population, focusing on a heart-healthy diet for all children age 2 and older. The second approach is for children with increased risk for premature CVD.

Population-based approach. With the population-based approach, a low–saturated fat (<10% of total calories), low–total fat (<30% of total calories), and low-cholesterol diet (<300 mg/d) with minimal *trans* fats is encouraged for all children age 2 and older.[20,21] Fruit juice and other sweetened beverages and foods, foods high in sodium, and fried and processed foods should be limited. Other lifestyle changes should be encouraged, including weight management, decreasing sedentary time, and increasing physical activity.

Individual-based approach. The focus of the individual-based approach is the child or adolescent who is at increased risk of premature CVD. Initially, the same diet as the population-based approach should be used. After 6 to 8 weeks of diet and lifestyle changes, a repeat fasting lipoprotein analysis should be obtained. If these laboratory values still reveal dyslipidemia, then a more restrictive diet is necessary, with further reduction of daily saturated fat to less than 7% of daily calories and reduction of dietary cholesterol to less than 200 mg/d. These dietary changes should be made in conjunction with a medical dietitian to ensure that all the requirements for protein, carbohydrates, and vitamins are met for appropriate growth and development.[17,20]

For dyslipidemia associated with overweight and obesity (ie, elevated TG and low HDL-C), treatment is weight loss and exercise. Increased exercise in conjunction with weight loss has been found to significantly improve the lipid profile in obese adolescents. Dietary changes are discussed earlier in the Obesity section.

Additional nonpharmacologic dietary interventions.
Adjunctive dietary therapies for cholesterol management in children may be useful prior to and/or in addition to pharmacologic therapy. These are summarized in Table 15-16.[21]

Pharmacologic therapy

Despite diet and lifestyle changes, it may be necessary to institute lipid-lowering medication to attain the LDL-C targeted goal. Medication should be considered in children 10 years of age or older (usually waiting until after menarche in females) who still have elevated LDL-C levels despite 6 to 12 months of a low-fat, low-cholesterol diet.[22] The LDL cut points for consideration of starting medication are outlined in Table 15-17.

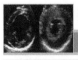

Dietary Supplements to Lower Cholesterol[21]

Product	Dose	Effect
Phytosterols/stanols	Up to 2 g/d	Lowers LDL-C
Fiber		
Total	Age + 5 to max dose 25 g	Lowers LDL-C
Soluble	5-10 g/d (adult dose)	
Nuts	Up to 1 oz/d	Lowers LDL-C
Omega-3 fatty acids	2-3 servings of fish/week	Shift lipoprotein subclasses to less atherogenic particles
	2-4 g/d	Lowers TG

DL-C, low-density lipoprotein cholesterol; TG, triglycerides.

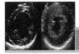

Recommendations for Starting Pharmacologic Treatment of Dyslipidemia in Children and Adolescents[1,22]

Risk Factor/Condition	Recommended LDL-C Cut Points
No other risk factors for CVD	LDL-C ≥ 190 mg/dL
Positive family history of premature CVD, or 1. High risk factor/condition or ≥ 2 other moderate risk factors/conditions (see Table 15-14)	LDL-C ≥ 160 mg/dL
2. High risk factors/conditions or 1 high + ≥ 2 moderate risk factors/conditions or clinical cardiovascular disease (see Table 15-14)	LDL-C ≥ 130 mg/dL

CVD, cardiovascular disease; LDL-C, low-density lipoprotein cholesterol.

There are some children who are at significantly increased risk of developing premature CVD.[18] With these patients, medication may be started before age 10 years, and these patients may have lower LDL-C cutoff levels, may need more aggressive intervention, and may require combination drug therapy to reach an appropriate target. These more complicated children should be referred to a lipid specialist for further evaluation and treatment.

There are 3 classes of drugs recommended for lowering LDL-C levels in the pediatric population as outlined in Table 15-18. The side effect profile should be reviewed carefully with patients and their family prior to initiation, and patients should be counseled appropriately. The medication should be started at the lowest recommended dose and titrated up slowly, following the fasting lipid profile to determine successful treatment.

Bile acid sequestrants.
Bile acid sequestrants act by binding bile acids in the intestine and decreasing their absorption. This leads to increased hepatic conversion of cholesterol to bile acids and improved clearance of LDL-C from the circulation. These agents can lower LDL-C by approximately 10% to 20%. However, gastrointestinal complaints and poor palatability makes compliance quite poor.

HMG-CoA reductase inhibitors (statins).
3-Hydroxy-3-methyl-glutaryl–coenzyme A (HMG-CoA) reductase inhibitors (statins) are considered first-line therapy for lowering LDL-C in the pediatric population.[18,22] Statins work by inhibiting the rate-limiting enzyme in endogenous cholesterol biosynthesis, HMG-CoA, which decreases the intracellular cholesterol

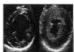

Medications for Lowering LDL-C in Children and Adolescents

Class	Names and Doses	Effect on Lipids	Possible Side Effects
Bile acid sequestrants	*Cholestyramine*: Not FDA approved for children 240 mg/kg/d ÷ BID Max dose 8 g/d *Colestipol*: Not FDA approved for children 5 g BID or 10 g daily *Colesevelam HCl*: Granules: 1 packet daily (3.75 g) mixed with water Tablets: 3 tablets QD or BID	Decrease LDL-C Increase TG	Gastrointestinal symptoms, bloating constipation, cramping
HMG-CoA reductase inhibitors (Statin)	*Atorvastatin*: 10-20 mg every evening (QHS) *Lovastatin*: 10-40 mg QHS *Pravastatin*: 20 mg QHS (8-13 years)* 20-40 mg QHS (14-18 years) *Simvastatin*: 5-40 mg QHS *Rosuvastatin*: 5-20 mg QHS	Decrease LDL-C Increase HDL-C Decrease TG	Myalgias, arthralgias, myopathy, rhabdomyolysis, elevated hepatic transaminase levels, gastrointestinal upset
Cholesterol absorption inhibitor	*Ezetimibe*: 10 mg daily	Decrease LDL-C	Elevated hepatic transaminases, gastrointestinal upset

BID, twice a day; FDA, Food and Drug Administration; HDL-C, high-density lipoprotein cholesterol; HMG-CoA, 3-hydroxy-3-methyl-glutaryl–coenzyme A; LDL-C, low-density lipoprotein cholesterol; TG, triglycerides; QD, every day.
* *Approved for prepubescent children (age 8 and older).*
Adapted with permission from Brothers JA, Daniels SR. When should children and adolescents be screened for dyslipidemia and how should they be treated? In: Toth PP, Sica DA, eds. Clinical Challenges in Lipid Disorders. *Ashland, OH: Clinical Publishing, 2008:66.*

levels and upregulates LDL receptors in the liver. This leads to increased hepatic clearance of LDL-C from the circulation. Statins also improve removal of VLDL and intermediate-density remnants, which accounts for their actions on reducing TG levels. Statins can reduce atherosclerotic progression in children as measured by carotid intimal-medial thickness, and age at initiation of statin therapy correlates positively with carotid intimal-medial thickness, suggesting that starting statins at a younger age may reduce the burden of atherosclerosis and premature CVD.[23,24]

Although statins are usually reserved for children with familial hypercholesterolemia, they may also be useful in children with FCHL or obesity-related dyslipidemia who cannot lower their LDL below the cut point (see Table 15-16) after dietary and other lifestyle changes.

The most common concern for patients and families is regarding statin safety, notably the possibility of liver and muscle toxicity. In a meta-analysis of statin safety in children and adolescents with HeFH, the prevalence of elevated alanine and aspartate aminotransferases greater than 3 times the upper limit of normal (ULN) and creatine kinase (CK) levels greater than 10 times the ULN were not significantly different from placebo.[25]

Monitoring patients while on statin therapy is important. Figure 15-12 outlines initiation, titration, and follow-up of a patient taking statin medication. When starting statin therapy, assess for contraindications to use, such as liver disease or potential for pregnancy. Patients should be instructed to report any adverse events, especially myopathy. If symptoms are reported, assess in relation to physical activity, stop the medication, and check the CK level. Concerning CK levels are 10 times the ULN. If a patient has a minor elevation in liver transaminase levels (<3 times the ULN), these should be checked again in 2 to 6 weeks; this is usually not an indication to stop therapy because these fluctuations are usually transient. Liver transaminase levels greater than 3 times the ULN require temporarily stopping the drug and rechecking levels in 2 weeks. Medication may be restarted when symptoms and/or laboratory abnormalities have normalized.

Teenage girls should be counseled that statins are potentially teratogenic. Physicians should document that female patients are not pregnant at the start of therapy and that patients are using adequate birth control if sexually active. In addition, drug interactions need to be discussed, notably that of statins with foods,

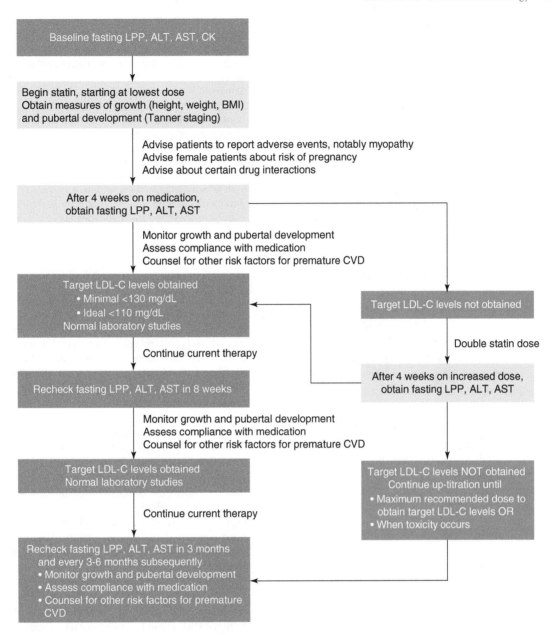

FIGURE 15-12 ■ Initiation, titration, and monitoring of children and adolescents using statins. ALT, alanine aminotransferase; AST, aspartate aminotransferase; BMI, body mass index; CK, creatine kinase; CVD, cardiovascular disease; LDL-C, low-density lipoprotein cholesterol; LPP, lipoprotein profile. (*Adapted with permission from McCrindle BW, Urbina EM, Dennison BA, et al. Drug therapy of high-risk lipid abnormalities in children and adolescents. A scientific statement from the American Heart Association Atherosclerosis, Hypertension, and Obesity in Youth Committee, Council of Cardiovascular Disease in the Young, with the Council on Cardiovascular Nursing. Circulation. 2007;115:1948-1967.*)

such as grapefruit, and drugs, such as fibrates, niacin, erythromycin, cyclosporine, nefazodone, azole antifungals, and several human immunodeficiency virus protease inhibitors.

Cholesterol absorption inhibitors. Cholesterol absorption inhibitors are a relatively new class of lipid-lowering medication that is indicated for reducing LDL-C and TC levels. In adults, 10 mg daily of ezetimibe affords a modest reduction in LDL-C levels as monotherapy; however, ezetimibe is often used in conjunction with a statin medication to lower LDL-C to obtain target levels.

SUMMARY

Children and adolescents with dyslipidemia are at increased risk for premature CVD, and it appears the earlier the treatment begins, the lower is the risk for developing atherosclerosis. Identification of children with dyslipidemia is of even greater significance in the current era of obesity, hypertension, poor diet, and sedentary behavior among today's youth. First-line therapy in all children with dyslipidemia is dietary and lifestyle changes. After these changes have been made, the majority of patients will not qualify for lipid-lowering medication; however, those with more severe dyslipidemia may require drug therapy. The main use of lipid-lowering medications in children and adolescents is for LDL-C lowering. Statins are the first-line treatment; other medications, such as ezetimibe or bile acid sequestrants, may also be needed. Treatment for obesity-related dyslipidemia with high TGs and low HDL-C generally involves diet, weight loss, and aerobic activity.

Indeed, the evidence is striking regarding the association between obesity, hypertension, and dyslipidemia and the development of premature CVD. Studies have shown that these risk factors begin in childhood and often track into adulthood. The behaviors leading to the development of obesity, hypertension, and dyslipidemia are usually acquired during childhood and include decreased physical activity, increased sedentary time, poor diet, and tobacco smoking. Lifestyle interventions to change these behaviors may be difficult for the child and family but can successfully lead to cardiovascular risk reduction. When lifestyle changes are not effective, pharmacologic intervention may be necessary. Primary prevention of risk factors for premature CVD has already been shown to alter the onset of atherosclerosis in adults. However, waiting until adulthood is too late for many of our nation's children. Given the overwhelming data that these same risk factors begin during childhood and adolescence, the time for primary preventive cardiology is now.

Clinical Pearls

- Body mass index (BMI = body weight in kilograms/ height in meters squared) should be calculated and plotted on growth charts at each well child visit. Those who are overweight (BMI ≥85th and <95th percentiles) and obese (BMI ≥95th percentile) are at risk for multiple medical comorbidities.
- Obesity prevention should begin during infancy. Irrespective of weight, patients and families should be counseled routinely to adopt and maintain healthy behaviors focused on improving physical activity and eating habits and decreasing sedentary behaviors.
- Blood pressure should be measured beginning at age 3 years and older at all medical visits. Any measurement of elevated blood pressure should be repeated several times in a single clinic visit and confirmed at follow-up visits.
- Primary hypertension is generally found in older children and adolescents who are overweight or obese and may have a strong family history of hypertension. There should be a high clinical suspicion of secondary hypertension in younger children and those with severe elevations in blood pressure.
- All patients with a new diagnosis of hypertension should be screened with basic serum chemistries, a complete blood count, urinalysis and culture, renal ultrasound, echocardiogram, and ophthalmic examination.

- Genetic dyslipidemias may be as common as 1 in 200 people and should be suspected in a child with a family history of high cholesterol or premature cardiovascular disease.
- Screening for dyslipidemia should occur between ages 9-11 years and again between 17-21 years. This can be done using either a fasting or a non-fasting lipid profile. The average of 2 fasting lipid profiles should be used for treatment decision making.
- The majority of children will not need lipid-lowering medication after diet and lifestyle intervention. Those with severe dyslipidemia may require medication, usually a statin for lowering LDL cholesterol. Medication is rarely needed in obesity-related dyslipidemia.

REFERENCES

1. Kavey REW, Simons-Morton DG, de Jesus JM and the Expert Panel. Expert panel on integrated guidelines for cardiovascular health and risk reduction in children and adolescents: summary report. *Pediatrics.* 22011;128:S1-44.
2. Skelton JA, Cook SR, Auinger P, et al. Prevalence and trends of severe obesity among US children and adolescents. *Acad Pediatr.* 2009;9:322-329.
3. Barlow SE; The Expert Committee. Expert Committee recommendations regarding the prevention, assessment, and treatment of child and adolescent overweight and obesity: summary report. *Pediatrics.* 2007;120:S164-S192.
4. Lee JM, Pilli S, Gebremariam A, et al. Getting heavier, younger: trajectories of obesity over the life course. *Int J Obes.* 2010;34:614-623.
5. Ogden CL, Flegal KM. Changes in terminology for childhood overweight and obesity. National Health Statistics Reports No. 25. Hyattsville, MD: National Center for Health Statistics, 2010.
6. Anderson SE, Whitaker RC. Prevalence and obesity among US preschool children in different racial and ethnic groups. *Arch Pediatr Adolesc Med.* 2009;163:344-348.
7. National High Blood Pressure Education Program Working Group on High Blood Pressure in Children and Adolescents. The fourth report on the diagnosis, evaluation, and treatment of high blood pressure in children and adolescents. *Pediatrics.* 2004;114:555-576.
8. Suresh S, Mahajan P, Kamat D. Emergency management of pediatric hypertension. *Clin Pediatr.* 2005;44:739-745.
9. Din-Dzietham R, Liu Y, Bielo MV, et al. High blood pressure trends in children and adolescents in national surveys, 1963 to 2002. *Circulation.* 2007;116:1488-1496.
10. Brady TM, Feld LG. Pediatric approach to hypertension. *Semin Nephrol.* 2009;29:379-388.
11. Falkner B, Gidding SS, Ramirez-Garnica G, et al. The relationship of body mass index and blood pressure in primary care pediatric patients. *J Pediatr.* 2006;148:195-200.
12. Varda NM, Gregoric A. A diagnostic approach for the child with hypertension. *Pediatr Nephrol.* 2005;20:499-506.
13. Stone NJ, Blum CB. Pathophysiology of hyperlipoproteinemias. In: *Management of Lipids in Clinical Practice.* 6th ed. Caddo, OK: Professional Communications, Inc., 2006:23-103.

14. Magnussen CG, Venn A, Thompson R, et al. The association of pediatric LDL-cholesterol and HDL-cholesterol dyslipidemia classifications and change in dyslipidemia status with carotid intima-media thickness in adulthood: evidence from the Cardiovascular Risk in Young Finns Study, the Bogalusa Heart Study, and the Childhood Determinants of Adult Health (CDAH) Study. *J Am Coll Cardiol*. 2009;53:860-869.

15. Fredrickson DS, Lees RS. Editorial: a system for phenotyping hyperlipidemias. *Circulation*. 1965;31; 321-327.

16. American Academy of Pediatrics. National Cholesterol Education Program (NCEP): report of the expert panel on blood cholesterol levels in children and adolescents. *Pediatrics*. 1992;89:525-584.

17. Daniels SR, Greer FR; Committee on Nutrition. Lipid screening and cardiovascular health in children. *Pediatrics*. 2008;122:198-208.

18. Kavey REW, Allada V, Daniels SR, et al. Cardiovascular risk reduction in high-risk pediatric patients: a scientific statement from the American Heart Association Expert Panel on Population and Prevention Science; the Councils on Cardiovascular Disease in the Young, Epidemiology and Prevention, Nutrition, Physical Activity and Metabolism, High Blood Pressure Research, Cardiovascular Nursing, and the Kidney in Heart Disease; and the Interdisciplinary Working Group on Quality of Care and Outcomes Research—endorsed by the American Academy of Pediatrics. *Circulation*. 2006;114:2710-2738.

19. Srinivasan SR, Myers L, Berenson GS. Distribution and correlates of non-high-density lipoprotein cholesterol in children: the Bogalusa Heart Study. *Pediatrics*. 2002;110:e29.

20. Gidding SS, Dennison BA, Birch LL, et al. Dietary recommendations for children and adolescents. A guide for practitioners. Consensus statement from the American Heart Association. Endorsed by the American Academy of Pediatrics. *Circulation*. 2005;112:2061-2075.

21. Nijjar PS, Burke FM, Bloesch A, Rader DJ. Role of dietary supplements in lowering low-density lipoprotein cholesterol: a review. *J Clin Lipid*. 2010;4:248-258.

22. McCrindle BW, Urbina EM, Dennison BA, et al. Drug therapy of high-risk lipid abnormalities in children and adolescents. A scientific statement from the American Heart Association Atherosclerosis, Hypertension, and Obesity in Youth Committee, Council of Cardiovascular Disease in the Young, with the Council on Cardiovascular Nursing. *Circulation*. 2007;115:1948-1967.

23. Wiegman A, Hutten BA, de Groot E, et al. Efficacy and safety of statin therapy in children with familial hypercholesterolemia: a randomized controlled trial. *JAMA*. 2004;292:331-337.

24. Rodenburg J, Vissers MN, Wiegman A, et al. Statin treatment in children with familial hypercholesterolemia. The younger the better. *Circulation*. 2007;116:664-668.

25. Avis HJ, Vissers MN, Stein EA, et al. A systematic review and meta-analysis of statin therapy in children with familial hypercholesterolemia. *Arterioscler Thromb Vasc Biol*. 2007;27:1803-1810.

CHAPTER 16

Pediatric Issues for Patients with Congenital Heart Disease

*Camila Londono-Obregon,
Lisa M. Montenegro, Therese Giglia,
V. Ramesh Iyer and Paul Farrell Jr*

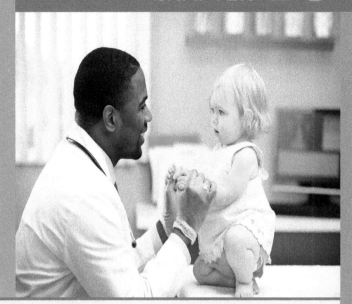

INTRODUCTION

Pediatric and young adult patients with congenital heart disease (CHD) represent a population with unique medical issues, who pose a challenge to the primary care physician (PCP). Advances in pediatric cardiology and cardiac surgery have resulted in an increasing number of survivors with CHD.[1] As a result, PCPs are now more likely to encounter patients with varying severity of CHD in their daily practice. In this chapter, we aim to discuss some common pediatric issues that may be encountered while taking care of this subset of patients.

DENTAL CARE

Oral health is an integral part of general health, and according to the Centers for Disease Control and Prevention, dental caries are the most prevalent infectious disease among U.S. children.[2] More than 40% of children have tooth decay by the time they reach kindergarten, and more than 52 million hours of school are lost each year because of dental problems.[2,3] Oral disease poses a significant burden in patients with CHD, not only by increasing the risk of acute and subacute endocarditis, but also by exposing these children to the risk associated with oral procedures. The morbidity and mortality of endocarditis is significant.[4,5] One important objective of the PCP caring for patients with CHD is to guide families to prevent oral pathology.[4,5] Oral disease increases morbidity and mortality in children with CHD by different mechanisms. The mouth is a portal of entry for microbial infection. Bacteremia may cause injury by directly damaging the epithelium and indirectly

by generating an inflammatory response. Through these mechanisms and potentially others, periodontitis may further increase the known risk of endocarditis. More recently, an association between periodontitis and increasing atherogenesis and thromboembolic phenomena has been described in adults.[4] In more severe cases, oral disease may also compromise nutrition, which in turn may have a deleterious effect on the course of the CHD.

Children with CHD have variable cardiovascular reserve; those with more tenuous hemodynamics are at higher risk of complications during dental intervention. For example, some local anesthetics with vasoconstrictors like epinephrine may be contraindicated in patients with refractory dysrhythmias. Some patients with CHD, such as patients with prosthetic valves or implanted devices, may require anticoagulation with agents like warfarin or aspirin. Stopping these agents to prevent severe bleeding may be appropriate during the much needed dental procedure but may increase the risk of valve or intracardiac thrombosis. Alternative strategies such as transition to heparin or enoxaparin and careful control of the coagulation profile before surgical intervention may be indicated. Consultation with hematology and coagulation experts may be essential in some of the complex cases. Stress and pain secondary to the dental procedure may generate catecholamine release enough to compromise hemodynamic stability. In the attempt to limit stress and pain in this vulnerable population, the clinician may have a lower threshold to use sedation; this poses other risks, some of which we will discuss later in this chapter.[4,5] Keeping these thoughts in mind, the PCP should target the higher risk populations to emphasize the importance of preventive care and oral health maintenance.

An oral health risk assessment should be administered periodically, and PCPs should apply the guidelines set by the American Academy of Pediatrics (AAP) regarding dental health.[2] Among these are dietary counseling for optimal oral health and administration of fluoride based on an individual's caries risk. The AAP has also introduced the concept of establishing a dental home by the first year of age. The term "dental home" alludes to a specialized primary dental care service expected to provide the following: (1) an accurate risk assessment for dental diseases and conditions; (2) an individualized preventive dental health program based on the risk assessment; (3) anticipatory guidance about growth and development issues (eg, teething, digit or pacifier habits, feeding practices); (4) a plan for emergency dental trauma and information about proper care of the child's teeth and gingival tissues; (5) information regarding proper nutrition and dietary practices, comprehensive dental care in accordance with accepted guidelines, and periodicity schedules for pediatric dental health; and (6) referrals to other dental specialists, such as endodontists, oral surgeons, orthodontists, and periodontists. Parents sometimes encounter significant difficulties accessing pediatric dental services. The PCP plays a crucial role in helping these families establish a "dental home."[1,3,6]

Once periodontal disease is present, interventions must be carefully planned to minimize risk. A significant concern is the risk of endocarditis. The efficacy of antibiotic prophylaxis as a preventive measure is debatable.[5] Newer strategies for better oral hygiene for the future include photodynamic therapy in which the inactivation of microorganisms is based on localization of a photosensitizer in bacteria. The photosensitizer, activated by low doses of visible light, reacts by generating free radicals that are toxic to bacteria.[7,8]

INFECTIVE ENDOCARDITIS PROPHYLAXIS

Prevention of infective endocarditis (IE) by appropriate administration of antibiotics prior to procedures known to cause bacteremia has been a subject of interest for decades. The initial recommendations regarding antibiotic prophylaxis for IE were made by the American Heart Association (AHA) in 1955.[5] Since then, 9 iterations of AHA recommendations for antibiotic prophylaxis have been made. The last statement was published in 2007[5] and was a revision of the statement that had been in place since 1997. The fundamental principles that the IE antibiotic prophylaxis guidelines were based on are as follows:

1. IE is uncommon, but it is associated with significant morbidity and mortality. Prevention is preferable.
2. Certain underlying cardiac conditions place the patient at increased risk for developing IE.
3. Bacteremia with certain organisms (such as streptococci, staphylococci, and enterococci) is more commonly associated with IE.
4. Certain invasive procedures, including dental, respiratory, gastrointestinal, and genitourinary (GU) tract procedures, have been associated with transient bacteremia.
5. Antimicrobial prophylaxis has proven to be effective for prevention of experimental IE in animals.[5,9,10]

Keeping these premises in mind and making the assumption that, in humans, antimicrobial prophylaxis may also be effective for prevention of IE associated with dental, respiratory, gastrointestinal, or GU tract procedures, antibiotic prophylaxis guidelines have been set forth.[7] Over the years, researchers have questioned the premises on which IE prophylaxis guidelines were based. The AHA appointed a multidisciplinary group, including members of the American Dental Association, the Infectious Disease Society of America, and the AAP, to regularly revise the recommendations as new literature was published.[5,9,10] The last IE prophylaxis guidelines published in 2007 reflect expert opinion based on relevant analysis of the literature published between 1950 and 2007 regarding (1) procedure-related bacteremia and IE; (2) in vitro susceptibility data of the most common microorganisms that cause IE; (3) results of prophylactic studies in animal models of experimental endocarditis; and (4) retrospective and prospective studies of prevention of IE. Most of the literature available was related to dental interventions.

The conclusions made were as follows:

1. The absolute risk for IE from dental procedures is impossible to measure precisely. Still, based on existing literature, it is estimated that if dental treatment causes 1% of all cases of Viridans streptococci IE annually in the United States, then the overall risk, in the general population, may be as low as 1 case of IE per 14 million.[5]
2. Estimates of absolute risk of IE from dental procedures in patients with heart disease indicate that IE is a very rare complication. It was estimated that in patients with mitral valve prolapse, the risk of IE was 1 in 1.1 million procedures; in patients with CHD, the risk was 1 in 475,000 procedures; and in patients with rheumatic heart disease, the risk was 1 in 142,000 procedures. The 2 populations with the highest estimated absolute risk were patients with prosthetic cardiac valves (absolute risk of 1 in 114,000 dental

Applying Classification of Recommendation and Level of Evidence for Antibiotic Prophylaxis	
Class of Recommendation	**Interpretation**
I: Benefit >>>> risk	Should be performed/administered
IIa: Benefit >> risk	Reasonable to perform/administer
IIb: Benefit ≥ risk	May be considered to be performed/administered
III: Risk ≥ benefit	Should not be performed/administered
Level of Evidence	**Recommendation Based on:**
A: Multiple populations evaluated	Randomized clinical trials and meta-analysis
B: Limited populations evaluated	Single randomized trial and non-randomized studies
C: Very limited populations evaluated	Expert opinion/consensus, case studies

Modified from Nishimura RA, Carabello BA, Faxon DP, et al. ACC/AHA 2008 guideline update on valvular heart disease: focused update on infective endocarditis: a report of the American College of Cardiology/American Heart Association Task Force on Practice Guidelines. Circulation. 2008;118;887-896.

procedures) and patients with previous IE (risk of 1 in 95,000 dental procedures).[5]

3. The efficiency of antibiotic prophylaxis in reducing bacteremia is questionable. Although it has been shown that dental procedures are associated with bacteremia, transient bacteremia is also common during daily activities like flossing and tooth brushing (20%-68%), use of wooden tooth picks (20%-40%), use of water irrigation devices (7%-50%), and chewing food (7%-51%). Because these activities are far more common causes of bacteremia than dental visits, it makes the premise of antibiotic prophylaxis for dental procedures questionable and highlights the importance of maintenance of good oral health in the prevention of IE.[5]

The antibiotic prophylaxis guidelines for IE from 2007 express the consensus of expert opinion on available literature and are designed to be interpreted based on class and level of evidence (LOE) (Table 16-1). When selecting the patient population eligible for IE prophylaxis, the 2007 recommendations shifted their focus to include a specific subset of patients with complex heart disease who were more likely to have the risk of increased mortality or long-term morbidity from IE (Table 16-2). This emphasis is in contrast to the 1997 recommendations that gave greater importance to increased risk of overall acquisition of IE in all complex and noncomplex CHD.

Antibiotic Regimens

Antibiotic regimens for IE prophylaxis are mainly targeted to patients undergoing dental procedures (Table 16-3). However, these recommendations may also be applied to patients undergoing other procedures (such

as GU interventions) when prophylaxis is indicated. In these cases, the choice of antibiotics may vary, and certain rules apply. The recommendation is that antibiotics should be administered in a single dose before the procedure. If this window is missed, antibiotics may still be given within 2 hours after the procedure. If the patient is febrile prior to the procedure, blood cultures should be considered. IE related to transient bacteremia, secondary to daily activities, such as flossing and tooth brushing, needs to be ruled out.

Cardiac Conditions Associated with the Highest Risk of Adverse Outcome From Endocarditis for Which Prophylaxis with Dental Procedures Is Reasonable[5]

- ■ Prosthetic cardiac valve or prosthetic material used for cardiac valve repair
- ■ Previous infective endocarditis
- ■ Congenital heart disease (CHD)[a]
- ■ Unrepaired cyanotic CHD, including palliative shunts and conduits
- ■ Completely repaired CHD with prosthetic material or device, whether placed by surgery or by catheter intervention, during the first 6 months after the procedure[b]
- ■ Repaired CHD with residual defects at the site of or adjacent to the site of a prosthetic patch or prosthetic device (which inhibit endothelialization)
- ■ Cardiac transplantation recipients who develop cardiac valvulopathy

[a]*Except for the conditions listed above, antibiotic prophylaxis is no longer recommended for other forms of CHD.*

[b]*Prophylaxis is reasonable because endothelialization of prosthetic material occurs within 6 months after the procedure.*

Antibiotic Prophylaxis Regimens[5,9]

Situation	Agent	Regimen: Single Dose 30-60 Minutes Before Procedure	
		Adults	Children
Oral	Amoxicillin	2 g	50 mg/kg
Unable to take oral medication	Ampicillin OR Cefazolin or ceftriaxone	2 g IM or IV 1 g IM or IV	50 mg/kg IM or IV 50 mg/kg IM or IV
Allergic to β-lactams; able to take oral medication	Cephalexin[a,b] OR Clindamycin OR Azithromycin or clarithromycin	2 g 600 mg 500 mg	50 mg/kg 20 mg/kg 15 mg/kg
Allergic to β-lactams or unable to take oral medication	Cefazolin or ceftriaxone[†] or Clindamycin	1 g IM or IV 600 mg IM or IV	50 mg/kg IM or IV 20 mg/kg IM or IV

IM, intramuscular; IV, intravenous.

[a]*Or other first- or second-generation oral cephalosporin in equivalent adult or pediatric dosage.*

[b]*Cephalosporins should not be used in an individual with a history of anaphylaxis, angioedema, or urticaria with penicillins or ampicillin.*

Modified with permission from Wilson W, Taubert KA, Gewitz M, et al. Prevention of infective endocarditis: guidelines from the American Heart Association: a guideline from the American Heart Association Rheumatic Fever, Endocarditis, and Kawasaki Disease Committee, Council on Cardiovascular Disease in the Young, and the Council on Clinical Cardiology, Council on Cardiovascular Surgery and Anesthesia, and the Quality of Care and Outcomes Research Interdisciplinary Working Group, and The Council on Scientific Affairs of the American Dental Association has approved the guideline as it relates to dentistry. Circulation. 2007;116:1736-1754.

Interventions for Which Antibiotic Prophylaxis Is Recommended

Dental procedures

Transient Viridans streptococcal bacteremia is the main concern during invasive dental procedures. Interventions for which IE prophylaxis is considered reasonable include all dental procedures that involve manipulation of gingival tissue or periapical region of teeth or perforation of the oral mucosa. Antibiotic prophylaxis is not recommended for mucosal bleeding associated with local anesthesia through noninfected tissue, dental radiographs, placement or removal of orthodontic appliances, tooth eruptions, or incidental trauma (class IIa, LOE C).

Strains of Viridans streptococci resistant to penicillin have increased significantly. Antibiotics such as vancomycin and fluoroquinolones are not recommended due to concerns of excessive use, increasing resistance, and a low risk–benefit ratio. The antibiotics of choice for prophylaxis for dental procedures are amoxicillin or cephalosporins and macrolides in special situations when antibiotic allergies are encountered (Table 16-3).[5]

Procedures involving the respiratory tract

IE antibiotic prophylaxis may be reasonable for respiratory tract procedures in which incision or biopsy of respiratory mucosa is made, for example tonsillectomy and adenoidectomy (class IIa, LOE C). Procedures like bronchoscopy, where there is no disruption of the respiratory mucosa expected, do not require antibiotic prophylaxis. Regimens detailed in Table 16-3 may be applied if underlying bacterial infection is suspected or confirmed; if organisms resistant to regimens detailed in Table 16-3 are suspected, alternative regimens should be used.[5]

Procedures involving the genitourinary tract

Antibiotics may be indicated in patients undergoing elective GU procedures, with the aim of eradicating enterococci in colonized patients or in patients with enterococci urinary tract infection (class IIb, LOE B). If the procedure is not elective, it may be reasonable to give antibiotic prophylaxis, including therapeutic antibiotic coverage for enterococci (class IIb, LOE B). Ampicillin and amoxicillin are the agents of choice. If the there is a contraindication to a β-lactam antibiotic, vancomycin can be used. Expert consultation should be obtained when prophylaxis is against multiresistant organisms.[5]

Procedures involving infected skin or musculoskeletal tissue

Antibiotic prophylaxis with a penicillin or a cephalosporin may be considered for procedures on infected skin or musculoskeletal tissue. Under these circumstances, the choice of antibiotics should include coverage against *Staphylococcus* and β-hemolytic *Streptococcus* (class IIb, LOE C). Vancomycin and clindamycin can be used as alternatives depending on bacterial resistance patterns and patient allergies.[5]

Patients who undergo cardiac surgery

Ideally, dental treatment should be completed before cardiac surgery because the absence of infective oral disease is preferred. Patients undergoing placement of prosthetic valves, intracardiac or intravascular prosthetic material, and transvenous pacemakers are candidates for perioperative antibiotic prophylaxis (class I, LOE B). Prophylaxis prior to surgery should be primarily targeted at *Staphylococcus aureus* species. Antibiotic choice should be based on the hospital's specific susceptibility patterns. Nonetheless, a first-generation cephalosporin is a class I, LOE A recommendation. If methicillin-resistant *S aureus* or *Staphylococcus epidermidis* species are highly prevalent, vancomycin may be considered (class IIb, LOE C).[5]

Special Considerations

Patients with CHD may have other comorbidities that merit special considerations:

1. Patients receiving long-term antibiotics for indications other than IE: Some patients may already be on daily antibiotics for issues such as rheumatic fever prophylaxis or urinary tract prophylaxis or because they are immunocompromised. If patients are undergoing a procedure for which prophylaxis is recommended, the suggestion of the AHA is to use an antibiotic from a different class instead of increasing the dose.[5,9]
2. Patients taking anticoagulation: Intramuscular injections as a mode of administering antibiotic prophylaxis should be avoided because of risk of hematoma (class I, LOE A). Oral administration is the preferred option. In patients who do not tolerate the enteric route, intravenous is the preferred alternative.[5]

Conditions for Which Antibiotic Prophylaxis Is No Longer Recommended

One of the significant changes in the 2007 AHA IE prophylaxis recommendations is that antibiotic prophylaxis is no longer recommended for patients undergoing gastrointestinal procedures (class III, LOE B). This change is based on new literature that indicates that normal gut

flora, including enterococci, and polymicrobial intra-abdominal infections are uncommon IE pathogens. The literature associating enterococci bacteremia to gastrointestinal procedures is scant, and reported cases are anecdotal. Alternatively, antibiotics may be recommended if a patient with an active gastrointestinal infection is undergoing a procedure. In this case, targeted antibiotic therapy should be considered, and coverage for enterococci is reasonable (class IIb, LOE B).[5,9]

PREGNANCY AND CONTRACEPTION

Education about pregnancy and contraception should be an integral part of the healthcare plan in the patient with CHD. Increasing survival in this patient population has resulted in more females with CHD reaching, and surviving beyond, childbearing years. Recent studies have shown that there needs to be a better effort in improving pregnancy and contraception counseling. As Vigil et al.[11] described in their study, which included 536 females with CHD, up to 43% of women reported they received no counseling regarding contraception. Forty-eight percent of women claimed they had not been informed of pregnancy-related risks before being seen by a specialist.[11] In addition, up to 45% of subjects in another study reported using or having used contraception methods that were contraindicated because of their cardiac diagnosis.[12] It is the responsibility of the healthcare team to work as an interdisciplinary group in educating this growing population regarding their fertility and the risks of pregnancy. The importance of education is specifically recognized in preventing unplanned pregnancy in females with more severe forms of CHD. In these patients, an unplanned pregnancy could lead to severe health consequences, including death, for both the mother and the fetus.

Counseling adolescents with CHD regarding pregnancy and contraception should begin early. This population is heterogeneous and includes females with simple cardiac lesions who can be counseled as healthy adolescents and women with more severe lesions who need individualized consideration. In counseling, the healthcare provider must take into account the risk of pregnancy to the patient and the unborn child, specific contraindications intrinsic to each contraception method and medications used by the patients, and the patient's capabilities and preferences.[12-14]

Pregnancy

Pregnancy imposes prohibitively high mortality to both mother and fetus in patients with Eisenmenger syndrome. In these patients, methods of contraception with the lowest failure rate need be considered. Other patients at high risk for complications during pregnancy include women with mechanical valves, Fontan circulation, or significant myocardial dysfunction. In these patients, contraception methods with low failure rates should also be recommended.[12]

The American College of Cardiology/AHA guidelines for adults with CHD emphasize the importance of these women being counseled regarding the genetics of their heart disease, the risk of offspring being affected, risks of fetal demise, prematurity, and maternal morbidity and mortality. All medications the patient is taking need to be reviewed, and the teratogenic potential for the fetus needs to be considered.[13]

Contraception

There are limited data on the safety of contraception methods in patients with CHD, so information is extrapolated from women with no CHD. The general categories of contraceptives and their risks are listed in Table 16-4.

Combined hormonal contraception

Estrogen-based formulations have been shown to increase risk of thromboembolism, have a negative impact on lipid profile (decreasing high-density lipoproteins and increasing low-density lipoproteins and triglycerides), increase the risk of glucose intolerance, and increase the risk of

Contraceptive Agents

Contraceptive Agent	Risks and Advantages
Combined hormonal contraception (estrogens and progestins)	↑ risk of thromboembolism ↑ LDL and triglyceride, ↓ HDL cholesterol ↑ glucose intolerance ↑ risk for hypertension
Progesterone-only formulations	No thrombosis risk
	Failure rate high (5%-10%) Fluid retention
Intrauterine device (IUD)	+/– ↑ risk of infection (IE)
Barrier methods	+/– efficacy is user dependent No specific contraindications
Sterilization	Most effective for high-risk patients
	Permanent Involves a surgical intervention, anesthesia

HDL, high-density lipoprotein; IE, infective endocarditis; LDL, low-density lipoprotein.

hypertension. Failure rate during the first year is 3% to 8%.[12] The 2008 American College of Cardiology/AHA guidelines for adults with CHD recommend that estrogen-containing oral contraceptive pills not be prescribed to patients at risk for thromboembolism (eg, patients who have undergone Fontan palliation), patients with significant cyanosis, patients with atrial fibrillation, and patients with pulmonary hypertension.[13] Although not included in the 2008 American College of Cardiology guidelines, patients who require anticoagulation are not ideal candidates for estrogen-based pills. This group includes patients just mentioned and patients with mechanical valves, due to the increased risk related to the known interaction of estrogen with warfarin.[12]

Progesterone-based contraceptive methods

Medroxyprogesterone and progesterone-only pills are an alternative to combined hormonal contraception. They have less effect on blood pressure, are not contraindicated in smokers, and do not increase the risk of thrombosis. Their most significant drawbacks are the high failure rates (5%-10% in the first year) and their association with increased fluid retention, which may compromise hemodynamic stability,[12,13] as in patients with Eisenmenger syndrome, other causes of pulmonary hypertension, severe cardiomyopathy, Marfan syndrome with dilated aorta, or severe aortic stenosis. If the decision is still to use progesterone-based contraception in these specific cardiac conditions, forms of slow-release contraception are preferred (intramuscular injections) because they are more reliable.[12] Per the AHA guidelines, levonorgestrel (Plan B), may be used in women with cyanotic CHD and with pulmonary hypertension.[13]

Intrauterine devices

The use of intrauterine devices should be individualized for patients with CHD. The suggested increased risk for endocarditis is controversial, so risk–benefit ratios should be considered based on the individual patient.[13] Intrauterine devices are not recommended in patients with Fontan circulation because they are at risk for severe vagal response during device placement.[12]

Barrier methods

Condoms, spermicidal products, and diaphragms are recommended as adjunctive methods. They have no specific contraindications, but efficiency and compliance are highly user dependent.

Permanent sterilization

Tubal ligation is the method of choice in women with prohibitively high risk for pregnancy. Procedure-related risks and long-term consequences need to be discussed. Sterilization of the male partner is controversial and should only be pursued after extensive counseling.[11–13]

Summary

In summary, it is mandatory that PCPs, cardiologists, and gynecologists caring for patients with CHD become proficient in educating this growing heterogeneous population of young adults regarding their fertility, pregnancy risk, and choice of contraception. We must strive to give these women the choice of making informed decisions regarding their reproductive years.

IMMUNIZATIONS

The Advisory Committee on Immunization Practices annually publishes an immunization schedule for persons age 0 through 18 years that summarizes recommendations for currently licensed vaccines. Healthcare providers are referred to the Centers for Disease Control and Prevention website[15] to review the most recent guidelines. Patients with CHD are subject to the same vaccination guidelines, with some extra requirements that are discussed in the following sections.

Respiratory Syncytial Virus Prophylaxis

Respiratory syncytial virus (RSV) is considered a significant cause of morbidity and mortality in some patients with CHD.[16,17] Candidates for RSV prophylaxis include children younger than 24 months with hemodynamically significant acyanotic congenital cardiac lesions and cyanotic heart disease. The AAP has come to the consensus that the patients most likely to benefit from RVS prophylaxis are infants younger than 12 months of age who are receiving medication to control congestive heart failure, infants with moderate to severe pulmonary hypertension, and infants with cyanotic heart disease.[16,17]

Patients who are candidates for RSV immunoglobulin should receive 5 doses (15 mg/kg/dose) of intramuscular palivizumab (class I evidence). Intramuscular palivizumab is preferred over the intravenous route because RSV intravenous immunoglobulin administration involves a 4-hour infusion, which may not be well tolerated by children with tenuous hemodynamics.[16–18]

Patients with CHD who do not qualify for RSV prophylaxis include children with CHD that does not significantly affect hemodynamic stability (atrial septal defect, small ventricular septal defect, pulmonic stenosis, mild aortic stenosis, and patent ductus arteriosus). Infants with lesions adequately corrected by cardiac surgery (who are not on anticongestive medication) and infants with mild cardiomyopathy also do not need RSV prophylaxis.

RSV immunoglobulin is not recommended for treatment of RSV infection. Nonetheless, the prophylaxis schedule should not be affected by breakthrough RSV infection (class III evidence). The administration of palivizumab does not affect the administration of other vaccines. The only described contraindication to palivizumab is a severe allergic reaction to prior doses.[16–18]

Influenza Vaccination

Influenza poses a large burden in patients with more severe forms of CHD. It is estimated that the virus causes up to 36,000 deaths and 225,000 hospitalizations a year in the United States.[19,20] Immunization against seasonal influenza is critical in decreasing morbidity and mortality in patients with CHD.

The 2010 Advisory Committee on Immunization Practices recommends all patients older than 6 months should be annually vaccinated against influenza.[20] In the United States, the ideal timing for influenza vaccination is September through November. If this window is missed, late vaccination is recommended because the peak influenza activity typically is between January and March.[19] Two forms of the vaccine exist, the trivalent inactivated vaccine (administered intramuscularly) and the live attenuated vaccine (administered intranasally). Patients with CHD should be immunized with the inactivated form. The live attenuated vaccine is currently not approved in this patient population.[19]

Contraindications to the administration of the intramuscular trivalent inactivated vaccine in patients with CHD are no different to those that apply to the general population. Patients with known anaphylactic hypersensitivity to eggs or other components of the influenza vaccine should not get this form, unless the recipient has been desensitized. Prophylactic use of antiviral agents is an option for preventing influenza among such patients. Persons with moderate to severe acute febrile illness usually should not be vaccinated until their symptoms have abated. Moderate or severe acute illness with or without fever is a precaution for trivalent inactivated vaccine administration. Guillain-Barré syndrome within 6 weeks following a previous dose of influenza vaccine is considered to be a precaution for use of influenza vaccines.[20]

Patients with CHD and Altered Immunocompetence

DiGeorge and heterotaxy syndromes, which are associated with a heterogeneous spectrum of CHDs, include different degrees of cellular and/or humoral immune compromise. Patients who undergo heart transplantation are also immunosuppressed due to their antirejection medications. The PCP needs to determine the degree of immunocompetence alteration and immunize these patients accordingly.

General rules set by the Advisory Committee on Immunization Practices include the following:

■ Severely immunocompromised individuals should receive the trivalent inactivated influenza vaccine, not the live attenuated vaccine.

■ Patients with functional asplenia, in the absence of hemodynamically significant heart disease, are candidates for the live attenuated influenza vaccine.

■ Immunocompromised patients should be immunized with polysaccharide-based vaccines (ie, pneumococcal conjugate vaccine [PCV], pneumococcal polysaccharide vaccine [PPV], meningococcal conjugated vaccine [MCV4], meningococcal polysaccharide vaccine [MPSV], and *Haemophilus influenzae* type b vaccine [Hib]); they seem to be more effective.

■ Household and other close contacts should receive all age-appropriate vaccines, with the exception of live oral polio vaccine and smallpox vaccine.[20]

■ Palivizumab prophylaxis has not been evaluated in randomized trials, so specific recommendations are not available.[18]

MEDICATION INTERACTIONS

QT Interval Prolongation

QT prolongation is associated with a potentially fatal form of polymorphic ventricular tachycardia called "torsades de pointes" (TdP). Long QT syndrome (LQTS) may be genetic or acquired. Genetic forms represent a wide spectrum of mild and severe diseases. The QT interval is usually corrected for heart rate to obtain the QTc interval, using the Bazett formula ($QTc = QT/\sqrt{RR}$ interval), when the heart rate is above 60 beats per minute. The classic, but relatively rare, genetic LQTS may be associated with substantial QTc prolongation and arrhythmic risk, even in the absence of additional risk amplifiers such as QTc-prolonging drugs. Acquired prolonged QT syndrome is most frequently drug induced.[21,22]

QT interval prolongation associated with medicines was first described in 1920; quinidine was one of the first recognized offenders. Since then, a better understanding of the myocardial action potential and interaction of different medications with the myocardial ion channels has been helpful. Understanding this interaction, we have recognized a wide variety of medicines that have an effect on the QT interval and thus may cause proarrhythmic side effects. It is important for the general practitioner to be familiar with medicines used in their daily practice that have this potential. A detailed and updated list of these can be found online at several websites including www.qtdrugs.org and www.azcert.org.[23,24]

Clinically relevant drug-induced QTc prolongation and arrhythmia occurrence are highly dependent on individual patient-specific factors, also called risk amplifiers. The identification of these risk amplifiers helps predict the given patient's arrhythmic risk. Specific factors to consider include genetic predisposition; various drug–drug interactions; female sex (70% of drug-associated TdP have been reported in women); age (elderly people are at higher risk); electrolyte imbalance such as hypokalemia and hypomagnesemia; bradycardia; and the presence of underlying structural heart disease, particularly ventricular hypertrophy and congestive heart failure.[21]

Most cases of drug-induced TdP present in the setting of significant QTc prolongation, typically beyond 500 ms.[21] Drugs that produce clinically relevant QT prolongation have been reported to do so by affecting the potassium channels encoded by a gene called *HERG*. Drugs for which *HERG* inhibition is part of the therapeutic mechanism of action place the patient at the highest risk for QT prolongation and TdP.[20] Among these drugs are class III antiarrhythmics including sotalol, dofetilide, ibutilide, and azimilide. The PCP does not commonly prescribe these medications but still may encounter patients using them. In much broader clinical use are a variety of noncardiac medicines, which may be part of the PCP's frequent practice. These include antibiotics, antipsychotics, antidepressants, and antihistamines, among others (Table 16-5).[21,25–28] Fatal arrhythmias are less commonly reported in association with these noncardiac medications than with class III antiarrhythmic agents. The risk of TdP is generally less than 0.01% to 0.1% for noncardiac medications, compared with greater than 1% with class III antiarrhythmics.[20] The Arizona Center for Education and Research on Therapeutics website[24] is a resource available to the public and healthcare providers and presents an up-to-date list of drugs that prolong the QT interval.

QT interval prolongation may also result from a drug–drug interaction. Reported interactions include:

■ Prescription of multiple agents with *HERG*-blocking properties.

■ Drug metabolism and pharmacokinetic drug interactions: Drugs that are metabolized by cytochrome P450 may be at higher risk of altering drug levels of concomitantly administered medicines and potentiate toxicity.

■ Drugs that affect electrolyte level: Examples are diuretics that can alter potassium and magnesium serum concentration and lower the threshold for TdP.

■ Drugs that affect excretion: If renal clearance is affected, *HERG*-blocking agents that are renally cleared, such as sotalol, may reach toxic levels.[21]

To avoid clinical TdP, medical personnel must correctly recognize a drug with the capacity to prolong the QTc interval and also assess that risk in each individual

Drugs with Risk of QT Interval Prolongation and Torsades de Pointes

Antiarrhythmics	Antipsychotics	Anti-infectives	Antiemetics	Analgesics
Amiodarone	Chlorpromazine	Chloroquine	Domperidone	Levomethadyl
Procainamide	Haloperidol	Clarithromycin	Droperidol	Methadone
Sotalol	Mesoridazine	Erythromycin		
	Pimozide	Pentamidine		

From Arizona Center for Education and Research on Therapeutics. QT drugs lists by risk group. Available at: http://www.QTdrugs.org. This table does not include drugs with possible risk or conditional risk of torsades de points. This list is updated on an ongoing basis, so the physician is advised to consult this site for up-to-date consultation.

patient. In an era in which pediatric patients more frequently visit healthcare providers of different subspecialties, the primary provider plays a crucial role in preventing polypharmacy and drug–drug interactions in patients with multiple comorbidities and risk factors for arrhythmia.

ATTENTION-DEFICIT HYPERACTIVITY DISORDER

Attention-deficit hyperactivity disorder (ADHD) is the most common neurodevelopmental disorder in childhood, and its prevalence seems to be even higher in patients with cyanotic CHD. For example, as many as 45% of patients with hypoplastic left heart syndrome have been found to have abnormal attention scores, and up to 39% have been found to have abnormal hyperactivity.[27] In addition, up to 50% of patients with total pulmonary venous return have been noted to have abnormal attention spans and hyperactivity.[27] For this reason, it is very important for the PCP to have information that facilitates treatment of ADHD in this patient population.

The use of stimulant medication in patients with structural heart disease or conditions associated with increased risk of sudden death is a subject of controversy.[27,28] Existing literature suggests that children with structural heart defects, cardiomyopathy, or heart rhythm disturbances may be at risk for adverse cardiac events, including sudden death. Suggestions have been made by the U.S. Food and Drug Administration to place a "black box" warning stating that patients with serious structural cardiac abnormalities, cardiomyopathy, heart rhythm abnormalities, or other serious cardiac problems may have increased vulnerability to the sympathomimetic effects of stimulant drugs.[27] This concern has made treatment of ADHD challenging.

Unless contraindicated by a cardiologist, it is reasonable to use stimulant medication for ADHD in most patients with structural heart disease (repaired or unrepaired), as long as they do not have significant hemodynamic or arrhythmic burden (class IIa, LOE C). It is also reasonable to start stimulant medications with caution in patients with ADHD and a cardiac diagnosis associated with increased risk of sudden cardiac death (Table 16-6)

Most Common Causes of Sudden Cardiac Death (SCD) in the United States[35]

Diagnosis	% of SCD Attributed to Specific Diagnosis
Hypertrophic cardiomyopathy	33%-50%
Long QT syndrome	15%-25%
Other cardiomyopathies, including arrhythmogenic right ventricular dysplasia and dilated cardiomyopathy	10%-20%
Coronary artery anomalies	10%-20%
Primary ventricular fibrillation or tachycardia	10%-15%
Wolff-Parkinson-White syndrome	3%-5%
Others, including aortic rupture	5%

The incidence of sudden cardiac death in the United States is 1000 to 7000 children annually.

when other methods like behavioral therapy have failed. In these patients, careful long-term monitoring is suggested.

The successful response rate to stimulant medication is as high as 70% compared with 12% with placebo.[27] Untreated ADHD in childhood is associated with increased risk of injuries, academic underachievement, and increased risk of poor social interaction. Adults with untreated ADHD have been found to attain lower occupational status and to be at higher risk for substance abuse, antisocial behavior, and automobile accidents than peers.[27,29] It is of crucial importance *not* to limit ADHD therapy in patients in whom it is not contraindicated.

Per the Scientific Statement by the AHA Council on Cardiovascular Disease in the Young, the Congenital Cardiac Defects Committee, and the Council on Cardiovascular Nursing published in April 2008, and revised May 16, 2008, by the AAP/AHA, medications that treat ADHD have not be found to cause heart disease and have not been shown to increase the risk of sudden cardiac death. Most recently Cooper et al. published a study including 1,200,438 children and young adults between the ages of 2 and 24 years. This large study adds evidence stating that use of ADHD medication is not associated with an increased risk of serious cardiovascular events.[30]

Nonetheless, some of these medications do increase or decrease heart rate and blood pressure (Table 16-7).[31] These side effects are not dangerous in most cases, but some patients with heart disease may not tolerate them well. It is reasonable to identify this population before starting stimulant medication and to monitor them during treatment. The committee recommends that before starting medication, the physician identify high-risk patients in whom long-term monitoring and possible cardiology consultation may be indicated.[27] A focused history and clinical examination are recommended to identify these individuals (Tables 16-8 to 16-10).

Once a focused examination has been attained, a 12-lead electrocardiogram (ECG) may be a reasonable part of the examination but is not mandatory (class IIa, LOE C). The decision whether to obtain an ECG is left to the individual physician. The ECG may help identify cardiac pathology such as hypertrophic cardiomyopathy, LQTS, and Wolff-Parkinson-White anomaly, but it is acknowledged that an ECG does not identify all individuals with these conditions (Table 16-11). Not being able to obtain an ECG is not a reason to withhold therapy.

Once this evaluation is completed, a cardiology consult (class I, LOE C) should be obtained before starting stimulant medications if structural heart disease,

ADHD Medications, Side Effects, and Follow-Up Plan[24]

Medication/Mechanism of Action	Cardiac Effects	First Visit Monitoring	Long-Term Monitoring
Methylphenidate (Ritalin, Ritalin SR, Concerta, Metadate, Methylin, Focalin, Daytrana) Amphetamine (dextroamphetamine, Dextrostat, Adderall, Vyvanse)/ increase catecholamines at synapse	Increased HR and BP, no ECG changes		
Atomoxetine (Strattera)/selective norepinephrine reuptake inhibitor	Increased HR and BP, adults may have palpitations, no ECG changes expected	ECG on first visit (class IIa, LOE C)[a]	BP and HR (class I, LOE C)
Guanfacine (Tenex)/α_2-adrenergic agonist	Decreased HR and BP, no ECG changes		
Bupropion (Wellbutrin, Zyban)/ decrease firing of norepinephrine- and serotonin-releasing neurons	Increased BP in adults, cardiotoxic if overdosed		
Clonidine (Catapres)/α_2-adrenergic agonist	Decreased HR and BP, rebound hypertension if discontinued suddenly, no ECG changes		BP and HR check in each visit, recheck if dose is changed (class I, LOE C)

ADHD, attention-deficit hyperactivity disorder; BP, blood pressure; ECG, electrocardiogram; HR, heart rate; LOE, level of evidence.

[a]*Cardiology consultation may be considered when abnormal intervals are present.*

Modified with permission from American Academy of Pediatrics/American Heart Association. American Academy of Pediatrics/American Heart Association clarification of statement on cardiovascular evaluation and monitoring of children and adolescents with heart disease receiving medications for ADHD. Endorsed by the American Academy of Child and Adolescent Psychiatry, the American College of Cardiology, Children and Adults with Attention-Deficit/Hyperactivity Disorder, the National Initiative for Children's Healthcare Quality and the Society for Developmental and Behavioral Pediatrics. J Dev Behav Pediatr. 2008;9:335-335.

Patient History That May Help Identify High-Risk Individuals in Whom Cardiology Consultation May Be Recommended Prior to Starting Stimulant Medication (Class I, LOE A)[27]

- Fainting or dizziness (especially during exercise)
- Seizures
- Rheumatic fever
- Chest pain, palpitations, increased heart rate, or extra or skipped heartbeats
- Shortness of breath with exercise, unexplained change in exercise tolerance
- High blood pressure
- Heart murmur (other than innocent or functional murmur)
- Viral illness with chest pains or palpitations (possible myocarditis)
- Current medications and health supplements should be reviewed

arrhythmias, or family history of sudden cardiac death in individuals less than 35 years of age is noted.

Long-Term Monitoring of Patients on Stimulant Medication

Individuals with ADHD and structural heart disease, arrhythmias, or family history of sudden cardiac death in individuals less than 35 years of age are candidates for long-term monitoring once they are started on stimulant medication. PCPs are recommended to do a targeted history and physical examination to monitor for potential cardiac symptoms during subsequent follow-up (class I, LOE C) (Table 16-7). Blood pressure and pulse should be recorded 1 to 3 months after starting therapy. Subsequently, patients may be monitored every 6 to 12 months (class I, LOE C). If cardiac symptoms are identified, the patient should be referred to a cardiologist (class I, LOE C). If the initial ECG

Family History That May Help Identify High-Risk Individuals in Whom Cardiology Consultation May Be Recommended Prior to Starting Stimulant Medication (Class I, LOE A)[27]

- Sudden or unexplained death in young individuals (people <35 years of age), sudden death during exercise
- Cardiac arrhythmias, long QT syndrome, short QT syndrome, Brugada syndrome, Wolff-Parkinson-White syndrome
- Cardiomyopathies
- Family history of Marfan syndrome should also be obtained

Physical Examination Findings That May Help Identify High-Risk Individuals in Whom Cardiology Consultation May Be Recommended Prior to Starting Stimulant Medication (Class I, LOE A)[27]

- Abnormal heart murmur
- Hypertension
- Irregular or rapid heart rhythm
- Physical findings suggestive of Marfan syndrome

was obtained before the child was 12 years of age, a repeat study may be recommended. If the patient has cardiovascular symptoms, an ECG is warranted.[27]

In summary, the treatment of ADHD should be individualized. Identifying and managing the underlying cardiac pathology may not eliminate the risks of serious cardiovascular events but may increase the safety of using the medication and may maximize treatment of the target population.

ANTICOAGULATION ISSUES

Disruptions in the balance of homeostasis, with resultant thrombosis or bleeding, are a significant cause of morbidity and mortality for some patients with CHD. The etiology is multifactorial and still not fully understood. Described anomalies include the following[32,33]:

1. Alterations in blood composition, including altered coagulation protein levels, decreased presence of endogenous inhibitors of coagulation, decreased fibrinolytic proteins, and genetic polymorphisms, all of which have been described in some children with CHD.[32]
2. Endothelial injury, such as endothelial dysfunction, graft material, and intravenous catheters.
3. Altered blood flow patterns, for example, nonpulsatile flow (Fontan physiology), valve or vessel stenosis, vascular and chamber dilatation, and immobility.

Depending on the variables affected, the individual patient may have higher risk of bleeding at certain times and increased risk of thromboembolic complications at others.

In the patient with CHD, beyond the immediate operative period, thromboembolic complications seem to be more frequent than hemorrhagic complications. Prophylactic antithrombotic agents are commonly used in specific high-risk patients.[32–36] Decreasing morbidity and mortality, resulting from altered homeostasis, is a difficult task. The PCP plays a crucial role in this regard, increasingly so when the patient meets criteria for

Normal and Abnormal Electrocardiogram (ECG) Variants and Their Management[24]

Normal ECG Variants	"Abnormal" ECG Findings That Do Not Preclude Stimulant Therapy*	Abnormal ECG Findings That May Correlate with Heart Disease and May Not Preclude Stimulant Therapy (Cardiology Consultation Suggested)
Sinus bradycardia	Isolated atrial enlargement	Left or right ventricular hypertrophy
Sinus arrhythmia	Biventricular hypertrophy with	Wolff-Parkinson-White syndrome
Sinus tachycardia	midprecordial voltages 45-50 mm	Left axis deviation/right axis deviation
Right ventricular conduction delay	Ectopic atrial arrhythmias at normal	>8 years old
without right ventricular hypertrophy	rates	Right atrial enlargement and right axis
or right axis deviation	Atrioventricular conduction delay	deviation
Isolated interventricular conduction		Right ventricular conduction delay and
delay		right axis deviation
Right axis deviation <8 years of age		Second- and third-degree atrioventricular
Early repolarization		block
Nonspecific ST-T wave changes		Right bundle-branch block, left bundle-
1. Juvenile T-wave pattern		branch block, wide QRS >120 ms
2. QTc >0.45 seconds by computer but		in >12 years and >100 ms in <8 years
normal by hand calculation		Long QTc
3. Borderline QTc 0.44-0.45 seconds		Abnormal T waves: inverted in V_5 and V_6,
		notched, biphasic, or flat
		ST-segment depression suggesting
		inflammation or ischemia
		Atrial junctional or ventricular
		tachyarrhythmias

*Cardiology consultation may be considered on individual basis. ECG changes should be interpreted in correlation to history and physical examination.

Modified with permission from American Academy of Pediatrics/American Heart Association. American Academy of Pediatrics/American Heart Association clarification of statement on cardiovascular evaluation and monitoring of children and adolescents with heart disease receiving medications for ADHD. Endorsed by the American Academy of Child and Adolescent Psychiatry, the American College of Cardiology, Children and Adults with Attention-Deficit/Hyperactivity Disorder, the National Initiative for Children's Healthcare Quality and the Society for Developmental and Behavioral Pediatrics. J Dev Behav Pediatr. 2008;9:335-335.

antithrombotic therapy or prophylaxis. In this section, we review which patients are eligible for antithrombotic prophylaxis, which medications are routinely used, how these medications are dosed and administered, which regimens require monitoring, and the more frequent side effects the PCP may encounter (Table 16-12).

In the prevention and treatment of thrombosis, anticoagulants (eg, unfractionated heparin, low molecular weight heparin [LMWH]), antiplatelet agents (eg, low-dose aspirin, clopidogrel), and fibrinolytic agents (eg, tissue plasminogen activator, alteplase) are available.[32] Most of these agents are used off label in children (Table 16-12).

Patients with CHD in whom prophylaxis is often recommended include the following:

1. *Patients status post systemic-to-pulmonary artery shunts:* Systemic-to-pulmonary shunts, for example the modified Blalock-Taussig shunt, are typically used as part of the first stage of palliation in patients with single-ventricle physiology or as a means to supply additional pulmonary blood flow in patients with right heart obstructive lesions

(eg, tetralogy of Fallot with pulmonary atresia). The incidence of thrombosis in patients with systemic-to-pulmonary shunts is 1% to 17%.[33] Complete shunt occlusion may require reinterventions in the catheterization laboratory or operating room.[37] Patients with aortopulmonary shunts are typically treated with intraoperative unfractionated heparin and are maintained postoperatively on low-dose aspirin.[33]

2. *Patients status post stage 1 Norwood procedure:* The Norwood procedure or stage 1 surgery is commonly used in patients with hypoplastic left heart syndrome. The usual practice is intraoperative unfractionated heparin and postoperative aspirin. High-risk patients may also be placed on clopidogrel in combination with aspirin; the safety and efficiency of this therapy are unproven.[33]

3. *Patients status post cavopulmonary anastomosis:* The cavopulmonary anastomosis, or Glenn operation, was first done in 1957. Initially, it was used as palliation for tricuspid atresia. Today, the bidirectional Glenn operation is commonly

Antithrombotic Agents Used for Prophylaxis and Treatment of Thromboembolic Complications in the Patient with Congenital Heart Disease (CHD)

Name/Mechanism of Action	Contraindications	Dose/Route of Administration	Monitoring	Target Range	Side Effects
Anticoagulant agents					
Unfractionated heparin (UFH); potentiates antithrombin inhibition of factors XIIa, XIa, Xa, IIa	1 Heparin-induced thrombocytopenia[36] 2 Poor venous access[28]	<12 months old = 28 U/kg/h ≥12 months old = 20 U/kg/h Low dose is commonly 10-15 U/kg/h Given IV	Minimum every 24 hours Gold standard anti-Xa PTT may also be used	Anti-Xa level 0.35-0.7 U/mL[a] or PTT 1.5-3× baseline PTT[28]	Hemorrhage (5.6%-30%) HIT (0%-2.3%) Osteoporosis[36,37,39]
Low molecular weight heparin; same as UFH, however greatest inhibition on factor Xa	1 High risk of bleeding 2 Renal insufficiency 3 Has to be held 24 hours prior to intervention	Age dependent and medication dependent Enoxaparin: <3 months old = 1.5 mg/kg/dose ≥3 months old = 1.0 mg/kg/dose Given SQ	Minimum every month once stability has been achieved Does not affect INR or PTT Levels must be obtained 4 hours after the dose	Anti-Xa level 0.5-1.0 U/mL	Hemorrhage (4.8%-8.1%)
Warfarin; inhibits γ-carboxylation of vitamin K–dependent proteins II, VII, IX, and X, and protein C, S, and Z	Relative: <1 year of age unless mechanical valve in situ[28] Absolute: pregnancy, bleeding diathesis	Load: 0.2 mg/kg/d Fontan patients: 0.1 mg/kg/d Maintenance: individualized dosing titrated to INR	INR daily until therapeutic then decreased frequency when stable; do minimum monthly INR; test INR with illness, medication, or diet change Point-of-care devices are available for in-office or at-home INR monitoring	Target INR range 2-3 Mechanical mitral valves 2.5-3.5 Point-of Care INR devices available for home or office monitoring	Hemorrhage Tracheal calcification, hair loss, decreased bone mineral density
Antiplatelet therapy					
Aspirin; inhibition of COX-1 and COX-2 activity	Ibuprofen within 4 hours of ASA dose increases risk of bleeding Varicella, fever due to risk for Reyes syndrome	Low dose: 1-5 mg/kg/d Maximum: 81-325 mg[28]	N/A	N/A	Bruising, confusion, vertigo, nausea, vomiting, tinnitus, abdominal pain, cramping, burning, fatigue, bleeding
Clopidogrel; inhibition of ADP-induced platelet aggregation	Genetic variability may alter cytochrome metabolism of clopidogrel and decrease antiplatelet effect[38]	0.2-1 mg/kg/d Ongoing study in CHD and shunts[28]	None studied	None	Fatigue, vertigo, stomach upset or pain, bruising, bleeding, diarrhea[28]

ADP, adenosine diphosphate; ASA, acetylsalicylic acid; IV, intravenous; HIT, heparin-induced thrombocytopenia; INR, international normalized ratio; N/A, not applicable; PTT, partial thromboplastin time; SQ, subcutaneous.

Data from Giglia T, et al. Prevention and treatment of thrombosis in children and adults with congenital heart disease and in children with acquired heart disease. Circulation. In press.

[a]Range may vary and should be based on individual lab normals.

used as the second stage of the single-ventricle palliation pathway. Thrombotic complications are seldom seen after this operation. There are no data to support anticoagulation or antiplatelet therapy in these patients; even so, aspirin is commonly used, and warfarin is rarely used.[33] A proposed rationale to treat these patients is to minimize the risk for recurrent pulmonary microemboli, which may compromise the hemodynamic success of the future Fontan operation.

4. *Patients status post Fontan procedure:* The Fontan procedure, which completes the diversion of systemic venous return from both the upper and lower body directly into the pulmonary arteries, is commonly used as the final stage of single-ventricle palliation. These patients are at high risk of venous thromboembolism (incidence as high as 16%). If there is a residual right-to-left shunt (ie, with the fenestrated Fontan modification), there is a significant risk of stroke (incidence as high as 19%).[33] Venous thromboembolism is a significant cause of morbidity. It may be fatal if there is complete or near-complete Fontan occlusion. There is a paucity of randomized clinical trials; consequently, a variety of regimens are used. Most commonly, patients are on low-dose aspirin. Warfarin or other anticoagulants are reserved for older or high-risk individuals, particularly those with prior thrombotic events, arrhythmias, ventricular dysfunction, immobilization, protein-losing enteropathy, and/or pleural effusions.[33,35]

5. *Patients with valve replacements:* Patients with tricuspid or pulmonary valve disease who meet criteria for valve replacement are often eligible for biologic prosthetic valves (tissue valves) and are typically treated with aspirin alone. Thrombotic or bleeding complications are rare in this patient population.[34,36] However, more commonly, we deal with patients with significant left-sided abnormalities of the aortic or mitral valves. Some of these patients who meet criteria for valve replacement may require a mechanical prosthetic heart valve and are treated with warfarin once the mechanical valve is placed. If a bioprosthetic valve is placed in the aortic position, then low-dose aspirin is often added to this regimen.[34,36]

6. *Other clinical indications:* The use of anticoagulation and antiplatelet therapy is variable in patients with intravascular stents. Patients are usually treated with low-dose aspirin for 6 months. Warfarin, LMWH, or clopidogrel may be added for high-risk patients, such as those with

prior thrombi or nonpulsatile flow through the stent.[34,38–41] Patients with cardiomyopathy and severe ventricular dysfunction are sometimes treated with low-dose unfractionated heparin, LMWH, or warfarin. The efficiency of this therapy is unclear. Studies suggest low-dose heparin may provide no benefit.[34] Patients with pulmonary arterial hypertension, especially those on intravenous medication to decrease pulmonary vascular resistance, are typically on anticoagulation therapy. The rationale is that thrombotic lesions (in situ pulmonary artery thromboses) and platelet dysfunction have been documented in patients with pulmonary vascular disease[42] and that anticoagulation may delay progression of disease.[34] Patients with atrial fibrillation are commonly on warfarin.[34,36]

ANESTHESIA AND SEDATION OF THE CARDIAC PATIENT

Over the past 20 years, the survival of children with CHD has increased substantially. These children are living longer, more active lives. As a result, children with many different cardiac diagnoses, ranging from physiologically insignificant to physiologically challenging complex CHD, are presenting for non–operating room diagnostic and interventional procedures requiring sedation or general anesthesia. Often, the need for sedation is related to evaluation of the underlying cardiac condition, such as cardiac catheterization, cardiac magnetic resonance imaging (MRI), or computed tomography (CT) imaging. Transthoracic echocardiography in infants and young children can be challenging, if not impossible, to accomplish without some form of sedation. Accurate information may best be gained by utilization of sedation.

These same children develop "common" pediatric conditions as well, such as otitis media, appendicitis, and limb fractures, which require operative intervention with sedation or general anesthesia. Dental health is essential in children with structural CHD. Children ranging in age from toddlers to adolescents can present for oral rehabilitation or oral surgery and require some form of sedation—ranging from mild sedation typically delivered in a dentist's office or clinic to general anesthesia in an operating room setting. Appreciation of an individual patient's physiology should guide the development of an appropriate sedation plan. Recent review articles have described these concerns in greater detail.[43]

The first guidelines for pediatric sedation were published in 1985 by the AAP in response to several sedation-related deaths in a dental office. Many other major organizations have followed with their own practice guidelines, including the AAP, the American Society of Anesthesiologists (ASA), the American College of Emergency Physicians, the American Academy of Pediatric Dentists, and the U.S. Joint Commission. The goals of these guidelines are simple: to share information among practitioners, to ensure the safe practice of pediatric sedation, and to create some standardization of care particularly relating to monitoring and management of pediatric sedation. Standardization of language has helped to decrease any confusion surrounding the use of these guidelines.[44] The ASA has defined sedation categories as "minimal," "moderate," or "deep" as well as "general anesthesia." These are clinical terms that have both level-of-consciousness guidelines as well as comments on the potential for physiologic disturbance rather than an absolute recommendation on specific drug administration (Table 16-13).

Children with cardiovascular disease, either structural or rhythm related, can pass through the stages of sedation more rapidly than an otherwise healthy child. The impact of a specific sedation regimen may also reduce the threshold to produce physiologic or rhythm abnormalities. The impact of even mild respiratory compromise in some patients, specifically those with pulmonary hypertension, can prove life threatening. Current ASA guidelines recommend that only personnel with training in the delivery of general anesthesia should administer deep sedation.[45]

Children 6 years of age and younger nearly always require deep sedation to successfully accomplish invasive procedures, and it should be assumed that this level of sedation will occur in this age group.[46] Many hospitals have developed pediatric sedation services using pediatric intensivists, hospitalists, and anesthesiologists to implement these guidelines, standardize care, and provide care to children in a variety of locations.

Goals of Sedation and Analgesia

The desired goals of each pediatric sedation encounter should be defined before initiation of any drug therapy. For instance, successful completion of most imaging studies requires only anxiolysis and sedation, not analgesia, whereas more painful procedures may require a deeper level of sedation or general anesthesia and administration of analgesics, including narcotics. For some imaging studies, the slightest movement may have a significant impact on the quality of information obtained, necessitating a general anesthetic to provide optimal imaging conditions. Involvement of child-life practitioners may be used initially to decrease anxiety in the child and parents before the procedure. Drug allergies should be reviewed. Careful attention to patient and parental preferences is important. Most patients with CHD have had multiple hospital experiences and, as a result, often have definitive preferences. Recognition

Levels of Sedation

Type	Description	Cardiovascular (CV) Effects	Airway
Minimal sedation	Responds normally and purposefully to verbal commands	Normal CV function	Normal respiratory function or respiratory state
Moderate sedation	Responds purposefully to verbal commands Older patients can be interactive Younger patients show age-appropriate behaviors	Normal CV function	No intervention needed to maintain a patent airway
Deep sedation	Not easily aroused Should respond purposefully to repeated painful or verbal stimuli	Normal CV function	May require assistance maintaining a patent airway Spontaneous ventilation may be inadequate Partial or complete loss of protective airway reflexes may occur (airway obstruction or aspiration)
General anesthesia	Medically controlled state of unconsciousness. Inability to respond purposefully to physical stimulation or verbal command	Cardiovascular function may be compromised	Loss of protective airway reflexes Inability to maintain a patent airway

of the primary goals of the patient and family, as well as the circumstance requiring sedation, will allow selection of the optimal drug regimen required to achieve satisfactory completion of the procedure with minimal patient risk.

Presedation Evaluation

A comprehensive presedation assessment is essential when planning the optimal timing, location, and magnitude of a procedure. This assessment can be particularly challenging given the wide spectrum of diagnoses and physiologies covered by CHD. For instance, children with unrepaired or palliated heart disease, especially infants and cyanotic patients, are often more fragile and require detailed assessment before even simple procedures. A child with a diagnosis of pulmonary hypertension may be particularly sensitive to changes in both cardiac and respiratory physiology. An understanding of the child's underlying lesion, clinical history, and current functional status, including recent changes in activity level and an assessment of the child's overall health status, is essential. Often, a cardiology consultation is necessary before proceeding, especially for noncardiac procedures. Open communication with the child's cardiologist, who may not be aware of an upcoming noncardiac procedure, may reveal ongoing concerns or planned cardiac procedures that may influence the timing and anesthetic management of the noncardiac procedure.

Careful note should be taken of current medications as well as any drug allergies or adverse reactions. Particular attention should be paid to anticoagulant medications, as these may need to be stopped or transitioned to other, shorter acting medications (eg, heparin infusion in hospital) prior to the procedure. Whenever appropriate, it is best to try to maintain the child's medication routine. The team should also review the cardiologist's recommendations and/or the recent AHA guidelines for bacterial endocarditis prophylaxis and ensure that appropriate prophylaxis is administered.

A physical examination is an important element of the presedation assessment, with particular attention being paid to the child's airway, chest, and heart. This assessment must be performed by an individual with training or experience evaluating an airway. Abnormalities such as micrognathia, macroglossia, and abnormal dentition should be noted and shared with the specific sedation/anesthesia provider because this may significantly influence the location of the planned procedure.

MEDICATIONS

There are several medications typically used for sedation and/or general anesthesia in children. The specific drug regimen chosen should be carefully tailored to meet the goals of sedation/anesthesia for a planned procedure.

Ketamine

Ketamine is an *N*-methyl-D-aspartate glutamate receptor antagonist that can provide sedation, amnesia, and profound analgesia with a minimum of negative side effects, especially in young children. Spontaneous ventilation and airway tone can generally be preserved. Ketamine has a favorable effect on hemodynamics in most patients; increased systemic vascular resistance, increased heart rate, and stable cardiac output are usually well tolerated. Although all sedative/anesthetic medications may have a negative effect on myocardial function, this effect is generally seen only in the catecholamine-depleted patient.

Benzodiazepines

Benzodiazepines are the most commonly used group of drugs in the pediatric sedation arsenal. They provide sedation, amnesia, and anxiolysis and have hypnotic and anticonvulsant properties.

Midazolam is short acting and water soluble and is the most commonly used benzodiazepine for premedication and procedural sedation in children. It can be administered orally, nasally, intramuscularly, or intravenously. Midazolam given orally (0.25-0.75 mg/kg to a maximum of 20 mg) has a predictable time to onset of 15 to 20 minutes after administration. Often, oral midazolam is administered before noxious stimulation such as intravenous line placement or induction of general anesthesia. Midazolam is a very effective anxiolytic and sedative but is rarely effective as the sole medication for invasive or lengthy procedures. Caution should be used when combining midazolam with opioids because adverse cardiovascular and respiratory effects are more likely to be seen in this circumstance. Rarely, midazolam administration can produce a paradoxical reaction. Respiratory depression, although rare, can occur as well. Flumazenil, a benzodiazepine antagonist, should always be available when these drugs are administered. Although flumazenil can reverse the respiratory depressant effects or dysphoria that can sometimes accompany benzodiazepine administration, it can also lower the seizure threshold and has a shorter half-life than midazolam, and as such, patients must be monitored closely after its administration for recurrence of midazolam-/benzodiazepine-induced respiratory depression.

Dexmedetomidine

Dexmedetomidine (Precedex) is a relative newcomer to the pediatric sedation/anesthesia drug armamentarium. It is a highly selective α_2-adrenoreceptor agonist with sedative, anxiolytic, and mild analgesic properties. Although not currently approved for infants and children in the United States, its use has been well described in multiple settings including the intensive care unit, operating room, cardiac catheterization laboratory, and radiology sedation units as a single sedative agent, an anesthetic adjuvant, and premedicant, as well as in other settings.

Dexmedetomidine is most commonly administered intravenously (IV) as follows: A loading dose of 0.5 to 1 µg/kg IV over 10 minutes, followed by an infusion of 0.2 to 2.0 µg/kg/h. Major advantages of dexmedetomidine include minimal risk of respiratory depression, rapid redistribution and elimination half-lives resulting in easy titration to effect, and relative physiologic stability. Decreases in heart rate and mean arterial blood pressure are the most commonly experienced cardiovascular side effects, especially at higher does over shorter infusion times. Hypertension may occasionally occur with rapid administration of the drug due to peripheral α_{2B}-receptor stimulation resulting in vasoconstriction. In most cases, cessation of the infusion terminates the bradycardia. Dexmedetomidine has been used as a sole sedative drug for both MRI and CT studies, although children may require a slightly higher infusion rate for satisfactory completion of MRI. Lower doses of dexmedetomidine have been used when administered in conjunction with a benzodiazepine. When compared with propofol, dexmedetomidine has a slightly longer time to onset but resulted in fewer episodes of hypotension and desaturation.[47] Dexmedetomidine has been used successfully in patients with tachyarrhythmias but should be used cautiously in children with known bradydysrhythmias or heart block.

Propofol

With the recent lack of availability of pentothal, propofol has become the most frequently used drug for the induction of general anesthesia in the United States. Propofol (Diprivan) is a potent hypnotic drug with sedative and amnestic properties. Its rapid onset, short duration of action, short recovery time, easy titratability, and antiemetic properties make it an appealing drug for procedures requiring sedation with a natural airway as well. It can be administered IV either as a bolus of 1 to 2 mg/kg (yielding 3-5 minutes of sedation; 5 minutes of sedation is ideal for CT scanning or fast procedures such as chest tube placement or dental extractions) or by infusion for longer procedures, such as MRI studies.

Propofol can have significant cardiorespiratory effects, including hypotension, myocardial depression, and respiratory depression and, as such, should be regarded deliberately in medically fragile patients. It is also associated with pain upon injection, particularly when injected through a small IV, making it a less desirable drug to be used in isolation in children. Premedication with intravenous lidocaine may obviate some of

this discomfort. Myoclonus may also be seen, especially after the infusion is terminated in older children.

In many institutions, the administration of both propofol and dexmedetomidine for sedation has not been restricted only to individuals trained in anesthesiology and airway management. This practice remains controversial because the continuum between "conscious sedation" or "mild sedation" and "deep sedation" or "general anesthesia" can be traversed rapidly, especially in medically fragile patients. The physiologic effects of respiratory compromise or myocardial depression must be recognized and treated quickly, especially in children with CHD. The ASA has consistently supported the practice that propofol administration be restricted to individuals trained in the practice of anesthesia and airway management or those closely supervised by these individuals.

As survival of patients with CHD continues to increase, there will be an increase in the demand for sedation and anesthesia both within and outside the "traditional" cardiac care environment. The specific goals for sedation and anesthesia in these venues continue to evolve, and there will remain significant variation in the physiologic status of patients carrying the same cardiac diagnosis. For these reasons, there must continue to be an emphasis on the presedation and preanesthetic evaluation, definition of the goals of sedation for a given procedure, active involvement of the cardiology services in evaluating and preparing patients for procedures, and open communication with the team providing the sedation services. This will allow deliberate preparation of a sedation plan, drug selection, and postsedation monitoring plan to maximize the potential for safe and successful completion of the planned procedure.

Clinical Pearls

- Maintenance of oral health is important in preventing endocarditis in patients with congenital heart disease (CHD).
- When advising on contraception and pregnancy, the risks of all medications taken by the patient should be considered, including possible teratogenic effects on the fetus.
- RVS prophylaxis is important for young patients who are receiving medication to control congestive heart failure or who have pulmonary hypertension or cyanotic heart disease. Immunization against seasonal influenza is critical in decreasing morbidity and mortality in patients with CHD.
- The immunocompromise seen in patients with DiGeorge or heterotaxy syndrome may affect what vaccines they are eligible for.
- The clinician must be familiar with medications that can prolong the QT interval to avoid potentially fatal arrhythmias. Drug–drug interactions and electrolyte anomalies should also be considered.

- Unless contraindicated by a cardiologist, it is reasonable to use stimulant medication for attention-deficit hyperactive disorder in most patients with structural heart disease (repaired or unrepaired), as long as they do not have significant hemodynamic or arrhythmic burden.
- Some patients require anticoagulation. The clinician needs to promote appropriate medication use and laboratory monitoring to avoid issues with thrombosis or bleeding.
- Patients with pulmonary hypertension, arrhythmias, or cyanotic heart disease may not tolerate sedation well. A presedation assessment is of great value, and trained personal must be available during procedures requiring sedation.

REFERENCES

1. Kaltman JR, Andropoulos DB, Checchia PA, et al. The Perioperative Working Group, report of the Pediatric Heart Network and National Heart, Lung, and Blood Institute Working Group on the perioperative management of congenital heart disease. *Circulation.* 2010;121:2766-2772.

2. Section on Pediatric Dentistry and Oral Health. Policy statement: preventive oral health intervention for pediatricians. *Pediatrics.* 2008;122:1387-1394.

3. Perce KM, Rozier RG, Vann WF Jr. Accuracy of pediatric primary care providers' screening and referral for early childhood caries. Department of Pediatric Dentistry, University of North Carolina at Chapel Hill, Chapel Hill, North Carolina, USA. *Pediatrics.* 2002;109:E82-E82.

4. Rose LF, Mealey B, Minsk L, et al. Oral care for patients with cardiovascular disease and stroke. *J Am Dent Assoc.* 2002;133:37S-44S.

5. Wilson W, Taubert KA, Gewitz M, et al. Prevention of infective endocarditis: guidelines from the American Heart Association: a guideline from the American Heart Association Rheumatic Fever, Endocarditis, and Kawasaki Disease Committee, Council on Cardiovascular Disease in the Young, and the Council on Clinical Cardiology, Council on Cardiovascular Surgery and Anesthesia, and the Quality of Care and Outcomes Research Interdisciplinary Working Group, and The Council on Scientific Affairs of the American Dental Association has approved the guideline as it relates to dentistry. *Circulation.* 2007;116: 1736-1754.

6. American Academy of Pediatrics. Policy statement: organizational principles to guide and define the child health care system and/or improve the health of all children, Section on Pediatric Dentistry Oral Health Risk Assessment Timing and Establishment of the Dental Home. *Pediatrics.* 2009;111:5.

7. Braun A, Dehn C, Krause F, Jepsen S. Short-term clinical effects of adjunctive antimicrobial photodynamic therapy in periodontal treatment: a randomized clinical trial. *J Clin Periodontol.* 2008;35:877-884.

8. Hajim KI, Salih DS, Rassam YZ. Laser light combined with a photosensitizer may eliminate methicillin-resistant strains of *Staphylococcus aureus. Lasers Med Sci.* 2010; 25:743-748.

9. Nishimura RA, Carabello BA, Faxon DP, et al. ACC/AHA 2008 guideline update on valvular heart disease: focused update on infective endocarditis: a report of the American College of Cardiology/American Heart Association Task Force on Practice Guidelines. *Circulation.* 2008;118; 887-896.

10. Baddour LM, Epstein AE, Erickson CC, et al. Update on cardiovascular implantable electronic device infections and their management, a scientific statement from the American Heart Association endorsed by the Heart Rhythm Society. *Circulation.* 2010;121;458-477.

11. Vigil M, Kaemmerer M, Medb C, et al. Contraception in women with congenital heart disease. *Am J Cardiol.* 2010;106:1317-1321.

12. Silversides CK, Sermer M, Siu SC. Choosing the best contraceptive method for the adult with congenital heart disease. *Curr Cardiol Rep.* 2009;11:298-305.

13. Warnes CA, Williams RG, Bashore TM. ACC/AHA 2008 guidelines for the management of adults with congenital heart disease. *J Am Coll Cardiol.* 2008;52:1-121.

14. Kovacs AH, Harrison JL, Colman JM, et al. Pregnancy and contraception in congenital heart disease: what women are not told. *J Am Coll Cardiol.* 2008,52:577-578.

15. Centers for Disease Control and Prevention. Vaccines and immunizations. Available at: http://www.cdc.gov/vaccines/2011. Accessed October 19, 2011.

16. Meissner HC, Long SS; Committee on Infectious Diseases, Committee on Fetus and Newborn. Revised indications for the use of palivizumab and respiratory syncytial virus immune globulin intravenous for the prevention of respiratory syncytial virus infections. *Pediatrics.* 2003;112: 1447-1452.

17. Committee on Infectious Diseases. Modified recommendations for use of palivizumab for prevention of respiratory syncytial virus infections. *Pediatrics.* 2009;124:1694-1701.

18. American Academy of Pediatrics. Policy statement—modified recommendations for use of palivizumab for prevention of respiratory syncytial virus infections. *Pediatrics.* 2009;124:1694-1701.

19. Davis MM, Taubert K, Benin AL, et al. Influenza vaccination as secondary prevention for cardiovascular disease: a science advisory from the American Heart Association/American College of Cardiology. *Circulation.* 2006;114:1549-1553.

20. Fiore AE, Uyeki TM, Broder K, et al. Prevention and control of influenza with vaccines: recommendations of the Advisory Committee on Immunization Practices (ACIP). *MMWR.* 2010;59:1-62.

21. Heist EK, Ruskin JN. Drug-induced arrhythmias. *Circulation.* 2010;122:1426-1435.

22. Benson AP, Al-Owais M, Holden AV. Quantitative prediction of the arrhythmogenic effects of de novo hERG mutations in computational models of human ventricular tissues. *Eur Biophys J.* 2011;40:627-639.

23. Arizona Center for Education and Research on Therapeutics. QT drugs by risk groups. Available at: http://www.qtdrugs.org. Accessed October 19, 2011.

24. Arizona Center for Education and Research on Therapeutics. Homepage. Available at: http://www.azcert.org. Accessed October 19, 2011.

25. Keller GA, Ponte ML, Di Girolamo G. Other drugs acting on nervous system associated with QT-interval prolongation. *Curr Drug Saf.* 2010;5:105-111.

26. Keller GA, Di Girolamo G. Antihistamines: past answers and present questions. *Curr Drug Saf.* 2010;5:58-64.

27. American Academy of Pediatrics/American Heart Association. American Academy of Pediatrics/American Heart Association clarification of statement on cardiovascular evaluation and monitoring of children and adolescents with heart disease receiving medications for ADHD. Endorsed by the American Academy of Child and Adolescent Psychiatry, the American College of Cardiology, Children and Adults with Attention-Deficit/Hyperactivity Disorder, the National Initiative for Children's Healthcare Quality and the Society for Developmental and Behavioral Pediatrics. *J Dev Behav Pediatr.* 2008;9:335-335.

28. Newcorn JH, Donnelly C. Cardiovascular safety of medication treatments for attention-deficit/hyperactivity disorder. *Mount Sinai J Med.* 2009;76:198-203.

29. Bukstein OG. Clinical practice guidelines for attention-deficit/hyperactivity disorder: a review. *Postgrad Med.* 2010;122:69-77.

30. William O. Cooper, Laurel A. Habel, Colin M. Sox, et al. ADHD Drugs and Serious Cardiovascular Events in Children and Young Adults. *N Engl J Med.* 2011; 365:1896-1904.

31. Elia J, Vetter VL. Cardiovascular effects of medications for the treatment of attention-deficit hyperactivity disorder: what is known and how should it influence prescribing in children? *Paediatr Drugs.* 2010;12:165-175.

32. Giglia TM, Massicotte P, Barst RJ. et al. Prevention and treatment of thrombosis in children and adults with congenital heart disease and in children with acquired heart disease. *Circulation.* In press.

33. Trenor CC III. Thrombosis and thrombophilia: principles for pediatric patients. *Blood Coagul Fibrinolysis.* 2010;21:S11-S15.

34. Monagle P, Chalmers E, Chan A, et al. Antithrombotic therapy in neonates and children: American College of Chest Physicians evidence-based clinical practice guidelines (8th edition). *Chest.* 2008;133:877S-986S.

35. Anderson PAW, Breitbart RE, McCrindle BW, et al. The Fontan patient: inconsistencies in medication therapy across seven pediatric heart network centers. *Pediatr Cardiol.* 2010;31:1219-1228.

36. Silva RL, De Sousa JC, Calisto C, et al. Oral anticoagulant therapy. Fundamentals, clinical practice and recommendations. *Rev Port Cardiol.* 2007;26:769-788.

37. O'Connor MJ, Ravishankar C, Ballweg JA, et al. Early systemic-to-pulmonary artery shunt intervention in neonates 5 with congenital heart disease. *J Thorac Cardiovasc Surg.* 2011;142:106-112.

38. Singer DE, Albers GW, Dalen JE, et al. Antithrombotic therapy in atrial fibrillation: American College of Chest Physicians evidence-based clinical practice guidelines (8th edition). *Chest.* 2008;133:546S-592S.

39. Otis SA, Zehnder JL. Heparin-induced thrombocytopenia: current status and diagnostic challenges. *Am J Hematol.* 2010;85:700-706.

40. Kuhle S, Eulmesekian P, Kavanagh B, et al. A clinically significant incidence of bleeding in critically ill children receiving therapeutic doses of unfractionated heparin: a prospective cohort study. *Haematologica.* 2007;92:244-247.

41. Holmes DR Jr, Dehmer GJ, Kaul S, et al. ACCF/AHA clopidogrel clinical alert: approaches to the FDA "boxed warning": a report of the American College of Cardiology Foundation Task Force on Clinical Expert Consensus Documents and the American Heart Association. *Circulation.* 2010;122:537-557.

42. Kawut SM, Bagiella E, Shimbo D, et al. The ASA-STAT Study Group: rationale and design of a phase II clinical trial of aspirin and simvastatin for the treatment of pulmonary arterial hypertension: ASA-STAT. *Contemp Clin Trials.* 2011;32:280-287.

43. Diaz LK, Jones L. Sedating the child with congenital heart disease. *Anesthesiol Clin.* 2009;27:301-319.

44. American Society of Anesthesiologists Task Force on Sedation and Analgesia by Non-Anesthesiologists. Practice guidelines for sedation and analgesia by non-anesthesiologists. *Anesthesiology.* 2002;96:1004-1017.

45. Statement on granting privileges to non-anesthesiologist practitioners for personally administering deep sedation or supervising deep sedation by individuals who are not anesthesia professionals. Approved by the American Society of Anesthesiologists House of Delegates on October 18, 2006. Available at: http://www.asahq.org/For-Healthcare-Professionals/Standards-Guidelines-and-Statements.aspxwww.asahq.org. Accessed October 19, 2011.

46. Cote CJ. Strategies for preventing sedation accidents. *Pediatr Ann.* 2005;34:625-633.

47. Koroglu A, Teksan H, Sagir O, et al. A comparison of the sedative, hemodynamic, and respiratory effects of dexmedetomidine and propofol in children undergoing magnetic resonance imaging. *Anesth Analg.* 2006;103:63-67.

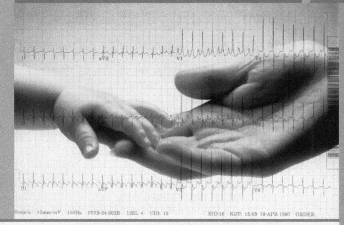

CHAPTER 17

Survival to Adulthood

Alex Davidson, Yuli Y. Kim,
Stephanie Fuller and
David Drajpuch

INTRODUCTION

Approximately 90% of children born with congenital heart disease (CHD) are expected to reach adulthood.[1] With advances in surgical and medical treatment, there are now more adults than children living with CHD,[2] with a current estimated 1.3 million adults with CHD in the United States.[3–5] This burgeoning population is accompanied by a set of specialized healthcare needs and quality-of-life concerns. Understanding what to expect for patients, parents, and their healthcare providers is essential for the well-being and adjustment of these children as they grow up into young adulthood and beyond.

The purpose of this chapter is to review the quality of life of survivors of CHD, their ongoing medical needs, and the setting and team needed to provide them with optimal care past the pediatric age group.

TRANSITION OF CARE

It is increasingly important to prepare the pediatric patient with CHD and their family for transition into the adult healthcare system. *Transition* is defined as the "purposeful and planned movement of adolescents and young adults with chronic physical and medical conditions from child-centered to adult-oriented healthcare systems."[6] Young adults are at risk for being lost to care during this time period; it is estimated that between one half and three quarters of adults with CHD do not have regular cardiology follow-up.[7,8] For those who are lost to follow-up, there is a 3-fold increase in the need for an urgent intervention such as cardiac catheterization or surgery.[8]

Although several models have been proposed for transition,[9] it is generally agreed that the goal is for the patient to enter the adult care environment and to establish accountability for their own medical care including communication, autonomy, self-care, and self-advocacy (Table 17-1).[10–12] The healthcare team, the family, and the patient must work together to achieve successful transition. The process should begin in childhood at an appropriate age for the individual child's psychosocial maturation and neurodevelopment.[13] Providers should begin early, age-appropriate education of the patient to encourage understanding of his or her disease process. As they develop into teenagers, patients should be given more autonomy, and a portion of the office visit should be conducted without the family present.[10] This should be framed in such a way that the family sees their role as one of encouragement and empowerment, but does not feel excluded from the patient's care. It is imperative that the family be prepared early in the transition process to allow increasing autonomy for the pediatric patient who will one day be responsible for his or her own care. The probability of a successful transition increases dramatically when pediatric providers set the stage for the following 2 fundamental transition goals: patient education about their medical condition and parental encouragement to allow their child the independence to take an active role in their own care.[14] A summary of the recommendations from the 32nd Bethesda Conference on key elements and strategies for successful transition can be found in Table 17-2.

Once the adolescent or young adult has successfully achieved accountability for his or her own care, then the patient is ready for transfer. *Transfer* is the period when the adolescent or young adult patient leaves the pediatric environment and enters the adult healthcare system. Most agree that the end of adolescence, around 18 years of age or at the completion of schooling, is the correct

Key Areas of Patient Mastery for Successful Transition

■ Understanding of cardiac anatomy and interventions
  performed
■ Exercise recommendations
■ Health maintenance and follow-up including making ap-
  pointments (cardiology, primary care, dental care, etc)
■ Insurance information
■ Medications
■ Genetic counseling
■ Occupation and education guidance
■ Fertility, contraception, and pregnancy

Data from Hudsmith LE, Thorne SA. Transition of care from paediatric to adult services in cardiology. Arch Dis Child. 2007;92:927-930; and Knauth A, Verstappen A, Reiss J, Webb GD. Transition and transfer from pediatric to adult care of the young adult with complex congenital heart disease. Cardiol Clin. 2006;24:619-629.

time to undergo this process.[7] Although an institutional policy should be developed stating when transfer is to take place, timing must be flexible to adjust to the social and mental development of the patient.

Who should the young adult with CHD see when transitioning to adult care? The American College of Cardiology (ACC)/American Heart Association (AHA) 2008 Guidelines for the Management of Adults With Congenital Heart Disease[12] have made recommendations for delivery of and access to care depending on the severity of underlying lesion (Table 17-3). Patients with moderate and complex CHD should be followed regularly at a regional adult CHD center. These quaternary referral centers are composed of a multidisciplinary team of healthcare practitioners experienced in the care of the adult with CHD. Patients with simple lesions should have at least 1 visit with a regional adult CHD center to formulate plans for future care and follow-up.

Finally, successful transition cannot be measured in a single appointment completed with an adult provider. Success occurs when the patient and family are able to transition their healthcare from a pediatric to an adult environment without disruption in care. Ultimately, this will enhance patients' physical and emotional health, resulting in improved quality of life.

BURDEN OF ONGOING CARE AND REINTERVENTION IN ADULT LIFE

As the adult CHD population continues to grow as the result of improvement in pediatric care, there will be an increasing number of adults who are dependent on specialists for their medical and interventional management. Adults with CHD may have symptoms related to residual defects and altered physiology. Complications may include arrhythmia, heart failure, endocarditis, psychosocial issues, and sudden death.[15]

The Euro Heart Survey on adult CHD assessed clinical and demographic characteristics of an adult CHD population over a 5-year period.[16] The information was extracted from charts of over 4000 patients

Summary of Recommendations for Transition

Key Elements for Effective Transition	Strategies for Successful Transition
A defined age for when patients will transfer care (with some flexibility)	The transition process begins before adolescence.
Education to prepare patients and families to function in an adult healthcare setting	There is a formal transition program.
Coordinated transfer plan including a transfer summary and a designated transfer provider in the adult clinic	Patients are not transferred to an adult program until they are mature enough and have the skills to thrive in that environment.
A competent adult cardiac provider/team	There is an identified provider for both the pediatric and adult teams to facilitate transition.
Administrative support	Management, financial, and contractual issues are worked out between the pediatric and adult institutions.
Primary care provider cooperation	Continual quality improvement of the process.
	Transfer occurs during a period of medical stability.
	Inclusion of the pediatric team after transfer has taken place.

Modified with permission from Foster E, Graham TP Jr, Driscoll DJ, et al. Task Force 2: special health care needs of adults with congenital heart disease. J Am Coll Cardiol. 2001;37:1176-1183.

Simple, Moderate, and Complex Adult CHD

Simple	Moderate	Complex
■ Congenital AS	■ Aorto-LV fistulae	■ Conduits, valved or nonvalved
■ Congenital mitral valve disease	■ PAPVR or TAPVR	■ Cyanotic congenital heart disease
■ PFO/ASD	■ AVC defects	■ Double-outlet ventricle
■ VSD	■ Coarctation of the aorta	■ Eisenmenger
■ Mild PS	■ Ebstein anomaly	■ Fontan
■ Previously ligated or occluded ductus arteriosus	■ Sub-PS	■ Mitral atresia
	■ PDA	■ Single ventricle
■ Repaired secundum or sinus venosus defect without residua	■ PR (mod-severe)	■ Pulmonary atresia
	■ PS (mod-severe)	■ Pulmonary vascular disease
■ Repaired VSD without residua	■ Sinus of valsalva fistula/aneurysm	■ Transposition
	■ Sinus venosus defect	■ Tricuspid atresia
	■ Sub- or supravalvar AS	■ Truncus arteriosus
	■ TOF	
	■ VSD with associated lesions	

AS, aortic stenosis; ASD, atrial septal defect; AVC, atrioventricular canal; LV, left ventricle; PAPVR, partial anomalous pulmonary venous return; PDA, patent ductus arteriosus; PFO, patent foramen ovale; PR, pulmonary regurgitation; PS, pulmonic stenosis; TAPVR, total anomalous pulmonary venous return; TOF, tetralogy of Fallot; VSD, ventricular septal defect.
Modified with permission from Clarizia NA, Chahal N, Manlhiot C, Kilburn J, Redington AN, McCrindle BW. Transition to adult health care for adolescents and young adults with congenital heart disease: Perspectives of the patient, parent and health care provider. Can J Cardiol. 2009;25:e317-e322.

from 1998 through 2003. Both quality of life and morbidity were highly related to the type of CHD. For example, mortality and deterioration of functional class were, not surprisingly, highest for patients with cyanotic or single-ventricle defects, whereas insertion of a permanent pacemaker was most frequent in patients with the diagnoses of transposition, Fontan circulation, and tetralogy of Fallot. Approximately 20% of the patients underwent surgery or a catheter-based intervention during the follow-up period. Arrhythmias were the most common cause for hospitalization in this population, particularly supraventricular tachycardia. Patients visited the outpatient clinic approximately 3 times in 2 years. More than one half of the patients were taking chronic medication, albeit some for prophylaxis. For example, Fontan patients are likely to be on antiarrhythmic medications as well as anticoagulants, whereas diuretics are more commonly used in patients with right-sided heart failure.

Adults with CHD who are referred for intervention, either percutaneous or surgical, fall into the following categories: those without previous reparative surgery or those with complete anatomic or physiologic repair returning for revisions because of residual defects or sequelae from their repairs. More common diagnoses in patients without previous surgery include atrial septal defect, aortic valve disease, coarctation of the aorta, and patent ductus arteriosus. For adults who have undergone surgical palliation during childhood, common conditions requiring reintervention include patch leaks, recurrent valvular or outflow tract stenoses, valve regurgitation, recurrent coarctation, arrhythmias, homograft valve stenosis, regurgitation, or aneurysm formation. Both primary repair and repeat operations are complex anatomically, and often patients suffer from abnormal physiology. Therefore, interventional care requires a multidisciplinary team experienced in both pediatric and adult cardiology and cardiac surgery.

Thorough evaluation of the patient is necessary as anatomic and physiologic complications evolve. Commonly, long-standing cyanosis and pressure or volume overload may result in uni- or biventricular dysfunction. Pulmonary vascular resistance may be affected by long-standing excessive flow and may make repair challenging and even impossible later in life. Therefore, a thorough and comprehensive plan of care must be established for each patient individually before consideration of repair and revision.

Preoperative planning begins with echocardiographic assessment. An additional imaging study such as magnetic resonance imaging or computerized tomography is useful in evaluating the proximity of vascular structures to the posterior sternum as well as providing flow-related and anatomic data. When performing repeat sternotomy, consideration is often given to femoral vessel access for institution of cardiopulmonary bypass. In many patients, however, previous cardiac catheterizations have resulted in femoral venous and/or arterial occlusion. Therefore, all patients need to have preoperative 4-extremity duplex imaging of the femoral, carotid, and jugular systems. Men age 35 years or older, premenopausal women age 35 years or older with risk factors for atherosclerosis, and postmenopausal women may need evaluation by cardiac catheterization and coronary angiography to rule out associated coronary artery disease before they undergo repeat cardiac surgery. Additional testing, such as exercise testing and nuclear perfusion scans for regional ischemia, are used as necessary.

Arrhythmias are common in patients with CHD and contribute to significant morbidity and medical burden. Treatment can involve surgical or catheter-based ablation, implantation of pacemakers, or antitachycardia devices. Most indications for treatment are derived from studies of acquired adult heart disease. However, special considerations must be given to the structurally abnormal heart with distorted anatomic landmarks, abnormal locations of the atrioventricular node, and a high incidence of multiple conduction pathways. In patients who cannot have transvenous pacemakers, such as single-ventricle Fontan patients, epicardial lead placement at the time of surgical reintervention must be considered.

Treatment of specific lesions is summarized in Table 17-4. Additionally, Table 17-5 summarizes the arrhythmias commonly encountered in different CHD conditions.

The incidence of atrial flutter is highest after the Senning, Mustard, or Fontan operations. Atrial fibrillation is controlled in some patients by drug therapy. For those undergoing concomitant surgery for revision, the maze procedure is performed. Ventricular tachycardia is most common in patients with a history of ventriculotomy such as those with repair of tetralogy of Fallot using a transannular patch. Treatment is usually an implantable cardioverter-defibrillator or catheter ablation. For patients with bradycardia and sinoatrial node dysfunction, pacemaker insertion is recommended for patients with resting heart rate of less than 40 beats per minute or sinus pauses longer than 3 seconds.[12] Clear knowledge of specific anatomy and review of all surgical records are important before pacemaker insertion because not all patients can undergo transvenous insertion.

EXERCISE

In discussing exercise in adult patients with CHD, we will review the contribution of exercise testing to the management of patients, the merits of exercise training in those patients, and guidelines for safe participation in sports activities.

Exercise testing is a valuable tool in the evaluation of patients with CHD. Assessment of a patient's functional status is prognostic and can predict risk of future adverse events and death. However, estimating functional capacity by subjective reporting is not reliable because patients

with CHD have developed lifelong physical and psychosocial adaptations to their condition and grossly overestimate their physical capabilities compared to aerobic capacity by exercise testing.[17] Even supposedly asymptomatic adult CHD patients (New York Heart Association [NYHA] functional class I), with minor defects like coarctation of the aorta and repaired atrial septal defects, had significantly lower peak oxygen uptake values (Vo_2) than healthy subjects of similar age.[18]

Multiple studies have demonstrated the prognostic value of various parameters of exercise testing in patients with CHD. Diller et al.[18] demonstrated that peak Vo_2 is reduced in adult CHD patients across all diagnostic groups compared to healthy subjects of similar age but is variable according to underlying lesion, with patients with complex lesions, such as congenitally corrected transposition of the great arteries, and Eisenmenger patients having the worst exercise capacity. Heart rate response, pulmonary arterial hypertension, cyanosis, pulmonary function, and underlying cardiac anatomy were important correlates of exercise capacity. Impaired peak Vo_2 predicted hospitalization and death over the year following exercise testing even after accounting for age, sex, NYHA class, laboratory parameters, and underlying cardiac lesions.

In addition to peak Vo_2, VE/Vco_2 slope, or the ventilatory cost of clearing a unit of carbon dioxide, is another exercise parameter that has been shown to be an important predictor of outcomes in adults with CHD. VE/Vco_2 slope has been shown to be elevated (ie, excessive ventilatory response to exercise) in adults with CHD with a variety of lesions, especially those that have associated cyanosis, which is a powerful stimulus for this response. An increased VE/Vco_2 slope is associated with increased mortality in noncyanotic patients, with slopes ≥ 38 identifying noncyanotic patients with a 10-fold increase in mortality.[19]

Abnormalities in *heart rate response* are common in adult CHD, affecting approximately 60% of all patients and greater than 80% of those with functional single-ventricle physiology.[20,21] In a study of 727 consecutive adults with CHD, an abnormal heart rate response to exercise, or chronotropic incompetence, was an independent risk factor for death. *Heart rate reserve*, or the rate of decrease in heart rate after cessation of exercise, was associated with greater mortality even after accounting for antiarrhythmic medication and exercise capacity.[20]

Thus, exercise testing is important in stratifying the functional status of adult CHD patients and evaluating their risk of adverse events and death. Exercise performance should be compared to measurements in other patients with similar heart disease. Figure 17-1 presents reference values of peak oxygen uptake for adult patients with various congenital cardiac conditions.[17,18,20,22-25]

Interventions for Specific Malformations Commonly Encountered in Adulthood

Diagnosis	Presentation in Adulthood	Treatment
Atrial septal defect	Syncope Embolic stroke Reduced exercise tolerance Atrial fibrillation Cyanosis and pulmonary hypertension with right ventricular failure Shunt >1.5:1	Percutaneous catheter-based device closure Open surgical repair using pericardial or synthetic patch Pulmonary vasodilator therapy for pulmonary hypertension Maze procedure for atrial fibrillation
Ventricular septal defect	Atrial or ventricular arrhythmia Endocarditis Aortic regurgitation Shunt >1.5:1	Surgical closure: direct suture repair if <3 mm vs patch closure if >3 mm Percutaneous catheter device closure for muscular VSDs
Atrioventricular septal defects	Atrial fibrillation Pulmonary hypertension with right ventricular failure Mitral regurgitation or stenosis	Primary surgical repair with pericardial patch, closure of mitral cleft, closure of VSD Repair or replacement of mitral valve
Patent ductus arteriosus	Pulmonary hypertension Endocarditis	Percutaneous catheter device closure Surgical closure for severely aneurysmal or calcified ductus
Coarctation of aorta	Hypertension Aortic aneurysm Systolic blood pressure gradient >30 mm Hg	Catheter-based stenting Surgical resection of coarctation and end-to-end anastomosis, extra-anatomic bypass, or interposition graft
Tetralogy of Fallot	Exercise intolerance Ventricular arrhythmia Residual right ventricular outflow tract stenosis (right ventricle/left ventricle pressure >2/3) Residual VSD Severe pulmonary insufficiency complicated by right ventricular dilatation or dysfunction Aortic root dilatation >5.5 cm	Percutaneous catheter-based stent placement for conduit stenosis or valve insertion in select patients Supraventricular or ventricular arrhythmia, which should be treated with catheter ablation[8] Surgical repair for small conduit, presence of aortopulmonary collateral vessels, or residual VSD
Transposition of great arteries	Exercise intolerance due to baffle obstruction or leak after atrial switch Atrial arrhythmias after atrial switch Aortic root dilation after arterial switch Pulmonary stenosis after arterial switch	Percutaneous catheter-based stent placement in baffles or leak occlusion if amenable, and dilation and stenting of pulmonary stenosis Surgical repair for aortic root dilation and for those lesions not amenable to catheter-based therapy
Single ventricle	Atrial arrhythmias Stroke or embolic events Pulmonary arteriovenous malformations Plastic bronchitis Protein-losing enteropathy	Fontan conversion from atriopulmonary to lateral tunnel or extracardiac Open maze procedure or epicardial pacemaker Percutaneous catheter-based intervention for occlusion of fenestration Heart transplantation

(Continued)

Interventions for Specific Malformations Commonly Encountered in Adulthood (Continued)

Ebstein anomaly	Cyanosis Decrease in exercise tolerance Refractory arrhythmias	Surgical repair or replacement of tricuspid valve

VSD, ventricular septal defect.

Data from the following references:

Stulak J, Burkhart H, Dearani J, et al. Reoperations after inital repair of complete atrioventricular septal defect. Ann Thorac Surg. 2009;87:1872-1878.

Birim O, van Gameren M, de Jong P, Witsenburgh M, van Osch-Gevers L, Bogers AJ. Outcome after reopeartion for atrioventricular septal defect repair. Interact Cardiovasc Thorac Surg. 2009;9:83-88.

Hanley FL, Fenton KN, Jonas RA, et al. Surgical repair of complete atrioventricular canal defects in infancy. Twenty-year trends. J Thorac Cardiovasc Surg. 1993;106:387-394.

Arakelyan V, Spiridonov A, Bockeria L. Ascending-to-descending aortic bypass via right thoracotomy for complex (re-) coarctation and hypoplastic aortic arch. Eur J Cardiothorac Surg. 2005;27:815-820.

Stulak J, Dearani J, Puga F, Zehr KJ, Schaff H, Danielson GK. Right-sided maze procedure for atrial tachyarrhythmias in congenital heart disease. Ann Thorac Surg. 2006; 81:1780-1785.

Murphy J, Gersh B, Mair D, et al. Long-term outcome in patients undergoing surgical repair of tetralogy of Fallot. N Engl J Med. 1993;329:593-599.

Nollert G, Fischlein T, Bouterwek S, Böhmer C, Klinner W, Reichart B. Long-term survival in patients with repair of tetralogy of Fallot: 36-year follow-up of 490 survivors of the first year after surgical repair. J Am Coll Cardiol. 1997;30:1374-1383.

Oechslin EN, Harrison DA, Harris L, et al. Reoperation in adults with repair of tetralogy of fallot: indications and outcomes. J Thorac Cardiovasc Surg. 1999;118:245-251.

Bacha EA, Scheule AM, Zurakowski D, et al. Long-term results after early primary repair of tetralogy of Fallot. J Thorac Cardiovasc Surg. 2001;122:154-161.

Therrien J, Provost Y, Merchant N, Williams W, Colman J, Webb G. Optimal timing for pulmonary valve replacement in adults after tetralogy of Fallot repair. Am J Cardiol. 2005;95:779-782.

de Ruijter RTH, Weenink I, Hitchcock FJ, Meijboom EJ, Bennink GB. Right ventricular dysfunction and pulmonary valve replacement after correction of tetralogy of Fallot. Ann Thorac Surg. 2002;73:1794-1800.

Williams WG, McCrindle BW, Ashburn DA, et al. Outcomes of 829 neonates with complete transposition of the great arteries 12-17 years after repair. Eur J Cardiothorac Surg. 2003;24:1-9.

Rhythm Disturbances in Adults with Congenital Heart Disease

Rhythm Disturbance	Associated Lesions
Wolff-Parkinson-White syndrome	Ebstein anomaly Congenitally corrected transposition
Intra-atrial re-entrant tachycardia (atrial flutter)	Postoperative Mustard Postoperative Senning Postoperative Fontan Tetralogy of Fallot
Atrial fibrillation	Mitral valve disease Aortic stenosis Tetralogy of Fallot Palliated single ventricle
Ventricular tachycardia	Tetralogy of Fallot Aortic stenosis
Sinus node dysfunction	Postoperative Mustard Postoperative Senning Postoperative Fontan Sinus venosus atrial septal defect Heterotaxy syndrome
Spontaneous atrioventricular block	Atrioventricular canal defects Congenitally corrected transposition
Surgically induced atrioventricular block	Ventricular septal defect closure Subaortic stenosis relief Atrioventricular valve replacement

Sports are important social and recreational activities that promote general health and self-esteem. The benefits of regular physical activity are myriad; exercise can reduce depression and anxiety, improve self-esteem, and be beneficial in chronic heart failure, obesity, and diabetes. Furthermore, exercise improves quality of life and has been shown to lower mortality. Walking remains the mainstay of exercise prescription for adult cardiac patients as part of home-based programs. In a prospective study, exercise training for 10 weeks increased

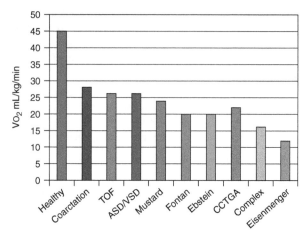

FIGURE 17-1 ■ Peak oxygen consumption (Vo₂) in adult congenital heart disease by underlying lesion. ASD, atrial septal defect; CCTGA, congenitally corrected transposition of the great arteries; TOF, tetralogy of Fallot; VSD, ventricular septal defect.

overall physical activity and treadmill test walking time and improved quality of life in adult CHD patients.[26]

Exercise can be divided into 2 types that represent the extremes of a continuum, with most physical activity having a component of both. Dynamic (isotonic) exercise involves changes in muscle length with rhythmic contractions that develop a relatively small intramuscular force. Static (isometric) exercise involves development of a large intramuscular force with little or no change in muscle length. Dynamic exercise causes a marked increase in oxygen consumption. Cardiac output, stroke volume, heart rate, and systolic blood pressure are increased. There is a smaller increase in mean blood pressure and a decrease in systemic vascular resistance and diastolic blood pressure. Dynamic exercise is a volume load to the heart. Static exercise causes only a small increase in oxygen consumption, cardiac output, and heart rate. It causes marked increases in systolic, diastolic, and mean blood pressure. Static exercise represents a pressure load to the heart. Dynamic exercise uses primarily aerobic muscle metabolism, whereas static exercise is mostly anaerobic.[27,28]

Guidelines exist for the participation of patients with cardiovascular disease in competitive sports.[27] Table 17-6 presents those guidelines in a modified format. No formal guidelines to participation in recreational sports exist. The exercise prescription for an individual patient should be based on his or her particular findings. The risk of bodily collision should be considered, especially for patients on anticoagulation therapy. Emotional involvement with the resultant sympathetic drive and possible increased risk of ischemia and arrhythmia should also be considered. The risk of injury if syncope occurs should be considered.

SEXUALITY AND REPRODUCTION

Adults with CHD often have concerns about their sexuality, the ability to bear children, and the risk of CHD in their offspring. These patients may lack basic education on these issues in part due to parental attitudes and pediatric care providers who may be uncomfortable broaching these subjects. Sexuality and family planning should be addressed proactively to educate patients so that they can make informed reproductive choices.

When pregnancy is being contemplated, consultation with an adult CHD specialist is recommended *prior to* conception.[12] Considerations to discuss during counseling include the risk of adverse maternal and fetal outcome, possible need for intervention or surgery prior to or during pregnancy, maternal life expectancy and ability to care for a child, and risk of CHD to the offspring. Determining risk of adverse outcome during pregnancy involves the consideration of multiple factors including underlying congenital heart defect, residual lesions, maternal functional status, and associated risk factors such as history of arrhythmia or

heart failure, cyanosis, systemic ventricular function, prosthetic valves, and medications. Although risk stratification of pregnancy in CHD is beyond the scope of this chapter, some lesions are generally accepted to be higher risk than others and are summarized in Table 17-7. It is emphasized that the process of guiding a patient with moderate to high risk through conception, pregnancy, labor, delivery, and the postpartum period is a multidisciplinary effort undertaken by an adult CHD specialist, high-risk obstetrician, geneticist, and anesthesiologist experienced in the care of women with CHD.[12]

Choice of contraception for women with CHD begins with understanding the risks of pregnancy itself, both maternal and fetal, the risks and benefits of the various options available, the failure rates of these methods, and the consequences of an unwanted pregnancy. There are limited data on the safety of various forms of contraception in adult CHD patients, but it is generally accepted that estrogen-containing medications are not recommended for those who are at increased risk for thromboembolism including cyanotic patients, Fontan patients, patients with certain types of mechanical heart valves, and patients with pulmonary hypertension. Disadvantages to the progesterone-only options, including the "mini-pill" and implantable subdermal form (Implanon; Schering-Plough, Kenilworth, NJ), are fluid retention and a higher failure rate compared to combined oral contraceptives. Other contraceptive options include intrauterine devices including a progesterone-releasing version (Mirena; Bayer, Leverkusen, Germany), levonorgestrel (ie, "Plan B"), barrier methods, and sterilization. Given the heterogeneity of CHD and strata of risk, various contraceptive options, and patient preferences, according to the 2008 ACC/AHA Guidelines for the Management of Adults With Congenital Heart Disease, "it is the duty of the ACHD specialist to provide or otherwise make available informed advice on contraception, including discussion of risks."[12]

A frequent concern for those contemplating starting a family is the risk of CHD in their children. When 1 parent has CHD, there is an increased risk of recurrence in the offspring, generally between 2% and 4%.[29,30] This is compared to 0.8% in the general population. However, there is significant variability depending on the lesion and mode of inheritance. Consultation with a genetics specialist should be offered prior to conception as a part of the prepregnancy assessment in conjunction with an adult CHD specialist and a high-risk obstetrician. Fetal echocardiography screening by a pediatric cardiologist is recommended if a parent is affected with CHD[12].

Many adults with CHD lack accurate information regarding contraception and pregnancy. It is the responsibility of the healthcare practitioner to initiate and continue the discourse on these subjects to empower the patient to make educated decisions about their sexual health and reproduction.

	Low Dynamic, Low Static	Moderate Dynamic, Low Static	High Dynamic, Low Static	Low Dynamic, Moderate Static	Moderate Dynamic, Moderate Static	High Dynamic, Moderate Static	Low Dynamic, High Static	Moderate Dynamic, High Static	High Dynamic, High Static
	Bowling, golf	Baseball/softball, table tennis, volley-ball	Running, soccer, tennis, cross-country skiing	Auto racing, motorcy-cling, diving, horse riding	American football, rugby, swimming, sprint running, figure skating	Basketball, ice hockey, lacrosse, swimming, cross country skiing	Weight lifting, gymnastics, water-skiing, windsurfing	Wrestling, downhill skiing, snow-boarding	Rowing, boxing, speed skating, cycling, speed skating, triathlon
ASD, VSD, PDA repaired and unrepaired (no pulmonary hypertension or arrhythmia)	Yes	Yes	Yes	Yes	Yes	Yes	Yes	Yes	Yes
Mild pulmonic stenosis (<40 mm Hg gradient)	Yes	Yes	Yes	Yes	Yes	Yes	Yes	Yes	Yes
Mild aortic stenosis (gradient: cath <30 mm Hg, mean echo <25 mm Hg. Normal ECG. Asymptomatic)	Yes	Yes	Yes	Yes	Yes	Yes	Yes	Yes	Yes
Moderate aortic stenosis (gradient cath <50, echo mean <40 mm Hg) Normal exercise test. No ECG strain	Yes	Yes	No	Yes	No	No	No	No	No
Mild to moderate aortic regurgitation, normal size LV	Yes	Yes	Yes	Yes	Yes	Yes	Yes	Yes	Yes
Mild or moderate aortic regurgitation. Modertae LV enlargement. No arrhythmia. Normal exercise test.	Yes	Yes	Yes	Yes	Yes	Yes	No	No	No
Severe aortic stenosis or regurgitation	No	No	No	No	No	No	No	No	No
Coarctation: <20 mm Hg arm–leg gradient, no aortic root dilatation. Exercise blood pressure <230 mm Hg	Yes	Yes	Yes	Yes	Yes	Yes	Yes	Yes	Yes

Condition								
Coarctation: >20 mm Hg arm-leg gradient, exercise blood pressure >230 mm Hg	Yes	No	No	No	No	No	No	No
Repaired coarctation. <20 mm Hg arm-leg gradient, normal exercise blood pressure	Yes	Yes	Yes	Yes	Yes	Yes	No	No
Significant aortic root dilatation or aneurysm	Yes	No	No	No	No	No	No	No
Ejection fraction 40%–50%	Yes	Yes	No	No	No	No	No	No
Ejection fraction <40%	No	No	No	No	No	No	No	No
Pulmonary hypertension, cyanotic heart disease	Need individual exercise prescription, usually only low-dynamic, low-static exercise							
Repaired tetralogy of Fallot, without a significant residual shunt, <50% systemic RV pressure, no arrhythmia	Yes	Yes	Yes	Yes	Yes	Yes	Yes	Yes
Repaired tetarology of Fallot with marked RV dilatation, >50% systemic RV pressure, arrhythmia	Yes	No	No	No	No	No	No	No
Transposition post atrial baffle repair, adequate RV function, no arrhythmia, normal exercise test	Yes	No	Yes	No	No	No	No	No
Transposition post arterial switch, normal ventricular function, normal exercise test, no arrhythmia	Yes	Yes	Yes	Yes	Yes	Yes	Yes	Yes
Transposition post arterial switch, ventricular dysfunction, normal exercise test	Yes	Yes	Yes	No	No	No	No	No
Congenitally corrected transposition of the great arteries (L-TGA)	Yes	No	No	No	No	No	No	No

(Continued)

Guidelines for the Participation of Patients with Cardiovascular Disease in Competitive Sports (Continued)

	Low Dynamic, Low Static	Moderate Dynamic, Low Static	High Dynamic, Low Static	Low Dynamic, Moderate Static	Moderate Dynamic, Moderate Static	High Dynamic, Moderate Static	Low Dynamic, High Static	Moderate Dynamic, High Static	High Dynamic, High Static
Fontan operation (single ventricle)	Yes	Yes If ventricular function and oxygen saturation are normal	No	No	No	No	No	No	No
Mild Ebstein, normal RV size, no arrhythmia	Yes	Yes	Yes	Yes	Yes	Yes	Yes	Yes	Yes
Ebstein with moderate tricuspid regurgitation, no arrhythmia	Yes	No	No	No	No	No	No	No	No
Severe Ebstein severe tricuspid regurgitation arrythmia	No	No	No	No	No	No	No	No	No
Coronary artery from the wrong sinus with a course in between the great arteries (unrepaired)	No	No	No	No	No	No	No	No	No
Repaired anomalous coronary artery. Normal maximal exercise test, no arrhythmia	Yes	Yes	Yes	Yes	Yes	Yes	Yes	Yes	Yes
Kawasaki without coronary abnormalities	Yes	Yes	Yes	Yes	Yes	Yes	Yes	Yes	Yes
Kawasaki with regressed aneurysms and normal exercise test with nuclear perfusion imaging	Yes	Yes	Yes	Yes	Yes	Yes	Yes	Yes	Yes
Kawasaki with medium-size aneurysms, normal exercise test with nuclear perfusion imaging	Yes	Yes	No	Yes	Yes	No	No	No	No
Kawasaki with large or complex aneurysms, normal yearly exercise tests with nuclear perfusion imaging	Yes	Yes	No	No	No	No	No	No	No

Hypertrophic cardiomyopathy	Yes	No	No	No	On individual basis	No	No	No	No
Long QT syndrome	Yes	Other sports on individual basis, based on presence of defibrillator, beta-blockade and past arrhythmia	No	No	No	No	No	No	No
Marfan syndrome	Yes	On individual basis	No	No	No	No	No	No	No

ASD, atrial septal defect; cath, catheter; ECG, electrocardiography; echo, echocardiography; LV, left ventricle; L-TGA, levo-transposition of the great arteries; PDA, patent ductus arteriosus; RV, right ventricle; VSD, ventricular septal defect.

Risk Stratification and Pregnancy in Congenital Heart Disease

Low risk
■ Small left-to-right shunts
■ Repaired lesions without residual cardiac dysfunction
■ Isolated mitral valve prolapse without significant regurgitation
■ Bicuspid aortic valve without stenosis
■ Mild to moderate pulmonic stenosis
■ Valvar regurgitation with normal ventricular systolic function

Intermediate risk
■ Palliated cyanotic congenital heart disease
■ Large left-to-right shunt
■ Uncorrected coarctation of the aorta
■ Mitral or aortic stenosis
■ Mechanical prosthetic valves
■ Severe pulmonic stenosis
■ Moderate systemic ventricular dysfunction
■ History of peripartum cardiomyopathy with no residual ventricular dysfunction

High risk
■ New York Heart Association (NYHA) class III or IV symptoms
■ Severe pulmonary hypertension
■ Marfan syndrome with aortic root or major valvar involvement
■ Severe aortic stenosis
■ History of peripartum cardiomyopathy with residual ventricular dysfunction
■ Severe systemic ventricular dysfunction
■ Cyanosis

Modified with permission from Siu SC, Colman JM. Heart disease and pregnancy. Heart. 2001;85:710-715.

INSURANCE AND EMPLOYMENT

The transition to adult years represents a particularly vulnerable time for those with CHD with regard to health insurance and access to care. It is estimated that 10% to 20% of adults with CHD are uninsured, and 67% have reported difficulty obtaining insurance coverage or have needed to change jobs to guarantee coverage.[31,32] Many lose coverage under their parents' plans as they enter young adulthood or are historically denied private insurance based on "pre-existing conditions." Some receive Social Security benefits for disability and obtain Medicaid coverage, and a number of adults with CHD live as dependents with relatives. It has been shown that the proportion of patients admitted to hospitals via the emergency department nearly doubles surrounding the transition period to adulthood; an independent risk factor for this finding is the lack of health insurance.[33]

Recent legislative policy efforts in healthcare reform will directly impact healthcare for adults with CHD. Under the Affordable Care Act, which was signed into law on March 23, 2010, young adults will be allowed to remain on their parents' plan until the age of 26 years regardless of their marital status or financial dependence on their parents and regardless of whether they are in school or are eligible to enroll in their employer's healthcare plan. The law also creates a new program, the Pre-Existing Condition Insurance Plan, to provide healthcare coverage to those who have been denied insurance by private companies due to a pre-existing condition. This is intended to provide coverage to those who have been locked out of the insurance market until 2014, at which time a new affordable healthcare insurance exchange will roll out that does not deny coverage based on prior medical history.[34] How these new policy changes will affect adults with CHD remains to be seen, but they represent a step toward eliminating barriers to care.

Adults with CHD have difficulty securing life insurance. Despite the heterogeneity of disease with patients with some lesions known to have near-normal or normal life expectancy compared to the general population, obtaining life insurance can still be elusive. A recent study found that more than one third of adults with CHD were denied life insurance compared to 4% of age-matched peers, regardless of CHD severity.[35]

Although most adults with CHD work, access to full employment is a significant problem for many, especially those with more complex CHD. In one study, there was a lower rate of job participation for those with complex CHD compared to those with milder forms of disease and to the general population. These adults with complex CHD were more likely to have job-related difficulties such as feeling restricted in choice of employment or being excluded from a job.[36] Although illegal, employers may not hire somebody with CHD for fear of rising health insurance premiums or future illness resulting in sick leave. As a result, many adults conceal their cardiac history from employers. Patients should be made aware of the Americans with Disability Act, which prohibits discrimination with respect to hiring, firing, or promoting based on disability, and that adults with CHD are not required to disclose their condition unless it interferes with the ability to fulfill the job description.

Insurability and employment are vital to the social and medical well-being of the adult with CHD. These issues ought to be addressed in adolescence with the involvement of healthcare providers to prepare the patient for these issues in adulthood.

QUALITY OF LIFE AND MENTAL HEALTH

Approximately one third of adults with CHD have mood or anxiety disorders, and depression is often underrecognized and undertreated. Studies have shown a high percentage of adult CHD patients with previous mental health treatment, but also many patients considered "well-adjusted" by their medical teams, who met diagnostic criteria for mood or anxiety disorders, yet who did not receive treatment.[37-39]

Multiple factors influence quality of life and mental health in this patient population. A significant number of patients with CHD have neurodevelopmental disorders related to genetic factors, abnormal cerebral perfusion during fetal life, and possible effects of surgical treatment. Chapter 11 in this book reviews neurodevelopment in depth. Children with chronic illness suffer from disruptions in their social interactions, are overprotected by parents, have a decreased self-image, and face other challenges that impact their psychological development and mental well-being. School absences and physical limitations that restrict participation with siblings and peers during childhood contribute to perceptions of social awkwardness and isolation. Many patients report that CHD was never openly discussed either within or outside the family.[40] Denial and minimization are frequently used and can be both adaptive and maladaptive. Denial can obscure mood disorders and foster loneliness and isolation. A protective adaptive denial during childhood can lead to unresolved mental health issues in adulthood. Perceived parental overprotection and heart defect complexity are associated with heart-focused anxiety in adults with CHD.[41,42]

Sexual dysfunction is not uncommon and influences mental health. In a study, men with CHD under the age of 40 engaged less frequently in sexual relationships than their peers, and 10% had erectile dysfunction. Compared to men with CHD without erectile dysfunction, those with erectile dysfunction had lower health-related quality-of-life scores and higher incidence of depressive symptoms.[43]

Hospitalizations of adult CHD patients occur either in pediatric units where the adult patient does not fit well or in adult units where caregivers are often unfamiliar with CHD. During hospitalizations of adults with CHD, divergence in expectations between patients, families, and healthcare providers can lead to friction and conflict in the experience of care. Role confusion and power struggles over control of care can occur between patients, spouses, parents, doctors, and nurses. This dissonance can result in interpersonal conflict, distrust, anxiety, and dissatisfaction with the care and the caretakers.[44]

Somewhat surprisingly, studies from Europe reported quality-of-life scores in adult patients with CHD that are comparable to those of the general population.[45] This is different from the experience in North America. It is unknown whether this discrepancy results from cultural differences and life expectations or is the result of superior healthcare access and social services.

Correlations between health-related quality of life and physical status are poor.[46] Some of the strongest

determinants of the quality of life of adult CHD patients were found to be family, job, education, friends, and leisure time.[47] Social adjustment and patient-perceived health status appear to be more predictive of depression and anxiety than medical variables.[39] These factors are modifiable and therefore a potential focus of intervention.

Given the high incidence of psychological issues in this patient population and that many of the responsible factors are potentially modifiable, it is important to offer mental health care to adult CHD patients. In a study, patients expressed preference for Internet-based mental health treatment.[37] This may represent an opportunity to help many potential patients while using limited resources. Children and adults with CHD should be screened for mental health issues, and psychological care should be incorporated into CHD programs. Primary care providers, who often have a privileged relationship with patients and parents, have an opportunity to explore unrecognized mental health challenges and refer the family to appropriate therapy.

Clinical Pearls

- Most babies born with CHD in the current era survive to adulthood.
- Surgery does not repair complex CHD; it only palliates it temporarily. Ongoing problems will require care by CHD specialists.
- As the survivors of complex CHD surgery age, they have more noncardiac medical issues requiring adult medical care and are best served in centers dedicated to adult CHD.
- Be alert for a high incidence of mental health issues and family tensions, which may require therapy.
- Individual counseling is required for these patients regarding reproduction and exercise.

REFERENCES

1. Moons P, Bovijn L, Budts W, Belmans A, Gewillig M. Temporal trends in survival to adulthood among patients born with congenital heart disease from 1970 to 1992 in belgium. *Circulation.* 2010;122:2264-2272.
2. Marelli AJ, Mackie AS, Ionescu-Ittu R, Rahme E, Pilote L. Congenital heart disease in the general population: changing prevalence and age distribution. *Circulation.* 2007;115:163-172.
3. Williams RG, Pearson GD, Barst RJ, et al. Report of the national heart, lung, and blood institute working group on research in adult congenital heart disease. *J Am Coll Cardiol.* 2006;47:701-707.
4. Warnes CA, Liberthson R, Danielson GK, et al. Task force 1: the changing profile of congenital heart disease in adult life. *J Am Coll Cardiol.* 2001;37:1170-1175.
5. Brickner ME, Hillis LD, Lange RA. Congenital heart disease in adults. First of two parts. *N Engl J Med.* 2000;342:256-263.

6. Blum RW, Garell D, Hodgman CH, et al. Transition from child-centered to adult health-care systems for adolescents with chronic conditions. A position paper of the Society for Adolescent Medicine. *J Adolesc Health*. 1993;14: 570-576.

7. Hilderson D, Saidi AS, Van Deyk K, et al. Attitude toward and current practice of transfer and transition of adolescents with congenital heart disease in the united states of america and europe. *Pediatr Cardiol*. 2009;30:786-793.

8. Yeung E, Kay J, Roosevelt GE, Brandon M, Yetman AT. Lapse of care as a predictor for morbidity in adults with congenital heart disease. *Int J Cardiol*. 2008;125:62-65.

9. Soanes C, Timmons S. Improving transition: a qualitative study examining the attitudes of young people with chronic illness transferring to adult care. *J Child Health Care*. 2004;8:102-112.

10. Hudsmith LE, Thorne SA. Transition of care from paediatric to adult services in cardiology. *Arch Dis Child*. 2007;92:927-930.

11. Knauth A, Verstappen A, Reiss J, Webb GD. Transition and transfer from pediatric to adult care of the young adult with complex congenital heart disease. *Cardiol Clin*. 2006;24:619-629.

12. Warnes CA, Williams RG, Bashore TM, et al. ACC/AHA 2008 guidelines for the management of adults with congenital heart disease: a report of the American College of Cardiology/American Heart Association Task Force on Practice Guidelines (Writing Committee to Develop Guidelines on the Management of Adults with Congenital Heart Disease). *Circulation*. 2008;118:e714-833.

13. Moons P, De Volder E, Budts W, et al. What do adult patients with congenital heart disease know about their disease, treatment, and prevention of complications? A call for structured patient education. *Heart*. 2001;86:74-80.

14. Clarizia NA, Chahal N, Manlhiot C, Kilburn J, Redington AN, McCrindle BW. Transition to adult health care for adolescents and young adults with congenital heart disease: Perspectives of the patient, parent and health care provider. *Can J Cardiol*. 2009;25:e317-e322.

15. Schultz AH, Wernovsky G. Late outcomes in patients with surgically treated congenital heart disease. *Semin Thorac Cardiovasc Surg*. 2005:145-156.

16. Engelfriet P, Boersma E, Oechslin EN, et al. The spectrum of adult congenital heart disease in Europe: morbidity and mortality in a 5 year follow-up period. *Eur Heart J*. 2005;26:2325-2333.

17. Gratz A, Hess J, Hager A. Self-estimated physical functioning poorly predicts actual exercise capacity in adolescents and adults with congenital heart disease. *Eur Heart J*. 2009;30:497-504.

18. Diller GP, Dimopoulos K, Okonko D, et al. Exercise intolerance in adult congenital heart disease: comparative severity, correlates, and prognostic implication. *Circulation*. 2005;112:828-835.

19. Dimopoulos K, Okonko DO, Diller GP, et al. Abnormal ventilatory response to exercise in adults with congenital heart disease relates to cyanosis and predicts survival. *Circulation*. 2006;113:2796-2802.

20. Diller GP, Dimopoulos K, Okonko D, et al. Heart rate response during exercise predicts survival in adults with congenital heart disease. *J Am Coll Cardiol*. 2006;48: 1250-1256.

21. Diller GP, Okonko DO, Uebing A, et al. Impaired heart rate response to exercise in adult patients with a systemic right ventricle or univentricular circulation: prevalence, relation to exercise, and potential therapeutic implications. *Int J Cardiol*. 2009;134:59-66.

22. Fredriksen PM, Chen A, Veldtman G, Hechter S, Therrien J, Webb G. Exercise capacity in adult patients with congenitally corrected transposition of the great arteries. *Heart*. 2001;85:191-195.

23. Fredriksen PM, Therrien J, Veldtman G, et al. Lung function and aerobic capacity in adult patients following modified fontan procedure. *Heart*. 2001;85:295-299.

24. Trojnarska O, Gwizdala A, Katarzynski S, et al. Evaluation of exercise capacity with cardiopulmonary exercise test and b-type natriuretic peptide in adults with congenital heart disease. *Cardiol J*. 2009;16:133-141.

25. Perloff JK, Child JS, Aboulhosen J. *Congenital Heart Disease in Adults*. New York, NY: Saunders Elsevier; 2009.

26. Dua JS, Cooper AR, Fox KR, Graham Stuart A. Exercise training in adults with congenital heart disease: feasibility and benefits. *Int J Cardiol*. 2010;138:196-205.

27. Maron BJ, Zipes DP. Introduction: eligibility recommendations for competitive athletes with cardiovascular abnormalities-general considerations. *J Am Coll Cardiol*. 2005;45:1318-1321.

28. Mitchell JH, Haskell WL, Raven PB. Classification of sports. *J Am Coll Cardiol*. 1994;24:864-866.

29. Nora JJ, Nora AH. Recurrence risks in children having one parent with a congenital heart disease. *Circulation*. 1976;53:701-702.

30. Gill HK, Splitt M, Sharland GK, Simpson JM. Patterns of recurrence of congenital heart disease: an analysis of 6,640 consecutive pregnancies evaluated by detailed fetal echocardiography. *J Am Coll Cardiol*. 2003;42:923-929.

31. Allen HD, Gersony WM, Taubert KA. Insurability of the adolescent and young adult with heart disease. Report from the Fifth Conference on Insurability, October 3-4, 1991, Columbus, Ohio. *Circulation*. 1992;86:703-710.

32. Skorton DJ, Garson A Jr, Allen HD, et al. Task Force 5: adults with congenital heart disease: access to care. *J Am Coll Cardiol*. 2001;37:1193-1198.

33. Gurvitz MZ, Inkelas M, Lee M, Stout K, Escarce J, Chang RK. Changes in hospitalization patterns among patients with congenital heart disease during the transition from adolescence to adulthood. *J Am Coll Cardiol*. 2007;49:875-882.

34. HealthCare.gov. Understand the affordable care act. Available at: http://www.Healthcare.Gov. Accessed October 23, 2011.

35. Crossland DS, Jackson SP, Lyall R, et al. Life insurance and mortgage application in adults with congenital heart disease. *Eur J Cardiothorac Surg*. 2004;25:931-934.

36. Kamphuis M, Vogels T, Ottenkamp J, Van Der Wall EE, Verloove-Vanhorick SP, Vliegen HW. Employment in adults with congenital heart disease. *Arch Pediatr Adolesc Med*. 2002;156:1143-1148.

37. Kovacs AH, Bendell KL, Colman J, Harrison JL, Oechslin E, Silversides C. Adults with congenital heart disease: psychological needs and treatment preferences. *Congenit Heart Dis*. 2009;4:139-146.

38. Bromberg JI, Beasley PJ, D'Angelo EJ, Landzberg M, DeMaso DR. Depression and anxiety in adults with congenital heart disease: a pilot study. *Heart Lung*. 2003;32:105-110

39. Kovacs AH, Saidi AS, Kuhl EA, et al. Depression and anxiety in adult congenital heart disease: predictors and prevalence. *Int J Cardiol.* 2009;137:158-164.

40. Horner T, Liberthson R, Jellinek MS. Psychosocial profile of adults with complex congenital heart disease. *Mayo Clin Proc.* 2000;75:31-36.

41. Brandhagen DJ, Feldt RH, Williams DE. Long-term psychologic implications of congenital heart disease: a 25-year follow-up. *Mayo Clin Proc.* 1991;66:474-479.

42. Ong L, Nolan RP, Irvine J, Kovacs AH. Parental overprotection and heart-focused anxiety in adults with congenital heart disease. *Int J Behav Med.* 2011;18:260-267.

43. Vigl M, Hager A, Bauer U, et al. Sexuality and subjective well-being in male patients with congenital heart disease. *Heart.* 2009;95:1179-1183.

44. Kools S, Tong EM, Hughes R, et al. Hospital experiences of young adults with congenital heart disease: divergence in expectations and dissonance in care. *Am J Crit Care.* 2002;11:115-125.

45. Loup O, von Weissenfluh C, Gahl B, Schwerzmann M, Carrel T, Kadner A. Quality of life of grown-up congenital heart disease patients after congenital cardiac surgery. *Eur J Cardiothorac Surg.* 2009;36:105-111.

46. Kamphuis M, Ottenkamp J, Vliegen HW, et al. Health related quality of life and health status in adult survivors with previously operated complex congenital heart disease. *Heart.* 2002;87:356-362.

47. Moons P, Van Deyk K, Marquet K, et al. Individual quality of life in adults with congenital heart disease: a paradigm shift. *Eur Heart J.* 2005;26:298-307.

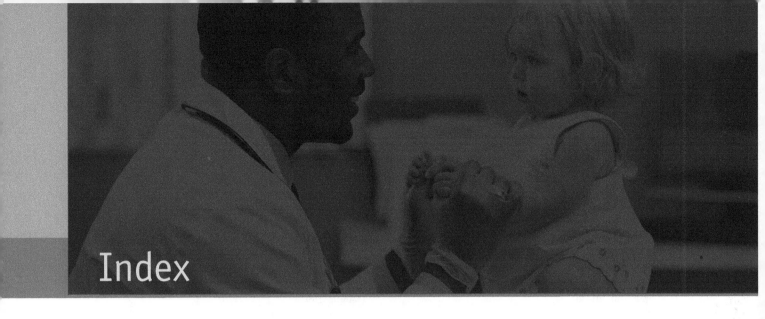

Index

Note: Page numbers followed by *f* or *t* indicate figures and tables.

C

Calcium channel blocker, 302
  for arrhythmia, 244
  for atrial fibrillation, 240
  for ectopic atrial tachycardia, 238
  for hypertension, 302
  for hypertrophic cardiomyopathy, 256
Cardiac anatomy, 1, 2*f*
Cardiac arrhythmias. *See* Arrhythmias
Cardiac asthma, 165
Cardiac catheterization
  Amplatzer septal occluder, 127, 128*f*
  in aortic coarctation, 173
  basics, 127
  complications, 130–131
  in dilated cardiomyopathy, 255
  in heart failure, 251
  Helex device, 127, 129*f*–130*f*
  interventional procedures, 127–130
  in peripheral pulmonary stenosis, 177
  in pulmonary atresia with intact ventricular septum, 209
  in pulmonary hypertension, 260
  in restrictive cardiomyopathy, 257
  in single-ventricle congenital heart disease, 201, 204–205
  in subvalvar aortic stenosis, 159
  in subvalvar pulmonary stenosis, 164
  in supravalvar aortic stenosis, 160
  in supravalvar pulmonary stenosis, 164
  transesophageal echocardiography, 46
  in valvar aortic stenosis, 158
  in valvar pulmonary stenosis, 163
Cardiac cycle, 1, 2*f*
Cardiac evaluation
  cardiac magnetic resonance, 46–56
    in congenital heart disease, 47–54
    future developments, 55–56
    indications of, 54–55
    overview, 46–47
  cardiopulmonary stress in/exercise testing in, 30–37
  echocardiography imaging in, 37–46
    pediatrics, 41–46
    principles, 37–41
    transesophageal, 46
  electrocardiography in
    cardiac rhythm detection, 27–30
    pediatric electrocardiogram, 23–27
Cardiac index, 2
Cardiac magnetic resonance (CMR)
  for anatomy, 47–49, 47*f*–49*f*
  in aortic coarctation, 174*f*
  in aortic regurgitation, 161
  in arrhythmogenic right ventricular cardiomyopathy, 258
  for blood flow, 49–53
  in chest pain, 53–54
  in congenital heart disease, 46–56
  in dilated cardiomyopathy, 255
  future developments, 55–56
  in hypertrophic cardiomyopathy, 256
  indications for, 54–55
    anatomy, 54*t*
    physiology/function, 55*t*
    tissue characterization, 55*t*
  in mitral regurgitation, 168
  in myocarditis, 279
  overview, 46–47
  in pulmonary regurgitation, 165
  in restrictive cardiomyopathy, 257
  in single-ventricle congenital heart disease, 201, 202*f*, 204–205

  for tissue characterization, 53–54
  in vascular rings, 176
  for ventricular function, 49
Cardiac murmur(s), 164
Cardiac output, 2, 20
  cardiac magnetic resonance, 53
  exercise testing, 31
Cardiac physiology, 1–3
Cardiac resynchronization therapy, 252–253
Cardiac rhythm detection, 30*t*
  additional testing, 29
  external cardiac ambulatory telemetry, 28–29, 29*f*
  fifteen-lead ECG with rhythm strip, 27
  Holter monitoring, 27, 28*f*
  insertable cardiac monitors, 29
  transtelephonic event recorders, 27–28, 28*f*
Cardioinhibitory syncope, 15
Cardiomyopathy, 254–258
  arrhythmogenic right ventricular, 258
  in children, 254–258
  definition, 254–255
  dilated, 255
  epidemiology, 254–255
  hypertrophic, 255–257
  left ventricular noncompaction, 258
  restrictive, 257–258
  secondary, 255
Cardiopulmonary bypass
  in children, 117–118
  in infant, 117–118
  in neonates, 117–118
  ultrafiltration, 118
Cardiopulmonary interactions, postoperative period, 121
Cardiopulmonary stress testing. *See* Exercise stress testing
Cardiovascular system
  fetal
    circulation in, 61, 62*f*
    extracardiac anomalies and, 67–69
Catecholaminergic medications
  hemodynamic monitoring, 119–120
  side effects, 120*t*
Catecholaminergic polymorphic ventricular tachycardia (CPVT), 244
Catheter ablation
  in arrhythmogenic right ventricular dysplasia/cardiomyopathy, 245
  in atrial fibrillation, 240
  in atrial flutter, 239
  in ectopic atrial tachycardia, 238–239
  in paroxysmal supraventricular tachycardia, 237
CAVCD. *See* Common atrioventricular canal defects
Cavopulmonary anastomosis, 326–328
CCAM (Congenital cystic adenomatoid malformation), 67–68
CCHB (Congenital complete heart block), 73–74
cCHD. *See* Complex congenital heart disease
CDH (Congenital diaphragmatic hernia), 68, 68*f*
Central nervous system injuries, 123–124
Char syndrome, 147
CHARGE syndrome, 86
CHD. *See* Congenital heart disease
Chest pain
  alphabetical pneumonic for evaluation, 18*t*
  cardiac causes, 19
  cardiac magnetic resonance, 53–54
  clinical presentation, 17
  definition of, 17
  diagnosis, 19, 20*f*
  differential diagnosis, 19
  epidemiology, 17
  gastrointestinal causes, 18